Essential
ORTHOPAEDICS

(Celebrating 25 Years of Publication)

Promoted by

Sports Injury Management Institute (SIMI)

Knee and Shoulder Clinic

New Delhi

Essential
ORTHOPAEDICS

(Celebrating 25 years of publication)

Based on Education Curriculum of NMC

Seventh Edition

J Maheshwari
MBBS (AIIMS), MS Orth (AIIMS)

Formerly
Additional Professor of Orthopaedics
All India Institute of Medical Sciences
New Delhi, India

Presently
Director
Knee and Shoulder Clinic
New Delhi, India

Vikram A Mhaskar
MS Orth, MCh Orth (UK)

Knee and Shoulder Clinic
New Delhi, India

Director
Sports Injury Management Institute (SIMI)
Sitaram Bhartia Institute of Science and Research
New Delhi, India

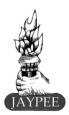

JAYPEE BROTHERS MEDICAL PUBLISHERS
The Health Sciences Publisher
New Delhi | London

Jaypee Brothers Medical Publishers (P) Ltd

Headquarter

Jaypee Brothers Medical Publishers (P) Ltd
EMCA House, 23/23-B
Ansari Road, Daryaganj
New Delhi - 110 002, India
Landline: +91-11-23272143,+91-11-23272703,
+91-11-23282021,+91-11-23245672
Email: jaypee@jaypeebrothers.com

Corporate Office

Jaypee Brothers Medical Publishers (P) Ltd
4838/24, Ansari Road, Daryaganj
New Delhi 110 002, India
Phone: +91-11-43574357
Fax: +91-11-43574314
Email: jaypee@jaypeebrothers.com

Overseas Office

J.P. Medical Ltd
83 Victoria Street, London
SW1H 0HW (UK)
Phone: +44 20 3170 8910
Fax: +44 (0)20 3008 6180
Email: info@jpmedpub.com

Website: www.jaypeebrothers.com
Website: www.jaypeedigital.com

Essential Orthopaedics

First Edition: 5 Reprints
Second Edition: 5 Reprints
Third Edition: Aug. 2001 (6 Reprints)
Third Edition (Revised): May 2005 (7 Reprints)
Fourth Edition: 2011
Reprint: 2014
Fifth Edition: 2015
Sixth Edition: 2019
Seventh Edition: 2022

Revised Reprint: **2023**

ISBN: 978-93-5465-376-6

Printed at Sanat Printers

Dedicated to

Our patients

for giving us an opportunity to make a difference in their lives
and *Our families and friends*
for continuous support at all times

Preface to the Seventh Edition

This book has completed 25 years of its publication and continues to remain a popular choice for medical and physiotherapy students. In these 25 years, a lot has changed in orthopaedics—some concepts have become outdated and new have taken roots. While revising a book, primarily aimed at an undergraduate medical student, it becomes a task to filter the information. One has to keep only what is required for an undergraduate. The book must maintain its basic character—a simple, readable and to-the-point book for an undergraduate. We kept reminding ourselves that there should not be even a single word more than what an undergraduate student needs.

Since over the years, our practice has got limited to knee and shoulder surgery, it was becoming difficult to update a book of general orthopaedics such as this. We decided that it was time to reach out to our colleagues from different subspecialities of orthopaedics, and seek their help. Our colleagues were readily forthcoming with their suggestions. For this, we would like to acknowledge the support of our colleagues—Dr HN Bajaj (Spine specialist), Dr Anil Jain (Prof of Orthopaedics, UCMS, New Delhi), Dr Kamal Dureja (Foot and Ankle specialist), Dr Vivek Trikha (Orthopaedic Trauma specialist, AIIMS), Dr Manoj Padman (Paediatric Orthopaedics specialist) and Dr Akshay Tiwari (Orthopaedic Oncologist).

With these changes in this edition, we are able to put the updated contents as of 2022. Hope students continue to enjoy reading the book. Comments and criticisms welcome.

Knee and Shoulder Clinic
Sports Injury Management Institute (SIMI)
Sitaram Bhartia Institute of Science and Research
New Delhi, India
dr.maheshwari@kneeandshoulderclinic.com

J Maheshwari
Vikram A Mhaskar

Preface to the First Edition

What was the thought behind this book in 1993

As an undergraduate, though exposed to orthopaedics only for a short period, I was impressed by the ease with which I could understand the wonderful texts I studied. The problems were that their contents did not exactly meet the requirements of an undergraduate, and most of these books, written by authors from developed countries, did not provide adequate information about diseases peculiar to tropical and underdeveloped countries. Above all, I thought that the concepts could be presented with still more clarity, and improved by way of presentation.

This feeling continued to haunt me everytime I was called upon to teach undergraduates. A couple of years later, an experience at home helped me give a practical shape to this feeling. My wife, who was preparing for PG entrance examination, expected me to teach her orthopaedics. I tried out my ideas on her, and the result was extremely gratifying. Soon after, many more such occasions of teaching undergraduates gave me further opportunities for refining the material. It was on the request of the students that I decided to give it the shape of a book.

The book is primarily addressed to undergraduates and those preparing for the postgraduate entrance tests. General practitioners, particularly in the early stage of their practice would find it useful reference. It would enable nurses and physiotherapists to understand the basic concepts in orthopaedics. Junior postgraduates would find it an enjoyable reading.

Following are the salient features of the book:
1. Most chapters begin with a brief review of the *relevant anatomy*. This is because by the time a student comes to clinical departments, he has forgotten most of the anatomy he had learnt in the dissection hall.
2. While discussing treatment of a condition, a brief mention of *principles* is made first, followed by various methods and their indications. This is followed by *treatment plan*; a practical plan of treatment which is either being followed or can be developed in an average hospital. A brief mention of recent developments is also made.
3. The book has three additional chapters. These are *"Approach to a Patient with Limb Injury"*, *"Approach to a Patient with Back Pain"*, and *"Recent Advances in Treatment of Fractures"*. The first two present a practical approach to handling these frequently encountered emergencies, and the third chapter updates the reader with the latest in this rapidly developing field. Due emphasis has been given to aspects of rehabilitation, considering the recent recommendations of Medical Council of India for including 'rehabilitation' in undergraduate curriculum.
4. *Simple line diagrams* have been used to supplement the text. Most of them have been developed by myself while teaching the undergraduates. Simplified line diagrams, rather than photographs, enable students understand the basic concepts better.
5. *Self-explanatory flow charts* are made use of wherever they would help to develop a concept in decision-making.
6. *Tables* have been used liberally. These serve two purposes: Firstly, they present the text matter in a concentrated form and allow review at a glance. Secondly, they permit quick and easily understandable comparison between related conditions.
7. Necessary information on instruments and implants commonly used in orthopaedics has been provided as an appendix, purely considering the requirement of such knowledge for final professional examination.

J Maheshwari

Contents

Competency Table

Number	COMPETENCY The student should be able to:	Domain K/S/A/C	Level K/KH/ SH/P	Core (Y/N)	Suggested Teaching Learning method	Suggested Assessment method	Chapter Number
OR1.1	Describe and discuss the principles of pre-hospital care and casuality management of a trauma victim including principles of triage	K/S/A/C	K/KH	Y	Lecture with video, Small group discussion	Written/Viva voce/OSCE/Simulation	3, 6
OR1.2	Describe and discuss the aetiopathogenesis, clinical features, investigations, and principles of management of shock	K/S	K/KH	Y	Lecture	Written/Viva voce/OSCE/Simulation	7
OR1.5	Describe and discuss the aetiopathogenesis, clinical features, investigations, and principles of management of dislocation of major joints, shoulder, knee, hip	K	K/KH	Y	Lecture, Small group discussion, Bed side clinic	Written/Viva voce/OSCE/Simulation	8, 13, 18
OR2.1	Describe and discuss the mechanism of injury, clinical features, investigations and plan management of fracture of clavicle	K/S	KH/SH	Y	Lecture, Small group discussion, Bed side clinic	Written/Viva voce/OSCE	13
OR2.2	Describe and discuss the mechanism of injury, clinical features, investigations and plan management of fractures of proximal humerus	K	K/KH/SH	Y	Lecture, Small group discussion, Bed side clinic	Written/Viva voce/OSCE	13
OR2.3	Select, prescribe and communicate appropriate medications for relief of joint pain	K	KH/SH	Y	Lecture, Small group discussion, Bed side clinic	Written/Viva voce/OSCE	12, 34
OR2.4	Describe and discuss the mechanism of injury, clinical features, investigations and principles of management of fracture of shaft of humerus and intercondylar fracture humerus with emphasis on neurovascular deficit	K/S	K/KH	Y	Lecture, Small group discussion, Bed side clinic	Written/Viva voce/OSCE	13
OR2.5	Describe and discuss the aetiopathogenesis, clinical features, mechanism of injury, investigation and principles of management of fractures of both bones forearm and Galeazzi and Monteggia injury	K	K/KH	Y	Lecture, Small group discussion, Bedside clinic	Written/Viva voce/OSCE	15
OR2.6	Describe and discuss the aetiopathogenesis, mechanism of injury, clinical features, investigations and principles of management of fractures of distal radius	K	KH	Y	Lecture, Small group discussion, Bedside clinic	Written/Viva voce/OSCE	15
OR2.7	Describe and discuss the aetiopathogenesis, mechanism of injury, clinical features, investigations and principles of management of pelvic injuries with emphasis on hemodynamic instability	K	K/KH/SH	Y	Lecture, Small group discussion, Bedside clinic	Written/Viva voce/OSCE	17

(Contd...)

(Contd...)

Number	COMPETENCY The student should be able to:	Domain K/S/A/C	Level K/KH/ SH/P	Core (Y/N)	Suggested Teaching Learning method	Suggested Assessment method	Chapter Number
OR2.8	Describe and discuss the aetiopathogenesis, mechanism of injury, clinical features, investigations and principles of management of spine injuries with emphasis on mobilisation of the patient	K	K/ KH	Y	Lecture, Small group discussion, Bedside clinic	Written/Viva voce/ OSCE	31, 32
OR2.9	Describe and discuss the mechanism of injury, clinical features, investigations and principle of management of acetabular fracture	K	K/ KH	Y	Lecture, Small group discussion, Bedside clinic	Written/Viva voce/ OSCE	17
OR2.10	Describe and discuss the aetiopathogenesis, mechanism of injury, clinical features, investigations and principles of management of fractures of proximal femur	K/S/ A/C	KH	Y	Lecture, Small group discussion, Bedside clinic	Written/Viva voce/ OSCE	18
OR2.11	Describe and discuss the aetiopathogenesis, mechanism of injury, clinical features, investigations and principles of management of: a. Fracture patella b. Fracture distal femur c. Fracture proximal tibia with special focus on neurovascular injury and compartment syndrome	K	K/ KH	Y	Lecture, Small group discussion, Bedside clinic	Written/Viva voce/ OSCE	20
OR2.12	Describe and discuss the aetiopathogenesis, clinical features, investigations and principles of management of fracture shaft of femur in all age groups and the recognition and management of fat embolism as a complication	K	K/ KH	Y	Lecture, Small group discussion, Bedside clinic	Written/Viva voce/ OSCE	19
OR2.13	Describe and discuss the aetiopathogenesis, clinical features, investigation and principles of management of: a. Fracture both bones leg b. Calcaneus c. Small bones of foot	K	K/ KH	Y	Lecture, Small group discussion, Bedside clinic	Written/Viva voce/ OSCE	21
OR2.14	Describe and discuss the aetiopathogenesis, clinical features, investigation and principles of management of ankle fractures	K/S/C	K/ KH	Y	Lecture, Small group discussion, Bedside clinic	Written/Viva voce/ OSCE	21
OR2.15	Plan and interpret the investigations to diagnose complications of fractures like malunion, non-union, infection, compartmental syndrome	K/S	SH	Y	Lecture, Small group discussion, Bedside clinic	Written/Viva voce/ OSCE	7
OR2.16	Describe and discuss the mechanism of injury, clinical features, investigations and principles of management of open fractures with focus on secondary infection prevention and management	K	K/ KH	Y	Lecture, Small group discussion, Bedside clinic	Written/Viva voce/ OSCE	3

(Contd...)

(Contd...)

Number	COMPETENCY The student should be able to:	Domain K/S/A/C	Level K/KH/ SH/P	Core (Y/N)	Suggested Teaching Learning method	Suggested Assessment method	Chapter Number
OR3.1	Describe and discuss the aetiopathogenesis, clinical features, investigations and principles of management of bone and joint infections: a. Acute osteomyelitis b. Subacute osteomyelitis c. Acute suppurative arthritis d. Septic arthritis and HIV infection e. Spirochaetal infection f. Skeletal tuberculosis	K/S	K/ KH/ SH	Y	Lecture, Small group discussion, Video assisted lecture	Written/Viva voce/ OSCE	22
OR4.1	Describe and discuss the clinical features, investigation and principles of management of tuberculosis affecting major joints (Hip, Knee) including cold abscess and caries spine	K	K/ KH	Y	Lecture, Small group discussion, Case discussion	Written/Viva voce/ OSCE	23
OR5.1	Describe and discuss the aetiopathogenesis, clinical features, investigations and principles of management of various inflammatory disorder of joints	K	K/ KH	Y	Lecture, Small group discussion, Bedside clinic	Written/Viva voce/ OSCE	34
OR6.1	Describe and discuss the clinical features, investigations and principles of management of degenerative condition of spine (Cervical spondylosis, Lumbar spondylosis, PID)	K	K/ KH	Y	Lecture, Small group discussion, Case discussion	Written/Viva voce/ OSCE	35
OR7.1	Describe and discuss the aetiopathogenesis, clinical features, investigation and principles of management of metabolic bone disorders in particular osteoporosis, osteomalacia, rickets, Paget's disease	K	K/ KH	Y	Lecture, Small group discussion, Case discussion	Written/Viva voce/ OSCE	37
OR8.1	Describe and discuss the aetiopathogenesis, clinical features, assessment and principles of management a patient with post polio residual paralysis	K	K/ KH	Y	Lecture, Small group discussion, Case discussion	Written/Viva voce/ OSCE	27
OR9.1	Describe and discuss the aetiopathogenesis, clinical features, assessment and principles of management of cerebral palsy patient	K	K/ KH	Y	Lecture, Small group discussion	Written/Viva voce/ OSCE	27
OR10.1	Describe and discuss the aetiopathogenesis, clinical features, investigations and principles of management of benign and malignant bone tumours and pathological fractures	K	K/ KH	Y	Lecture, Small group discussion, Video assisted interactive lecture	Written/Viva voce/ OSCE	28
OR11.1	Describe and discuss the aetiopathogenesis, clinical features, investigations and principles of management of peripheral nerve injuries in diseases like foot drop, wrist drop, claw hand, palsies of radial, ulnar, median, lateral popliteal and sciatic nerves	K	K/H	Y	Lecture, Small group discussion, case discussion	Written/Viva voce/ OSCE	10

(Contd...)

(Contd...)

Number	COMPETENCY The student should be able to:	Domain K/S/A/C	Level K/KH/ SH/P	Core (Y/N)	Suggested Teaching Learning method	Suggested Assessment method	Chapter Number
OR12.1	Describe and discuss the clinical features, investigations and principles of management of congenital and acquired malformations and deformities of: a. Limbs and spine - Scoliosis and spinal bifida b. Congenital dislocation of hip,torticollis, c. Congenital talipes equino varus	K	KH	Y	Lecture, Small group discussion	Written/Viva voce/ OSCE	25, 26, 33

Orthopaedic Trauma: Introduction

Learning Objectives

- ❖ How do you classify fractures and what is its clinical relevance?
- ❖ What is a pathological fracture, its causes, and approach to treatment?

An injury to the musculoskeletal system may result in damage to bones, joints, muscles and tendons. In addition, the neurovascular bundle of the limb may be damaged. This chapter will outline the broad principles used in the diagnosis and management of these injuries. These principles can be applied with suitable modifications, in the management of any musculoskeletal injury.

CLASSIFICATION OF FRACTURES

A fracture is a break in the continuity of a bone. It can be classified on the basis of etiology, the communication between the fracture and external environment, the displacement of the fracture, and finally, the pattern of the fracture.

ON THE BASIS OF ETIOLOGY

Traumatic fracture: A fracture sustained due to trauma is called a traumatic fracture*. Normal bone can withstand considerable force, and breaks only when subjected to excessive force. Most fractures seen in day-to-day practice fall into this category, e.g., fractures caused by a fall, road traffic accident, fight, etc.

Pathological fracture: A fracture through a bone which has become weak due to some underlying

disease is called pathological fracture. A trivial or no force may be required to cause such a fracture, e.g., a fracture through a bone weakened by metastasis. *Although, traumatic fractures have a predictable and generally successful outcome, non-traumatic (pathological) fractures often go into non-union.*

Stress fracture: This is a special type of fracture sustained due to chronic repetitive injury. Repeated stress results in breakage if bony trabeculae. Such a fracture may not be visible on X-rays, and may present only as pain in the bone. These are often difficult to diagnose, and may only be picked up on MRI or bone scan.

ON THE BASIS OF DISPLACEMENTS

Fractures are described as per their pattern of displacement. This is also important in understanding the fracturing force and management. It can be one of the following:

Undisplaced fractures: These fractures are easy to identify by the absence of significant displacement.

Displaced fracture: A fracture may be displaced. The factors responsible for displacement are: (i) the fracturing force; (ii) the muscle pull on the fracture fragments and (iii) the gravity. While describing the displacements of a fracture, *conventionally, it is the displacement of the distal fragment in relation to the*

---

* An unqualified word 'fracture' usually means a traumatic fracture.

proximal fragment which is mentioned. The displacement can be in the form of shift, angulation or rotation (Fig. 1.1). A combination of displacements occur.

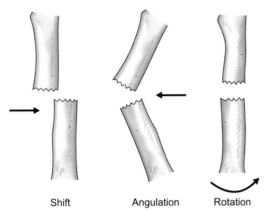

Shift   Angulation   Rotation

Fig. 1.1: Displacements in fractures.

ON THE BASIS OF COMMUNICATION WITH EXTERNAL ENVIRONMENT

Closed* fracture: A fracture not communicating with the external environment, i.e., the overlying skin and other soft tissues are intact, is called a closed fracture.

Open fracture: A fracture with break in the overlying skin and soft tissues, leading to the fracture communicating with the external environment, is called an open fracture. It is also called compound fracture. A fracture may be open from within or outside, the so called internally or externally open (compound) fracture, respectively.

a. *Internally open* (internal compounding - compounding from within): The sharp fracture end pierces the skin from within, resulting in an open fracture. It commonly occurs in bones which are subcutaneous. One common site of such a fracture is fracture lower end of the tibia.

b. *Externally open* (external compounding - compounding from outside): The object causing the fracture lacerates the skin and soft tissues over the bone as it breaks the bone, resulting in an open fracture. One example of such a fracture is open fracture of ulna sustained as a result of hit by a stick.

Exposure of an open fracture to the external environment makes it prone to infection. This risk is higher in externally open fracture.

* Terms, simple fracture for closed fracture, and compound fracture for open fracture is being dropped, as it is confusing.

ON THE BASIS OF COMPLEXITY OF TREATMENT

Simple fracture: A fracture in two pieces, usually easy to treat, is called simple fracture, e.g., a transverse fracture of humerus.

Complex fracture: A fracture in multiple pieces, usually difficult to treat, is called complex fracture, e.g., an intercondylar fracture of tibia.

ON THE BASIS OF QUANTUM OF FORCE CAUSING FRACTURE

High-velocity fractures: These are fractures sustained as a result of severe trauma force, as in traffic accidents. In these fractures, there is severe soft tissue injury (periosteal and muscle injury). There is extensive devascularisation of fracture ends. Such fractures are difficult to treat as they are often unstable, and heal slower. *Most complications occur in these type of fractures.*

Low-velocity fractures: These fractures are sustained as a result of mild trauma force, as in a fall while walking, for example. There is little associated soft tissue injury, and hence these fractures often heal predictably. *Lately, there is a change in the pattern of fractures due to shift from low-velocity to high-velocity injuries. The latter gives rise to more complex fractures, which are difficult to treat.*

ON THE BASIS OF PATTERN

Transverse fracture: In this fracture, the fracture line is perpendicular to the long axis of the bone. Such a fracture is caused by a tapping or bending force (Fig. 1.2).

Oblique fracture: In this fracture, the fracture line is oblique. Such a fracture is caused by a bending force which, in addition, has a component of force along the long axis of the bone.

Spiral fracture: In this fracture, the fracture line runs spirally in more than one plane. Such a fracture is caused by a primarily twisting force.

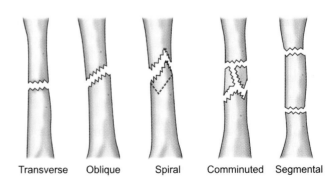

Transverse   Oblique   Spiral   Comminuted   Segmental

Fig. 1.2: Patterns of fractures.

Comminuted fracture: This is a fracture with multiple fragments. It is caused by a crushing or compression force along the long axis of the bone.

Segmental fracture: In this type, there are two fractures in one bone, but at different levels.

A fracture may have a combination of two or more patterns. For example, it may be a comminuted but primarily a transverse fracture.

FRACTURES WITH EPONYMS

Some fractures are better known by names, mostly of those who first described them. Some such fractures are as follows:

- *Monteggia fracture-dislocation:* Fracture of the proximal third of the ulna, with dislocation of the head of the radius (page 107–108).
- *Galeazzi fracture-dislocation:* Fracture of the distal third of the radius with dislocation of the distal radioulnar joint (page 108).
- *Nightstick fracture:* Isolated fracture of the shaft of the ulna, sustained while trying to ward off a stick blow.
- *Colles' fracture:* A fracture occurring in adults, at the corticocancellous junction of the distal end of the radius with *dorsal* tilt and other displacements (page 109).
- *Smith's fracture:* A fracture occurring in adults, at the corticocancellous junction of the distal end of the radius with *ventral* tilt and other displacements (reverse of Colles').
- *Barton's fracture* (marginal fracture): Intra-articular fractures through the distal articular surface of the radius, taking a margin, anterior or posterior, of the distal radius with the carpals, displaced anteriorly or posteriorly (page 112).
- *Chauffeur fracture:* An intra-articular, oblique fracture of the styloid process of the radius.
- *Bennett's fracture-dislocation:* It is an oblique, intra-articular fracture of the base of the first metacarpal with subluxation of the trapeziometacarpal joint (page 115).
- *Boxers' fracture:* It is a ventrally displaced fracture through the neck of the 5th metacarpal, usually occurs in boxers.
- *Side-swipe fracture:* It is an elbow injury sustained when one's elbow, projecting out of a car, is 'side-swept' by another vehicle. It has a combination of fractures of the distal end of the humerus with fractures of proximal ends of radius and/or ulna. It is also called baby car fracture.
- *Bumper fracture:* It is a comminuted, depressed fracture of the lateral condyle of the tibia.

- *Pott's fracture:* Bimalleolar ankle fracture.
- *Cotton's fracture:* Trimalleolar ankle fracture.
- *Massonaise's fracture:* It is a type of ankle fracture in which fracture of the *neck* of the fibula occurs.
- *Pilon fracture:* It is a comminuted intra-articular fracture of the distal end of the tibia.
- *Aviator's fracture:* Fracture of neck of the talus.
- *Chopart fracture-dislocation:* A fracture-dislocation through inter-tarsal joints.
- *Jone's fracture:* Avulsion fracture of the base of the 5th metatarsal.
- *Rolando fracture:* Fracture of the base of the first metacarpal (extra-articular).
- *Jefferson's fracture:* Fracture of the first cervical vertebra.
- *Whiplash injury:* Cervical spine injury where sudden flexion followed by hyperextension takes place.
- *Chance fracture:* Also called seat belt fracture, the fracture line runs horizontally through the body of the vertebra, through and through, to the posterior elements.
- *March fracture:* Fatigue fracture of the shaft of 2nd or 3rd metatarsal.
- *Burst fracture:* It is a comminuted fracture of the vertebral body where fragments "burst out" in different directions (page 264–265).
- *Clay-Shoveller fracture:* It is an avulsion fracture of spinous process of one or more of the lower cervical or upper thoracic vertebrae.
- *Hangman's fracture:* It is a fracture through the pedicle and lamina of C_2 vertebra, with subluxation of C_2 over C_3, sustained in hanging.
- *Dashboard fracture:* A fracture of posterior lip of the acetabulum, often associated with posterior dislocation of the hip.
- *Straddle fracture:* Bilateral superior and inferior pubic rami fractures.
- *Malgaigne's fracture:* A type of pelvis fracture in which there is a combination of fractures, pubic rami anteriorly and sacroiliac joint or ilium posteriorly, on the *same* side.
- *Mallet finger:* A finger flexed at the DIP joint due to avulsion or rupture of extensor tendon at the base of the distal phalanx.

PATHOLOGICAL FRACTURES

A fracture is termed pathological when it occurs in a bone made weak by some disease. Often, the bone breaks as a result of a trivial trauma, or even spontaneously.

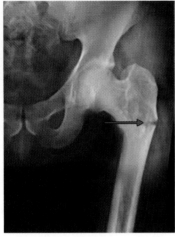

Fig. 1.3: X-ray of the hip showing destruction of the bone, which lead to a pathological fracture through the weak portion.

CAUSES

A bone may be rendered weak by a disease localised to that particular bone (Fig. 1.3), or by a generalised bone disorder. Table 1.1 gives some of the common causes

Table 1.1: Causes of pathological fractures.
Localised Diseases
■ *Neoplastic*
- Benign tumours
• Giant cell tumour, Enchondroma
• Malignant tumours
• Primary
- Osteosarcoma, Ewing's tumour
- Secondary
- In males: lung, prostate, kidney
- In females: breast, lung, genitals
■ *Inflammatory*
- Pyogenic osteomyelitis
- Tubercular osteomyelitis
■ *Miscellaneous*
- Simple bone cyst
- Aneurysmal bone cyst
- Monostotic fibrous dysplasia
- Eosinophilic granuloma
- Bone atrophy secondary to polio, etc.
Generalised Diseases
■ *Hereditary*
- Osteogenesis imperfecta
- Dyschondroplasia (Ollier's disease)
- Osteopetrosis
■ *Acquired*
- Osteoporosis
- Osteomalacia
- Rickets
- Scurvy
- Disseminated malignancy in bones
• Multiple myeloma
• Diffuse metastatic carcinoma
- Miscellaneous
• Paget's disease
• Polyostotic fibrous dysplasia

of pathological fractures. Osteoporosis is the *commonest* cause of pathological fracture. The bones most affected are the vertebrae (thoracic and lumbar). Other common fractures associated with osteoporosis are fracture of the neck of the femur and Colles' fracture.

A local or circumscribed lesion of the bone, responsible for a pathological fracture, may be due to varying causes in different age groups (Table 1.2). In children, it is commonly due to chronic osteomyelitis or a bone cyst. In adults, it is often due to a bone cyst or giant cell tumour. In elderly people, metastatic tumour is a frequent cause.

Table 1.2: Causes of pathological fractures - age wise.	
Age	**Causes**
At birth	Osteogenesis imperfecta
0–5 years	■ Osteogenesis imperfecta ■ Osteomyelitis
5–20 years	■ Osteomyelitis ■ Simple bone cyst ■ Primary bone malignancy
20–50 years	■ Cystic lesions of the bone ■ Malignancy ■ Osteomalacia ■ Giant cell tumour
After 50 years	■ Osteoporosis ■ Multiple myeloma ■ Secondaries in the bone

DIAGNOSIS

A fracture sustained without a significant trauma should arouse suspicion of a pathological fracture. Often the patient, when directly questioned, admits to having suffered from some discomfort in the region of the affected bone for some time prior to the occurrence of the fracture. In quite a few cases, the patient may be a diagnosed case of a disease known to produce pathological fractures, thus making the diagnosis of a pathological fracture simple. For example, a known case of malignancy may present with a fracture through a bony metastasis. At other times, the patient may present with a pathological fracture, and it is only on detailed work up that one comes to know about a hidden primary tumour.

TREATMENT

Treatment of a pathological fracture consists of: (i) finding the underlying pathology (cause of the fracture), and (ii) making an assessment of the capacity of the fracture to unite, based on the nature of the underlying disease.

A fracture in a bone affected by a generalised disorder, such as Paget's disease, osteogenesis imperfecta and osteoporosis, is expected to unite with conventional methods of treatment. A fracture at the site of a bone cyst or a benign tumour will also generally unite, but the union may be delayed. Fractures occurring in osteomyelitic bone often take a long time to unite, and sometimes fail to unite at all. Healing in fractures through a metastatic bone lesion depends upon the aggressive nature of the primary tumour. If the primary tumour can be brought under control, healing occurs. When the primary tumour is aggressive, it eats up the bone, and fracture does not heal at all.

With the availability of facilities for internal fixation, more and more pathological fractures are now treated operatively with an aim to: (i) enhance the process of union by bone grafting (e.g., in bone cyst or benign tumour); or (ii) mobilise the patient by surgical stabilisation of the fracture. Achieving stable fixation in these fractures is difficult because of the bone defect caused by the underlying pathology. The defect may have to be filled using bone grafts or bone cement. Quite a few juxta-articular pathological fractures are treated by primary joint replacement.

INJURIES TO JOINTS

Joint injuries may be either a subluxation or a dislocation. A joint is subluxated when its articular surfaces are *partially displaced* but retain some contact between them (Fig. 1.4). A joint is dislocated when its articular surfaces are so much displaced that all contact between them is lost. A dislocated joint is an emergency, and should be treated at the earliest. Shoulder is the most common joint to dislocate.

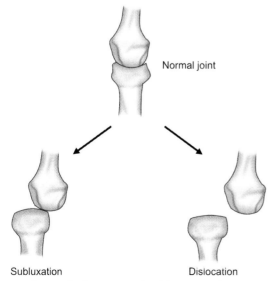

Fig. 1.4: Dislocation and subluxation of joints.

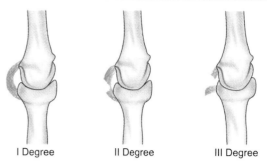

Fig. 1.5: Degrees of ligament sprain.

INJURIES TO LIGAMENTS

An injury to a ligament is termed as a sprain. This is to be differentiated from the term 'strain' which means stretching of a muscle or its tendinous attachment.

CLASSIFICATION

Sprains are classified into three degrees (Fig. 1.5):

First-degree sprain is a tear of only a few fibres of the ligament. It is characterised by minimal or no swelling, localised tenderness, but little functional disability.

Second-degree sprain is the one where, anything from a third to almost all the fibres of a ligament are disrupted. The patient presents with pain, swelling and inability to use the limb. Joint movements are restricted due to pain. The diagnosis can be made on performing a stress test as discussed subsequently.

Third-degree sprain is a complete tear of the ligament. There is swelling and pain over the torn ligament. Contrary to expectations, often the pain in such tears is minimal as also the swelling. This is because torn tissues fall apart and haematoma seeps into the surrounding soft tissues. There is often significant ecchymosis. Diagnosis can be made clinically by performing a stress test (page 347–348).

PATHOLOGY

A ligament may get torn in its substance (mid-substance tear) or at either end. The latter is called avulsion. Usually, avulsion occurs as simple tearing off of the ligament from the bone (soft-tissue avulsion), but often ligament avulses with a small piece of bone from its attachment (Fig. 1.6). This is called bony avulsion.

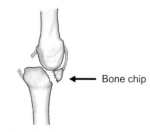

Fig. 1.6: Ligament avulsion with bone chip.

DIAGNOSIS

A detailed history eliciting the exact mechanism of injury, often indicates the ligament likely to be injured. The examination helps in finding the precise location and severity of the ligament injury, which can then be confirmed by investigations.

Clinical examination: A localised swelling, tenderness, and ecchymosis over a ligament indicates injury to that ligament. Usually, a haemarthrosis is noticed in second and third-degree sprains within 2 hours. Haemarthrosis may be absent despite a complete tear, or if the torn ligament is covered by synovium (e.g., intra-synovial tear of anterior cruciate ligament).

Stress test (Fig. 1.7): This is a very useful test in diagnosing a sprain and judging its severity. The ligament in question is put to stress by a certain manoeuvre. The manoeuvre used for testing individual ligaments will be discussed in respective chapters. When a ligament is stressed, in first and second-degree sprains, there will be pain at the site of the tear but little or no opening may be appreciated. In third-degree sprain, the joint will 'open up' as well.

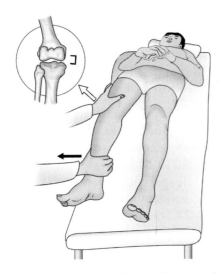

Fig. 1.7: Stress test for medial collateral ligament of the knee.

INVESTIGATIONS

A plain X-ray of the joint is usually normal. Sometimes, a chip of bone may be seen in the region of the attachment of the ligament to the bone.

Stress X-rays: These are special X-rays done where the injured ligament is put to stress by a particular manoeuvre (e.g., valgus stress for medial collateral ligament of the knee). This can help in deciding the grade of injury in doubtful cases. Doing stress X-rays may need sedation or general anaesthesia.

The investigation of choice is MRI. Arthroscopy may be done in doubtful cases.

TREATMENT

There has been a significant change in the treatment of sprains. All sprains are treated initially with rest, ice therapy, compression bandage, elevation (RICE). Suitable analgesics and anti-inflammatory medication is given. This is enough for first-degree sprains. Second and third-degree sprains are immobilised in a brace or a plaster cast for a period of 1-2 weeks, mainly for pain relief. *No longer is plaster immobilisation advised for long periods as was the trend in the past.* In fact, it is now understood that early mobilisation and walking with support (what is called functional rehabilitation) enhances healing of ligaments. In some third-degree sprain, surgery may be required.

INJURIES TO MUSCLES AND TENDONS

Muscles are ruptured more often than tendons in young people, while the reverse is true in the elderly. The most frequent cause of partial or complete rupture of a muscle or a tendon is sudden vigorous contraction of a muscle. It may be by over-stretching of a muscle at rest. *Such an injury to muscle is termed strain (and not sprain, which is ligament injury).* A muscle or tendon injury may also be produced by a sharp object such as a sword.

PATHOLOGY

A rupture occurs within a tendon only if it is abnormal and has become weak, either due to degeneration or wear and tear. Degenerative tendon ruptures commonly occur in rheumatoid arthritis, systemic lupus erythematosus (SLE), age-related degeneration, etc. Tendon rupture related to wear and tear commonly occurs in the supraspinatus, and in extensor tendons of hand. Some tendons known to rupture commonly are as given in Table 1.3. Diagnosis of a ruptured tendon is usually easy. The patient complains of pain and inability to perform the movement for which the tendon is meant.

DIAGNOSIS

Diagnosis of a muscle strain can be made by clinical examination. In sprains at superficial locations such as hamstring sprain, pain and swelling is common. In deeper muscle ruptures, often clinical examination

Table 1.3: Common sites of tendon rupture.
• Supraspinatus tendon
• Achilles tendon
• Biceps tendon – long head
• Extensor polices longus tendon
• Quadriceps tendon
• Patellar tendon

alone may not be adequate, and one may need to do investigations. Investigation if choice is MRI.

TREATMENT

Muscle ruptures in the belly of the muscle heal spontaneously. The resultant fibrous tissue may make it weak and the muscle may lose its stretchability. A long period of rehabilitation is often required. A muscle rupture through its tendinous portion, if fresh, is best treated with end-to-end repair. When the gap is too much, it can be filled with the help of a tendon graft. In cases where the repair is not possible, a tendon transfer may be performed. Some tendon ruptures, with degeneration in the background, may not be best suited for repair. These are best treated with rehabilitation alone. In some old tendon ruptures, especially in the elderly, there may be only a minimal functional disability. These patients do well without treatment.

 What have we learnt?

When we see a fracture, we must find out:
- Is it purely a traumatic fracture or is there an underlying pathology (weak bone)?
- What is the pattern of the fracture, so as to know the inherent stability of the fracture. Stable fractures can generally be treated non-operatively, unstable fractures often need surgery.
- What is the force causing the fracture. Is it a 'high-velocity' injury where fracture is likely to be unstable with lot of associated injury or a 'low-velocity' injury. The type of force producing the injury has bearing on healing of the fracture.
- It is a simple or complex fracture? The latter may be a badly comminuted fracture as a result of a bad trauma, and hence may be associated with lot of soft tissue damage. Such fractures often need surgical treatment.
- An open fracture has additional problem of getting infected. Hence, appropriate care in the early part of management is important.
- Sprain and strain are not interchangeable terms. MRI is the investigation of choice for diagnosing soft tissue injuries such as ligament and muscle injuries.
- A 'no bony injury' on X-ray does not mean no injury. Look for ligament or muscle injuries.

Additional information: From the entrance exams point of view

Best diagnostic test for a suspected stress fracture is MRI. The most common cause of pathological fracture is osteoporosis.

Anatomy of Bone, Fracture Healing

Learning Objectives

❖ Describe the anatomy of a typical long bones and its blood supply.
❖ Describe the mechanism of healing of bones.

ANATOMY OF BONE

Bones may be classified into four types on the basis of their shape, i.e., long, short, flat and irregular. Anatomy of a typical long bone only is being discussed here.

Structure of a typical long bone: A typical long bone in children (e.g., femur) has two ends or *epiphyses* (singular epiphysis) and an intermediate part called the shaft or *diaphysis* (Fig. 2.1). The part of the shaft which is adjoining the epiphysis is called the *metaphysis.* There is one metaphysis

next to each epiphysis. Separating the epiphysis from the metaphysis, there is a thin plate of growth cartilage, one at each end, called the *epiphyseal plate.* The bone grows at epiphyseal plates. At maturity, the epiphysis fuses with the metaphysis and the epiphyseal plate (also called growth plate) is replaced by bone. Epiphysis which does not contribute to the growth of length of the bone is called *apophysis* (Fig. 2.1). The articular ends of the epiphyses are covered with articular cartilage and remain so all life. Rest of the bone is covered with periosteum which provides attachment to tendons, muscles, ligaments, etc. The strands of fibrous tissue connecting the bone to the periosteum are called *Sharpey's fibres.*

Microscopically, bone can be classified as either woven or lamellar. *Woven bone or immature bone* is characterized by *random arrangement* of bone cells and collagen fibres. Woven bone is formed at periods of rapid bone formation, as in the initial stages of fracture healing. *Lamellar bone or mature bone* has an *orderly arrangement* of bone cells and collagen fibres. Both, cortical and cancellous bones are made up of lamellar bone, the only difference being the way lamellar bone is arranged—loosely v/s compactly.

The *basic structural unit* of the bone is the *osteon.* It consists of a series of concentric laminations or lamellae surrounding a central canal, the *Haversian*

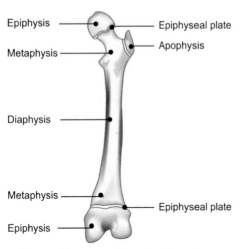

Epiphysis — Epiphyseal plate
Metaphysis — Apophysis
Diaphysis
Metaphysis — Epiphyseal plate
Epiphysis

Fig. 2.1: Structure of a typical long bone.

canal. These canals run longitudinally and connect freely with each other and with *Volkmann's canals.* The latter run horizontally from endosteal to periosteal surfaces of the bone. The shaft of a bone is made up of cortical bone, and the ends mainly of cancellous bone. The junction between the two, i.e., cortical bones of the shaft and cancellous bone-ends is termed the *corticocancellous junction.* It is a common site of fractures (Fig. 2.2).

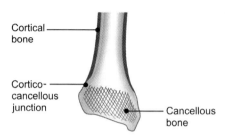

Fig. 2.2: Corticocancellous junction.

Structural composition of bone: The bone is made up of bone cells and extracellular matrix. The matrix consists of two types of materials—organic and inorganic. The organic matrix is formed by the collagen, which forms 30–35 percent of dry weight of a bone. The inorganic matrix is primarily calcium and phosphorus salts, especially *hydroxyapatite* $[Ca_{10}(PO_4)_6(OH)_2]$. It constitutes about 65–70 percent of dry weight of a bone.

Bone cells: There are three main cell types in the bone. These are:
a. *Osteoblasts:* Concerned with ossification, these cells are rich in alkaline phosphatase, glycolytic enzymes and phosphorylases.
b. *Osteocytes:* These are mature bone cells. These vary in activity, and may assume the form of an osteoclast or a reticulocyte. These cells are rich in glycogen and PAS positive granules.
c. *Osteoclasts:* These are multi-nucleate mesenchymal cells concerned with bone resorption. These have glycolytic acid hydrolases, collagenases and acid phosphatase enzymes.

GROWTH OF A LONG BONE

All long bones (except clavicle) develop from cartilaginous model (endochondral ossification). This type of ossification commences in the middle of the shaft before birth. This is called *primary* centre of ossification. The *secondary* centres of ossification appear at the ends of the bone (epiphysis), mostly* after birth.

The bone grows in length by a continuous growth at the epiphyseal plate. The increase in the girth of the bone is by subperiosteal new bone deposition.

At the end of the growth period, the epiphysis fuses with the diaphysis, and the growth stops. Presence of epiphysis, its time of appearance and fusion with metaphysis has clinical relevance in deciding the true age (bone age) of a child. An epiphyseal plate may sometimes be wrongly interpreted as a fracture.

Remodelling of bone: Bone has the ability to alter its size, shape and structure in response to stress. This happens throughout life though is not perceptible. According to *Wolff's law* of bone remodelling, bone hypertrophy occurs in the plane of stress.

BLOOD SUPPLY OF BONES

There is a standard pattern of the blood supply of a typical long bone. Blood supply of individual bones will be discussed wherever considered relevant. The blood supply of a typical long bone is derived from the following sources (Fig. 2.3):

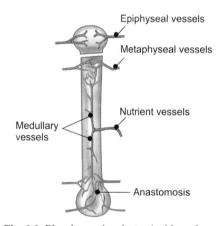

Fig. 2.3: Blood supply of a typical long bone.

a. **Nutrient artery:** This vessel enters the bone around its middle and divides into two branches, one running towards either end of the bone. Each of these further divide into a leash of parallel vessels which run towards the respective metaphysis.
b. **Metaphyseal vessels:** These are numerous small vessels derived from the anastomosis around the joint. They pierce the metaphysis along the line of attachment of the joint capsule.
c. **Epiphyseal vessels:** These are vessels which enter directly into the epiphysis.
d. **Periosteal vessels:** The periosteum has a rich blood supply, from which many little vessels enter the bone to supply roughly the *outer-third* of the cortex of the adult bone.

Blood supply to the inner two-thirds of the bone comes from the nutrient artery and the outer one-

---

* The epiphysis of distal end of the femur is present at birth.

third from the periosteal vessels. Knowledge of blood supply of the bone comes handy in explaining some orthopaedic diseases such as avascular necrosis, as also explanation for reason for delayed and non-union of certain fractures.

FRACTURE HEALING

The healing of fractures is in many ways similar to the healing of soft tissue, except that end result of a soft tissue healing is fibrous tissue, but that of a bone healing is *mineralised mesenchymal tissue*, i.e., bone. Fracture healing means, the way a fracture heals in a natural or non-operative way. This happens through a continuous series of stages described in Table 2.1. It is relevant to understand the stages of fracture healing as this has bearing on fracture management. There is a stage (stage of soft callus) till when one can 'play' with a fracture, change its alignment etc. But after a certain stage this is not possible to do so. Any further desired change in position can occur only by intervention - by breaking the healing fracture (osteoclasis) or by formal opening the fracture and cutting it with instruments, a procedure called osteotomy.

Fracture healing occurs in the following stages:
- Stage of haematoma
- Stage of fibrocartilaginous callus formation
- Stage of bony callus formation
- Stage of bone remodelling

STAGE OF HAEMATOMA (DAYS 1 TO 5)

This stage begins immediately following the fracture. The blood vessels supplying the bone and periosteum are ruptured causing a haematoma around the fracture site. The injury results in marginal necrosis of fracture-end, and surrounding tissues. It is for this reason that, often the *gap between what was a 'crack fracture' appears increased after a few days.* It should not be a cause for concern. Dead tissues lead to secretion of pro-inflammatory cytokines like tumour necrosis factor-alpha (TNF-α), bone morphogenetic proteins (BMPs), and interleukins (IL-1, IL-6, IL-11, IL-23). These cytokines stimulate essential cellular response, attracting macrophages, monocytes, and lymphocytes. These cells do the job of scavenging, and remove damaged, necrotic tissue. The cells also secrete cytokines-like vascular endothelial growth factor (VEGF) to stimulate healing at the site. *The fracture is very much mobile at this stage.*

STAGE OF SOFT CALLUS (DAYS 5 TO 11)

The release of VEGF leads to angiogenesis at the site. Within the haematoma, fibrin-rich granulation tissue begins to develop. Further mesenchymal stem cells are recruited to the area and they begin to differentiate to fibroblasts, chondroblasts, and osteoblasts. As a result, laying down a *collagen-rich fibrocartilaginous tissue* spanning the fracture ends occurs. At the same time, adjacent to the periosteal layers, a layer of woven

Table 2.1: Stages of fracture healing.		
Stage of healing	**Approximate time**	**Essential features**
Stage of haematoma	Less than 5 days	■ Fracture end necrosis occurs. Cytokines liberated ■ Sensitisation of precursor cells ■ Fracture is mobile
Stage of soft (fibrocartilaginous) callus	5–11 days	■ Proliferation and differentiation of precursor cells into vessels, fibroblasts, chondroblasts and osteoblasts ■ Early callus becomes visible (2 weeks). Fracture *is sticky*
Stage of hard (bony) callus	11–28 days	■ Ossification of fibrocartilaginous tissue ■ *Callus* radiologically visible ■ Fracture clinically united, *no more mobile*
Stage of remodelling	18 days to many years	Modelling of endosteal and periosteal surfaces so that the fracture site becomes indistinguishable from the parent bone

bone is laid down. Visibility of this bone, a cloud-like image on a rays, is the *earliest sign of fracture healing*. It typically appears in 2 weeks from fracture. It happens much earlier in children. This is the stage where the fracture starts becoming 'sticky'. *It is still possible to change the alignment of the bone by gentle manipulation.*

STAGE OF BONY CALLUS (DAYS 11 TO 28)

The cartilaginous callus (soft callus) begins to undergo endochondral ossification. In this process, the cartilaginous callus starts resorbing and begins to calcify. Subperiosteally, woven bone continues to be laid down. The newly formed blood vessels continue to proliferate, allowing further migration of mesenchymal stem cells. At the end of this phase, a hard, calcified callus of immature bone forms between the fracture ends, what is commonly referred to as *bridging callus* (Fig. 2.4). This is a sign of progressive bone healing, and can be clearly seen on X-rays. Over a period of time, the bridging callus becomes more and more solid. By this time, the fracture has gained enough strength, and *to change the alignment now may not be easy.* One will have to 'break' the healing bone, what is called *osteoclasis.*

BONE REMODELLING (DAY 18 ONWARDS, LASTING MONTHS TO YEARS)

With the continued migration of osteoblasts and osteoclasts, the hard callus undergoes repeated remodelling. The process of remodelling happens in block-by-block manner, termed *'coupled remodelling'*. This is a balance of coupled process - resorption by osteoclasts and new bone formation by osteoblasts. The centre of the callus is ultimately replaced by compact bone, while the callus edges become replaced by lamellar bone. *This can be seen on X-rays as what was callus, turning into dense white bone, akin to normal bone.* Wolff's law plays an important role here - 'bone changes its shape according to the stresses it is subjected to'. The process of bone remodelling lasts for many months, ultimately resulting in the regeneration of the normal bone structure. So effective is the remodelling in some cases that *it is often impossible to detect an old fracture after a few years.* Remodelling is much quicker and much more in children.

This process of bone healing (ossification) is also called *endochondral ossification.* In this, first collagen rich cartilage cells are formed. The cartilage cells are subsequently replaced by immature bone. This process (endochondral ossification) also occurs during the formation of long bones in the fetus, where the cartilage model of the skeleton is replaced by bony skeleton. There is another type of ossification involved

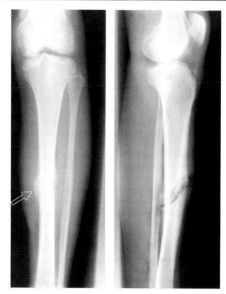

Fig. 2.4: X-ray of the fracture of the tibial shaft showing callus formation.

in skeletal development in fetus—*intramembranous ossification.* This is a process by which mesenchymal tissue (primitive connective tissue) is converted directly to the bone, with no cartilage intermediate. This process takes place in the formation of flat bones of the skull.

HEALING OF CANCELLOUS BONES

The healing of fractured cancellous bone follows a different pattern. The bone is of uniform spongy texture and has no medullary cavity so that there is a large area of contact between the trabeculae. Union can occur directly between the bony trabeculae. Subsequent to haematoma and granulation formation, mature osteoblasts lay down woven bone in the intercellular matrix, and the two fragments unite.

PRIMARY AND SECONDARY FRACTURE HEALING (Table 2.2)

Primary bone healing or direct healing: In this type, the fracture heals bone-to-bone *without callus formation.*

Table 2.2: Primary and secondary healing of fractures.	
Primary healing	**Secondary healing**
Direct healing—bone to bone, no callus formation	Callus formation, followed by bone to bone healing
Rigid immobilization (absolute stability) a pre-requisite	Relative immobilisation (relative stability) only possible
Possible only by surgical fixation of fracture	Most fractures treated non-operatively, and others which can not be fixed rigidly (e.g., comminuted fracture)

Pre-requisite for this is: (a) bone ends have been anatomically reduced; (b) there is no gap at the fracture site and (c) the fracture has been rigidly fixed surgically; and there is no micro-motion at the fracture. This type of fixation is called fixation with *absolute stability*. Due to absence of callus, it is often difficult to assess fracture union in such cases. Absolute stability is essential for healing of some fractures, and hence resort to operative intervention is common in these fractures.

Secondary fracture healing or indirect healing: It is a process of natural bone healing, the way most fractures heal. Here they heal *by callus formation*. This occurs in fractures where bone ends are well-aligned, not necessarily anatomically reduced. Once these fractures are immobilised, there is some micro-motion between the ends. This is called providing *relative stability*. Healing with callus formation occurs in fractures treated non-operatively (in plaster for example). It also occurs in cases treated operatively where though the fracture has been fixed surgically, but not necessarily reduced anatomically or fixed rigidly, accepting a certain amount of micromobility. In some operated fractures, it may not be possible to fix the fracture absolutely rigidly (e.g., comminuted fractures), and there may be micro-motion at the fracture site. Such fractures heal by *secondary healing*.

FACTORS AFFECTING FRACTURE HEALING

A number of factors affect fracture union. They can be divided into three categories:

PATIENT FACTORS

- **Age of the patient:** Fractures unite faster in children. In younger children, callus is often visible on X-rays as early as *two weeks* after the fracture. On an average, bones in children unite in *half* the time compared to that in adults. Failure of union is uncommon in fractures of children.
- **Nutritional status**
- **Metabolic disorder**, such as diabetes, hypothyroidism
- **Smoking and alcoholism**

FRACTURE FACTORS

- **Type of bone:** Flat and cancellous bones unite faster than tubular and cortical bones.
- **Pattern of fracture:** Spiral fractures unite faster than oblique fractures, which in turn unite

faster than transverse fractures. Comminuted fractures are usually result of a severe trauma or occur in osteoporotic bones, and thus heal slower.

- **Mechanism of injury:** We tend to differentiate fractures into *low-velocity* and *high-velocity*, depending upon severity of injury that has resulted it. Low-velocity injury, for example, just fall at home. High-velocity injury, for example that sustained in a traffic accident. Why these two fractures behave differently is due to associated soft tissue injury—extend of soft tissue stripping due to injury. Fractures with more soft tissue stripping loose blood supply of a larger segment of bone, and hence it takes time for the bone ends to revascularise, and hence for the bone to unite.
- **Disturbed pathoanatomy:** Following a fracture, changes may occur at the fracture site, and may hinder the normal healing process. These are: (i) soft tissue interposition; and (ii) ischaemic fracture ends. In the former, the fracture ends pierce through the surrounding soft tissues, and get stuck. This causes soft tissue interposition between the fragments, and prevents the callus from bridging the fragments. In the latter, due to anatomical peculiarities of blood supply of some bones (e.g., scaphoid), vascularity of one of the fragments is cut off. Since vascularised bone ends are important for optimal fracture union, these fractures unite slowly or do not unite at all.
- **Open fractures:** Open fractures often go into delayed union and non-union (discussed subsequently on page 21).

SURGEON FACTORS

- **Type of reduction:** Good apposition of the fracture results in faster union. At least half the fracture surface should be in contact for optimal union in adults. In children, a fracture may unite even if bones are only side-to-side in contact (bayonet reduction).
- **Immobilisation:** It is not necessary to immobilise all fractures (e.g., fracture ribs, scapula, etc.). They heal anyway. Some fractures need strict immobilisation and may still not heal.
- **Stable fixation:** Whenever surgery is done, stable fixation is important. This could be rigid fixation wherever possible and hence aim at primary healing, or at least a stable fixation and achieve union by secondary healing.

What have we learnt?

- There are different parts of a long bone such as diaphysis, metaphysis and epiphysis. There are diseases which typically affect only some parts of the bones
- Growing skeleton is identified by presence of growth plate
- The structure of the bone is complex, made of the basic structural unit called osteon
- Different bone cells have different functions
- Fracture healing follows a series of stages. The understanding helps in treatment of fracture
- Difference between endochondral and intramembranous ossification
- Difference between primary and secondary bone healing
- Fracture healing depends upon a number of factors.

Additional information: From the entrance exams point of view

Pathognomonic sign of traumatic and fresh fracture is crepitus. Most common cause of non-union is inadequate immobilisation.

Markers of bone formation: Serum bone specific alkaline phosphatase
Serum osteocalcin
Serum peptide of type 1 collagen

Markers of bone resorption: Urine and serum cross-linked 'N' telopeptide
Urine and serum cross-linked 'C' telopeptide
Urine total free deoxypyridinoline

Rate of mineralisation determined by labelled tetracycline

Competencies

- ❖ **OR1.1:** Describe and discuss the principles of pre-hospital care and casualty management of a trauma victim including principles of triage.
- ❖ **OR2.16:** Describe and discuss the mechanism of injury, clinical features, investigations and principles of management of open fractures with focus on secondary infection prevention and management.

Treatment of a fracture can be considered in three phases:

- Phase I - Emergency care
- Phase II - Definitive care
- Phase III - Rehabilitation

PHASE I - EMERGENCY CARE

At the site of accident: Emergency care of a fracture begins at the site of the accident. In principle, it consists of RICE, which means:

- **R**est to the part, by splinting.
- **I**ce therapy, to reduce occurrence of swelling
- **C**ompression, to reduce swelling
- **E**levation, to reduce swelling

Rest to the part is done by splinting - 'Splint them where they lie'. Before applying the splint, remove ring or bangles worn by the patient. Almost any available object at the site of the accident can be used for splinting. It may be a folded newspaper, a magazine, a rigid cardboard, a stick, an umbrella, a pillow, or a wooden plank. Any available long piece of cloth can be used for tying the made up splint. Some of the examples of splinting a fractured extremity at the site of the accident are shown in Figure 3.1. One may correct any gross deformity by gentle traction.

It may be a little painful, but desirable. Feel for distal pulses, and do a quick assessment of nerve supply before and after splinting. Absence of pulse is a *dire emergency* and a consideration has to be made to shift the patient to a facility equipped for taking care of vascular injury.

The advantages of splinting are:

- Relief of pain, by preventing movement at the fracture.
- Prevention of further damage to skin, soft tissues and neurovascular bundle of the injured extremity.
- Prevention of complications such as fat embolism and hypovolaemic shock.
- Transportation of the patient made easier.

Ice therapy: An immediate application of ice to injured part helps in reducing pain and swelling. Icing can be done by taking crushed ice in a polythene bag and covering it with a wet cloth. Commercially available ice packs can also be used. Any wound, if present, has to be covered with sterile clean cloth.

Compression: A crepe bandage is applied over the injured part, making sure that it is not too tight.

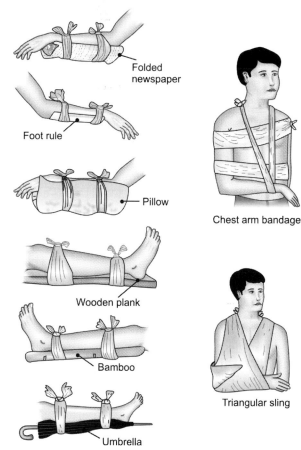

Fig. 3.1: Some of the commonly available articles used for splintage of fractures.

this is done before taking any further action such as doing X-rays, etc.

It is important to check the bandaging and splintage done elsewhere, as it may be too tight. Some of the splints used in the emergency department are as shown in Figure 3.2. In addition to splintage, the patient should be made comfortable by giving him intramuscular analgesics. In a case with suspected head injury, narcotic analgesics should be avoided. A broad spectrum antibiotic may be given to those with open fractures. It is only after the emergency care has been given, and it is ensured that the patient is stable, he should be sent for suitable radiological and other investigations.

In a case of multiple injuries, orthopaedic treatment takes back seat over more serious visceral injuries. Here, the goal of orthopaedic treatment is to *damage control*, by appropriate splintage, which may involve using an interim external fixator.

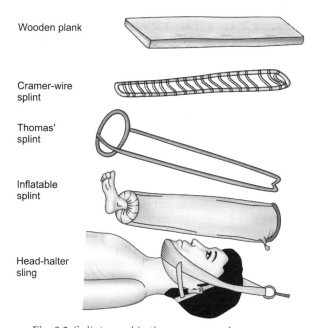

Fig. 3.2: Splints used in the emergency department.

Elevation: The limb is elevated so that the injured part is above the level of the heart. For lower limb, this can be done using pillows. For upper limb, a sling and pillow can be used.

In the emergency department: Soon after a patient with musculoskeletal trauma is received in an emergency department, one has to act in a coordinated way. First principle is to *save life by quick assessment and providing basic life support (BLS)*, wherever required.

Second principle is to make a *quick assessment of possibly life-threatening injuries* such as head injury, chest injury and abdominal injury. These can be cause of early fatality. Any bleeding is recognised and stopped by local pressure. The fractured limb is examined to exclude injury to nerves or vessels. If the patient is in shock, which is common in major skeletal injuries such as femur fracture and pelvis fracture, the shock is appropriately managed and patient stablised. All

PHASE II - DEFINITIVE CARE

Philosophy of fracture treatment: Over the years, treatment of fractures has undergone change in philosophy. In the past, the aim of treatment was a mere fracture union. This could be achieved in most cases by immobilisation of some kind. With this, though the fracture would heal in most circumstances, there would be residual joint stiffness, muscle wasting, etc., and this may result in less than optimal functional recovery of the limb as a whole. The aim in modern days is to get the limb functions back to pre-injury level. For this, early functional use of the limb, as far as possible, is desirable.

Perfect anatomical reduction and stable fixation is preferred for intra-articular fractures, as only then early mobilisation can be done. This is most often possible only by operative methods. In diaphyseal fractures, the aim is to achieve union in good alignment and maintaining length. This can be achieved by non-operative methods if the fracture is stable. In case the fracture is unstable, or sometimes as a matter of comfort of early mobility, operative treatment is preferred. With currently available techniques of surgery, the trend is towards treating more and more fractures operatively as this gives more predictable results, early recovery and better functions. The discussion that follows will give the reader a guideline.

Fundamental principles of fracture treatment: The three *fundamental principles* of treatment of a fracture are: (i) reduction; (ii) immobilisation; and (iii) preservation of functions.

Reduction is the technique of 'setting' a displaced fracture to proper alignment. This may be done non-operatively or operatively—so-called closed and open reduction respectively.

Immobilisation is necessary to maintain the bones in reduced position. This may be done by external immobilisation such as plaster, etc., or by internal fixation of the fracture using rods, plates, screw, etc.

To *preserve the functions* of the limb, by physiotherapy all through the treatment, even when the limb is immobilised, and thereafter.

Methods of treatment: Not all the three fundamental treatment principles mentioned above apply to all fractures. Treatment of a particular fracture can fall in one of the following categories:

a. *Treatment by functional use of the limb*: This means one can simply ignore the fracture and continue to use the limb. There are fractures such as fractured ribs, scapula, etc., which need no reduction or immobilisation. These fractures unite despite functional use of the part. Simple analgesics and splinting are needed for the initial few days, basically for pain relief.

b. *Treatment by immobilisation alone*: In some fractures, mere immobilisation of the fracture in whatever position, is good enough. Accurate anatomical reduction is not a must in these fractures. Fractures which are not displaced in the first place, or even if they are, the displacement is of no consequence in terms of eventual outcome (e.g., some fractures of surgical neck of the humerus).

c. *Treatment by closed reduction followed by immobilisation:* This is required for most displaced fractures treated non-operatively. The reduction could be done under mild sedation or under anaesthesia. Immobilisation is usually in a plaster cast. There is trend towards use of a special video X-rays machine called 'image intensifier' (page 33) to aid. Once acceptable reduction is achieved, it is prudent to keep a close watch on position of the fracture in the plaster by taking frequent X-rays.

d. *Closed reduction and percutaneous fixation:* There are fractures, which though can be reduced by closed manipulation but are unstable, and have potential to get displace subsequently. These fractures are reduced under image intensifier, and fixed with percutaneous devices such as K-wire, rush pins, etc. These devices can be put without opening the fracture, percutaneously. These hold the fracture good enough till it heals. External support of a plaster or splint for a limited period is usually required, in addition.

e. *Open reduction and internal fixation (ORIF):* There are some fractures, such as intra-articular fractures, where accurate reduction, stable fixation and early mobilisation are very important to regain joint functions. Such fractures are best treated by open reduction and internal fixation. Some unstable juxta-articular fractures are also treated by ORIF. The scope of using this method has expanded over the years.

f. *Minimally invasive open surgery (MIS):* For the fractures which need operation, there is trend towards using with minimally invasive techniques. In the past, in order to fix a fracture, the whole bone used to be exposed, and then fixed. Though it was technically easier for surgeons to do surgery, but this would often lead to extensive soft tissue damage and also damage to blood supply of the bone. Often the X-rays would look good but the bone would fail to heal as extensive damage would be cause to blood supply of the bones by these rather liberal open surgeries.

In modern days, trend is to do these operations by minimal exposure, and hence minimal damage to soft-tissues. Image intensifier is of great use in doing so as it as possible to achieve reduction by indirect methods by manipulating under image intensifier vision. The fracture is stabilised internally using special devices such as rods, plates, etc. These devices are introduced through small incisions using special instrumentation. MIS has the advantage that the blood supply of the bone is preserved, and thus early union occurs. Less pain, early recovery and cosmesis are other advantages.

g. *Primary joint replacement:* There are fractures in which results of trying to achieve union are little, and hence the broken part of the bone is replaced with artificial part (prosthesis). This is commonly used for hip fractures and shoulder fractures.

Which of the above method is used in a particular fracture depends upon a number of factors such as patient's profession, whether the injured limb is dominant or not, surgeon's experience, availability of facilities, patient's affordability, etc. It is therefore common to see differing opinions by different surgeons, on the treatment of the same fracture.

Discussed below are the three fundamental principles of fracture treatment - reduction, immobilisation and preservation of functions.

REDUCTION OF FRACTURES

Indications: Not all fractures require reduction, either because there is no displacement or because the displacement is immaterial to the final outcome. For example, a child's clavicle fracture does not need reduction because normal function and appearance will be restored without any intervention.

In general, imperfect apposition of fragments can be accepted more readily than imperfect angulatory alignment or rotational mal-alignment. Perfect anatomical reduction is desirable in some fractures, even if for this an operation is required (e.g., intra-articular fractures).

Methods: Reduction of a fracture can be carried out by one of the following methods:

a. *Closed manipulation:* This is the standard initial method of reducing most of the common fractures. It is usually carried out under general anaesthesia* and requires experience. It is an art of realigning a displaced bone by feeling through the soft tissues. The availability of an image intensifier has greatly added to the skills of closed reduction. It is not necessary that perfect anatomical reduction be achieved in all cases. Displacements compatible with normal functions are considered 'acceptable'. Most fractures reduced by closed manipulation

need some kind of immobilisation (PoP, brace, bandaging, etc.) (page 18).

b. *Continuous traction:* It is used to counter the forces which may not allow reduction to happen or forces that would cause re-displacement. These are muscle forces and the force of gravity. A common example is that of an inter-trochanteric fracture, in which the muscles attached to different fragments cause displacements. A continuous traction can counter this force, and bring the bones in proper alignment. Once maintained in good position in traction, the fracture heals predictably.

Though continuous traction is easily available and cost-effective, it has its own problems. These are problems of keeping the patient in bed for long time with associated complications such as bedsores, etc. It is for this reason that one often practices a hybrid policy, which means, keep the patient in traction as long as it takes to become sticky, and once it so happens, and there is little possibility of re-displacement, the traction is discontinued and the fracture supported in a plaster cast till healing occurs. Many of these fractures which were earlier treated in traction, are now treated operatively, due to uncertainty of result and need for long periods of in-bed immobilization. Different methods of applying traction are discussed in Chapter 4.

c. *Open reduction:* In this method, the fracture is surgically exposed, and the fragments are reduced under vision. Once reduced, some form of internal fixation is used to maintain the position. This is commonly referred as 'open reduction and internal fixation' or ORIF. This is one area of fracture treatment which is continuously evolving. There used to be times when orthopaedic wards used to be full of patients in traction and huge plaster casts for months. Today, with the advancement in surgical treatment, the paradigm has shifted to operative treatment. The big deciding factor for adopting ORIF as the treatment of choice is the facilities available and training of the surgeon. Operative treatment of fractures, though has become a preferred method these days, but has to be done with care as potential risks of surgery are sometimes worse than the disadvantages of non-operative treatment.

One clear reason to do open reduction is when other methods of achieving reduction have failed. There are fractures which are so unstable that one knows that these fractures will re-displace in due course. In such fractures, open reduction and secure internal fixation is carried out in the first instance.

---

* For reasons of practicality, sometimes closed reduction is carried out under sedation.

Table 3.1: Indications for open reduction.

Absolute
- Failure of closed reduction
- Displaced intra-articular fractures
- Some displaced epiphyseal injuries (types III and IV)
- Major avulsion fractures, e.g., fracture of patella
- Non-union

Relative
- Delayed union and malunion
- Multiple fractures
- Pathological fractures
- Where closed reduction is known to be ineffective, e.g., fracture of the neck of the femur
- Fractures with vascular or neural injuries

Some of the widely accepted indications of ORIF are given in Table 3.1.

IMMOBILISATION OF FRACTURES

Indications: Not all fractures require immobilisation. The reasons for immobilising a fracture may be:

a. To *prevent displacement or angulation:* In general, if reduction has been necessary, immobilisation will be required.

b. To *prevent movement that might interfere with the union:* Persistent movement might tear the delicate early capillaries bridging the fracture. More strict immobilisation is necessary for some fractures (e.g., scaphoid fracture).

c. *To relieve pain:* This is the most important reason for the immobilisation of most fractures. As the fracture become pain free and feels stable, guarded mobilisation may be started.

Methods: Immobilisation of a fracture can be done by non-operative or operative methods.

NON-OPERATIVE METHODS

Most fractures can be immobilised by one of the following non-operative methods:

- **Strapping:** The fractured part is strapped to an adjacent part of the body, e.g., a phalanx fracture, where one finger is strapped to the adjacent normal finger (see Fig. 16.3 on page 117).
- **Sling:** A fracture of the upper extremity is immobilised in a sling. This is mostly to relieve pain in cases where strict immobilisation is not necessary, e.g., triangular sling used for a fracture of the clavicle.
- **Cast immobilisation:** This is the most common method of immobilisation. Plaster-of-Paris casts have been in use for a long time. Lately, fibreglass casting tapes have become popular. The latter provide durable, light-weight, radiolucent casts.

Plaster of Paris (Gypsum salt) is $CaSO . \frac{1}{2} H_2O$ in dry form, which becomes $CaSO_4.2H_2O$ on wetting. This conversion is an *exothermic reaction* and is *irreversible*. The plaster sets in the given shape on drying. The setting time of a plaster varies with its quality, and temperature of the water. Names of some of the plaster casts commonly used are given in Table 3.2.

Types of plaster bandages: There are two types of plaster bandages in use—one prepared by impregnating rolls of starched cotton bandages with plaster powder (home-made bandages), which were widely used in the past. These have been replaced by readymade plaster bandages available as a proprietary bandage.

Use of plaster of Paris: It can be applied in two forms, i.e., slab or a cast.

Table 3.2: Plaster casts and their uses.	
Name of the cast	**Use**
Minerva cast	Cervical spine disease
Risser's cast	Scoliosis
Turn-buckle cast	Scoliosis
Shoulder spica*	Shoulder immobilisation
U-slab	Fracture of the humerus
Hanging cast	Fracture of the humerus
Colles' cast	Colles' fracture
Hip spica	Fracture of the femur
Cylinder cast	Fracture of the patella
PTB cast	Fracture of the tibia

* A spica is a cast where a limb and a part of the trunk are included, e.g., hip spica, shoulder spica.

A plaster slab covers only a part of the circumference of a limb. It is made by unrolling a plaster bandage to and fro on a table. An average slab is about twelve such thicknesses. The slab is used for the immobilisation of soft tissue injuries and for reinforcing plaster casts. A plaster cast covers the whole of the circumference of a limb. Its thickness varies with the type of fracture and the part of the body on which it is applied. Some of the fundamental principles to be remembered while applying a plaster cast are as follows:

- Immobilise the joints above and below the fracture.
- Immobilise joints in a functional position*.
- Pad the limb adequately, especially over bony prominences.

---

* There are exceptions: the important one being Colles' fracture where the elbow is not immobilised; and also the wrist is not immobilised in 'functional' position.

After care of a plaster: This involves noticing any crack in the plaster, avoiding wetting the plaster, and graduated weight-bearing for lower limb fractures. Exercising the muscles within the plaster and moving the joints not in the plaster, is necessary to ensure early recovery.

Complications of plaster treatment: The following are some of the common complications of plaster treatment:

- **Impairment of circulation (*tight cast*) (Fig. 3.3):** A plaster cast is a closed compartment. Haematoma and tissue oedema following a fracture can result in increased pressure inside the cast, leading to impaired circulation of the extremity. If not diagnosed early, this can result in disastrous complications such as gangrene. Key to early diagnosis is: (a) high index of suspicion; (b) unrelenting pain, not settling with usual dose of analgesics; (c) swelling over the fingers or toes, and inability to move them; (d) stretch pain (see page 48); (e) hypoesthesia or bluish discolouration of the digits. A tight cast can be prevented by adequately padding the cast and elevating the extremity for the first 2-3 days following a cast application.

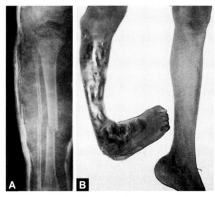

Fig. 3.3: Disastrous complication of plaster cast: (A) X-ray of a child with rather simple fracture; (B) Ischaemic and deformed foot due to tight plaster.

- **Plaster sores:** These are caused by inadequate padding, irregularity of the inner surface of the cast, or foreign bodies in the plaster. A sore formation within a plaster cast can be suspected by the following:
  - Pain, out of proportion to fracture
  - Fretfulness
  - Disturbed sleep
  - Recurrence of swelling over toes or fingers
  - Low grade fever
  - Patch of blood/soakage over the cast.

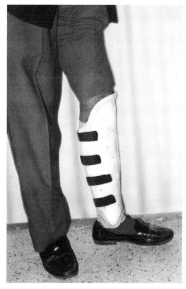

Fig. 3.4: A plastic brace is used for a sticky fracture of the tibia. The patient is up and about, can put on shoes and go to work.

A plaster sore can be prevented by examination of the suspected area through a window in the cast. It is possible to dress a small sore through this window. Occasionally, the plaster has to be removed and reapplied.

- **Blisters inside the plaster:** Sometimes, when a plaster cast or a slab is applied for a fresh injury, due to ensuing oedema and skin stretching blistered develop inside the plaster. Prevention by adequate padding and opening us the plaster if too much pain is the way out.

- **Functional bracing (Fig. 3.4):** A brace is a type of cast where the joints are not included, so that while the fracture is kept in position, the joints can also be mobilised. This method is commonly used for stable fractures of the tibia and humerus. It is based on the principle that continuous use of the affected limb while the fracture is kept adequately supported, rather encourages union and prevents joint stiffness. The brace is usually applied after the fracture becomes 'sticky'. In experienced hands, the rate of fracture healing by this method is comparable to other methods (see details on page 34). It is a useful option at places where facilities for surgical treatment are not available.

Splints and traction: Splints of various designs are used for the definitive treatment of fractures. Thomas splint is still very popular for the treatment of fractures of the lower limb. Disadvantages of this method of treatment are prolonged hospitalisation and confinement to the bed. This can be hazardous, especially in elderly people who develop complications secondary to recumbency (e.g., bed sores, chest infection, etc.). For details about splints, see Chapter 4.

OPERATIVE METHODS

Wherever open reduction is performed, fixation (internal or external) should also be used. External fixation is usually indicated in situations where for some reason, internal fixation cannot be done.

Internal fixation: In this method, the fracture once reduced, is held internally with the help of some metallic or non-metallic device (implant), such as steel wire, screw, plate, Kirschner wire (K-wire), intramedullary nail, etc. These implants are made of high quality medical grade stainless steel, to which the body is inert.

Indications: Internal fixation of fractures may be indicated under the following circumstances:

a. When a fracture is so unstable that it is difficult to maintain it in an acceptable position by non-operative means. This is the most frequent indication for internal fixation.

b. As a treatment of choice in some fractures, in order to secure rigid immobilisation and to allow early mobility of the patient.

c. When it has been necessary to perform open reduction for any other reason such as an associated neurovascular injury.

Methods: A fracture can be fixed internally by any one or combination of implants given in Table 3.3.

a. *Steel wire:* A gauge 18 or 20 steel wire is used for internal fixation of small fractures (e.g., fracture of the patella, comminuted fragments of large bones, etc.).

b. *Kirschner wire:* It is a straight stainless steel wire, 1–3 mm in diameter. It is used for the fixation of small bones of the hands and feet.

c. *Intramedullary nail:* It is erroneously called 'nail', but in fact is a hollow rod made of stainless steel. This can be introduced into the medullary cavity of the long bones such as femur and tibia. They can be inserted into the medullary canal from proximal to distal (antegrade nail) or from distal to proximal (retrograde nail). Different shapes and sizes of these nails are available.

d. *Screws:* These can be used for fixing small fragments of bone to the main bone (e.g., for fixation of medial malleolus).

e. *Plate and screws:* These devices which can be fixed on the surface of a bone with the help of screws. Different thicknesses, shapes and sizes are available.

Table 3.3: Some implants used in treatment of fractures.	
Intramedullary nails	
PFN, DFN, PHN, Recon nail	
▪ Kuntscher's nail	Fracture shaft femur
▪ Talwalkar's nail	Fracture forearm bones
▪ V-nail	Fracture tibia
▪ Ender's nail	Intertrochanteric fracture
▪ Rush nail	General purpose
▪ Hartshill rectangle	Spine injuries
▪ GK nail	Fracture shaft femur
▪ Gamma nail	Intertrochanteric fracture
Plates and screws	
▪ Compression plate	Transverse and oblique fractures of any long bone
▪ Neutralisation plate	Comminuted fractures
▪ Buttress plate	Condylar fracture of tibia
▪ Locking compression	Peri-articular fractures plate
Special implants	
▪ Dynamic hip screw (DHS)	Intertrochanteric fracture
▪ PHILOS plate	Proximal humerus fractures
▪ Condylar blade-plate	Condylar fracture of femur
▪ Spoon plate	Fracture of lower end of tibia
▪ Cobra plate	Hip arthrodesis
Others	
▪ Steel wire	Fracture of patella
▪ K-wire	Fracture of small bones

f. *Special, fracture specific implants:* These are used for internal fixation of some fractures (Table 3.3).

g. *Combination:* A combination of the above-mentioned implants can be used for a given fracture.

For details about commonly used implants, refer to Annexure III, page 362.

Advantages of internal fixation: With the use of modern techniques and implants, there is minimal need for external immobilisation. It allows early mobility of the patient out of bed and hospital. Joints do not get stiff and the muscle functions remain good. The complications associated with confinement of a patient to bed are also avoided.

Disadvantages: The disadvantages of internal fixation are infection and non-union. It needs a trained orthopaedic surgeon, free availability of implants and a good operation theatre; failing which, the results of internal fixation may not only be poor but disastrous.

External fixator: It is a device (Fig. 3.5) by which the fracture is held in a steel frame *outside the limb.* For this, pins are passed percutaneously to hold the bone, and are connected outside to a bar with the help of clamps. This method is useful in the treatment of open fractures where internal fixation cannot be carried out due to risk of infection. These are of the following type:

i. *Tubular fixators:* In these, 3–4 mm size steel pins are passed through the bone percutaneously, and are held outside with the help of a variety of tubular rods and clamps [Fig. 3.5(A)].

ii. *Ring fixators:* In this, thin 'K' wires (1–2 mm) are passed through the bone. The same are held outside the bone with rings [Fig. 3.5(B)], (For details, page 35).

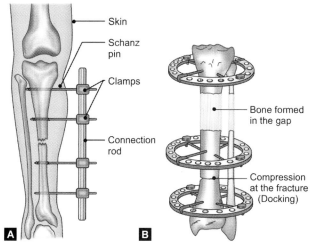

Fig. 3.5: External fixator: (A) Tubular fixator; (B) Ring fixator.

PHASE III - REHABILITATION OF A FRACTURED LIMB

Rehabilitation of a fractured limb begins at the time of injury, and goes on till maximum possible functions have been regained. It consists of joint mobilisation, muscle re-education exercises and instructions regarding gait training.

Joint mobilisation: The joint adjacent to an injured bone tends to get stiff due to: (i) immobilisation; (ii) inability to move the joints due to pain; and (iii) associated injury to the joint as well. To prevent stiffness, the joint should be mobilised as soon as possible. This is done initially by *passive mobilisation* (some one else does it for the patient). Once the pain reduces, patient is encouraged to move the joint himself with assistance (active assisted), or move the joint by himself (active mobilisation). Motorized devices which slowly move the joint through a predetermined range of motion can be used. These are called *continuous passive motion (CPM) machines*. Techniques such as hot fomentation, gentle massage and manipulation aid in joint mobilisation.

Muscle re-education exercises: Because of lack of use, the muscles get wasted quickly. Hence, it is desirable that muscle activity be maintained all through the treatment. This can be done even during immobilisation (static contractions) or after removal of external immobilisation (dynamic contractions), as discussed below:

a. *During immobilisation:* Even while a fracture is immobilised, the joints which are out of the plaster, should be moved to prevent stiffness and wasting of muscles. Such movements do not cause any deleterious effect on the position of the fracture. The muscles working on the joints inside the plaster can be contracted without moving the joint (static contractions). This maintains some functions of the immobilised muscles.

b. *After removal of immobilisation:* After a limb is immobilised for some period, it gets stiff. As the plaster is removed, the following care is required:
  - The skin is cleaned, scales removed, and some oil applied.
  - The joints are moved to regain the range of motion. Hot fomentation, active and active-assisted joint mobilising exercises are required for this (page 52).
  - The muscles wasted due to prolonged immobilisation are exercised.

Functional use of the limb: Once a fracture is on way to union, at a suitable opportunity, the limb is put to use in a guarded way. For example, in lower limb injuries, gradual weight-bearing is started—partial followed by full. One may need to support the limb in a brace, caliper, cast, etc. Walking aids such as a walker, a pair of crutches, stick, etc., may be necessary.

A general plan of management for a usual fracture is shown in Flowchart 3.1 on next page.

MANAGEMENT OF OPEN FRACTURES

A fracture is called open (compound) when there is a break in the overlying skin and soft tissues, establishing communication between the fracture and the external environment. Three specific consequences may result from this.

a. **Infection of bone:** Contamination of the wound with bacteria from the outside environment may lead to infection of the bone (osteomyelitis).

b. **Inability to use traditional methods:** A small wound can be managed through a window in a plaster cast. But, it may not be possible to manage a big wound through a window. The presence of a wound may also be a deterrent to operative fixation of the fracture.

Flowchart 3.1: General plan for treatment of fractures.

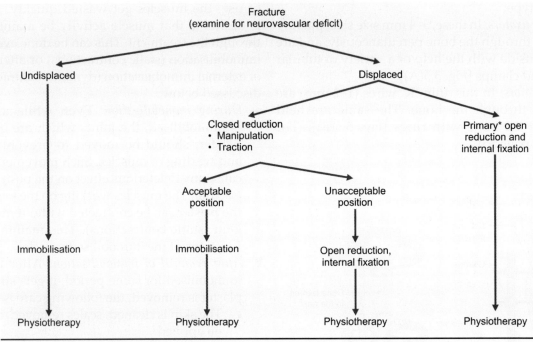

* Open reduction straightaway is required for some fractures

c. **Problems related to union:** Non-union and malunion occur commonly in open fractures. This may be because of one or more of the following reasons: (i) a piece of bone may be lost from the wound at the time of the fracture, the gap thus created predisposes to non-union; (ii) the fracture haematoma, which is supposed to have osteogenic potential, is lost from the wound; (iii) the 'vascular' cover by the overlying soft tissues, so important for fracture union, may be missing; and (iv) the bone may get secondarily infected, and thus affect union.

It is because of these possible consequences that open fractures deserve utmost care throughout their management. Open fractures have been classified into three types, depending upon the extent of soft tissue injury (Table 3.4).

TREATMENT

The principle of treatment is to convert an open fracture into a closed fracture by meticulous wound care. Thereafter, the treatment of open fracture is essentially on the lines of closed fractures. The following discussion emphasises the points pertinent to the treatment of open fractures.

Phase I - Emergency Care

At the site of accident: The following measures are taken at the site of the accident:

a. The bleeding from the wound is stopped by applying firm pressure using a clean piece of cloth. At times it may be necessary to use a tight

Table 3.4: Modified Gustilo and Anderson classification for open fractures.	
Type	**Description**
I	<ul><li>Skin wound less than 1 cm</li><li>Clean</li><li>Simple fracture pattern</li></ul>
II	<ul><li>Skin wound more than 1 cm</li><li>Soft-tissue damage not extensive</li><li>No flaps or avulsions</li><li>Simple fracture pattern</li></ul>
III	High-energy injury involving extensive soft-tissue damage Or multi-fragmentary fracture, segmental fractures, or bone loss irrespective of the size of skin wound Or severe crush injuries Or vascular injury requiring repair Or severe contamination including farmyard injuries A later modification subdivided type III injuries based on the degree of contamination, the extent of periosteal stripping and the presence of vascular injury. IIIA. Adequate soft-tissue cover of bone despite extensive soft-tissue damage IIIB. Extensive soft-tissue injury with periosteal stripping and bone exposure. Major wound contamination IIIC. High-energy injury involving extensive soft-tissue damage

circular bandage proximal to the wound in order to stop bleeding.

b. The wound is washed with clean tap water or saline, and covered with a clean cloth.

c. The fracture is splinted.

At times, a piece of bone devoid of all soft tissue attachments may be lying out of the wound. It should be washed and taken to the hospital in a clean cloth. It may be useful in reconstruction of the fracture.

In the emergency department: Open fractures are known to be associated with neurovascular injuries more often than the simple fractures. Hence, one should carefully look for these associated injuries.

The following treatment is performed in the emergency department:

Wound care: Care in the emergency room consists of washing the wound under strict aseptic conditions and covering it with sterile dressing. Sometimes, the bone may be jetting out of the skin, causing stretching of the skin around the wound. Replacing the projecting bone is necessary in order to prevent devascularisation of the skin. A piece of bone with intact soft tissue attachments hanging out of the wound, should be washed and put back in the wound. All this is done under proper aseptic conditions.

a. *Splintage* as described on page 15.

b. *Prophylactic antibiotics* should be given to all patients. Cephalexin is a good broad-spectrum antibiotic for this purpose. In serious compound fractures, a combination of third generation cephalosporins and an amino-glycoside is preferred.

c. *Tetanus prophylaxis* is given after evaluating the tetanus immunisation status of the patient.

d. *Analgesics* to be given parenterally to make the patient comfortable.

e. *X-rays* are done to evaluate the fracture in order to plan further treatment.

Phase II - Definitive Care

Definitive care of an open fracture is possible at a place equipped with a high class aseptic operation theatre, plenty of orthopaedic instruments and implants, and a competent orthopaedic surgeon. In some compound fractures, the damage to soft tissues is so much that it is wise to consult a plastic surgeon right at the beginning. The patient may need plastic surgery techniques such as flap reconstruction at the time of the first operation itself, or subsequently. Longer a bone is exposed to outside environment, more it gets desiccated, resulting in subsequent non-union.

In principle, in the treatment of open fractures, care of the wound goes hand in hand with that of the fracture.

Wound care: This consists of early wound debridement and subsequent care.

a. *Wound debridement:* Wound debridement is needed in all cases. There may be only a puncture wound, needing minimal debridement, irrigation and wound closure; or the limb may be so badly crushed that repeated debridement may be required. While debriding the wound, the skin should be excised as little as necessary. The muscles and fascia can be excised liberally. The most reliable indicator of the viability of a muscle is its contractility, on pinching it with a forceps. Only badly lacerated tendons are excised. The ends of a cut tendon are approximated with non-absorbable sutures so that they can be identified at a later date, and a definitive repair performed. Bone ends are cleaned thoroughly with normal saline. The margins of the fractured ends may be nibbled. A bone fragment with attached soft tissues is re-placed at the fracture site. Small fragments without soft tissue attachments can be discarded.

Sometimes, the limb is so badly injured that the prospects of salvaging the limb to a reasonable function is poor. In such cases, amputation, straight away, may be a better option. It is recommended that opinion of at least one more surgeon be taken before taking such a drastic decision.

b. *Definitive wound management:* Once the wound is debrided, decision regarding its closure is to be made. *Primary* closure by suturing the skin edges or by raising a flap, is okay for clean wounds. In all wounds debrided after 6-8 hours, immediate closure should not be done. The wound, in such cases should be covered with sterile dressings, and subsequently treated by delayed primary closure or be allowed to heal by secondary intention. Whenever in doubt, it is best to leave the wound open. A plan of wound closure in open fractures is shown in Flowchart 3.2.

Fracture management: In spite of the best debridement, an open fracture is a potentially infected fracture. Non-operative methods of treatment, as in closed fractures, usually give good results. In case an operative reduction of the fracture is considered necessary, it is safer to wait for the wound to heal before intervening. In cases where there is extensive damage to soft tissues, external fixation provides fixation of the fracture

Flowchart 3.2: Plan of wound closure in open fractures.

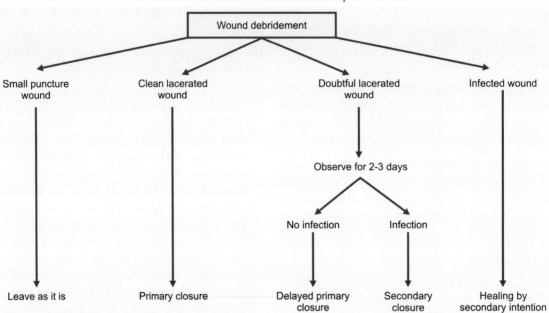

and allows good care of the wound. Some of the commonly used methods in the definitive care of an open fracture are as follows:

a. *Immobilisation in plaster:* For cases with moderate size wound, where a stable reduction of the fracture can be achieved, treatment by Plaster of Paris cast is as appropriate as for closed fractures. Care of the wound is possible through a window in the cast. Once the wound heals, the window is closed and the fracture treated on the lines of closed fractures.

b. *Pins and plaster:* For cases where the wound is moderate in size and is manageable through a window in a plaster cast, but reduction is unstable; the fracture can be stabilised by passing pins in the proximal and distal fragments, achieving reduction, and applying plaster cast with pins incorporated in it. This method is useful in open, unstable tibial fractures (Fig. 3.6).

c. *Skeletal traction:* In cases where there is circumferential loss of skin or the wound is big, it may not be possible to treat them in plaster. In such cases, skeletal traction can be used to keep the fracture in good alignment until the wound heals. After healing of the wound, one can continue traction until the fracture unites, or change over to some other form of immobilisation such as plaster cast.

d. *External skeletal fixation:* It provides stability to fracture and permits access to virtually the whole circumference of the limb (see also page 35).

e. *Internal fixation:* Conventionally, open fractures are not treated internal fixation as theoretically, a foreign implant in a not so healthy environment increases the risk of infection. But, lately, the approach to management of open fractures has become aggressive, and more and more open fractures are being treated with internal fixation. This is based on a premise that providing a stable environment to healing tissues, reduces the chances of infection. Closed methods of intramedullary fixation and minimally invasive plating techniques have been a big boon in success of this approach. Such facilities are fast becoming available in most centres in India and other developing countries.

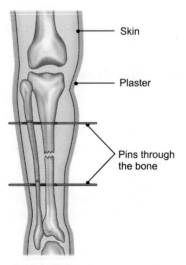

Fig. 3.6: Pin and plaster method.

Phase III - Rehabilitation

Rehabilitation of a limb with an open fracture is along the lines of a simple fracture as discussed on page 21. It consists of joint mobilisation, muscle exercises during immobilisation, after removal of immobilisation, and advice regarding mobilisation of the injured limb.

Recent trend is towards operative treatment of fractures. This has been possible due to better implants, operative techniques and safe surgical environment. Benefit is early rehabilitation, and no immobilization-related complications. For healing of fractures, there is requirement of both - adequate fixation, and good biological healing environment. Hence, the trend in recent times is to fix fractures with minimally invasive surgical (MIS) techniques such as closed nailing and MIPO (Minimally Invasive Plate Osteosynthesis) techniques.

What have we learnt?

- Fracture has to be splinted as soon as possible.
- Fracture treatment consists of keeping the fracture in acceptable position till union. This can be done by non-operative methods or operative methods.
- Non-operative methods consists of bandaging, plaster application, use of brace, traction, etc.
- Operative treatment consists of reduction of the fracture and holding it in position by internal fixation or external fixation.
- Open fractures are serious injuries, as they are more prone to complications. Adequate wound care and fracture treatment is required.

Additional information: From the entrance exams point of view

Securing the airway is the first step in treatment of polytrauma.

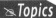Topics

❖ Splints ❖ Tractions

Learning Objectives

❖ Describe various types of splits and tractions used in orthopaedics. Discuss the daily care of the patient in traction and splint.

SPLINTS

OBJECTIVES

Splints are used for immobilising fractures; either temporarily during transportation or for definitive treatment. They are also used in other orthopaedic conditions like infection, congenital dislocation of the hip, etc.

TYPES

Some of the splints used in orthopaedic practice, and the conditions for which they are used are given in Table 4.1. The following are a few examples of common splints:

- **Cramer-wire splint:** This splint is used for temporary splintage of fractures during transportation. It is made up of two thick parallel wires with interlacing wires (Fig. 4.1). It can be bent into different shapes in order to immobilise different parts of the body.
- **Thomas knee-bed splint (Thomas splint):** It is one of the most common splints used in orthopaedic practice. It was devised by HO. Thomas, initially for immobilisation for tuberculosis of the knee. It is now commonly used for the immobilisation of hip and thigh injuries.

  Parts of a Thomas splint (Fig. 4.2): A Thomas splint has a ring and two side bars joined distally. The ring is at an angle of 120° to the inside bar. The

Table 4.1: Common splints/braces and their uses.	
Name	**Use**
Cramer-wire splint	Emergency immobilisation
Thomas splint	Fracture femur - anywhere
Bohler-Braun splint	Fracture femur - anywhere
Aluminium splint	Immobilisation of fingers
Dennis Brown splint	Congenital talipes equinovarus (CTEV)
Cock-up splint	Radial nerve palsy
Knuckle–Bender splint	Ulnar nerve palsy
Toe-raising splint	Foot drop
Volkmann's splint	Volkmann's ischaemic contracture (VIC)
Four-post collar	Neck immobilisation
Aeroplane splint	Brachial plexus injury
SOMI brace	Cervical spine injury
ASHE (anterior spinal hyper extension)	Dorso-lumbar spinal injury brace
Taylor's brace	Dorso-lumbar immobilisation
Milwaukee brace	Scoliosis
Boston brace	Scoliosis
Lumbar corset	Backache

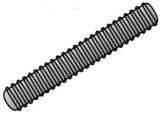

Fig. 4.1: Cramer-wire splint.

outside bar has a curvature near its junction with the ring to accommodate the greater trochanter.

Size of a Thomas splint: This is measured by finding the ring size and the length of the splint. The ring size is found by addition of 2 inches to the thigh circumference at the highest point of the groin. The length of a Thomas splint is the measurement from the highest point on the medial side of the groin up to the heel plus 6 inches.

Uses: A Thomas splint is used for immobilisation of the lower limb. The ring of the Thomas splint is introduced around the limb. The thigh and leg are supported on slings tied over the side bars.

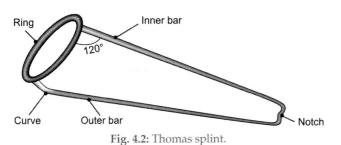

Fig. 4.2: Thomas splint.

- **Bohler-Braun splint:** This is a frame as shown in Figure 4.3. It has a number of pulleys (1–3) over which the traction cord passes while giving traction for different fractures. It is more convenient than Thomas splint since it has no ring. The ring of a

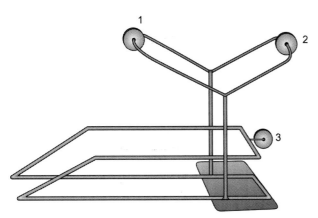

Fig. 4.3: Bohler-Braun splint (pulleys 1-3 for traction).

Thomas splint is a common cause of discomfort, especially in elderly people. A Bohler-Braun splint has no inbuilt system of countertraction, hence it is not suitable for transportation.

CARE OF A PATIENT IN A SPLINT

A patient in splint needs the following care:

a. The splint should be properly applied, well-padded at bony prominences and at the fracture site.

b. The bandage of the splint should not be too tight as it may produce sores; nor too loose, lest it becomes ineffective.

c. The patient should be encouraged to actively exercise the muscles and the joints inside the splint as much as permitted.

d. Any compression of nerve or vessel, usually due to too tight a bandage or lack of adequate padding, should be detected early and managed accordingly.

e. Daily checking and adjustments, if required, should be made. Regular portable X-rays may be taken to ensure good position of the fracture.

Now-a-days, readymade braces are available for immobilising different joints. These are available in small to extra large (XL) sizes. Common ones in use are knee immobiliser, wrist immobiliser, and ankle support.

TRACTIONS

OBJECTIVES

Traction is used for: (i) reduction of fractures and dislocations, and their maintenance; (ii) for immobilising a painful, inflamed joint; (iii) for the prevention of deformity, by counteracting the muscle spasms associated with painful joint conditions; and (iv) for the correction of soft tissue contractures by stretching them out.

TYPES OF TRACTION

For effectiveness of any traction, a countertraction is necessary. Depending upon what acts as countertraction, a traction can be fixed or sliding.

- **Fixed traction:** In this type, countertraction is pro-vided by a part of the body, e.g., in Thomas splint fixed traction, the ring of the splint comes to lie against the ischial tuberosity and provides coun-tertraction (Fig. 4.4A).

- **Sliding traction:** In this type, the weight of the body acts as countertraction; e.g., traction given for a pelvic fracture, where the weight of the

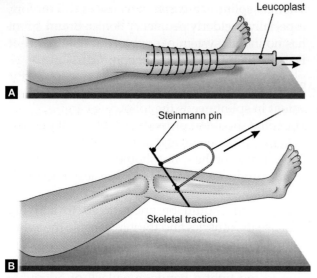

Fig. 4.4: (A) Skin traction; (B) Skeletal traction.

Table 4.3: Traction systems and their uses.	
Name	**Use**
Gallow's traction	Fracture shaft of the femur in children below 2 years
Bryant's traction	Same
Russell's traction	Trochanteric fractures
Buck's traction	Conventional skin traction
Perkin's traction	Fracture shaft of femur in adults
90°-90° traction	Fracture shaft of femur in children
Well-leg traction	Correction of adduction or abduction deformity of hip
Dunlop traction	Supracondylar fracture of humerus
Smith's traction	Supracondylar fracture of humerus
Calcaneal traction	Open fractures of ankle or leg
Metacarpal traction	Open forearm fractures
Head-halter traction	Cervical spine injuries
Crutchfield traction	Cervical spine injuries
Halo-pelvic traction	Scoliosis

body acts as countertraction; made effective by elevating the foot-end of the bed (Fig. 4.4B).

METHODS OF APPLYING TRACTION

There are two methods of applying traction - skin and skeletal (Fig. 4.4).

- **Skin traction:** An adhesive strap is applied on the skin and traction applied. The traction force is transmitted from the skin through the deep fascia and intermuscular septae to the bone. These days, readymade foam traction kits are available for this purpose.
- **Skeletal traction:** The traction is applied directly on the bone by inserting a K-wire or Steinmann pin through the bone.

Some of the differentiating features of skin and skeletal tractions are given in Table 4.2.

Table 4.2: Comparison between skin and skeletal tractions.		
Point	**Skin traction**	**Skeletal traction**
Required for	Mild to moderate force	Moderate to severe force
Age used for	Children	Adults
Applied with	Adhesive plaster	Steinmann pin, K-wire
Applied	On skin	Through bone
Common site	Below knee	Upper tibial pin traction
Weight permitted	Up to 3-4 kg	Up to 20 kg
Used for	Short duration	Long duration

Common traction systems used are given in Table 4.3.

DAILY CARE OF A PATIENT IN TRACTION

A patient in traction can develop serious complications and needs the following care:

a. The traction should be as comfortable as possible.

b. Proper functioning of the traction unit must be ensured. Traction weights should not be touching the ground. See that the ropes are in the grooves of the pulleys. The foot of the patient or the end of the traction device should not be touching the pulley, as it makes traction ineffective.

c. One must see that terminal part of the limb in traction (hand or foot) is warm and of normal colour. Sensations over toes and fingers should be normal. Any numbness or tingling may point to a traction palsy of a nerve.

d. Any swelling over the fingers or toes may point to a tight bandage or slipped skin traction.

e. A pin tract infection in skeletal traction can be detected early by eliciting pain on gentle tapping at the site of the pin insertion.

f. The proper position of the fracture should be ensured by taking check X-rays in traction.

g. Physiotherapy of the limb in traction should be continued to minimise muscle wasting.

h. A watch must be kept on general complications of recumbency, i.e., bed sores, chest congestion, UTI, constipation, etc.

i. Diversion therapy is important for any patient confined to bed for a long period of time. This may be done by suggesting the patient to do things he likes - such as reading, craft, games, watching television, net surfing, etc.

Lately, with modern methods of treatment having evolved, tractions are sparingly used in orthopaedic practice. There was a time a few decades ago when orthopaedic ward were recognized by patients in traction. That is a rare site now-a-days. Traction used to be prepared with Leucoplast tape and other stuff, but now, readymade traction kits are available. There have been significant developments in usage of splints. Readymade splints are available for every part of the body, and have replaced plaster slab which were used for splinting in the past. Lighter and mouldable plastic splints are available, making the whole experience of splintage pleasurable.

 What have we learnt?

- Splints are useful and readily available methods of immobilising a limb. Due care is required while treating a patient in splint.
- There are two types of traction—fixed and sliding.
- There are two methods of applying traction—skin and skeletal.
- Skeletal traction is more convenient for giving traction for longer duration. Also, more weight can be applied by skeletal traction. Skin traction is suitable for short-term traction only.
- How to take proper care of a patient in traction?

Additional information: From the entrance exams point of view

Skin traction is contraindicated in skin damage, deep vein thrombosis, significant vascular deficit and neurological deficit.

Recent Advances in the Treatment of Fractures

Learning Objectives

❖ What are the principles of AO method of fracture treatment?
❖ What is functional bracing and how does it help in fracture healing?
❖ Describe Ilizarov technique of treating fractures.

AO METHOD OF FRACTURE TREATMENT

The AO (Arbeitsgemeinschaft für Osteosynthese fragen, a Swiss term meaning association for osteosynthesis) and its English counterpart, the ASIF (Association for the Study of Internal Fixation) advocated the internal fixation of fractures based on principles laid down by them. The basic guiding principle is that *by achieving stable fixation of fractures, a limb can be mobilised early*, thereby avoiding the disadvantages of immobilisation, i.e., stiffness of joints, muscle wasting, etc. All of these disadvantages have been termed *'fracture disease'* by them. The following principles are used to achieve stable fixation (Fig. 5.1):

a. *Interfragmentary compression,* i.e., achieving compression between different fracture fragments.
b. *Splinting,* i.e., splinting the fracture internally or externally.
c. *Combination* of a and b.

INTERFRAGMENTARY COMPRESSION

Mechanically, a fracture fixed with interfragmetary compression is best fixed—so called rigidly fixed (called *absolute stability*). In this, the fracture fragments are not merely in contact, but are compressed against each other. Compression improves the strength of

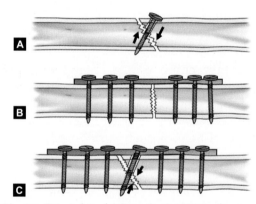

Fig. 5.1: Principles of AO method: (A) Interfragmentary compression; (B) Splintage; (C) Combination of A and B.

the fixation. Compression between fragments can be produced at the time of surgery, and is called *static* compression. It can also occur between fragments as a result of muscle action once the limb is put to use, the so called *dynamic* compression.

Methods of producing static compression: It can be produced by the following methods:

a. *Lag* screw fixation:* In this, a screw is passed across the fracture site in such a way that as

---

* Lag screw is no special screw. It is just the way a screw is used. Partially threaded screws are used to produce lag-screw effect. Even a fully threaded screw can be used as a lag screw by 'over drilling' the near cortex.

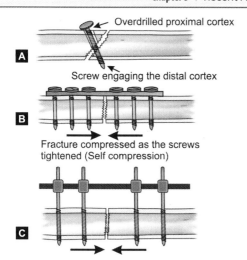

Fig. 5.2: Methods of producing compression: (A) A lag screw; (B) A self compression plate; (C) An external fixator.

the screw is tightened, the fracture surfaces are compressed against each other. How it is done is as shown in Figure 5.1A. First (a) the fracture is reduced and held with a clamp; (b) a hole is drilled across the fracture; (c) the near cortex hole is 'over-drilled'. As the screw is passed, it slides through the near cortex (having been over-drilled), and its threads catch the far cortex (Fig. 5.2A). The head of the screw pushes the near cortex to the far cortex, producing inter-fragmentary compression. This technique is suitable for achieving compression across a short oblique or a spiral fracture.

b. *Compression plating* (Fig. 5.2B): Plating is a technique of using a thick metallic strip (a plate), on the surface of the bone. The two fragments of a transverse or short oblique fracture can be compressed against each other using the plate. Compression across the fracture can be achieved by a special device called Muller's compression clamp (Fig. 5.2B) or by the use of a specially designed, compression plates (Fig. 5.2B). In the latter, the screw holes of the plate are so designed that as the screws are tightened, compression is produced.

c. *External fixator* (Fig. 5.2C): It can also be used to produce compression between the fragments at the time of its application or later by gradually tightening the sliding mechanism of the fixator.

Methods of producing dynamic compression: A fractured bone has a tension side - the side which is subjected to a distracting force once a fracture occurs, in a way it tends to 'open up' on that side (Fig. 5.3A). The opposite side, naturally, comes under compression. If this distracting force is countered by

some device fixed on the tension side the fracture, overall, comes under compression. This principle of converting a tension (distracting) force into a compression force is called *tension-band principle*.

Dynamic compression can be achieved by the following methods:

a. *Tension-band wire* (Fig. 5.3A): This can be used for producing dynamic compression in fractures of the patella and olecranon.

b. *Tension-band plate* (Fig. 5.3B): This can be used for fractures of the humerus and tibia by applying the plate on tension surface.

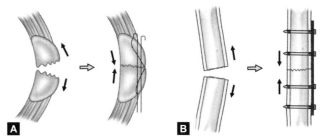

Fig. 5.3: Tension-band principle: (A) Wiring; (B) Plating.

SPLINTING

Not all fractures can be rigidly fixed (e.g., a comminuted fracture), and hence stable enough fixation can be achieved by mere splintage (relative stability). There are various methods of 'splinting' the fracture surgically. These do not provide 'rigid' fixation, but the fixation is good enough to support fracture healing. Following are some such methods (Fig. 5.4).

a. **Intramedullary splintage (nailing):** This is useful for fixation of fractures of the long bones, e.g., fracture of the shaft of the femur. A long hollow rod, called 'nail' is inserted in the medullary cavity of the long bone (Fig. 5.4A).

b. **Extramedullary splinting (plating):** This can be done for any fracture by applying a plate on the surface of the bone. This plate, being used just to 'splint' the fracture, without producing compression, is called a *neutralisation plate* (Fig. 5.4B). Sometimes, the plate may just be buttressing the fracture, without really 'fixing' it (*buttress plating*), as is done for fixing tibial condyle fractures (Fig. 5.4C).

c. **Splintage from outside the body:** Pins are inserted through the skin into the bone, and the same are held outside with clamps and rod (external fixators). This is used to hold the fragments, for example, that of an open fracture (Fig. 5.4D).

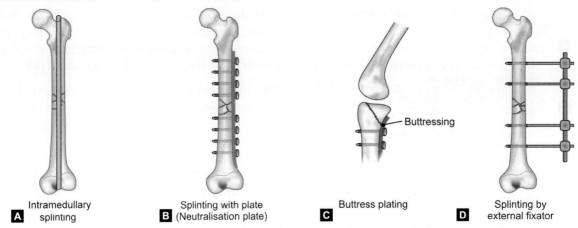

Fig. 5.4: Various methods of splinting the fracture surgically.

COMBINATION OF COMPRESSION AND SPLINTING

A compression screw fixation by itself may not produce good stability, and has to be combined with a neutralization or buttress plate, in addition. This combination of principles is required in achieving stable fixation in most fractures, e.g., a spiral fracture of the shaft of the femur can be stabilised by using interfragmentary screws across the fracture, and a neutralisation plate to add to fixation (Fig. 5.5).

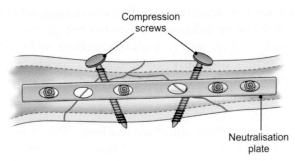

Fig. 5.5: An example of use of combination of compression screws and a neutralisation plate, used for a spiral fracture.

CHANGING AO CONCEPTS

Before 50's, fractures were treated primarily non-operatively. The healing of fractures occurred as per stages described in Chapter 2. Callus formation was an important stage in the healing of fractures. Non-operative treatment required immobilisation of the limb, which lead to stiffness of joints, wasting of muscles, etc. (the so-called *fracture disease*). Operative techniques were primitive, and were associated with unacceptable complications.

EARLY AO CONCEPTS

In the late 50's, AO group brought revolution in the treatment of fractures. They proposed *anatomical*

reduction of the fracture, which meant, putting each and every bone fragment back to where it belonged. The fragments were rigidly fixed using AO principles (as explained earlier). The aim of rigid fixation was to achieve bone-to-bone healing, without callus formation (*primary bone healing*). In an attempt to achieve anatomical reduction and rigid fixation, it became necessary to widely expose the fracture, and thus damage to its blood supply. It was soon realised that, although this method is mechanically superior, it does not respect the biological environment of the fracture. Hence, though well-fixed, fractures will often fail to unite. The importance of preserving biology while mechanically achieving a good fixation was appreciated.

CURRENT AO CONCEPTS

Hence, in the 90's, the concept changed from rigid fixation to a term 'stable fixation'. By stable fixation it meant that the fixation should be good enough to achieve union. It could be rigid fixation in certain situations, intra-articular fractures, for example, where exact anatomical reduction and rigid fixation (absolute stable fixation) was a must for getting the fracture to heal well and also mobilise the fracture early. On the other hand, for diaphyseal fractures, anatomical reduction is not a must. Just functional reduction (achieving length and overall alignment), and a more biological (preserving blood supply of fragments), and a less-than-rigid (*relative stable*) fixation is good enough. For example, recommendations in the past for a comminuted fracture of the femur was to reconstruct the femur, fixing each and every small piece of bone to where it belonged using small screws and plates. It was more like solving a jig-saw puzzle. It caused a lot of damage to blood supply of individual fragments, and hence produced delayed and non-union. I current perspective, the same fracture is 'stabilised' by using a bridging plate (Fig. 5.6), or a nail where the length of the bone and its alignment is restored, without exposing the comminuted segment of the bone. The *'relative stability'* provided by these devices, is good enough to allow early mobilisation, but since the blood supply of the bone is preserved, the chances of fracture healing are better. Stable fixation does not mean less than optimum fixation, as that will lead to implant failure in early phase of healing. Choosing the right method of fixation for a particular fracture is the art of operative fracture treatment.

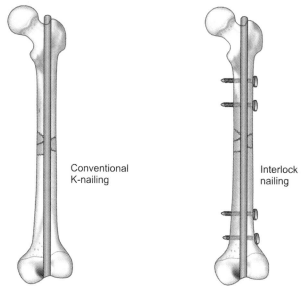

Fig. 5.7: Interlock nailing.

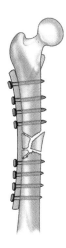

Fig. 5.6: Biological fixation: The fracture is stabilized without touching the small comminuted pieces of bone (bridging plate).

In order to preserve the blood supply of the fracture, emphasis has shifted from *direct reduction* where fragments are exposed and directly reduced, to *indirect reduction* where reduction is achieved by manipulating the limb without touching the fracture.

In general, intramedullary nailing has been considered a mechanically superior device compared to plating. This is because a nail is a *load sharing device* (the load is shared by nail and bone). Intramedullary nailing is a preferred option for fractures of long bones. The only disadvantage of the conventional nailing was that it did not provide rotational stability to the fracture. For this, the conventional nail has been modified. Holes have been made at the two ends of the nail. After the nail is inserted into the medullary canal, it is locked in place with the help of two bolts (Fig. 5.7). This gives rotational stability to the fixation, and results in improved stability. The technique of 'interlock nailing' is state-of-the-art treatment for fixation of long bone diaphyseal fractures. An image intensifier (Fig. 5.8), a special fracture table and surgical experience are prerequisites for this technically demanding procedure.

There has been a change in the design of the conventional plates too. The new plates are so designed that they are in contact with the bone at minimum surface (low contact dynamic compression plates - LCDCP). This allows better vascularisation of the fracture under the plate.

The latest development in plating technique is *Locking Compression Plate (LCP)*. This plate has a mechanism where the screw head is 'locked' into the plate. There are many methods of locking the screw to the plate. One popular one is using 'combination' screw hole. In this, the screw hole has two half; one half is like a conventional DCP hole (unthreaded), whereas the

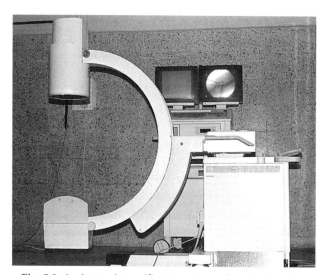

Fig. 5.8: An image intensifier is an integral part of modern fracture treatment.

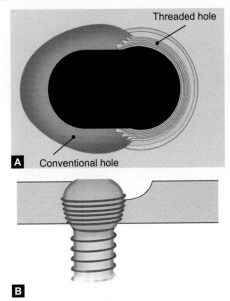

Fig. 5.9: Screw hole of a locking compression plate.

other half is threaded (Fig. 5.9A). The screw head also has threads so that as the screw is tightened, the head gets 'locked' in the plate (Fig. 5.9B). This provides a rigid plate-screw construct, which has been found to be mechanically superior to a conventional plate. LCP is a versatile plate which can be used in different modes - a compression plate, a neutralisation plate, a buttress plate, a bridging plate and as a internal fixator. Locking principle is particularly suitable for periarticular fractures and fractures in osteoporotic bones. Further development in plating technology is *anatomically pre-contoured plates* - specific for specific region of the body (Fig. 5.10). These have made fixation of metaphyseal region of the bones, surgeon friendly.

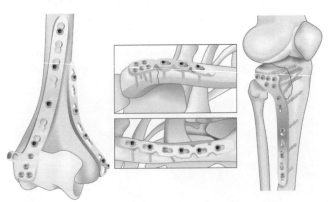

Fig. 5.10: Anatomically pre-contoured plates, specific to specific parts of the body.

Carbon plates and biodegradable* implants also came into use. Though biodegradable screws are used widely, used of biodegradable plates did not catch

* These are implants made of special plastic, which 'dissolves' over a period of time.

up due to some issues. The advantage is that they do not show up on the X-rays, and biodegradable ones get 'absorbed' after sometime.

FUNCTIONAL BRACING

Sarmiento (1973) popularized functional bracing technique for treating fractures. In principle, the technique consists of applying an external contraption (called a brace) to a fractured limb. The brace provides adequate support to the fracture while permitting use of that limb until the union is complete. Bracing is done if the reduction of the fracture is satisfactory and the swelling has subsided - usually 2–3 weeks after the injury.

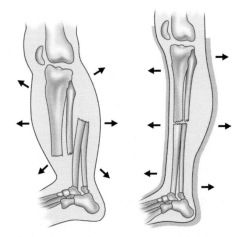

Fig. 5.11: Functional bracing—the principle. The hydraulic pressure generated within the braced compartment immobilises the fracture.

It seems likely that the brace works by supporting the soft tissues in a tight compartment (Fig. 5.11). As the limb is put to use, the axial pressure on the limb (caused by weight bearing or due to muscle contraction) tends to shorten the bone segment, producing a 'bulging effect' on the soft tissues. Since the whole leg is enclosed in a confined space (the brace), there develops a sort of hydraulic pressure within the brace, which helps in maintaining the fracture alignment. In long series of cases treated this way, it was found that shortening and angulation was not a significant problem.

Bracing may not reduce the time taken by the fracture to unite, but it markedly reduces the stiffness and wasting of muscles caused by immobilisation in traction or plaster. It also drastically reduces the length of rehabilitation. Functional bracing is used for simple fractures where the reduction is stable. It is also useful for a fracture fixed internally where internal fixation is inadequate. In such cases, a guarded mobilisation may be done using a brace, and thus strain on the implant is avoided. In severely compound fractures, after initial treatment with external fixator or traction, if internal fixation is not possible, brace can be used to allow functional use of the limb.

Overall, bracing is most popular for fractures of the shaft of the tibia, humerus, and forearm bones.

ILIZAROV'S TECHNIQUE
(Ring Fixator)

Gavriil A Ilizarov, a Russian surgeon revolutionised the application of external fixation in the management of difficult non-unions and limb lengthening (Fig. 5.12). These used to be some of the most difficult orthopaedic problems before the advent of Ilizarov's technique.

The basic premise of Ilizarov's technique is that *osteogenesis requires dynamic state*. The dynamic state means that the site of osteogenesis (e.g., a fracture) requires either a controlled distraction or a controlled compression. This dynamic force, when properly applied, causes the dormant mesenchymal cells at the non-union site to differentiate into functioning osteoblasts. This results in bone synthesis and fracture healing. The concept that compression enhances bone healing, was known even prior to Ilizarov, but the concept of *distraction osteogenesis* was put on a sound footing by Ilizarov. According to his theory in wider perspective, *any living tissue when subjected to constant stretch under biological conditions, can grow to any extent.* The biological conditions are provided by: (i) aligning the fracture with minimal damage to its vascularity, and (ii) performing an 'osteotomy' of the bone (e.g., in limb lengthening surgeries), without damaging its periosteal and endosteal blood supply. Such an 'osteotomy' was termed *corticotomy* by Ilizarov.

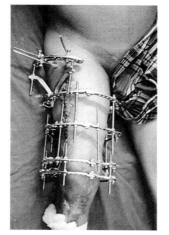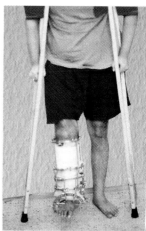

Fig. 5.12: Ilizarov's fixation applied to thigh and leg.

The whole segment of the limb is stabilised by a specially designed fixation system called *ring fixator*. This protects the growing tissues from bending or shearing forces, but permits loading in the long axis of the limb. Distraction or compression can be applied at the fracture or corticotomy site by twisting nuts on the fixation system (Fig. 5.13). Distraction or compression is carried out at the rate of 1 mm per day. This is done in four sittings -¼ mm, four times a day. Ring fixator application consists of inserting thin (1.5 or 1.8 mm) stainless steel wires through the bone. Outside the limb, the wires are attached to steel rings with the help of bolts. Before fixing the wire to the ring, the wire is put under tension so as to make it 'stiff', and thus impart stability to the fixator. The rings are interconnected with the help of threaded rods with nuts on either ends. It is by twisting these nuts that the rings can be moved up or down, and the fracture distracted or compressed. The use of external fixators has undergone ultimate sophistication where computers are used to programme the application and sequencing of distraction and compression.

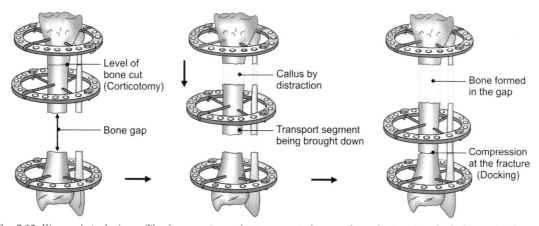

Fig. 5.13: Ilizarov's technique: The fragments can be transported up or down by turning the bolts on the fixator.

Ilizarov technique is useful in the management of the following conditions:

a. Limb lengthening, especially when the shortening is associated with deformity. In this situation the fixator assembly is so designed that it corrects the deformity and produces lengthening at the same time. Massive limb lengthening (even up to 18 inches) have been performed by using this technique. The fixator provides a stable biological environment to the new bone at the site of lengthening (Fig. 5.14).

b. Non-union, especially those resistant to conventional methods of treatment or those associated with deformity or shortening. By this method, non-union, deformity as well-shortening can be treated by one-stage fixator application. Non-unions requiring skin cover and bone grafting operations can be managed by using Ilizarov technique without subjecting the patient to staged surgeries.

c. Deformity correction, which may be congenital or acquired can be corrected by Ilizarov's technique.

d. Osteomyelitis can be treated, as this technique offers the possibility of liberal excision of necrotic bone. The gap thus created can subsequently be made up by transporting a segment of bone from either end.

e. Arthrodesis can be performed by "crushing" the articular surfaces against each other, and thus stimulating union between opposite bones.

ADVANTAGES OF ILIZAROV'S TECHNIQUE

• Immediate load bearing
• A healthy viable bone in place of de-vascularised bone

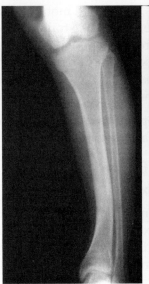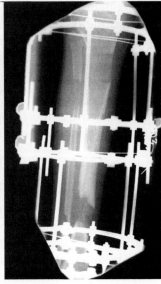

Fig. 5.14: Correction of a deformity and lengthening done simultaneously.

• Correction of more than one problem by one-stage operation.

DISADVANTAGES OF ILIZAROV'S TECHNIQUE

• Inconvenience, as the external fixator hampers normal activity
• Long duration of treatment
• Pin tract infection
• Nerve palsy by pin insertion or traction
• Joint stiffness caused by transfixation of the soft tissues by the external fixator.

 What have we learnt?

■ The AO methods of internal fixation are based on achieving interfragmentary compression or splintage or both. Plates and screws can be used to achieve this. Nailing is a splintage device, interlock nailing being a recent modification.

■ In the treatment of diaphyseal fracture, emphasis has shifted from rigid (absolute) stability to relative stability. Anatomical reduction has been replaced by functional reduction.

■ Plate fixation has undergone changes to make it a more 'biological' implant. Locking compression plate (LCP) is a recent addition to plating techniques.

■ Functional bracing is a non-operative method of treating fractures of the long bones.

■ Ilizarov method is a type of external fixator system which is versatile in its application, particularly suited for difficult non-unions, malunions and limb length discrepancies.

Approach to a Patient with Limb Injury

Competency

- ❖ **OR1.1:** Describe and discuss the Principles of pre-hospital care and Casualty management of a trauma victim including principles of triage.

While examining a case of injury to the musculoskeletal system, answers to the following questions are sought:

- Is there a fracture*?
- Is it a closed or an open fracture?
- Is it a traumatic or a pathological fracture?
- Are there any complication associated with the fracture?

CLINICAL EXAMINATION

With widespread availability of X-ray facilities, diagnosis of fractures and dislocations has become easy. But the clinical examination still continues to be important, especially in the following situations:

a. To decide whether an X-ray examination is needed. This is particularly relevant when a patient has to travel to far off places for X-ray.

b. To ascertain whether the injury under consideration needs a special view. For example, an oblique view of the wrist best shows a scaphoid fracture.

c. To avoid making a wrong diagnosis, by correlating the clinical findings with the radiological findings. This way, some artifacts

otherwise likely to be diagnosed as 'fracture', are recognised.

d. To detect complications associated with a fracture, e.g., injury to the neurovascular bundle.

This will be missed if a clinical examination is not carried out.

Thus, a thorough clinical examination must *precede* an X-ray in all cases of musculoskeletal injury. The following questions should be kept in mind while performing the clinical examination:

IS THERE A FRACTURE?

Most often a fracture can be diagnosed on the basis of history and clinical examination. The following points in clinical examination need to be considered:

Age of the patient: *Fractures occur at all ages but dislocations are uncommon in children**.* Some fractures are common in a particular age group, as shown in the Table 6.1.

Mechanism of injury: The mechanism by which the patient sustains the injury often gives an idea about the expected fracture/dislocation. For example, in a fall from some height onto the heels, one is likely

---

*For ease of discussion, the term 'fracture' is used for both, fracture and dislocation.

**In children, force around a joint produces an epiphyseal injury through the epiphyseal plate, and not a dislocation.

Table 6.1: Common fractures at different ages.

Age group	Fractures
At birth	Clavicle, humerus
In children	▪ Supracondylar fracture of humerus ▪ Epiphyseal injuries
In adults	Fractures of shafts of long bones
In elderly people	▪ Colles' fracture ▪ Fracture neck of femur

to sustain a fracture of the calcaneum, fracture of lumbar vertebrae and fracture of pubic rami. Some common injuries and mechanisms involved are shown in Table 6.2.

Table 6.2: Mechanisms of injury and fractures/dislocations.

Mechanism	Common injuries
▪ Fall on an outstretched hand	▪ Fracture clavicle ▪ Fractures around the elbow
▪ Fall with spine forced in a particular direction	▪ Flexion injuries ▪ Extension injuries, etc.
▪ Slipping in the bathroom (trivial trauma)	▪ Fractures neck of the femur
▪ Dashboard injury	▪ Posterior dislocation of hip
▪ Fall onto the heel	▪ Fracture calcaneum
▪ Hit by a stick	▪ Fracture ulna

Presenting complaints: A patient with suspected fracture may present with the following complaints:
- *Pain:* It is the most common presenting complaint in cases of musculoskeletal injury. The severity of pain has no bearing on the diagnosis. Sprains and strains can be as painful as fracture.
- *Swelling:* Fractures are usually accompanied with swelling. The swelling may be slight if patient presents immediately after the injury; but in those presenting late, the whole limb may be swollen, mostly because of gravitational oedema.
- *Deformity:* A fractured bone may result in deformity of that part of the body.
- *Loss of function:* Following a fracture, the patient may* be unable to use the affected limb.

Examination: A proper exposure of the body part is crucial to an accurate examination. At times the findings are subtle, and comparison of the injured

limb with the opposite, normal, extremity may be useful. Joints proximal and distal to the injured bone should always be examined. In a patient of road traffic accident with multiple injuries, it is wise to expose the patient completely and examine each body part in a systematic manner. One should look for the following signs:
- *Swelling:* Though most fractures are accompanied with swelling at the site, it can be a misleading sign as there may be minimal visible swelling in the presence of a serious fracture (e.g., fracture of the neck of the femur); on the other hand, a massive swelling may be present in the absence of a fracture (e.g., in cases of ligament sprain and muscle injuries). The swelling may be due to a haematoma, prominence of the bone ends or passive oedema.
- *Deformity:* An obvious deformity of a body part is a very specific sign of a fracture or dislocation. So characteristic is the deformity in some fractures and dislocations that a diagnosis can be made just by looking at the deformity (Table 6.3). Deformity may be absent if there is an impacted fracture.
- *Tenderness:* Pain elicited by direct pressure at the fracture site or by indirect pressure may suggest a fracture.
  Direct pressure: A localised tenderness on a subcutaneous bone, elicited by gently running the back of the thumb (Fig. 6.1A) may suggest an underlying fracture. The site of maximum tenderness helps in differentiating ligament injuries from that of fractures around a joint (e.g., ankle injuries). One may feel or hear a crepitus while eliciting tenderness.
  Indirect pressure: It may be possible to elicit pain at the fracture site by applying pressure at a site

Table 6.3: Injuries with characteristic deformities.

Deformity	Injury
▪ Flattening of shoulder	▪ Shoulder dislocation (anterior)
▪ Dinner fork deformity	▪ Colles' fracture
▪ Mallet finger	▪ Avulsion of the insertion of the extensor tendon from the distal phalanx
▪ Flexion, adduction and internal rotation of the hip	▪ Posterior dislocation of the hip
▪ Abduction, external rotation of the hip	▪ Anterior dislocation of the hip
▪ External rotation of the leg	▪ Fracture neck of femur Trochanteric fracture

*Ability to keep using the limb after an injury is not conclusive of 'no fracture', especially in children.

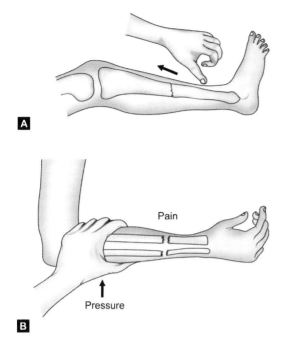

Fig. 6.1: Eliciting tenderness: (A) With back of the thumb; (B) Springing of forearm.

away from the fracture. Some examples are given below:
- *Springing test:* It may be possible to elicit pain from a fracture of the forearm bones by pressing the two bones towards each other at a distance away from the fracture (Fig. 6.1B).
- *Axial pressure:* An axial pressure along the second metacarpal may elicit pain in the scaphoid fossa, in a case of scaphoid fracture.
- *Bony irregularity:* It is possible to feel bony elevations and depressions in fractures of subcutaneous bones such as the tibia. This is a definite sign of fracture.
- *Abnormal mobility:* In any limb, movements occur only at joints. If one can elicit mobility at sites other than the joints (say in the middle of the arm), or an abnormal range of movement at a joint, a fracture or dislocation is *definite*. One may hear or feel a crepitus while doing this.
- *Absence of transmitted movements:* Normally, if a bone is moved holding it at one end, the movement can be felt at the other end. This transmitted movement will be absent in case of a displaced fracture. In case the fracture is undisplaced or impacted, the movement will be transmitted even in the presence of a fracture.

IS IT AN OPEN FRACTURE?

Whenever there is a wound in the vicinity of a fracture, it is important to ascertain whether the wound is communicating with the fracture. This is done by examination of the wound under aseptic conditions. One may see the bone under the wound. Sometimes it may be difficult to say whether a wound is communicating with the fracture or not, in which situation, it should be considered an 'open fracture', to be on the safe side. It must be ascertained whether the compounding is from inside (internal) or from outside (external).

IS IT A PATHOLOGICAL FRACTURE?

A pathological fracture must be suspected if: (i) the force producing the fracture is insignificant (trivial trauma); (ii) there is a history of pain or swelling in the affected bone prior to the occurrence of fracture; (iii) there is history suggestive of frequent fractures in the past (e.g., osteogenesis imperfecta); and (iv) the patient is suffering from a debilitating systemic illness known to weaken bones (e.g., rheumatoid arthritis).

ANY ASSOCIATED COMPLICATION?

Complications such as injuries to the nerves and vessels, etc., may be associated with a fracture. These can be diagnosed on clinical examination (see Chapter 10).

RADIOLOGICAL EXAMINATION

A radiological examination helps in: (i) diagnosis of a fracture or dislocation; (ii) evaluation of displacements, if any; and (iii) studying the nature of the force causing fracture. The following are some of the points to be remembered in a radiological examination of a case of skeletal injury:

ASKING FOR AN X-RAY

Before asking for an X-ray, the following points should be kept in mind:
- *At least two views* (AP and lateral, for example) should be requested in most situations.
- Joint above and below should be included in the X-ray.
- *Special views* show fractures better in some cases (Table 6.4).
- X-ray requisition must *specify* the area of suspicion, e.g., if an injury to D_{12} vertebra is suspected, ask for an X-ray of the dorsolumbar spine *focussing* D_{12}.

Table 6.4: Some commonly used special views.	
Deformity	**Injury**
▪ Oblique view wrist	▪ Scaphoid fracture
▪ Judet view	▪ Acetabular fracture
▪ Merchant view	▪ Patellofemoral joint
▪ Skyline view	▪ Calcaneum fracture

- X-ray of the *pelvis wtih both hips* should be asked for in all cases of suspected pelvic injury. Major injuries of the thigh are often associated with fractures of the pelvis, hence an X-ray of the pelvis must be taken as a routine in cases with major fractures of the leg.
- For an X-ray evaluation of the hands and feet, antero-posterior and *oblique* views (not lateral) are required.

READING AN X-RAY

An X-ray view box should be used in all cases. If a fracture is obvious, one must make a note of the following points:

- *Which bone* is affected?
- *Which part* of the bone is affected?, e.g., shaft, etc.
- *At what level* is the fracture?, i.e., whether the fracture is in the upper, middle or lower third.
- What is the *pattern* of the fracture?, i.e., whether the fracture is transverse, oblique, etc.
- Is the fracture displaced? If yes, in what direction, i.e., whether it is a shift (anteroposterior, sideways), a tilt, or angulation in any direction, or a rotational displacement. Rotational displacement is sometimes not visible on X-rays, and can only be diagnosed clinically.
- Is the fracture line *extending* into the nearby joint?
- Does the underlying bone appear pathological?, e.g., a cyst, abnormal texture of the whole bone, etc.
- Is it a fresh or an old fracture? An X-ray of a fresh fracture shows a soft tissue shadow resulting from haematoma, and the fracture ends are sharp. An old fracture shows callus formation and disuse osteoporosis and the fracture ends are smoothened.

If the fracture is not obvious immediately, all the bones and joints seen on the X-ray must be examined systematically for a break in the cortex or loss of joint congruity.

X-ray findings should be correlated with clinical findings, so as to avoid error because of some artifacts which may mimic a fracture. Also one must ensure that the part under question is visible on X-ray. An X-ray of a bone must include the joints proximal and distal to the bone. Do look for an associated injury to all the other bones and joints visible on the X-ray.

One must be aware of some normal X-ray findings which are often *misinterpreted* as fracture, e.g., epiphyseal lines, vascular markings on bones, accessory bones, etc. A comparison with the X-ray of the opposite limb helps in clearing any doubt.

Table 6.5: Fractures commonly missed.

Upper Limb
- Greater tuberosity: In AP view of the shoulder, fracture of greater tuberosity is missed, as the fragment gets displaced behind the head of humerus.
- AC joint subluxation
- Posterior dislocation of shoulder
- Head of radius, neck of the radius
- Capitulum
- Medial epicondyle fracture
- Scaphoid

Lower Limb
- Fracture neck of femur (impacted)
- Acetabulum
- Patella
- Hoffa's fracture (posterior condyle femur)
- Calcaneum
- Dislocation of foot (Lisfranc injury)

Other
- Epiphyseal injuries
- Compression fracture of spine

There are some injuries particularly liable to be missed by a novice (Table 6.5). Before an X-ray is passed as normal, one must carefully look for these injuries.

A diagrammatic presentation of approach to a patient with a limb injury is as shown in Flowchart 6.1.

OLD FRACTURE

After 2-3 weeks, signs of a fresh fracture like pain, soft tissue swelling, tenderness, etc., diminish markedly. On X-ray examination, the fracture ends will not appear sharp. Callus may be present. When a patient with fracture presents late after injury, to decide further treatment, it is important to ascertain: (i) whether the position of the fracture fragments is acceptable; and (ii) at what stage of union is the fracture?, e.g., united, uniting or non-union (Fig. 6.2).

APPROACH TO A POLYTRAUMA PATIENT

An isolated skeletal injury rarely poses any threat, but in association with multiple injuries, musculoskeletal injuries assume great significance in terms of morbidity and mortality. Proper, well-articulated, early management plays a vital role in improving the outcome of these patients. The following constitute the key points in the management.

FIELD TRIAGE

Ideally, the management of a multiple injured should begin at the scene of accident where the medical

Flowchart 6.1: Approach to a patient with limb injury.

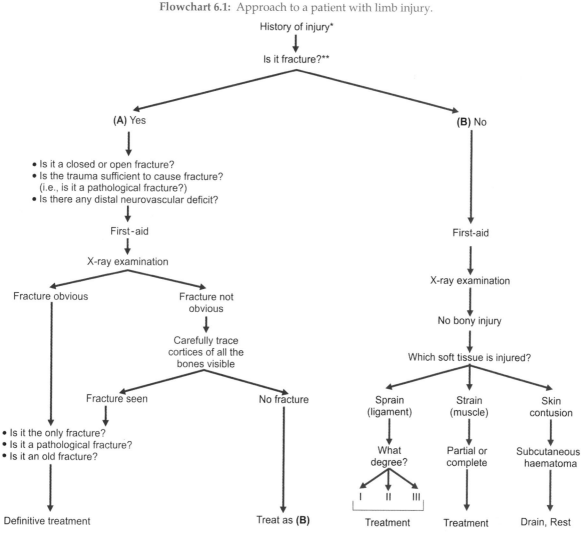

* History of injury may not be present in pathological fractures.

** The term 'fracture' includes dislocation (for ease of presentation).

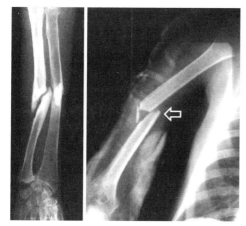

Fig. 6.2: X-rays showing old fractures
(Note smoothening of the ends).

technician should be able to work in coordination with the doctors. He should be able to provide basic life support and help in transportation. He should be able to decide, on the basis of the level of injury, whether the victim needs to be transferred to the local hospital or a hospital with developed trauma services. In the present day context, trauma services are not so well developed in countries like India, but this is something to aspire for.

TREATMENT IN THE EMERGENCY DEPARTMENT

Once the patient reaches the emergency department, management consists of the following:

- **Primary survey:** This constitutes rapid assessment of vitals of the patient and ensuring patent airway, adequate breathing, circulation and control of external bleeding.

- **Resuscitation:** This is conducted on established lines of ABCDE (please refer to book on Anaesthesia for details).

- **Secondary survey:** Once the patient is stable, proper neurologic assessment, thoracoabdominal assessment, genitourinary assessment and musculoskeletal assessment is carried out. As is obvious from the above sequence, musculoskeletal assessment is *not* high on priority. The only injuries related to musculoskeletal system which are important at this stage are: (i) vascular injuries—so check all peripheral pulses and capillary circulation; (ii) nerve injuries—check peripheral nerves and correct malposition of the fractures to relieve pressure or stretch on the affected nerve and (iii) dislocation or subluxation—these need to be corrected early. All other orthopaedic injuries can be treated once other systems have been stabilised.

- **Definitive treatment:** From orthopaedic view point, this consists of planning whether some fractures need internal fixation. Those being treated conservatively, need to be reduced and immobilised. Current trend is to internally fix as many fractures as possible in a polytrauma patient, often in one sitting. This has been shown to help in nursing care, and has resulted in *decrease* in mortality and morbidity.

What have we learnt?

- When evaluating a fracture, a correlation between clinical findings and X-ray findings is a must.
- Wherever possible take AP and lateral X-rays.
- Think of the possibility of a background pathological process which may have contributed to the fracture.
- Proper X-ray requisition can prevent a lot of problems.
- Comparative X-ray of the normal, opposite side may help in diagnosing a doubtful fracture.

Competencies

- **OR1.2:** Describe and discuss the aetiopathogenesis, clinical features, investigations, and principles of management of shock.
- **OR2.15:** Plan and interpret the investigations to diagnose complications of fractures like malunion, non-union, infection, compartmental syndrome.

Complications inevitably occur in a proportion of fractures. With early diagnosis and treatment, the disability caused by these complications can be greatly reduced.

CLASSIFICATION

Complications of fractures can be classified into three broad groups depending upon their time of occurrence. These are as follows:

a. *Immediate* complications—occurring at the time of the fracture.
b. *Early* complications—occurring in the initial few days after the fracture.
c. *Late* complications—occurring a long time after the fracture.

Some of the complications of the fractures seen in day-to-day practice are given in Table 7.1.

HYPOVOLAEMIC SHOCK

Hypovolaemic shock is the most common cause of death following fractures of major bones such as the pelvis and femur. Its frequency is on the increase due to a rise in the number of patients with multiple injuries.

Cause: The cause of hypovolaemia could be external haemorrhage or internal haemorrhage. External haemorrhage may result from a compound fracture with or without an associated injury to a major vessel of the limb. Internal haemorrhage is more difficult to diagnose. It is usually massive bleeding in the body cavities such as chest or abdomen. Significant blood loss may occur in fractures of the major bones like the pelvis (1500–2000 mL), and femur (1000–1500 mL).

Management: This begins even before the cause can be ascertained. An immediate step is to put in at

Table 7.1: Complications of fractures.

Immediate complications
- *Systemic*
  - Hypovolaemic shock
- *Local*
  - Injury to major vessels
  - Injury to muscles and tendons
  - Injury to joints
  - Injury to viscera

Early complications
- *Systemic*
  - Hypovolaemic shock
  - Acute respiratory distress syndrome (ARDS)
  - Fat embolism syndrome
  - DVT and pulmonary embolism
  - Aseptic traumatic fever
  - Septicaemia (in open fractures)
  - Crush syndrome
- *Local*
  - Infection
  - Compartment syndrome

Late complications
- *Imperfect union of the fracture*
  - Delayed union
  - Non-union
  - Malunion
  - Cross union
- *Others*
  - Avascular necrosis
  - Shortening
  - Joint stiffness
  - Sudeck's dystrophy (reflex sympathetic dystrophy)
  - Osteomyelitis
  - Ischaemic contracture
  - Myositis ossificans
  - Osteoarthritis

least two *large* bore intravenous cannulas (No. 16 or No. 14). If there is peripheral vasoconstriction, no time should be wasted in performing a cut down. 2000 mL of crystalloids (preferably Ringer lactate), should be infused rapidly, followed by colloids (Haemaccel) and blood. At the earliest opportunity, effort is made to localize the site of bleed—whether it is in the chest or in the abdomen. Needle aspiration from the chest, and diagnostic peritoneal lavage provide quick information to this effect. If possible, a plain X-ray chest, and X-ray abdomen may be done. A chest tube for chest bleeding, laparotomy for abdominal bleeding, may be required.

Excessive blood loss from fractured bone may be prevented by avoiding moving the patient from one couch to another. For fractures of the pelvis, temporary stabilisation with an external fixator has been found useful in reducing haemorrhage. In advanced trauma centres, an emergency angiography and embolisation of the bleeding vessel is performed to control bleeding from deeper vessels.

ADULT RESPIRATORY DISTRESS SYNDROME

Adult respiratory distress syndrome (ARDS) can be a sequelae of trauma with subsequent shock. The exact mechanism is not known, but it is supposed to be due to release of inflammatory mediators which cause disruption of microvasculature of the pulmonary system. The onset is usually *24 hours* after the injury. The patient develops tachypnoea and laboured breathing. X-ray chest shows diffuse pulmonary infiltrates. Arterial PO_2 falls to less than 50. Management consists of 100 per cent oxygen and assisted ventillation. It takes from 4–7 days for the chest to clear, and the patient returns to normal. If not detected early, patient's condition deteriorates rapidly, he develops cardiorespiratory failure and dies.

FAT EMBOLISM SYNDROME

This is one of the most serious complications, the essential feature being occlusion of small vessels by fat globules.

Causes: The fat globules may originate from bone marrow or adipose tissue. Fat embolism is more common following severe injuries with multiple fractures and fractures of major bones. The pathogenesis of the syndrome is not clear, but it seems likely that two events occur: (i) release of free fatty acids (by action of lipases on the neutral fat), which induces a toxic vasculitis, followed by platelet-fibrin thrombosis and (ii) actual obstruction of small pulmonary vessels by fat globules.

Consequences: Symptoms are evident a day or so after the injury. Presenting features are in the form of two, more or less distinct types: (i) cerebral and (ii) pulmonary. In the cerebral type, the patient becomes drowsy, restless and disoriented and gradually goes into a state of coma. In the pulmonary type, tachypnoea and tachycardia are the more prominent features. The other common feature of fat embolism is a petechial rash, usually on the front of the neck, anterior axillary folds, chest or conjunctiva. If untreated, and sometimes despite treatment, the patient develops respiratory failure and dies.

Diagnosis: In a case with multiple fractures, early diagnosis may be possible by strong suspicion. In addition to the classic clinical features, signs of retinal artery emboli (striate haemorrhages and exudates) may be present. Sputum and urine may reveal the presence of fat globules. X-ray of the chest may show a patchy pulmonary infiltration (snow-storm appearance). Blood PO of less than 50 mmHg may indicate impending respiratory failure.

Treatment: This consists of respiratory support, heparinisation, intravenous low molecular weight dextran (Lomodex-20) and corticosteroids. An intravenous 5 per cent dextrose solution with 5 per cent alcohol helps in emulsification of fat globules, and is used by some.

DEEP VEIN THROMBOSIS (DVT) AND PULMONARY EMBOLISM

Deep vein thrombosis (DVT) is a common complication associated with lower limb injuries and with spinal injuries.

Causes: Immobilisation following trauma leads to venous stasis which results in thrombosis of veins. DVT proximal to the knee is a common cause of life-threatening complication of pulmonary embolism. DVT can be recognised as early as 48 hours after the injury. Embolism occurs, usually 4-5 days after the injury.

Consequences: DVT can be diagnosed early with high index of suspicion. The group of patients 'at risk' include the elderly and the obese patients. Leg swelling and calf tenderness are usual signs. The calf tenderness may get exaggerated by passive dorsiflexion of the ankle (Homan's sign). Definitive diagnosis can be made by venography. One should keep a patient of DVT on constant watch for development of pulmonary embolism. This can be suspected if the patient develops tachypnoea and dyspnoea, usually 4-5 days after the accident. There may be chest pain or haemoptysis.

Treatment of DVT is elevation of the limb, elastic bandage and anticoagulant therapy. For pulmonary embolism, respiratory support and heparin therapy is to be done. Early internal fixation of fractures, so as to allow early, active mobilisation of the extremity is an effective means of prevention of DVT, and hence of pulmonary embolism.

CRUSH SYNDROME

This syndrome results from massive crushing of the muscles, commonly associated with crush injuries sustained during earthquakes, air raids, mining and other such accidents. A similar effect may follow the application of tourniquet for an excessive period.

Causes: Crushing of muscles results in entry of *myohaemoglobin* into the circulation, which precipitates in renal tubules, leading to acute renal tubular necrosis.

Consequences: Acute tubular necrosis produces signs of deficient renal functions such as scanty urine, apathy, restlessness and delirium. It may take 2-3 days for these features to appear.

Treatment: In a case with crushed limb, first aid treatment may necessitate the application of a tourniquet, which is gradually released, so that deleterious substances are released into the circulation in small quantities. If oliguria develops, the patient is treated as for acute renal failure.

INJURY TO MAJOR BLOOD VESSELS

Blood vessels lie in close proximity to bones, and hence are liable to injury with different fractures and dislocations (Table 7.2). The popliteal artery is the most frequently damaged vessel in musculoskeletal injuries.

Causes: The artery may be damaged by the object causing the fracture (e.g., bullet) or by a sharp edge of a bone fragment (e.g., supracondylar fracture of the humerus). The damage to the vessel may vary from just a pressure from outside to a complete rupture.

Consequences: Obstruction to blood flow will not always lead to gangrene. Where the collateral circulation is good, the following may result:
- *No effect:* If collateral circulation of the limb around the site of vascular damage is good, there will be no adverse effect of the vascular injury.
- *Exercise ischaemia:* The collaterals are good enough to keep the limb viable but any further demand on the blood supply during exercise, causes ischaemic pain (vascular claudication).
- *Ischaemic contracture:* If the collaterals do not provide adequate blood supply to the muscles, there results an ischaemic muscle necrosis. This is followed by contracture and fibrosis of the necrotic muscles, leading to deformities (e.g., Volkmann's ischaemic contracture, see page 47).

Table 7.2: Vascular injuries and skeletal trauma.	
Vessel injured	**Trauma**
Femoral	Fracture lower third of femur
Popliteal	Supracondylar fracture of the femur
Posterior tibial	Dislocation of the knee, fracture tibia
Subclavian	Fracture of the clavicle
Axillary	Fracture-dislocation of the shoulder
Brachial	Supracondylar fracture of the humerus

Flowchart 7.1: Management of vascular injury to limb.

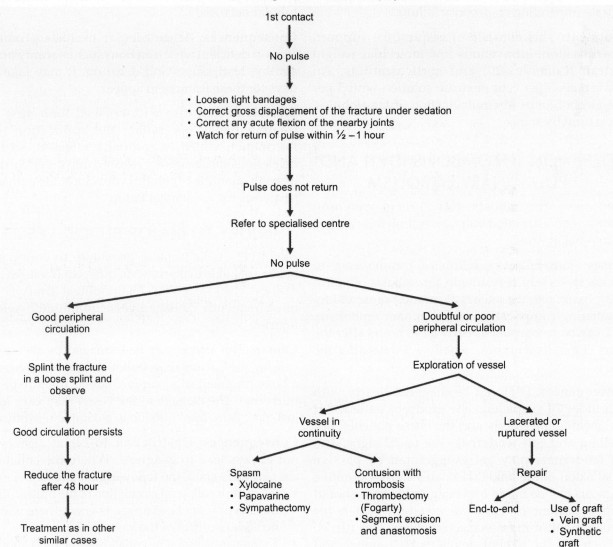

- *Gangrene:* If the blood supply is grossly insufficient, gangrene occurs.

Diagnosis: The pulses distal to the injury should be examined in every case of a fracture or dislocation. Some of the features which suggest a possible vascular injury of a limb are listed below:

a. *Signs at the fracture site:* The following signs may be present at the fracture site:
   - Rapidly increasing swelling
   - Massive external bleeding (in open fractures)
   - A wound in the normal anatomical path of the vessel

b. *Signs in the limb distal to the fracture:* The following signs may be present in the limb distal to the fracture (five P's):
   1. Pain – cramp like
   2. Pulse – absent
   3. Pallor

4. Paraesthesias
5. Paralysis

As a matter of *rule,* absent peripheral pulses in an injured limb should be considered to be due to vascular damage unless proved otherwise. The confirmation of obstruction to blood flow in a vessel and its site can be easily done by Doppler study. In the absence of such a facility, one there is no need to waste crucial time by ordering an angiogram merely for confirmation of diagnosis. An angiogram may be justified in cases with multiple fractures in the same limb, where it may help in localising the site of the vascular injury.

Treatment: Early diagnosis and urgent treatment are of paramount importance because of the serious consequences that may follow. Correct treatment at the site of first contact (Flowchart 7.1), followed by referral to a centre equipped with facilities to treat vascular injuries is essential. In case exploration of the vessel is required, the fracture should be suitably stabilised using internal or external fixation.

INJURY TO NERVES

Nerves lie in close proximity to bones, and hence are liable to damage in different fractures or dislocations (Table 7.3). The radial nerve is the most frequently damaged nerve in musculoskeletal injuries. Nerves and vessels lie together in limbs, and so are often injured together.

Causes: A nerve may be damaged in one of the following ways:
• By the agent causing the fracture (e.g., bullet).
• By direct pressure by the fracture ends at the time of fracture or during manipulation.
• Traction injury at the time of fracture, when the fracture is being manipulated or during skeletal traction.
• Entrapment in callus at the fracture site.

Consequences: Damage to the nerve may be neurapraxia, axonotmesis, or neurotmesis. It may result in a variable degree of motor and sensory loss along the distribution of the nerve (see Chapter 10, Peripheral Nerve Injuries).

Treatment: This depends upon the type of fracture, whether it is closed or open. When the nerve injury is associated with a closed fracture, the type of damage is generally neurapraxia or axonotmesis, and nerve recovery is good with conservative treatment. In case the fracture *per se* needs open reduction for other reasons, the nerve should also be explored.

When associated with an open fracture, the type of nerve damage is often neurotmesis. In such cases, the nerve should be explored and repaired as per need, and the fracture fixed internally with nail, plate, etc.

INJURY TO MUSCLES AND TENDONS

Some degree of damage to muscles and tendons occurs with most fractures. It may result from the object causing the fracture (e.g., an axe), or from the sharp edge of the fractured bone. Often these injuries are overshadowed by more alarming fractures, and are detected only late, when the joint distal to the fracture becomes stiff and deformed due to scarring of the injured muscle.

Rest to the injured muscle and analgesics is enough in cases with partial rupture. A complete rupture requires repair. Rarely, if rupture of a tendon or muscle is detected late, reconstruction may be required.

INJURY TO JOINTS

Fractures near a joint may be associated with subluxation or dislocation of that joint. This combination is becoming more frequent due to high-velocity traffic accidents. Early open reduction and stabilisation of the fracture to permit early joint movements has improved the results.

INJURY TO VISCERA

Visceral injuries are seen in pelvic and rib fractures. Their management is discussed in Surgery textbooks.

INFECTION – OSTEOMYELITIS

Causes: Infection of the bone is an early complication of fractures. It occurs more commonly in open fractures, particularly in those where compounding occurs from outside (external compounding). The increasing use of operative methods in the treatment of fractures is responsible for the rise in the incidence of infection of the bone, often years later. Infection may be superficial, moderate (osteomyelitis), or severe (gas gangrene).

Treatment: Proper care of an open fracture can prevent osteomyelitis. Once infection occurs, it should be adequately treated.

COMPARTMENT SYNDROME

The limbs contain muscles in compartments enclosed by bones, fascia and interosseous

Table 7.3: Nerve injuries and skeletal trauma.		
Nerve	**Trauma**	**Effect**
Axillary nerve	Dislocation of the shoulder	Deltoid paralysis
Radial nerve	Fracture shaft of the humerus	Wrist drop
Median nerve	Supracondylar fracture of humerus	Pointing index
Ulnar nerve	Fracture medial epicondyle humerus	Claw hand
Sciatic nerve	Posterior dislocation of the hip	Foot drop due to weakness of dorsiflexors of the foot
Common peroneal nerve	Knee dislocation Fracture of neck of the fibula	Foot drop

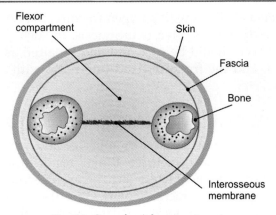

Fig. 7.1: Osseofascial compartment.

membrane (Fig. 7.1). A rise in pressure within these compartments due to any reason may jeopardize the blood supply to the muscles and nerves within the compartment, resulting in what is known as "compartment syndrome".

Causes: The rise in compartment pressure can be due to any of the following reasons:

- Any injury leading to oedema of muscles.
- Fracture haematoma within the compartment.
- Ischaemia to the compartment, leading to muscle oedema.

Consequences: The increased pressure within the compartment compromises the circulation leading to further muscle ischaemia. A *vicious cycle* is thus initiated (Fig. 7.2) and continues until the total vascularity of the muscles and nerves within the compartment is jeopardized. This results in ischaemic muscle necrosis and nerve damage. The necrotic

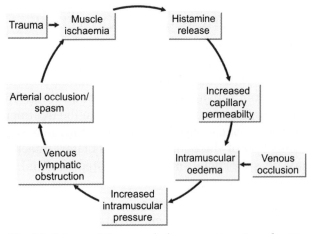

Fig. 7.2: Eaton and Green cycle for compartment syndrome.

muscles undergo healing with fibrosis, leading to contractures. Nerve damage may result in motor and sensory loss. In an extreme case, gangrene may occur.

Diagnosis: Compartment syndrome can be diagnosed early by high index of suspicion. Excessive pain, not relieved with usual doses of analgesics, in a patient with an injury known to cause compartment syndrome must raise an alarm in the mind of the treating doctor. Injuries with a high risk of developing compartment syndrome are as follows:

- Supracondylar fracture of the humerus
- Forearm bone fractures
- Closed tibial fractures
- Crush injuries to leg and forearm.

Stretch test: This is the earliest sign of impending compartment syndrome. The ischaemic muscles, when stretched, give rise to pain. It is possible to stretch the affected muscles by passively moving the joints in direction opposite to that of the damaged muscle's action. (e.g., passive extension of fingers produces pain in *flexor* compartment of the forearm).

Other signs include a tense compartment, hypoaesthesia in the distribution of involved nerves, muscle weakness, etc. Compartment syndrome can be confirmed by measuring compartment pressure. A pressure higher than 40 mm of water is indicative of compartment syndrome. Pulses may remain palpable till very late in impending compartment syndrome, and should not provide a false sense of security that all is well.

Treatment: A close watch for an impending compartment syndrome and effective early preventive measures like limb elevation, active finger movements, etc., can prevent this serious complication. Early surgical decompression is necessary in established cases. This can be performed by the following methods:

- *Fasciotomy:* The deep fascia of the compartment is slit longitudinally (e.g., in forearm).
- *Fibulectomy:* The middle third of the fibula is excised in order to decompress all compartments of the leg.

DELAYED AND NON-UNION

When a fracture takes more than the usual time to unite, it is said to have gone in *delayed union.* A large percentage of such fractures eventually unite. In some, the union does not progress, and they fail to unite. These are called *non-union.* Conventionally, it is not before 6 months that a fracture can be declared as non-union. It is often difficult to say whether the fracture is in delayed union, or has gone into non-union. Only progressive evaluation of the X-rays over a period of time can solve this issue. Presence of mobility at the fracture after a reasonable period is surely a sign of non-union. Presence of pain at the fracture site on using the limbs also indicates non-union. Non-union may be painless if pseudo joint forms between the fracture ends (pseudoarthrosis).

Causes: Some of the factors responsible for delayed union are given in Table 7.4. In any given case, there may be one or more factors operating.

Types of non-union: There are two main types of non-union (Fig. 7.3):
1. Atrophic, where there is minimal or no attempt at callus formation.
2. Hypertrophic, where though the callus is present, it does not bridge the fracture site.

Common sites: Sites where non-union occurs commonly are neck of the femur, scaphoid, lower third of the tibia, lower third of the ulna and lateral condyle of the humerus.

Consequences: Delayed and non-union can result in persistent pain, deformity, or abnormal mobility at the fracture site. A fracture in delayed union, if stressed, can lead to refracture.

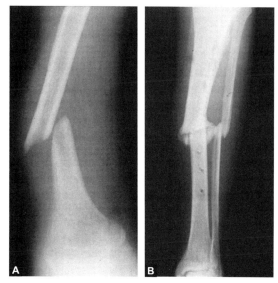

Fig. 7.3: Types of non-union: (A) Atrophic; (B) Hypertrophic.

Table 7.4: Causes of delayed and non-union, and their common sites.

Causes related to the patient
- *Age: Common in old age*
- *Associated systemic illness: Malignancy, osteomalacia*

Causes related to fracture
- *Distraction at the fracture site*
  - Muscle pulling the fragments
    - Fracture patella
    - Fracture olecranon
  - Gravity
    - Fracture shaft of humerus
- *Soft tissue interposition*
  - Fracture shaft of humerus
  - Fracture shaft of femur
  - Fracture medial malleolus (abduction type)
- *Bone loss at the time of fracture*
  - Fracture tibia (open type)
  - Fracture ulna (open type)
- *Infection from an open fracture*
  - Fracture tibia
- *Damage to blood supply of fracture fragments*
  - Fracture neck of femur
  - Fracture lower third of tibia
- *Pathological fracture*
  - Fracture of the shaft of the femur
  - Fracture of humerus

Causes related to treatment
- *Inadequate reduction*
  - Fracture shafts of long bones
- *Inadequate immobilisation*
  - Fracture shafts of long bones
  - Fracture neck of femur
- *Distraction during treatment*
  - Fracture shaft of femur

Diagnosis: Delayed union is a diagnosis in relation to time. The fracture may not show any abnormal sign clinically, but X-rays may fail to show bony union. The following are some of the clinical findings which suggest delayed union and non-union:
- Persistent pain
- Pain on stressing the fracture
- Mobility (in non-union)
- Increasing deformity at the fracture site (in non-union).

The following are some of the radiological features suggestive of these complications:
- *Delayed union:* The fracture line is visible. There may be inadequate callus bridging the fracture site.
- *Non-union:* The fracture line is visible. There is little bridging callus. The fracture ends may be rounded, smooth and sclerotic. The medullary cavity may be obliterated.

It is sometimes very difficult to be sure about union of a fracture where internal fixation has been used. Evaluation of serial X-rays may help detect subtle angulation, non-progress of bridging callus, resorption of callus, loosening of screws and bending of the nail or plate. Excessive rotation may be the only abnormal mobility in a case with intramedullary rod in situ. Oblique views, done under fluoroscopy may show an unhealed fracture better than conventional AP and lateral X-rays. It may be possible to demonstrate mobility at the fracture by stress X-rays or weight bearing X-rays. 3-D CT scan is sometimes helpful in differentiating between delayed and non-union.

Treatment: Most fractures in delayed union unite on continuing the conservative treatment. Sometimes, this may not occur and the fracture may need surgical intervention. Bone grafting with or without internal fixation may be required. Treatment of non-union depends upon the site of non-union and the disability caused by it. The following possibilities of treatment should be considered, depending upon the individual cases.

- *Open reduction, internal fixation and bone grafting:* This is the most common operation performed for non-union. The grafts are taken from iliac crest. Internal fixation is required in most cases.
- *Excision of fragments:* Sometimes, achieving union is difficult and time-consuming compared to excision of one of the fragments. This can only be done where excision of the fragment will not cause any loss of functions. An excision may or may not need to be combined with replacement with an artificial mould (prosthesis). For example, the lower-end of the ulna can be excised for non-union of the fracture of the distal-end of the ulna without much loss. In non-union of fracture of the neck of femur in an elderly, the head of the femur can be replaced by a prosthesis (replacement arthroplasty).
- *No treatment:* Some non-unions do not give rise to any symptoms, and hence require no treatment, e.g., some non-unions of the fracture scaphoid.
- *Ilizarov's method:* Prof Ilizarov from the former USSR designed a special external fixation apparatus for treating non-union (see page 35).

MALUNION

When a fracture does not unite in proper position, it is said to have malunited. A slight degree of malunion occurs in a large proportion of fractures, but in practice the term is reserved for cases where the resulting disability is of clinical significance.

Causes: Improper treatment is the most common cause. Malunion is therefore preventable in most cases by keeping a close watch on position of the fracture during treatment. Sometimes, malunion is inevitable because of unchecked muscle pull (e.g., fracture of the clavicle), or excessive comminution (e.g., Colles' fracture).

Common sites: Fractures at the ends of a bone always unite, but they often malunite, e.g., supracondylar fracture of the humerus, Colles' fracture, etc.

Consequences: Malunion results in deformity, shortening of the limb, and limitation of movements.

Treatment: Each case is treated on its merit. A slight degree of malunion may not require any treatment,

but a malunion producing significant disability, especially in adults, needs operative intervention. The following treatment possibilities can be considered:

a. *Treatment required:* Malunion may require treatment because of deformity (e.g., supracondylar fracture of the humerus), shortening (e.g., fracture of the shaft of the femur) or functional limitations (e.g., limitation of rotations in malunion of forearm fractures). Some of the methods for treating malunion are as follows:

- *Osteoclasis* (refracturing the bone): It is used for correction of mild to moderate angular deformities in children. Under general anaesthesia the fracture is recreated, the angulation corrected, and the limb immobilised in plaster.
- *Redoing the fracture surgically:* This is the most commonly performed operation for malunion. The fracture site is exposed, the malunion corrected and the fracture fixed internally with suitable implants. Bone grafting is also performed, in addition, in most cases, e.g., malunion of long bones.
- *Corrective osteotomy:* In some cases, redoing the fracture, as discussed above may not be desirable due to variety of reasons such as poor skin condition, poor vascularity of bone in that area, etc. In such cases, the deformity is corrected by osteotomy at a site away from the fracture as the healing may be quicker at this new site, e.g., supramalleolar corrective osteotomy for malunion of distal-third tibial fractures.
- *Excision of the protruding bone*: In a fracture of the clavicle, a bone spike protruding under the skin may be shaved off. Same may be required in a spikey malunion of fracture of the shaft of the tibia.

b. *No treatment:* Sometimes malunion may not need any treatment, either because it does not cause any disability, or because it is expected to correct by remodelling. Remodelling of a fracture depends on the following factors:

- *Age:* Remodelling is better in children.
- *Type of deformity:* Sideways shifts are well-corrected by remodelling. Five to ten degrees of angulation may also get corrected, but *malrotation does not get corrected.*
- *Angulation in the plane* of movement of the adjacent joint is remodelled better than that in other planes, e.g., posterior angulation in a fracture of the tibial shaft remodels better.
- *Location of fracture:* Fractures near joints remodel better.

Cross union is a special type of malunion which occurs in fractures of the forearm bones, wherein the two bones unite with each other. For details please refer to page 107.

SHORTENING

Causes: It is a common complication of fractures, resulting from the following causes:

- *Malunion*: The fracture unites with an overlap or marked angulation, e.g., most long bone fractures.
- *Crushing*: Actual bone loss, e.g., bone loss in gunshot wounds.
- *Growth defect*: Injury to the growth plate may result in shortening (see Salter-Harris classification of epiphyseal injuries, page 58).

Treatment: A little shortening in upper limbs goes unnoticed, hence no treatment is required. For shortening in lower limbs, treatment depends upon the amount of shortening.

- Shortening *less than 2 cm* is not much noticeable, hence can be compensated by a shoe raise.
- Shortening *more than 2 cm* is noticeable. In elderly patients, it may be compensated for by raising the shoe on the affected side. In younger patients, correction of angulation or overlap by operative method is necessary. Limb length equalisation procedure is required to correct shortening in an old, healed, remodelled fracture.

AVASCULAR NECROSIS

Blood supply of some bones is such that the vascularity of a part of it is seriously jeopardized following fracture, resulting in necrosis of that part.

Common sites: Some of the sites where avascular necrosis commonly occurs are given in Table 7.5.

Consequences: Avascular necrosis causes deformation of the bone. This leads to secondary osteoarthritis a few years later, thus causing painful limitation of joint movement.

Diagnosis: Avascular necrosis should always be suspected in fracture where it is known to occur. Pain

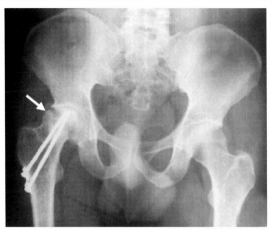

Fig. 7.4: Avascular necrosis of the femoral head after a neck fracture fixed with screws.

and stiffness appear rather late. Radiological changes as given below appear earlier (Fig. 7.4).

Sclerosis of necrotic area: The avascular bone is unable to share disuse osteoporosis as occurs in the surrounding normal bones. Hence, it stands out densely on the X-ray.

Deformity of the bone occurs because of the collapse of necrotic bone.

Osteoarthritis supervenes giving rise to diminished joint space, osteophytes (lipping of bone from margins), etc.

It is possible to diagnose avascular necrosis on bone scan before changes appear on plain X-rays. It is visible as 'cold area' on the bone scan.

Treatment: Avascular necrosis may be prevented by early, energetic reduction of susceptible fractures and dislocations. Once it has occurred, the following treatment options remain:

- *Delay weight bearing* on the necrotic bone until it is revascularised, thereby preventing its collapse. It takes anywhere from 6–8 months for the bone to revascularise.
- *Revascularisation procedure* by using vascularised bone grafts (e.g., vascularised bone pedicle graft from greater trochanter in an avascular femoral head in fracture of the neck of the femur).
- *Excision* of the avascular segment of bone where doing so does not hamper functions, e.g. fracture of the scaphoid.
- *Excision* followed by replacement, e.g., in fracture of the neck of the femur, the avascular head can be replaced by a prosthesis.
- *Total joint replacement* or arthrodesis may be required once the patient is disabled because of pain from osteoarthritis secondary to avascular necrosis.

Table 7.5: Common sites of avascular necrosis.	
Site	**Cause**
Head of the femur	▪ Fracture neck of the femur ▪ Posterior dislocation of the hip
Proximal pole of scaphoid	Fracture through the waist of the scaphoid
Body of the talus	Fracture through neck of the talus

STIFFNESS OF JOINTS

It is a common complication of fracture treatment. Shoulder, elbow and knee joints are particularly prone to stiffness following fractures.

Causes: The following are some of the causes of joint stiffness:

- Intra-articular and peri-articular adhesions secondary to immobilisation, mostly in intra-articular fractures.
- Contracture of the muscles around a joint because of prolonged immobilisation.
- Tethering of muscle at the fracture site (e.g., quadriceps adhesion to a fracture of femoral shaft).
- Myositis ossificans (refer page 52).

Consequences: Stiff joints hamper normal physical activity of the patient.

Treatment: The treatment is heat therapy (hot fomentation, wax bath, diathermy, etc.) and exercises. Sometimes, there may be a need for manipulating the joint under general anaesthesia. Surgical intervention is required in the following circumstances:

- To excise intra-articular adhesions, preferably arthroscopically.
- To excise an extra-articular bone block which may be acting as a 'door stopper'.
- To lengthen contracted muscles.
- Joint replacement, if there is pain due to secondary osteoarthritis.

REFLEX SYMPATHETIC DYSTROPHY (SUDECK'S DYSTROPHY)

This is a term given to a group of vague painful conditions observed as a sequelae of trauma. The trauma is sometimes relatively minor, and hence symptoms and signs are out of proportion to the trauma.

Consequences: Clinical features consist of pain, hyperaesthesia, tenderness and swelling. Skin becomes red, shiny and warm in early stage. Progressive atrophy of the skin, muscles and nails occur in the later stage. Joint deformities and stiffness ensues. X-ray shows characteristic spotty rarefaction.

Treatment: It is a difficult condition to explain to the patient, and also the treatment is prolonged. Physiotherapy constitutes the principle modality of treatment. Further trauma in the form of an operation or forceful mobilisation is detrimental. In some cases, beta-blockers have been shown to produce good response. In resistant cases, sympathetic blocks may aid in recovery. Prolonged physiotherapy and patience on the part of the doctor and the patient is usually rewarding.

MYOSITIS OSSIFICANS (POST-TRAUMATIC OSSIFICATION)

This is ossification of the haematoma around a joint, resulting in the formation of a mass of bone restricting joint movements, often completely.

Causes: It occurs in cases with severe injury to a joint, especially when the capsule and the periosteum have been stripped from the bones by violent displacement of the fragments. It is common in children because in them the periosteum is loosely attached to the bones. It is particularly common around the elbow joint. There is also a relatively high incidence in patients with prolonged or permanent neuronal damage from head injury, and in patient with paraplegia. Massage following trauma is a factor known to aggravate myositis.

Consequences: The bone formation leads to stiffness of the joint, either due to thickening of the capsule or due to the bone blocking movement.

In extreme cases, the bone bridges the joint resulting in complete loss of movements (extra-articular ankylosis).

Radiologically, an active myositis and a mature myositis have been identified. In the former, the margins of the bone mass are fluffy (Fig. 7.5); in the latter the bone appears trabeculated with well-defined margins.

Treatment: Massage following injury is strictly prohibited. In the early active stage of myositis the limb should be rested, and NSAID is given. In

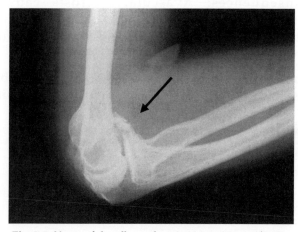

Fig. 7.5: X-ray of the elbow showing myositis ossificans.

late stages, it is possible to regain movement by physiotherapy. In some cases, once the myositis mass matures, surgical excision of the bone mass may help regain movement.

 What have we learnt?

- A neurovascular examination of the limb distal to the fracture is a must in every patient with fracture. It is a disastrous complication, if not attended to in time.
- Not all delayed union, non-union and malunion need surgical treatment. Some are quite compatible with normal functions. Treatment has to be tailored to patient's need.
- Active joint mobilisation is necessary to prevent joint stiffness.
- No massage after a fracture or joint injury. It can lead to myositis ossificans.

Additional information: From the entrance exams point of view

- Basic pathology in myositis ossificans lies in the muscle fibres.
- Most common location for myositis ossificans is elbow, next common is hip.
- In myositis ossificans mature bone is seen in the periphery and immature bone in the centre.
- Myositis ossificans progressiva (fibrodysplasia): The life expectancy decreases and the most common cause of death is lung disease. It affects children before the age of 6 and involves deformities of spine, hands and feet.
- Bone scan (Tc99 three-phase scan) is the most sensitive for early detection of heterotopic ossification.
- Alkaline phosphatase and 24 hours PGE_2 urinary excretion are screening tests for heterotopic ossification.

Injury to Joints: Dislocation and Subluxation

Competency

- ❖ **OR1.5:** Describe and discuss the aetiopathogenesis, clinical features, investigations, and principles of management of dislocation of major joints, shoulder, knee, hip.

RELEVANT ANATOMY

It is important to first understand the factors responsible for the stability of a joint in order to understand why a particular joint dislocates more often than another. Normally, a joint is held in position because of the inherent stability in its design, by the ligaments, and by the surrounding muscles, as discussed below:

The shape of a joint: The shape of the articulating surfaces in themselves may provide great security against displacement, e.g., the hip joint with its deep socket (the acetabulum) and an almost spherical ball (the femoral head) is a good design from the stability viewpoint. On the other hand, the shoulder joint with its shallow socket (the glenoid) and a large ball (the humeral head) is a poor design and therefore dislocates more easily than the hip joint.

The ligaments: These prevent any abnormal mobility of a joint and are called *static stabilisers.* The role of the ligaments in providing stability to a joint is variable. In some joints (e.g., the knee and finger joints), ligaments form the main stabilising structures, whereas in others (e.g., the hip or shoulder) they do not play an important role.

The muscles: A strong muscle cover around a joint gives it stability. Muscles may also provide a supporting function to the ligaments by reflexly contracting to protect the ligaments, when the latter come under harmful stresses. These are, therefore, called the *dynamic stabilisers* of a joint.

DEFINITIONS

Dislocation: A joint is dislocated when its articular surfaces are *completely displaced,* one from the other, so that all contact between them is lost (see Fig. 1.4, page 5).

Subluxation: A joint is subluxated when its articular surfaces are only *partly displaced* and retain some contact between them.

CLASSIFICATION

Dislocations and subluxations may be classified on the basis of etiology into congenital or acquired. Congenital dislocation is a condition where a joint is dislocated at birth, e.g., congenital dislocation of the hip (CDH). Acquired dislocation may occur at any age. It may be traumatic or pathological as discussed below.

Traumatic dislocation: Injury is by far the most common cause of dislocations and subluxations at almost all joints (Table 8.1). The force required to dislocate a particular joint varies from joint to joint.

Table 8.1: Common dislocations at different joints.	
Spine	Cervical spine (anterior C_5 over C_6)
Hip	*Posterior*, anterior
Shoulder	*Anterior (most common overall)*, posterior
Elbow	*Posterior*, postero-lateral
Wrist	Lunate, perilunate
MP joint	Dorsal (index finger)
Knee	Posterior
Patella	Lateral
Ankle	Antero-lateral
Foot ■ Intertarsal ■ Tarsometatarsal	■ Chopart's dislocation ■ Lisfranc's dislocation

The following are the different types of traumatic dislocations seen in clinical practice:

a. *Acute traumatic dislocation:* This is an episode of dislocation where the force of injury is the main contributing factor, e.g., shoulder dislocation.

b. *Old unreduced dislocation:* A traumatic dislocation, not reduced, may present as an old unreduced dislocation, e.g., old posterior dislocation of the hip.

c. *Recurrent dislocation:* In some joints, proper healing does not occur after the first dislocation. This results in weakness of the supporting structures of the joint so that the joint dislocates repeatedly, often with trivial trauma. Recurrent dislocation of the shoulder and patella are common.

d. *Fracture-dislocation:* When a dislocation is associated with a fracture of one or both of the articulating bones, it is called fracture-dislocation. A dislocation of the hip is often associated with a fracture of the lip of the acetabulum.

Pathological dislocation: The articulating surfaces forming a joint may be destroyed by an infective or a neoplastic process, or the ligaments may be damaged due to some disease. This results in dislocation or subluxation of the joint without any trauma, e.g., dislocation of the hip in septic arthritis.

PATHOANATOMY

Dislocation cannot occur without damage to the protective ligaments or joint capsule. Usually the capsule and one or more of the reinforcing ligaments are torn, permitting the articular end of the bone to escape through the rent. Sometimes, the capsule is not torn in its substance but is stripped from one of its bony attachments (Fig. 8.1). Rarely, a ligament

may withstand the force of the injury so that instead of ligament rupture, a fragment of bone at one of its attachments may be chipped off (avulsed).

At the time of dislocation, as movement occurs between the two articulating surfaces, a piece of articular cartilage with or without its underlying bone may be 'shaved off' producing an *osteochondral fragment* within the joint. This fragment may lie loose inside the joint and may cause symptoms long after the dislocation is reduced (Fig. 8.2).

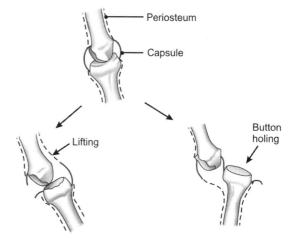

Fig. 8.1: Pathoanatomy of dislocations.

DIAGNOSIS

Clinical examination: In most cases of dislocation, the clinical features are sufficiently striking and make the diagnosis easy. Nevertheless, a dislocation or subluxation is sometimes overlooked, especially in a multiple injury case, an unconscious patient or in a case where the bony landmarks are obscured by severe swelling or obesity. Some dislocations, which are particularly notorious for getting overlooked are:

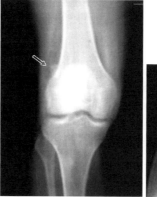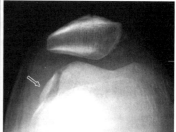

Fig. 8.2: X-ray showing osteochondral fragment.

Table 8.2: Typical deformities in dislocations.	
Joint (dislocation)	**Deformity**
Shoulder (anterior)	Abduction
Elbow (posterior)	Flexion
Hip ■ Posterior ■ Anterior	■ Flexion, adduction, internal rotation ■ Abduction, external rotation
Knee	Flexion, external rotation
Ankle	Varus

(i) posterior dislocation of the shoulder especially in an epileptic; and (ii) dislocation of the hip associated with a fracture of the shaft of the femur on the same side. The classic deformity of a hip dislocation does not occur, and the attention is drawn on the more obvious injury—the femoral shaft fracture. Some of the salient clinical features of dislocation are as follows:

- *Pain:* Dislocations are very painful.
- *Deformity:* In most dislocations the limb attains a classic attitude (Table 8.2).
- *Swelling:* It is obvious in the dislocation of a superficial joint, but may not be so in a joint located deep.
- *Loss of movement* because of severe pain and muscle spasm and loss of articulation.
- *Shortening of the limb* occurs in most dislocations *except* in anterior dislocation of the hip where lengthening occurs.
- *Telescopy:* In this test, it is possible to produce an abnormal to and fro movement in a dislocated joint (see Annexure I).

As with all limbs injuries, specific tests to establish the integrity or otherwise of major nerves and vessels of the extremity must be established in all cases of dislocation.

Radiological examination: In doubtful cases, the diagnosis must finally depend on adequate X-ray examination. The following principles should be remembered:

- X-ray should always be taken in two planes at right angles to each other, because a dislocation may not be apparent on a single projection.
- If in doubt, X-rays of the opposite limb may be taken for comparison. CT scan may also be of help.

- An associated fracture or an osteochondral fragment must always be looked for.

COMPLICATIONS

As with a fracture, complications following a dislocation can be immediate, early or late. Immediate complication is an injury to the neurovascular bundle of the limb. Early complications are: (i) recurrence; (ii) myositis ossificans; (iii) persistent instability; and (iv) joint stiffness. Late complications are: (i) recurrence; (ii) osteoarthritis; and (iii) avascular necrosis.

TREATMENT

Treatment of a dislocation or subluxation depends upon its type, as discussed below:

Acute traumatic dislocation: In acute traumatic dislocation, an urgent reduction of the dislocation is of paramount importance. Often it is possible to do so by conservative methods, although sometimes operative reduction may be required.

a. *Conservative methods:* A dislocation may be reduced by closed manipulative manoeuvres. Reduction of a dislocated joint is one of the most gratifying jobs an orthopaedic surgeon is called upon to do, as it produces instant pain relief to the patient. Prolonged traction may be required for reducing some dislocations.

b. *Operative methods:* Operative reduction may be required in some cases. Following are some of the indications:
  - Failure of closed reduction, often because the dislocation is detected late.
  - Fracture-dislocation: (i) if the fracture has produced significant incongruity of the joint surfaces; (ii) a loose piece of bone is lying within the joint; and (iii) the dislocation is difficult to maintain by closed treatment.

Old unreduced dislocations: This often needs operative reduction. In some cases, if the function of the dislocated joint is good, nothing needs to be done. These are discussed in the respective chapters.

Recurrent dislocations: An individual episode is treated like a traumatic dislocation. For prevention of recurrences, reconstructive procedures are required. These are discussed in the respective chapters.

What have we learnt?

- Dislocation means complete loss of contact between articulating bones.
- Treatment of acute dislocation is an emergency.
- Shoulder is the joint to dislocate most often.

Fractures in Children

Learning Objectives

- ❖ Discuss classification of epiphyseal injuries, and their relevance in management.
- ❖ Discuss how treatment of fractures in children varies from that in adults.

RELEVANT ANATOMY

Fractures in children are different from those in adults, mostly because of some anatomical and physiological differences between a child's and an adult's bone. Some of these are discussed below:

- **Growing skeleton:** Bones in children are growing. At each end of major long bones, and usually at only one end of short bones, there is a cartilaginous growth plate. This is a potential weak point giving rise to different types of epiphyseal injuries. In some injuries through the epiphyseal plate, growth of the limb may be affected.
- **Springy bones:** Bones in children are more resilient and springy, withstanding greater deformation without fracture. This characteristic is responsible for 'greenstick' fractures in children. Such fractures do not occur in adults.
- **Loose periosteum:** The periosteum is attached loosely to the diaphysis in a child's bones. This results in easy stripping of the periosteum over a considerable part following fracture. The haematoma soon gets calcified to become callus, therefore a child's fracture unites with a lot of callus.
- **Site of fractures:** Some fractures are more common in children than in adults as given in Table 9.1.

Table 9.1: Fractures* common in children.

- Forearm bones fractures
- Supracondylar fracture of the humerus
- Fracture of lateral condyle of the humerus
- Epiphyseal injuries
- Spiral fracture of tibial shaft

* Dislocations are uncommon in children. Fractures of hands and feet are also uncommon in children.

- **Healing of fractures:** Fractures unite quicker in children, taking almost half the time taken in adults.
- **Remodelling:** Fractures in children have greater remodelling potential, so much so that any evidence of a past fracture may be absent after a few months. The remodelling potential varies with: (i) age of the child; (ii) location of the fracture; and (iii) degree and type of angulation.

TYPES OF FRACTURES

Fractures in children can be conveniently considered under four headings: (i) birth fractures and related injuries; (ii) epiphyseal injuries; (iii) fractures of shafts of long bones in older children and (iv) pathological fractures.

Birth fractures: Three types of fractures may occur in a newborn. These are as follows:

a. Fracture or epiphyseal separation *sustained during a difficult delivery:* These are the most common fractures seen at birth. Fracture of the shaft of the humerus occurs most frequently; others are fracture of the shaft of the femur, fracture clavicle, etc. Simple strapping of the fracture may be sufficient. Union occurs rapidly with a lot of callus. Remodelling occurs during the first few years of life.

b. Multiple fractures *associated with the congenital fragility* of bones, e.g., osteogenesis imperfecta (see page 307–308).

c. *Pseudoarthrosis of tibia:* This is a pathological entity, very different from a simple fracture or birth injury mentioned above. In this type, there is an inherent indolence of the fracture to unite.

Epiphyseal injuries: This is a group of injuries seen in a growing skeleton. An injury involving the growth plate may result in deformities due to irregular growth. Shortening may occur because of premature epiphyseal closure.

Salter and Harris classification (Fig. 9.1): Epiphyseal injuries have been classified into 5 types based on their X-ray appearance. The higher the classification, the more severe the injury. The incidence of growth disturbance is common in types III, IV and V (Table 9.2).

Shaft fractures in older children: Although, fractures of the shaft of long bones have many similarities in children and adults, the following are some of the features peculiar to children:

a. *Displacement is less:* Fractures of the shaft of long bones in children often do not displace much. A

Table 9.2: Essential features of epiphyseal injuries (Salter and Harris classification).

Type	Example	Treatment	Prognosis
I	Radial neck epiphysis separation	Closed reduction	Good
II	Lower end radius epiphysis	Closed reduction	Good
III	Medial malleolus epiphysis	Open reduction	Growth disturbance can occur
IV	Lateral condyle of humerus	Open reduction	Growth disturbance common
V	Lower tibial epiphysis injury	Conservative	Growth disturbance always

special type called 'greenstick fracture' occurs only in children. In this type, the bones being resilient, do not break completely. The inner cortex bends, while the outer cortex breaks (Fig. 9.2). Such fractures occur commonly in the shafts of forearm bones.

b. *Alignment:* Perfect, *end-to-end alignment is not mandatory*. Some amount of 'malalignment' gets corrected with growth.

c. *Union:* Fractures unite faster in children.

d. *Treatment:* Fractures in children can usually be treated by conservative methods. An operation is sometimes necessary.

Pathological fractures: These are uncommon in children. However, there are some diseases which are particularly common in children and result in pathological fractures. These are: (i) fractures through

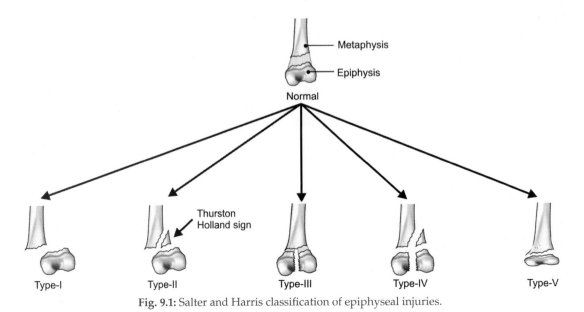

Fig. 9.1: Salter and Harris classification of epiphyseal injuries.

infected bones; (ii) fractures through cysts; and (iii) fractures associated with osteogenesis imperfecta.

DIAGNOSIS

Diagnosis of fractures in children is often missed for the following reasons:

a. History of trauma is either concealed, or the child is not old enough to communicate.
b. The more dramatic signs of fracture may be absent, especially in incomplete fractures. Thus, there may be no deformity, no abnormal mobility, no crepitus, etc.
c. Parents may attempt to conceal the fact that an infant has been injured, especially when there has been abuse (battered baby syndrome).
d. Undisplaced fractures are often missed on X-ray, unless carefully looked for.

Therefore, irrespective of the history, possibility of an injury should always be considered whenever marked loss of function, pain and tenderness, and unwillingness to use a limb occurs in children. On the other hand, trauma may be falsely implicated as a cause, in some non-traumatic diseases. In such cases, a clear gap between occurrence of trauma and onset of symptoms can be elicited by careful history.

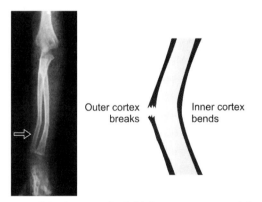

Fig. 9.2: X-ray of the forearm of a child showing a greenstick fracture. (Note that the outer cortex breaks, and the inner cortex bends).

TREATMENT

Conservative: Most fractures in children can be successfully treated by non-operative methods like plaster immobilisation, traction, sling, etc.

Following are some facts about fractures in children:
- Fractures in children heal faster.
- Fractures close to the joint heal faster.
- Sideways displacement will remodel.
- Reasonable angulation in the plane of the movement at an adjacent joint is acceptable.
- Rotational malalignment will not remodel, hence not acceptable.
- Epiphyseal plate, subjected to compressive forces, inhibits growth.

Operative: Operative intervention is necessary in some fractures, as listed below:
- Displaced fracture of the neck of the femur.
- Displaced fracture of lateral condyle of the humerus (Type IV epiphyseal injury).
- Fracture of the shaft of the femur, particularly in an adolescent.
- Wherever operation is considered necessary for some other reason such as vascular injury, the fracture is also fixed internally.

With the availability of image intensifier (a video X-ray machine in the OT) and development of techniques of percutaneous fixation (with minimal or no cutting), more and more fractures in children, which were hitherto treated by plaster immobilization, are being treated operatively. The reason for this change is: (a) reduced acceptability of 'malunion' by non-operative methods in a hope that remodelling will take care; (b) early and better recovery by operative methods; (c) availability of minimally invasive methods using newer fixation devices such as TENS nails or rush nails.

COMPLICATIONS

Fractures in children are associated with few complications. Union of a fracture is generally not a problem; non-union being very rare. Some complications relatively important in children's fractures are:
- Growth disturbances in epiphyseal injuries.
- Brachial artery injury in supracondylar fracture of the humerus.
- Myositis ossificans in injuries around the elbow.
- Avascular necrosis in fracture of the neck of the femur.

What have we learnt?

- Fractures in children are easier to treat.
- A special category, i.e., epiphyseal injuries, occur in children, and can lead to growth disturbances.
- History of injury has to be carefully probed, as often non-traumatic problems such as infection or tumour, may be erroneously linked to an unrelated episode of 'injury'.

Additional information: From the entrance exams point of view.

- Distal radius and ulna are the most common fracture locations in children followed by the clavicle.
- Most common bone fractured during birth is the clavicle.
- Injury to the perichondrial ring is type VI Salter Harris fracture or Rang's injury.
- Multiple fractures at various stages of healing in a child, always consider battered baby syndrome.
- Epiphyseal enlargement seen in haemophilia.
- Epiphyseal dysgenesis seen in hypothyroidism.

Peripheral Nerve Injuries

Competency

- ❖ **OR11.1:** Describe and discuss the aetiopathogenesis, clinical features, investigations and principles of management of peripheral nerve injuries in diseases like foot drop, wrist drop, claw hand, palsies of radial, ulnar, median, lateral popliteal and sciatic Nerves.

RELEVANT ANATOMY

Structure of a peripheral nerve: A peripheral nerve consists of masses of axis cylinders (axons), each with a neurilemma tube (Fig. 10.1). An individual nerve fibre is enclosed in a collagen connective tissue known as *endoneurium*. A bundle of such nerve fibres are further bound together by fibrous tissue to form a fasciculus. The binding fibrous tissue is known as *perineurium*. A number of fasciculi are bound together by a fibrous tissue sheath known as *epineurium*. An individual nerve, therefore, is a bundle of a number of fasciculi.

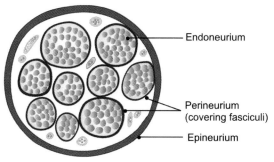

Endoneurium

Perineurium
(covering fasciculi)

Epineurium

Fig. 10.1: Structure of a nerve.

Formation of a peripheral nerve: These are formed from nerves arising from the spinal cord (spinal nerves). There are 31 pairs of spinal nerves in the body, each representing a segment of the spinal cord. These, either through direct branching or through a network of nerves (plexus), give rise to peripheral nerves. Peripheral nerves are mixed nerves carrying motor, sensory and autonomous supply to the limbs. The anatomy of individual nerves will be discussed in respective sections.

Motor innervation of limb muscles: A knowledge of motor innervation of different muscles in the limb is essential for diagnosis of a nerve injury. The following knowledge of anatomy is often required when dealing with a case of nerve injury, and is discussed subsequently in the sections on individual nerve injuries:

a. What is the nerve supply of a particular muscle?
b. What are the different muscles supplied by a nerve?
c. What is the action of a muscle and by what manoeuvre can one appreciate its action *in isolation*? Only such muscles, whose action can be elicited in isolation are suitable for testing.

Sensory innervation of limbs: The area of hypoaesthesia resulting from a nerve injury may be less than the area of skin innervated by that nerve because of the overlap of sensory supply by different nerves. A relatively small area supplied exclusively by a single nerve, called autonomous zone, is found in

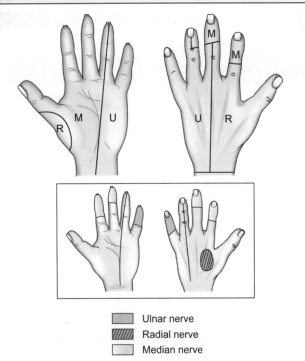

	Ulnar nerve
	Radial nerve
	Median nerve

Fig. 10.2: Sensory innervation of the hand. The picture in the box shows autonomous sensory zones in the hand.

all nerve injuries (Fig. 10.2). The sensory innervation by different nerves of the limbs is discussed in the section on individual nerve injuries.

Anatomical features relevant to nerve injuries: There are some features related to the anatomy of a nerve which make a particular nerve more prone to injury. These are as follows:

a. *Relation to the surface*: Superficially placed nerves are more prone to injury by external objects, e.g., the median nerve at the wrist often gets cut by a piece of glass.

b. *Relation to bone*: Nerves in close proximity to a bone or a joint are more prone to injury, e.g., radial nerve injury in a fracture of the shaft of the humerus.

c. *Relation to fibrous septae*: Some nerves pierce fibrous septae along their course. They may get entrapped in these septae (entrapment neuropathies).

d. *Relation to major vessels*: Nerves in close relation to a major vessel run the risk of ligation during surgery, or damage by an aneurysm.

e. *Course in a confined space*: A nerve may travel in a confined fibro-osseous tunnel and get compressed if there is a compromise of the space, e.g., median nerve compression in carpal tunnel syndrome.

f. *Fixation at points along the course*: Nerves are relatively fixed at some points along their course and do not tolerate the stretch they may be subjected to, e.g., the common peroneal nerve is relatively fixed over the neck of the fibula, and any stretching of the sciatic nerve often leads to isolated damage to this component of the nerve.

PATHOLOGY

Nerve degeneration: The part of the neurone distal to the point of injury undergoes secondary or Wallerian degeneration; the proximal part undergoes primary or retrograde degeneration upto a single node.

Nerve regeneration: As regeneration begins, the axonal stump from the proximal segment begins to grow distally. If the endoneural tube with its contained Schwann cells is intact, the axonal sprout may readily pass along its primary course and reinnervate the end-organ. The rate of recovery of axon is 1 mm per day. The muscle nearest to the site of injury recovers first, followed by others as the nerve reinnervates muscles from proximal to distal, the so-called motor march. If the endoneural tube is interrupted, the sprouts, as many as 100 from one axonal stump, may migrate aimlessly throughout the damaged area into the epineural, perineural or adjacent tissues to form an end-neuroma or a neuroma in continuity (Fig. 10.3). An end-neuroma may form when the proximal-end is widely separated from the distal-end. A side neuroma usually indicates a partial nerve cut.

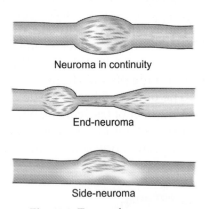

Neuroma in continuity

End-neuroma

Side-neuroma

Fig. 10.3: Types of neuromas.

MECHANISM OF INJURY

Fractures and dislocations are the most common cause of peripheral nerve injuries. Some other mechanisms by which a nerve may be damaged are: (i) direct injury–cut, laceration; (ii) infections–leprosy; (iii) mechanical injury–compression, traction, friction and shock wave; (iv) cooling and freezing– 'frost bite', etc.; (v) thermal injury; (vi) electrical injury–lectric shock; (vii) ischaemic injury–Volkmann's ischaemia; (viii)

Table 10.1: Seddon's classification of nerve injuries.

Type of injury	Pathology	Degeneration	Neuroma	Prognosis
Neurapraxia	Physiological interruption, anatomically normal	Nil	Nil	Recovery complete within 6 weeks
Axonotmesis	Axons broken, nerve intact	Proximally + distally	Neuroma in continuity	Recovery +/- Motor march +
Neurotmesis	Axons as well as nerve broken	Proximally + distally	End or side neuroma	Recovery poor

toxic agents–injection tetracycline resulting in radial nerve palsy; and (ix) radiation–for cancer treatment.

CLASSIFICATION

Seddon's classification: Seddon classifies nerve injuries into three types: (i) neurapraxia; (ii) axonotmesis; and (iii) neurotmesis.

- *Neurapraxia*: It is a physiological disruption of conduction in the nerve fibre. No structural changes occur. Recovery occurs spontaneously within a few weeks, and is complete.
- *Axonotmesis*: The axons are damaged but the internal architecture of the nerve is preserved. Wallerian degeneration occurs. Recovery may occur spontaneously but may take many months. Complete recovery may not occur.
- *Neurotmesis*: The structure of a nerve is damaged by actual cutting or scarring of a segment. Wallerian degeneration occurs. Spontaneous recovery is not possible, and nerve repair is required.

Most nerve injuries are a combination of these. Table 10.1 compares the essential features of the three types of nerve injuries.

DIAGNOSIS

In a case of peripheral nerve injury, the following information should be obtained by careful history and examination:
a. Which nerve is affected?
b. At what level is the nerve affected?
c. What is the cause?
d. What type of nerve injury (neurapraxia, etc.) is it likely to be?
e. In case of an old injury, is the nerve recovering?

History: A patient with a nerve injury commonly presents with complaints of inability to move a part of the limb, weakness and numbness. The cause of nerve injury may or may not be obvious.

In case the *cause is obvious*, say a penetrating wound along the course of a peripheral nerve (e.g., glass cut

injury to the median nerve), the nerve affected and its level is easy to decide. Similarly, nerve injury may occur during an operation as a result of stretching or direct injury.

When the *cause is not obvious*, an inquiry must be made regarding any history of injection in the proximity of the nerve. Neurotoxic drugs such as quinine and tetracycline are known to damage nerves. Medical causes of nerve affection like leprosy, diabetes should be considered in patients who do not give a history of injury.

Examination: Often, the clinical findings in a case of nerve palsy are very few. Therefore, it is essential to perform a systematic motor and sensory examination of the involved limb. Classic deformities may not be present in an early case or in a case with partial nerve injury. A combination of nerve injuries and anatomical variation in the nerve supply may distort the clinical picture of a classic nerve lesion. The following observations must be made during examination:

WHICH NERVE IS AFFECTED?

Attitude and deformity: Patients with some peripheral nerve injuries present with a classic attitude and deformity of the limb. Some such attitudes in different nerve injuries are as follows:
- *Wrist drop*: The wrist remains in palmar flexion due to weakness of the dorsiflexors. It is seen in radial nerve palsy.
- *Foot drop*: The foot remains in plantar flexion due to weakness of the dorsiflexors. It occurs in common peroneal nerve palsy.
- *Winging of scapula*: The vertebral border of the scapula becomes prominent when the patient tries to push against a wall. It occurs in paralysis of the serratus anterior muscle in long thoracic nerve palsy.
- *Claw hand (Main-en-griffe)*: Claw hand means hyperextension at the metacarpophalangeal joints and flexion at the proximal and distal

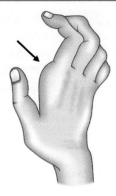

Fig. 10.4: Claw hand (hyperextension at the MP joint).

interphalangeal joints (Fig. 10.4). This occurs due to paralysis of the lumbricals, which flex the metacarpophalangeal joints and extend the interphalangeal joints. Paradoxically, clawing is more marked in low ulnar nerve palsy than in high ulnar nerve palsy. This is because in the latter, flexors of the fingers (both profundus and superficialis), which cause clawing affect are also paralysed. In ulnar nerve palsy, only the medial two fingers develop clawing while all the four fingers develop clawing in combined median and ulnar nerve palsies. Clawing may not become apparent in the early post-injury period.

- *'Ape thumb' deformity:* In this deformity the thumb is in the same plane as the wrist. It occurs due to paralysis of the opponens pollicis muscle in median nerve palsy.
- *'Pointing index':* On asking the patient to make a fist, it is noticed that the index finger remains straight. This is due to paralysis of both the flexors (digitorum superficialis and lateral half of the digitorum profundus) of the index finger, which occurs in median nerve palsy at a level proximal to the elbow. The other fingers can be flexed by the functioning medial side of the flexor digitorum profundus, supplied by the ulnar nerve.
- *'Policeman tip' deformity:* In this deformity, the arm hangs by the side of the body with elbow extended and forearm fully pronated. This is because of the paralysis of the abductor and external rotators of the shoulder alongwith flexors and supinators of the elbow.

Wasting of muscles: This will be obvious some time after the paralysis. It may be slight and become apparent only on comparing the affected limb with the sound limb. Some examples of this are given in Table 10.2.

Skin: The skin becomes dry (there is no sweating due to the involvement of the sympathetic nerves), glossy

and smooth. In partial lesions, there may be vasomotor changes in the form of pallor, cyanosis, or excessive sweating. There may be trophic disturbances such as ridged and brittle nails, shiny atrophic skin, trophic ulcers, etc.

Temperature: A paralysed part is usually colder and drier because of loss of sweating, best appreciated by comparing it with normal skin.

Sensory examination: The different forms of sensation to be tested in a suspected case of nerve palsy are touch, pain, temperature and vibration. The area of sensory loss may be smaller than expected. If it is so, look for sensation in the autonomous zone (see Fig. 10.2).

Reflexes: Reflexes in the area of nerve distribution are absent in cases of peripheral nerve injuries.

Table 10.2: Muscle wasting in nerve injuries.	
Muscle wasting	**Nerve**
Flat shoulder (Deltoid muscle)	Axillary nerve
Thenar eminence (Thenar muscle)	Median nerve
Hypothenar eminence (Hypothenar muscle)	Ulnar nerve
Hollowing between metacarpals (Interossei muscle)	Ulnar nerve
Thigh wasting (Quadriceps muscle)	Femoral nerve
Calf wasting (Gastrosoleus muscle)	Sciatic nerve

Sweat test: This is a test to detect sympathetic function in the skin supplied by a nerve. Sympathetic fibres are among the *most resistant* to mechanical trauma. The presence of sweating within an autonomous zone of an injured peripheral nerve reassures the examiner that complete interruption of the nerve has not occurred. Sweating can be determined by the *starch test or ninhydrin print test*. In these tests, the extremity is dusted with an agent that changes colour on coming in contact with sweat.

Motor examination: For evaluation of motor functions, clear concepts about the anatomy, as to which nerve supplies which muscle is essential. The muscles which are exclusively supplied by a particular nerve are most suitable for motor examination. The tests are nothing but manoeuvres to make a muscle contract. One must carefully watch for trick movements—the movement produced by the adjacent muscles, often substituting for the paralysed muscle. The contraction of the muscle must be appreciated, wherever possible, by feeling its belly or its tendon getting taut. Motor examination conducted for different nerves is discussed below.

RADIAL NERVE

Anatomy: This nerve is a continuation of the posterior cord of the brachial plexus. In the axilla, it gives off a branch to the long head of triceps, and enters the arm.

Course in the arm: As it comes into the arm, the radial nerve gives off the posterior cutaneous nerve of the arm and a branch to the medial head of the triceps. It now travels inferolaterally into the groove for the radial nerve on the posterior surface of the humerus, winding spirally around the bone. In the groove, it gives branches to the lateral head of triceps and anconeus muscles, and cutaneous branches to the arm and forearm. After winding around the humerus, the nerve pierces the lateral intermuscular septum from behind, at the junction of the middle and lower-third of the arm. In the distal-third of the arm it comes to lie in the anterior compartment, between the brachialis muscle on the medial side and brachioradialis and extensor carpi radialis longus on the lateral side.

Before it crosses the elbow in front of the lateral condyle, it divides into two branches—superficial and deep. The *superficial branch* is primarily sensory and travels along side the radial artery into the forearm. The *deep branch* is primarily motor. It gives branches to the extensor carpi radialis brevis and the supinator. It then pierces the supinator and emerges in the posterior compartment of the forearm to become the *posterior interosseous nerve*, which divides immediately into branches supplying the extensor muscles of the forearm. Branches of the radial nerve are as given in Table 10.3.

Tests: Various muscles supplied by the radial nerve will be affected according to the level of radial nerve injury, i.e., high or low.
a. **High radial nerve palsy:** This occurs if the nerve is injured in the radial groove. In this type, all

the muscles supplied by radial nerve except the triceps and anconeus are paralysed. Occasionally, the radial nerve may be injured still higher up, in which case even the triceps may be paralysed. This is called very high radial nerve palsy.
b. **Low radial nerve palsy:** This occurs if the nerve is injured around the elbow so that the muscles supplied by the radial nerve in the distal arm (brachioradialis, extensor carpi radialis longus and brevis) are spared.

From proximal to distal, the following muscles can be examined:
- *Triceps:* The patient is asked to extend his elbow against resistance applied by the examiner, whose other hand feels for triceps contraction.
- *Brachioradialis:* The patient is asked to flex the elbow from 90° onwards, keeping the forearm midprone. As he does so against resistance, the brachioradialis stands out, and can be felt.
- *Wrist extensors:* The patient with paralysed wrist extensors has 'wrist drop'. In case the paralysis is partial, the contraction of the extensor carpi radialis and extensor carpi ulnaris muscle can be felt, though actual movement may not occur.
- *Extensor digitorum*: It causes extension at the metacarpo-phalangeal joints. The patient cannot do so if it is paralysed (finger drop). The examiner should not be misled by the ability of the patient to 'extend the fingers' at the interphalangeal joints (function performed by the lumbricals).
- *Extensor pollicis longus*: This causes extension at the inter-phalangeal joint of the thumb. It is examined by stabilising the metacarpophalangeal joint of the thumb, while the patient is asked to extend the interphalangeal joint.

MEDIAN NERVE

Anatomy: This nerve is formed by the joining of branches from the lateral and medial cords of brachial plexus. In the arm, the median nerve descends adjacent to the brachial artery.

Course in the forearm: The nerve enters the forearm between the two heads of the pronator teres. It then passes deep to the tendinous bridge of the origin of the flexor digitorum superficialis, in the proximal-third of the forearm. In the mid-forearm it descends between the flexor digitorum superficialis and flexor digitorum profundus. About 5 cm above the wrist, it comes to lie on the lateral side of the flexor digitorum superficialis. It becomes superficial just above the wrist, where it lies between the tendons of the flexor digitorum superficialis and flexor carpi radialis.

Table 10.3: Major motor branches of radial nerve.	
Before the radial groove	Long and medial heads of triceps
After the radial groove, before crossing the elbow	Lateral head of triceps, anconeus, brachioradialis, extensor carpi, radialis longus
After crossing the elbow, before piercing the supinator	Extensor carpi radialis brevis, the supinator
After piercing the supinator	Other extensor muscles of the forearm and hand

Course in the hand: The nerve passes deep to the flexor retinaculum and enters the palm. Here a short and stout muscular branch from it supplies the muscles of the thenar eminence (abductor pollicis brevis, opponens pollicis and flexor pollicis brevis). The median nerve finally divides into 4 to 5 palmar digital branches supplying the area of skin shown in Figure 10.2. Also, motor branches are given to the first and second lumbrical muscles at this level. The nerve supply to various muscles by the median nerve along its course is given in Table 10.4.

Table 10.4: Major motor branches of the median nerve.	
In the arm	Nil

In the forearm
   Proximal
   Distal
	All the flexor muscles of the forearm, *except* the flexor carpi ulnaris and medial-half of the flexor digitorum profundus
	Nil

In the hand	Thenar muscles* (three) First two lumbricals

*The three muscles are flexor pollicis brevis, opponens pollicis and abductor pollicis. Adductor pollicis is not supplied by median nerve.

Tests: The various muscles supplied by the median nerve will be affected according to the level of median nerve injury, i.e., high or low.

a. *High median nerve palsy (injury proximal to the elbow):* This will cause paralysis of all the muscles supplied by the median nerve in the forearm and hand. In addition, there will be sensory deficit in the skin of the hand.

b. *Low median nerve palsy (injury in the distal-third of the forearm):* There will be sparing of the forearm muscles, but the muscles of the hand will be paralysed. In addition, there will be anaesthesia over the median nerve distribution in the hand.

From proximal to distal, the following muscles can be examined:

- *Flexor pollicis longus:* The patient is asked to flex the terminal phalanx of the thumb against resistance while the proximal phalanx is kept steady by the examiner.

- *Flexor digitorum superficialis and lateral half of flexor digitorum profundus:* If the patient is asked to clasp his hand, the index finger will remain straight, the so-called 'pointing index'. This occurs because both the finger flexors, superficialis as well as the profundus of the index finger are paralysed; though the available medial-half of the flexor digitorum profundus (supplied by the ulnar nerve) makes flexion of the other fingers possible.

- *Flexor carpi radialis:* Normally, the palmar flexion at the wrist occurs in the long axis of the forearm. In a patient with paralysed flexor carpi radialis, the wrist deviates to the ulnar side while palmar flexion occurs. In addition, one cannot feel the tendon of the flexor carpi radialis getting taut.

- *Muscles of the thenar eminence:* Out of the three muscles of the thenar eminence, only two can be examined for their isolated action. These are as follows: (i) abductor pollicis brevis (Fig. 10.5): The action of this muscle is to draw the thumb forwards at right angle to the palm. The patient is asked to lay his hand flat on the table with palm facing the ceiling. A pen is held above the thumb and the patient is asked to touch the pen with tip of his thumb. This is called the '*pentest*'; (ii) opponens pollicis: The function of this muscle is to appose the tip of the thumb to other fingers. Apposition is a swinging movement of the thumb across the palm and not a simple adduction. The latter movement is by the adductor pollicis muscle supplied by the ulnar nerve.

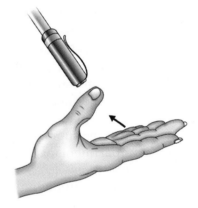

Fig. 10.5: The pen test.

ULNAR NERVE

Anatomy: This nerve arises from the medial cord of the brachial plexus. In the arm, it lies on the medial side of the axillary artery. At the junction of the middle and lower-third of the arm, it pierces the medial intermuscular septum and comes to lie in the posterior compartment. It becomes more and more superficial as it approaches the elbow, where it lies behind the medial epicondyle.

Course in the forearm: The ulnar nerve enters the forearm between the two heads of the flexor carpi ulnaris, and descends along the medial side of the forearm. Here it lies anterior to the flexor digitorum profundus, along with the ulnar vessels.

Course at the wrist: It passes in front of the flexor retinaculum just lateral to the pisiform bone. On entering the palm, the ulnar nerve finally divides into superficial and deep terminal branches supplying the hand muscles. The nerve supply to various muscles by the ulnar nerve along its course are given in Table 10.5.

Table 10.5: Major motor branches of the ulnar nerve.	
In the arm	Nil
In the forearm Proximal Distal 1/3	Flexor carpi ulnaris, medial half of flexor digitorum profundus Nil
In the hand Superficial branch Deep branch	Hypothenar muscles Adductor pollicis, all interossei and medial two lumbricals

Tests: Various muscles supplied by ulnar nerve will be affected according to the level of ulnar nerve injury, i.e., high or low.

a. *High ulnar nerve palsy* (injury proximal to the elbow): This will cause paralysis of all the muscles supplied by the ulnar nerve in the forearm and hand. In addition, there will be a sensory deficit in the skin of the hand.

b. *Low ulnar nerve palsy* (injury in distal-third of forearm): There will be sparing of forearm muscles but the muscles of the hand will be paralysed. Sensory deficit will be same as in high ulnar nerve palsy.

Individual muscles which could be examined in a case of ulnar nerve palsy are given below:

- *Flexor carpi ulnaris:* The patient is asked to palmar flex the wrist against gravity. In doing so, the hand deviates towards the radial side. The tendon of flexor carpi ulnaris just above the pisiform, does not stand out. On performing the same test against resistance, the tendon cannot be felt.

- *Abductor digiti minimi:* The patient is asked to abduct the little finger against resistance while keeping the hand flat on the table (in order to avoid action of flexors of the finger).
- *Interossei:* Palmar interossei do adduction (PAD), the dorsal interossei do abduction (DAB) of the fingers at metacarpo-phalangeal joints. These can be tested as follows:
  - Egawa's test (Fig. 10.6A): This is for dorsal interossei (abductors) of the middle finger. With the hand kept flat on a table palmar surface down, the patient is asked to move his middle finger sideways.
  - Card test (Fig. 10.6B): This is for palmar interossei (adductors) of the fingers. In this test, the examiner inserts a card between two extended fingers and the patient is asked to hold it as tightly as possible while the examiner tries to pull the card out. The power of adductors can thus be judged. In case of weak palmar interossei, it is easy to pull out the card. First dorsal interosseous muscle can be separately examined by asking the patient to abduct the index finger against resistance (Fig. 10.6C).
- *The lumbricals:* These are mainly responsible for flexion at the metacarpophalangeal joints but their isolated action cannot be tested.
- *Adductor pollicis:* The patient is asked to grasp a book between the thumb and index finger. Normally, a person will grasp the book firmly with thumb extended, taking full advantage of the adductor pollicis and the first dorsal interosseous muscles. If the ulnar nerve is injured, the adductor pollicis will be paralysed and the patient will hold the book by using the flexor pollicis longus (supplied by median nerve) in place of the adductor. This produces flexion at the interphalangeal joint of the

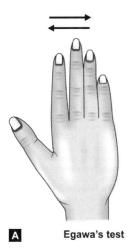

A Egawa's test

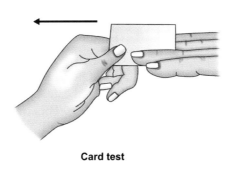

Card test

B

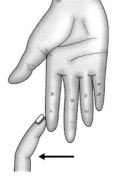

C Test for 1st dorsal interosseous

Fig. 10.6: Tests for ulnar nerve.

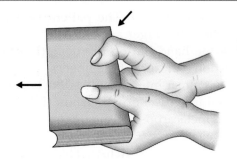

Fig. 10.7: Froment's sign (book test).

thumb (Fig. 10.7). This becomes more pronounced if the examiner tries to pull the book out while the patient tries to hold it. This sign is known as 'Froment's sign' or the 'book test.'

ACCESSORY NERVE

This supplies the trapezius muscle.

Test: The trapezius muscle is tested by asking the patient to elevate his shoulder against resistance. One can see and feel the trapezius belly stand out. Similarly, the patient is asked to brace his shoulder backward and depress it to examine middle and lower part of the muscle.

LONG THORACIC NERVE

Anatomy: The nerve arises from the ventral rami of C_5, C_6 and C_7. It descends behind the brachial plexus on the lateral surface of the serratus anterior, which it supplies.

Test: The serratus anterior muscle can be examined by asking the patient to push against a wall with both hands. The medial border of the scapula on the affected side will become prominent (*winging of scapula*, Fig. 10.8).

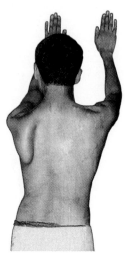

Fig. 10.8: Winging of the scapula.

AXILLARY NERVE

Anatomy: The axillary nerve arises from the posterior cord of the brachial plexus and curves backwards on the lower border of the subscapularis. It crosses the quadrangular space and comes to lie on the medial side of the surgical neck of the humerus, medial and inferior to the capsule of the shoulder joint. Here it divides into anterior and posterior branches. The posterior branch supplies the teres minor and posterior part of the deltoid and terminates as the cutaneous nerve which supplies the skin over the lower-half of the deltoid. The anterior branch continues horizontally between the deltoid and the surgical neck of the humerus, and supplies the rest of the deltoid.

Test: The surgeon stabilises the scapula with one hand while the other hand is kept on the deltoid to feel for its contraction. The patient is asked to abduct his shoulder. Inability to abduct the shoulder, and the absence of the deltoid becoming taut indicates deltoid paralysis.

SCIATIC NERVE

Anatomy: The sciatic nerve consists of two anatomically distinct components - the tibial and common peroneal nerves. The common peroneal component is more frequently affected than the tibial. Complete lesion of the sciatic nerve is rare.

Tests: The common peroneal nerve supplies the extensors and the evertors of the foot. Paralysis of these muscles results in foot drop. The patient walks with a 'high-step gait', i.e., while walking he has to lift the foot high in order to clear the ground. The plantar flexors of the foot are normal.

The tibial nerve supplies the plantar flexors of the foot. One can test for weakness of these muscles by asking the patient to plantar-flex the ankle and toes. The function of the hamstring group of muscles, also supplied by the sciatic nerve, can be tested by flexing the knee against resistance.

THE CAUSES OF INJURY

Once it is decided on clinical examination, which nerve is affected and at what level, one must look for a tell tale signs along the course of the nerve for the cause. This may be in the form of an injury such as displaced bone fragments or a scar to suggest an old external injury. The nerve may be thickened (e.g., leprosy). If no such exteral evidence is present, the paralysis could be due to some medical cause such as neuropathy, myelopathy, etc. (Refer to a Textbook of Medicine).

THE TYPE OF INJURY

Once the cause of nerve injury is established, one must make an attempt to evaluate the predominant type of nerve injury (Seddon's classification). The nature of the causative factor, a period of observation and electrodiagnostic studies may help in deciding this.

SIGNS OF REGENERATION

Whenever a case of nerve injury is seen some time after the injury or following a repair, signs of regeneration of the nerve should be looked for during examination. These are as follows:

• *Tinel's sign:* On gently tapping over the nerve along its course, from *distal to proximal,* a pins and needle sensation is felt in the area of the skin supplied by the nerve. A distal progression of the level at which this occurs, suggests regeneration.

• *Motor examination:* The muscle supplied nearest to the site of injury is the first to recover, noticed clinically by the ability of the muscle to contract. The muscles in the more distal area begin to contract as they are reinnervated one after another (motor march). This phenomenon is absent in neuropraxia where all muscles recover together.

• *Electrodiagnostic test:* This can help in predicting nerve recovery even before it is apparent clinically.

ELECTRODIAGNOSTIC STUDIES

Electromyography: Electromyography (EMG) is a graphic recording of the electrical activity of a muscle at rest and during activity.

Normal muscle: A normal muscle at rest shows no electrical activity. With voluntary contraction, action potentials develop in the motor units. In a weak contraction, these may be recordable as single motor unit potentials in the vicinity of the recording electrode. In a strong contraction, impulses of a number of motor units firing simultaneously are superimposed, giving rise to an *interference pattern* (Fig. 10.9)

Denervated muscle: The denervated muscle has spontaneous electrical activity at rest. This is called *denervation potentials.* These potentials represent the embryonic electrical activity of a muscle, which is normally suppressed by stronger nerve action potentials. These appear at around 15-20 days after the muscle denervation. As nerve degeneration progresses, more and more denervation potentials appear. If these potentials have not appeared by the end of the 2nd week after a nerve injury, it is a good prognostic sign.

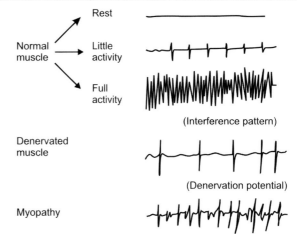

Fig. 10.9: Electromyography.

Electromyography is useful in deciding the following:

a. *Whether or not a nerve injury is present:* It helps in differentiating a muscle paralysis because of nerve injury from that due to other causes such as myopathy.

b. *Whether it is a complete or incomplete nerve injury:* If the nerve supply of a muscle is partially cut, there will be evidence of residual innervation of the muscles. This may be too small to produce any clinically detectable muscle contraction, but can be picked up on the EMG. Also, if a group of muscles supplied by a nerve do not show signs of denervation, it indicates a preserved nerve supply to these muscles, hence an incomplete nerve injury.

c. *Whether any regeneration occurring:* The earliest evidence of reinnervation of a muscle is the appearance of reinnervation potentials on attempted voluntary contraction of the muscle. These potentials appear weeks before a contraction can be noticed clinically. The progress of a nerve recovery can thus be monitored.

d. *Level of nerve injury:* By performing an EMG of all the muscle supplied by a nerve, one can decide the level of nerve injury. Muscles supplied distal to the site of nerve injury would show changes of denervation.

Strength-duration curve: This is a graphic representation of the excitability of muscle and nerve tissue under test. A small strength of current can excite a normal muscle. This occurs by excitation of the muscle through neuromuscular junction, which needs a weaker current. In a denervated muscle, the excitation is possible only on direct stimulation of the muscle fibres, which need a higher strength of current.

A very low-strength current is given for a duration of 300 milliseconds and its response noted. The strength of the current is gradually increased until a minimal visible contraction of the muscle is observed. This minimal current strength, required to elicit muscle contraction, is called the *Rheobase*, and is measured in milliamperes. The *Chronaxie* is the duration of current required to excite a muscle with a current-strength of double the rheobase. It is measured in milliseconds. These two are the basic parameters of excitability of a muscle.

For knowing excitability of a muscle in relation to current-strength and its duration, the muscle is stimulated by reducing the duration of the current from 300 milliseconds, gradually to a 1 millisecond or even lower. A corresponding increase in strength of the current required is detected. A graph is plotted between current-duration and corresponding current-strength. This is called a strength-duration curve (Fig. 10.10).

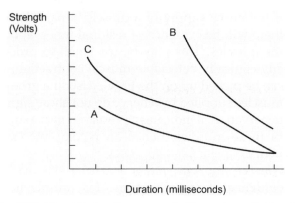

Fig. 10.10: Strength-duration curve: A. Nerve curve, B. Muscle curve, C. Partial denervation.

Interpretation: The pattern of the strength-duration curve of an innervated muscle is different from that of a denervated muscle or regenerating muscle, as discussed below:

- *Normal strength-duration curve:* A normal muscle will respond to stimuli varying in duration from 300 milliseconds to as low as 3 or even 1 millisecond without any increase in the strength of the current. If the duration of current is decreased beyond it, a progressive increase in the strength of current is required in order to produce a contraction. A strength-duration curve plotted from such a muscle is termed a *nerve curve*, because the muscle contraction is caused by stimulation of the motor nerve entering the muscle.
- *Denervated muscle:* A totally denervated muscle will need current either of more strength or for

a longer duration. A curve from such a muscle is termed a *muscle curve*.

- *A partially denervated muscle:* The curve of a partially denervated muscle or a muscle recovering after nerve injury lies between the normal and the curve of denervation, and is characterised by an upward kink. The kink denotes the superimposition of the two basic types of curves.
- *Assessment of recovery by the strength-duration curve:* If progressive recovery is occurring the curve will, on serial examination, become flatter with a shift to the left. On the other hand, if the process of denervation is progressive, the curve will become steeper and will shift to the right.

Nerve conduction studies: It is a measure of the velocity of conduction of impulse in a nerve. A stimulating electrode is applied over a point on the nerve trunk and the response is picked up by an electrode at a distance or directly over the muscle. The velocity of the conduction of the impulse between any two points of the nerve can be calculated. The normal nerve conduction velocity of motor nerve is 70 metres/second. This conduction study helps in the following:

a. *Whether a nerve injury is present:* If a nerve injury is present there will be no conduction of the impulse across the suspected level.
b. *Whether it is a complete or partial nerve injury:* Absence of any transmitted impulse across the suspected site is an indicator of a complete nerve injury.
c. *Compressive lesion:* The conduction velocity may simply be delayed in compressive nerve lesions such as carpal tunnel syndrome, etc.

TREATMENT

General consideration: In fresh nerve injuries, the general condition of the patient must be evaluated before undertaking a nerve repair. Arterial, bone and joint repair takes precedence over nerve repair. The treatment of nerve injuries may be conservative or operative. Though conservative treatment yields good results, in selected cases an operation should not be delayed in the hope of spontaneous recovery.

CONSERVATIVE TREATMENT

This alone or in addition to operative treatment is required in all types of nerve injuries. The aim of conservative treatment is to preserve the mobility of the affected limb while the nerve recovers.

The following are the essential components of conservative treatment:

- *Splintage of the paralysed limb*: The first procedure to be adopted in every case of nerve injury is to

Table 10.6: Splints used for various nerve injuries.	
Nerve injured	**Splint**
Axillary nerve (deltoid paralysis)	Aeroplane splint
Radial nerve palsy (extensors of wrist and MP joints paralysed)	Cock-up splint
Ulnar nerve palsy (lumbricals paralysis)	Knuckle-bender splint
Sciatic nerve palsy or common peroneal nerve palsy	Foot drop splint

splint the limb in the position which will most effectively relax the affected muscles. The type of splints used for common nerve injuries are as given in Table 10.6.

- *Preserve mobility of the joints*: Every joint of the affected limb must be put through full range of movement at least once every day.
- *Care of the skin and nails*: Since the skin is anaesthetic, it should be protected from trauma, burn or pressure sores. Trophic ulcers should be meticulously treated. Nails should be cleaned and cut with care.
- *Physiotherapy*: Physiotherapeutic measures consist of: (i) massage of the paralysed muscles; (ii) passive exercises to the limb; (iii) building up of the recovering muscles; and (iv) developing the unaffected or partially affected muscles. Attempts were made in the past to preserve tone and functions of denervated muscles by electrical stimulation, but it has been found to be of no use.
- *Relief of pain*: Suitable analgesics are prescribed for relief of pain.

OPERATIVE TREATMENT

Operative procedures for nerve injuries consist of nerve repair, neurolysis, and tendon transfers.

Nerve repair: It may be performed within a few days of injury (primary repair) or later (secondary repair).

Primary repair: It is indicated when the nerve is cut by a sharp object, and the patient reports early. In such cases an immediate primary repair is the best. One needs experience in the use of the fine sutures and operative microscope for this kind of surgery. In case the wound is contaminated or the patient reports late, a delayed primary repair is better. In this, in the first stage, the wound is debrided and the two nerve ends approximated with one or two fine silk sutures so as to prevent retraction of the cut ends. This also makes identification of the cut ends easy at a later date. After

two weeks, once the wound heals, a definitive repair is done. Some surgeons routinely perform a delayed primary repair because they feel that the epineurium gets thickened in two weeks and sutures hold better.

Secondary repair: It is indicated for the following cases:
a. *Nerve lesions presenting some time after injury*: Often nerve injuries are missed at the time of injury, or it may not have been possible to treat them early for reason, such as poor general condition of the patient.
b. *Syndrome of incomplete interruption*: If no definite improvement occurs in 6 weeks in cases with an apparently incomplete nerve injury, nerve exploration, and if required secondary repair should be carried out.
c. *Syndrome of irritation*: Cases with signs of nerve irritation need exploration and sometimes a secondary repair.
d. *Failure of conservative treatment*: If a nerve injury is treated conservatively and no improvement occurs within 3 weeks, one should proceed to electrodiagnostic studies, and if required, nerve exploration.

Techniques of nerve repair: Nerve repair can be either end-to-end or by using a nerve graft.
a. *Nerve suture:* When the nerve ends can be brought close to each other, they may be sutured by one of the following techniques (Fig. 10.11):
   - Epineural suture
   - Epi-perineural suture
   - Perineural suture
   - Group fascicular repair

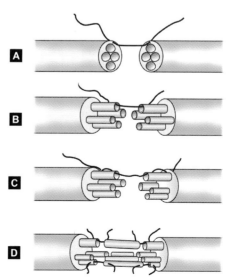

Fig. 10.11: Techniques of nerve repair: (A) Epineural; (B) Perineural; (C) Epi-perineural; (D) Nerve grafting.

Methods of closing nerve gaps: Sometimes, the loss of nerve tissue is so much, that an end-to-end suture cannot be obtained. In such a situation, the following measures are adopted to gain length and achieve an end-to-end suture:

- Mobilisation of the nerve on both sides of the lesion.
- Relaxation of the nerve by temporarily positioning the joints in a favourable position.
- Alteration of the course of the nerve, e.g., the ulnar nerve may be brought in front of the medial epicondyle (*anterior transposition*).
- Stripping the branches from the parent nerve without tearing them.
- Sacrificing some unimportant branch if it is hampering nerve mobilisation.

b. *Nerve grafting:* When the nerve gap is more than 10 cm or end-to-end suture is likely to result in tension at the suture line, nerve grafting may be done. In this, an expandable nerve (the sural nerve) is taken and sutured between two ends of the original nerve as shown in Figure 10.11D.

Neurolysis: This term is applied to the operation where the nerve is freed from enveloping scar (perineural fibrosis). This is called external neurolysis. In many cases, the nerve sheath may be dissected longitudinally to relieve the pressure from the fibrous tissue within the nerve (intraneural fibrosis). This is called internal neurolysis.

Reconstructive surgery: These are operations performed when there is no hope of the recovery of a nerve, usually after 18 months of injury. After this time even if the nerve recovers, transmission of impulses across the neuromuscular junction does not occur because the neuromuscular function itself has degenerated. Operations included in this group are tendon transfers, arthrodesis and muscle transfer. Rarely, an amputation may be justified for an anaesthetic limb or the one with causalgia.

DECISION MAKING IN NERVE INJURIES

It is often difficult to decide when to operate in a case of nerve injury. This is especially so if there is a partial lesion or partial recovery has taken place. Electrodiagnostic studies are helpful in these cases.

Unless the nature of the nerve injury is known before the operation, the appearance of the involved nerve is often the best guide to deciding on the type of operative procedure. Where the nerve ends are visibly apart, nerve repair is the only choice. Where the nerve is in continuity, it is often difficult to decide the further course. A fusiform thickening of a nerve (neuroma in continuity) indicates a partial cut. A nerve stimulator may be used to find if there is any continuity of the nerve. If there is a brisk response in the muscles supplied by the nerve on stimulating the nerve proximal to the neuroma, there is no need for nerve suture; neurolysis may suffice. In case there is little or no response, the neuroma should be excised and the nerve repaired.

A practical plan for management of nerve injury is shown in Flowchart 10.1.

PROGNOSIS

The following factors dictate recovery following a nerve repair:

a. **Age:** The lower the age, the better the prognosis.
b. **Tension at the suture line:** The more the tension, the poorer the prognosis.
c. **Time since injury:** After 18 months only sensory functions can be expected.
d. **Location of injury:** The more proximal the injury, the worse the prognosis.
e. **Type of nerve:** A primarily motor nerve, like radial nerve, has a better prognosis than a mixed nerve.
f. **Condition of the nerve ends:** The more the crushing and infection, the poorer the prognosis.
g. **Associated conditions:** Infection, ischaemia, etc. indicate poor prognosis.

Flowchart 10.1: Treatment plan for management of peripheral nerve injury.

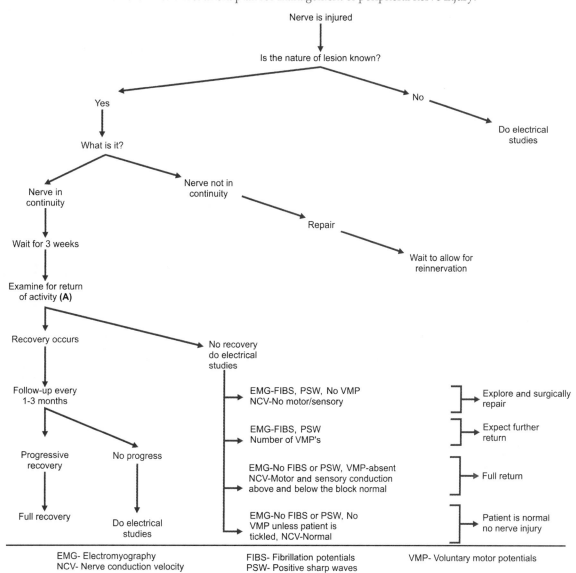

EMG- Electromyography
NCV- Nerve conduction velocity

FIBS- Fibrillation potentials
PSW- Positive sharp waves

VMP- Voluntary motor potentials

What have we learnt?

- There are three types of nerve injuries: Neurapraxia, Axonotmesis, Neurotmesis.
- Nerve recovers at the rate of 1 mm/day.
- How to diagnose a nerve injury, clinical signs and their explanation.
- How to monitor nerve regeneration, and role of electrodiagnostic studies.
- Methods of nerve repair.
- Decision making in nerve injury.
- How to predict whether a nerve will recover or not?

Additional information: From the entrance exams point of view

- Tinel's sign indicates regeneration of nerves.
- Prognosis after nerve suturing: radial nerve > ulnar nerve > peroneal nerve> sciatic nerve> femoral nerve.
- Erb's palsy is the most common neurological deficit in the upper limb.
- Erb's palsy is injury to upper C5, 6 roots of brachial plexus.
- Klumpke's palsy is injury to the lower trunk C8 and partially T1.
- Crutch palsy is injury to the radial nerve.
- Claw hand due to leprosy is classified as Grade II WHO grading.
- Sudden hyperflexion of the thigh over the abdomen (McRobert's procedure) done on the mother for delivery of babies with shoulder dystocia leads to injury to the lateral cutaneous nerve of thigh (meralgia paresthetica).

Deformities and Their Management

Learning Objectives

❖ Discuss causes of deformities and principles and techniques of deformity correction.

CAUSES

Deformities may arise from an abnormality in the bone (e.g., a malunited fracture), joint (e.g., tuberculosis of the knee), or soft tissues (e.g., clubfoot). These may be either congenital or acquired.

CONGENITAL DEFORMITIES

These are deformities or malformations present at birth (e.g., clubfoot). Some of these malformations, though present at birth, may become apparent only later in life (e.g., spina bifida). The deformity may be severe and incompatible with life (e.g., osteogenesis imperfecta congenita), and can only be found in stillborn infants. On the other hand, it may be very minor and have no practical significance.

The underlying causative factors may be: (i) a genetic abnormality (e.g., diaphyseal aclasis, mongolism, etc.); (ii) environmental factors (e.g., phocomelia); and (iii) combined—genetic and environmental factors (e.g., congenital dislocation of the hip, clubfoot).

ACQUIRED DEFORMITIES

Deformities acquired later in life may be divided into those arising at a joint or in a bone (Fig. 11.1), as discussed below:

Deformities arising at a joint: A joint may become deformed because of any of the following factors:

a. *Dislocations and subluxations:* These may be traumatic (e.g., most dislocations and subluxations

seen in day-to-day practice) or pathological (e.g., following acute septic arthritis). Classic deformities are produced in some subluxation or dislocation (Table 8.2, page 56).

b. *Muscle imbalance:* All joints are spanned by two opposing groups of muscles. Normally, these muscles maintain a balance so that the joint can be kept in any position. In some diseases, an unbalanced action of the muscles may hold the joint in a particular position. With time the other soft tissues around the joint (the capsule, ligaments, etc.) also contract and prevent the joint from returning to its neutral position. The muscle imbalance may arise from paralysis of a group (e.g., polio) or overactivity (e.g., spasticity in cerebral palsy).

c. *Tethering or contracture of muscles and tendons:* Joint movement is associated with contraction of a group of muscles and elongation of opposing group. To and fro gliding of tendons also happens in this process. If by some disease, these functions are interrupted, the joint is prevented from moving full range. For example, the muscles or tendons, may get tethered to the underlying bone (e.g., tethering of the quadriceps to the femur in a fracture). The muscle may get contracture (e.g., Volkmann's ischaemic contracture of the flexor muscles of forearm, leading to flexion deformity of the wrist and fingers).

d. *Contracture of soft tissues other than muscles:* Apart from muscles, contracture of other soft-tissues like skin, deep fascia, etc., may account for the deformity. For example, contracture of palmar aponeurosis may pull the metacarpophalangeal and *proximal* interphalangeal joints of one or more fingers (Dupuytren's contracture). Similarly, contracture of the scarred skin on the flexor aspect of the elbow or knee following a burn, may result in a flexion deformity of the respective joint.

e. *Arthritis:* Joint deformity may result from arthritis. This may occur: (i) because of sustained spasm of a group of muscles in response to pain; or (ii) as a result of damage to important structures like ligaments, cartilage, etc., by the arthritic process.

f. *Posture:* The habitual keeping of a joint in a deformed position may result in a deformity, for example, lateral deviation of the great toe (hallux valgus) is seen in women who wear narrow pointed high-heeled shoes.

g. *Unknown factors:* Some deformities of joints result from no apparent reason. For example, knock-knees deformity (genu valgum) commonly seen in children, often has no cause.

Deformities arising in a bone: Three major causes of deformity arising in a bone are fractures, bone diseases and abnormally growing bones.

a. *Fracture:* This is the most common cause of deformity of a bone. This results when a fracture unites in a malaligned position. Some of the

Table 11.1: Deformities due to fractures.	
Deformity	**Fracture**
■ Gun stock deformity of (cubitus varus)	■ Supracondylar fracture the humerus
■ Cubitus valgus	■ Fracture of lateral condyle of humerus
■ Dinner fork deformity	■ Colles' fracture
■ Mallet finger	■ Avulsion of the extensor tendon from base of distal phalanx
■ Coxa vara	■ Intertrochanteric fracture
■ Genu valgum	■ Condylar fractures of tibia (e.g., bumper fracture)
■ Varus-valgus at ankle	■ Ankle injuries

common deformities resulting from malunion of fractures are given in Table 11.1.

b. *Bone diseases:* Some diseases of the bone result in a softening and bending of the bones. Most of these are generalised disorders where several or all of the bones are affected. The following are some examples:
   ▪ Metabolic disorders—rickets, osteomalacia.
   ▪ Endocrine disorders—parathyroid osteodystrophy, Cushing's syndrome.
   ▪ Disorder of unknown etiology—Paget's disease, fibrous dysplasia, senile osteoporosis.

c. *Abnormal bone growth:* Bone deformity may result from uneven growth occuring at the epiphyseal

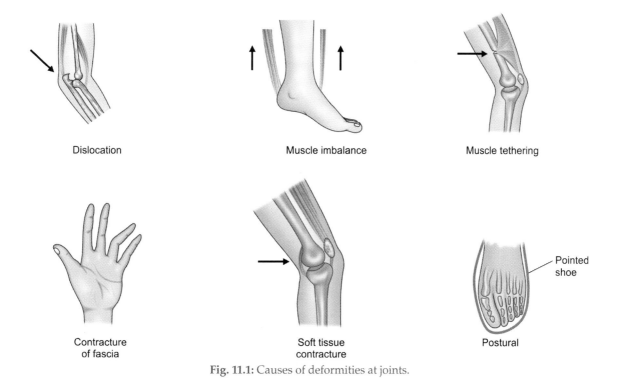

Dislocation   Muscle imbalance   Muscle tethering

Contracture of fascia   Soft tissue contracture   Postural

Fig. 11.1: Causes of deformities at joints.

plate. Unequal growth of one of the two bones in a part of the limb with two bones (e.g., forearm or leg), may result in deformity at the joint adjacent (e.g., wrist or ankle). The common causes of uneven growth at the epiphyseal plate are as follows:

- Crushing fracture involving the epiphyseal plate (Grade-V, Salter and Harris epiphyseal injury).
- Infection from a nearby osteomyelitis or arthritis, spreading to the epiphyseal plate, and damaging it.
- A tumour may retard the growth of a nearby epiphyseal plate (e.g., enchondroma as in Ollier's disease). Occasionally, the tumour may stimulate uneven growth of the adjacent plate by causing local hyperaemia (e.g., haemangioma).
- Dysplasia: In some epiphyseal dysplasias, abnormal growth at the epiphysis results in joint deformities.

TREATMENT

Many deformities do not need treatment, as they are of no significant functional or cosmetic concern. A simple reassurance and watchful neglect may be appropriate in these cases. Most other deformities cause functional impediment or cosmetic concerns, and have to be corrected. Some deformities (e.g., bow legs), may not be of immediate functional concern, but may cause problem in long-term, and thus may need to be corrected. The methods used for correction of deformities may be non-operative or operative.

NON-OPERATIVE METHODS

Wherever possible, non-operative methods are attempted first. These are suitable for deformities due to soft tissue contracture. The method essentially consists of stretching the contracted soft tissue, and then maintaining the correction by splints. The disadvantage of this method is that the treatment is long drawn, and an equally prolonged effort at maintenance is required. Recurrence of deformity is common. Correction of deformity by non-operative methods is done by the following ways:

a. **Manipulative correction:** The contracture is gently manipulated, so as to stretch it. Once corrected, it is maintained in the corrected position in a plaster cast or splint. An example of use of this method is treatment of a club foot by manipulation and PoP.

b. **Wedging cast:** In this technique, a cast is applied on the limb with deformed joint. A wedge of plaster is cut out on the convex side of the deformity, the wedge closed by forcing the part, thus achieving correction.

c. **Traction:** Gradual traction can stretch out contracted soft tissues. The correction is subsequently maintained in a splint or calipers.

d. **Splints:** These are special splints which permit gradual stretching of the soft tissues, leading to the correction of deformities (e.g., turn-buckle splint for VIC, see page 99).

OPERATIVE METHODS

In cases where the non-operative methods fail or the deformity is primarily bony, operative correction may be required. The following methods are used:

a. **Soft tissue release:** The contracted soft tissues are released. Tethering of soft tissues is removed.

b. **Osteotomy (Fig. 11.2):** It is used for correcting bony deformity. The deformed bone is cut and suitably realigned in a corrected position (e.g., for genu varum and genu valgum).

c. **Arthrodesis (fusion of joint):** This method is adopted where a joint is not only deformed, but also its articulating surfaces damaged beyond repair. Arthrodesis is suitable for joints where loss of motion at the joint does not produce

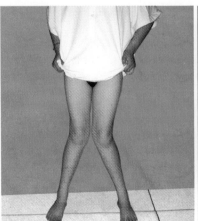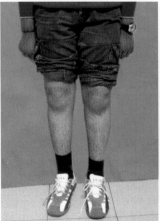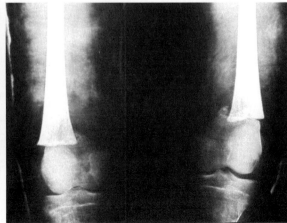

Fig. 11.2: A child with bilateral genu valgum corrected by supracondylar osteotomy on both the sides.

Flowchart 11.1: Plan of management of a deformed joint.

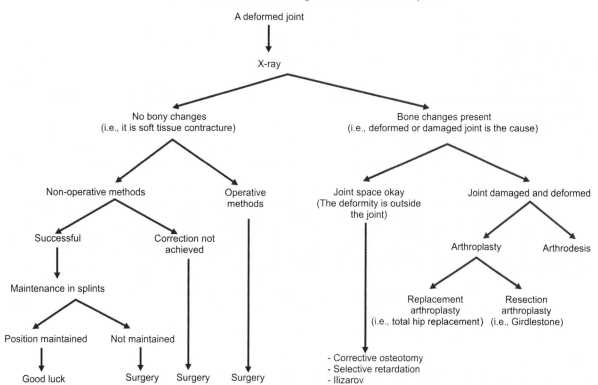

much functional disability (e.g., wrist). In other situations, such as hip and knee, joint replacement is a better option. With the availability and better longevity of artificial joints, arthrodesis has become less popular. There are situations where joint replacement cannot be done (e.g., joint infection, paralysed limb), and arthrodesis remains the only option. The procedure involves opening up the joint, removing its cartilage, and immobilizing it in functional position. The raw bone ends unite (as in a fracture), resulting in fusion.

d. **Arthroplasty:** The term arthroplasty means 'reconstructing a joint'. Reconstruction can be done by two methods: (i) by excising a part of the deformed joint, thereby relaxing the surrounding soft tissues, and thus correcting deformity or (ii) by replacing the joint with artificial components. The former is called *excision arthroplasty*, and is done for joints damaged due to infection. The latter is called *replacement arthroplasty* (joint replacement), and is done for most other damaged and deformed joints (e.g., osteoarthritis knee). See also Chapter 42.

Correction of deformity by selective retardation of epiphyseal growth (growth modulation): This is useful in cases where the cause of deformity is unequal epiphyseal growth, and the child has residual growth potential. Here, the faster growing side of the epiphysis is temporarily or permanently stopped by surgical means (stapling, direct damage, etc.). Over a period of time, the slower growing side keeps growing, while the stapled side does not, resulting in correction of the deformity. This is performed in selected cases of genu varum or valgum in a growing child. It is a minimally invasive operation, but a little unpredictable.

Ilizarov's technique: This is a versatile technique of correcting deformity. Its utility is more when the deformity is associated with shortening, or if the deformity is in more than one plane. The apparatus provides an opportunity for correcting the deformity very accurately (see also page 35). A comprehensive plan of management of a deformed joint is given in Flowchart 11.1.

What have we learnt?

- Deformities may be since birth, or develop later.
- The cause of deformity may be bone (e.g., malunion), joint (e.g., OA knee), or soft tissue contracture (e.g., Volkmann's contracture).
- Initial treatment of deformity is by non-operative methods, and thereafter operative methods.
- Different operative methods of correction of deformity exist.

Treatment of Orthopaedic Disorders: A General Review

Competency
❖ **OR2.3:** Select, prescribe and communicate appropriate medications for relief of joint pain.

Orthopaedic treatment can be broadly divided into two types: non-operative (conservative) or operative. A lot of times a patient needs no definite treatment except reassurance. One interesting paradigm in *orthopaedics is that it is a functional speciality, and outcome has to be in alignment with functional requirement of the patient.* As functional requirements vary from person to person, the treatment of the same problem will also vary from person to person. For example, treatment of a wrist fracture in a tennis player will be different from that in a housewife. Broadly speaking, it is preferable to try non-operative methods first, though there are occasions when early or an immediate operation must be advised.

NON-OPERATIVE METHODS OF TREATMENT

REST

Since olden times, rest has been the mainstay of orthopaedic treatment. It helps in reducing inflammation and pain. The word 'rest' could mean complete inactivity or immobility of the affected part, as is sometimes required in acute inflammatory conditions such as acute osteomyelitis. But, more often than not, rest may mean only 'relative rest', implying, simply a reduction of activity and avoidance of strain. This is called 'functional treatment', meaning, treatment going on without affecting the working

of the part much. This has been possible due to advances in orthopaedic treatment, whereby more and more methods have been devised by which the period of rest could be reduced significantly. Some of these advances are in the field of bracing and surgical fixation of fractures.

SUPPORT

A limb or a joint not capable of functioning because of inadequate muscle power needs support (e.g., a polio limb). Temporary support may be given with a splint made from Plaster of Paris or other plastic splinting material. Use of a walking aid such as a stick is a form of support to damaged part. A permanent or prolonged support may be required in some cases (e.g., polio), in the form of life-time appliances called *orthoses* (see page 323).

PHYSIOTHERAPY

This includes a variety of treatment modalities based on physical methods of treatment such as heat therapy, exercises, etc. It may be aimed at alleviation of pain, restoration of functions, or both. It may be used as a primary treatment modality (e.g., for backache, etc.) or in conjunction with other methods of treatment (e.g., post-operative physiotherapy).

When appropriately prescribed and adequately pursued under the supervision of a skilled physiotherapist, it can achieve wonders. On the other hand, an unskilled physiotherapist by his overenthusiastic approach may retard rather than hasten patient's recovery. The following are the common methods used in physiotherapy:

Ice therapy: Ice therapy is beneficial during the first 24-72 hours after injury. It may be used for longer time in chronic inflammation. It causes relief in pain, reduces haematoma formation and reduces inflammation. The pain relieving effect of cold therapy is appreciated more after the application than during it.

Heat therapy: Heat produces a soothing effect on many aches and pains, probably by increasing the blood flow, or possibly by some other mechanism. It is to be done for chronic cases with pain, and act more by principle of counter-irritation.

Heat application is done for 15 to 20 minutes 2 or 3 times a day. Heat must not be applied to insensitive or ischaemic skin, and if there is underlying acute infection or neoplastic tissue. Depending upon the depth of penetration of the heat, it can be either surface heat, i.e., only the skin and subcutaneous tissues are heated, or deep heat, i.e., deeper structures are heated.

a. *Surface heat:* This can be provided by: (i) hot water bottle (rubber-bottle); (ii) warm bath; (iii) hot soaks or compresses; (iv) infra-red lamp; and (v) wax bath.

b. *Deep heat:* This can be provided by: (i) shortwave diathermy—heat generated by a high frequency alternating current (frequency 27 mega hertz or cycles/second) using a shortwave diathermy emitter; (ii) ultrasonic therapy—these waves (a million cycles/second) are projected as a beam from a transducer; and (iii) microwave. The ultrasonic waves and microwaves penetrate to a considerable depth. When the waves strike the tissues, energy is converted into heat. It is most useful for localised tender fibrous nodules.

Exercise therapy: These are given for three purposes: (i) to mobilise joints; (ii) to strengthen muscles; and (iii) to improve coordination and balance.

a. *Joint mobilising exercises:* The following exercises may be advised:
   - *Passive joint movements:* These are used to preserve joint mobility when the patient is unable to move the joint himself (e.g., when the muscles are paralysed).
   - *Active joint movements:* The patient moves his joints actively so as to gain more and more range of movement. Sometimes, a patient's active efforts may be assisted by gentle pressure from the physiotherapist.

   - *Continuous passive mobilisation (CPM):* The joint is fitted in a machine which moves the joint slowly through a predetermined arc of motion. Since the motion produced is very slow, it is tolerated by the patient in even the very early post-operative period.

b. *Muscle strengthening exercises:* These are used to preserve or improve the strength of the muscles. These may be of the following types:
   - Static or isometric exercises i.e., the muscle contracts while its length remains the same, e.g., muscle contraction while pushing a wall.
   - Dynamic or isotonic exercises, i.e., the muscle contracts and produces movement. These exercises could be: (i) active—the patient does the movements himself; (ii) active-assisted—the patient does the movement while the physiotherapist helps; or (iii) active-resisted—the patient does the movement against resistance. The last is the most effective in gaining muscle strength.

c. *Exercises to improve coordination:* These are special exercises, useful in polio and cerebral palsy patients.

Tractions: In physiotherapy, traction is applied: (i) to separate joint surfaces while giving passive movements to a joint; (ii) to obtain the relaxation of muscles which are in spasm (e.g., by giving cervical or lumbar traction); or (iii) to correct deformities by gentle continuous traction. For details please refer to Chapter 4.

Massage: This is a systematic and scientific manipulation of the skin and the underlying soft tissues which gives rise to relief of pain and the relaxation of muscles. Most massage and manipulations are soothing except for frictions which are painful, and are used to breakdown adhesions.

Hydrotherapy: The principles of buoyancy help to reduce pain by relaxation of the muscles, mobilisation of stiff joints, and thereby assist in the development of muscle power. This is useful as it produces a general sense of well-being.

Occupational therapy: Occupational therapy aims at enabling the person to become as independent as possible, despite the disability he may have. A person needs independence in following day-to-day activity.

a. *Activities of daily living (ADL):* These constitute activities such as self-care—bathing, eating, wearing clothes, etc.

b. *Work-related activities:* These constitute employment related and home management related activities.

c. *Leisure time activities:* These constitute sports and social activities.

Initial emphasis in rehabilitation is on restoring the abilities of the person by physiotherapy measures such as exercises, positioning, etc. Even during this period, occupational therapy helps the patient to be as independent as possible. When it is not possible to achieve any further improvement, adaptation is done in the patient's environment, so that he is able to maintain independence. Psychological adaptation constitutes an important part of this. Use of adaptive devices such as walking aids, adaptive clothing, etc., is encouraged. The person is also trained to perform purposeful activities of daily living (ADL), and activities related to work and play environment. All these make him independent despite his disability.

DRUGS

Drugs have a limited role in orthopaedic disorders. Those used may be placed in five categories as given below:

a. **Pure analgesics or anti-inflammatory medicines:** These are the most important group of drugs used for pain relief. They are broadly divided into primarily pain relievers (e.g., Tramadol), or primarily anti-inflammatory drugs (e.g., Diclofenac). Anti-inflammatory drugs are further divided into non-steroidal anti-inflammatory drugs (NSAIDs) and steroids. Depending upon the need, the choice varies from a primarily analgesic to a mainly anti-inflammatory drug. In long-standing illnesses, it is desirable to use single daily-dose drugs, e.g., Coxibs and slow release (SR) formulations.

b. **Antibacterial drugs:** These drugs are of immense value in acute infective conditions such as septic arthritis, acute osteomyelitis, etc. It is important to start with a broad-spectrum drug and change over to specific antibiotics after a culture-sensitivity report.

c. **Hormones:** The main drugs in this group are parathyroid hormone, anabolic steroids, oestrogens (for osteoporosis) and stilbestrol (for metastasis from prostate).

d. **Specific drugs:** These are used in certain specific disorders, e.g., vitamin D for rickets, vitamin C for scurvy, etc.

e. **Cytotoxic drugs:** These are used in the treatment of malignant bone tumours.

f. **Local injections** of a depot preparation of hydrocortisone or methylprednisolone are used to control non-specific inflammation of a joint

or an extra-articular lesion like tennis elbow. Hyaluronidases injection is considered as joint lubrication injection (viscosupplementation). Newer agents in this group are biologics such as platelet rich plasma (PRP), stem cells injections.

MANIPULATION

This is a term used for a manoeuvre whereby passive movements of joints, bones or soft tissues are carried out to break adhesions or stretch capsule and muscles. It may be done with or without an anaesthesia. It may be done for: (i) correction of deformity; (ii) improving the range of movement of a stiff joint; or (iii) relief of chronic pain in or about a joint.

a. **Manipulation for the correction of a deformity:** In this category, manipulation has its most obvious application in the reduction of fractures and dislocations. It is also used to correct a deformity due to contracted soft tissues, as in CTEV.

b. **Manipulation for stiff joints:** In the treatment of stiff joints, while effort is being made to achieve movements, manipulation under anaesthesia may speed up the process of recovery. The joints where this modality is used most often are, knee and shoulder. Manipulation is *strictly contraindicated* in the elbow because it may lead to increased stiffness due to 'myositis'.

c. **Manipulation for the relief of pain:** The role of manipulation in some chronic painful conditions is empirical. It has been shown to be effective in some conditions like tennis elbow, low backache, etc.

RADIOTHERAPY

Radiotherapy is useful in the following orthopaedic disorders:

a. **Malignant tumours:** Ewing's sarcoma is a highly radiosensitive malignant bone tumour. Radiotherapy is also used for other malignant tumours, either pre- or post-surgery.

b. **Benign tumours:** Giant cell tumours of the bone which are unsuitable for excision, can be irradiated.

c. **Other conditions:** Myositis ossificans.

OPERATIVE METHODS OF TREATMENT

An operation is a useful yet serious undertaking. A trained surgeon, modern operation theatre and adequate instruments are essential before one ventures to perform an orthopaedic operation. Failing this, one may have to face serious complications like

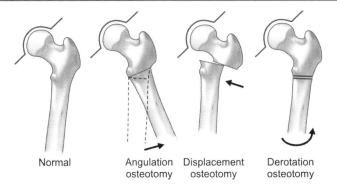

Fig. 12.1: Types of osteotomies.

Normal | Angulation osteotomy | Displacement osteotomy | Derotation osteotomy

Table 12.1: Common osteotomies and their indications.	
Name	**Indication**
McMurray's osteotomy	Fracture neck of femur
Pauwel's osteotomy	Osteoarthritis of the hip Fracture neck of femur
High tibial osteotomy	Osteoarthritis of the knee
French osteotomy	Correction of cubitus varus deformity
Spinal osteotomy	Ankylosing spondylitis

osteomyelitis, etc. The following are some of the common orthopaedic operations:

OSTEOTOMY

It means the cutting of a bone (Fig. 12.1). Indications for performing osteotomy are as follows:
- To correct excessive angulation, bowing or rotation of long bone.
- To correct malalignment of a joint.
- To permit elongation or shortening of a bone in cases of leg length inequality.
- Special indications where osteotomy is performed for purposes other than above, e.g., McMurray's osteotomy.

ARTHRODESIS

Arthrodesis is arthro+desis, which means fusing the joint. Fusion is achieved between the bones so as to eliminate any motion at the joint (Fig. 12.2). Although fusing a joint is, in a way, an unnatural way of treating a joint problem considering that a joint is meant for movement. But in certain situations, taking away the joint movements better than keeping the joint mobility. For example, a stiff and painful ankle may be more disabling than an arthrodesed (fused) ankle which is painless though stiff. An arthrodesis is used most often for a painful and stiff joint where any kind of repair or replacement of the joint is not possible. It is also performed for grossly unstable joints in polio.

Table 12.1 gives some of the commonly performed osteotomies and their indications.

Types of arthrodesis: An arthrodesis may be intra-articular, extra-articular or combined (Fig. 12.3). In an *intra-articular arthrodesis,* the articulating bone surfaces are made raw and the joint immobilised. Immobilisation is done in the position of optimum function until there is union between the opposing surface. In an *extra-articular arthrodesis*, a bridge of

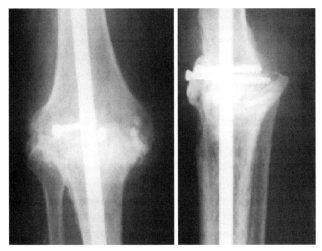

Fig. 12.2: X-rays of the knee, AP and lateral views, showing arthrodesis of the knee.

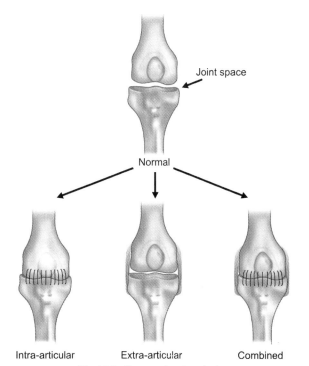

Joint space

Normal

Intra-articular | Extra-articular | Combined

Fig 12.3: Types of arthrodesis.

bone is created between the articulating bones, outside the joint. This bridge acts as a block to movement. Triple arthrodesis (talo-calcaneal, calcaneo-cuboid and talonavicular) is one of the most commonly performed arthrodesis.

Position of arthrodesis of different joints: The best position of arthrodesis of a joint is the one that conforms to the requirements of the patient's work. Table 12.2 gives positions in which common joints are fused.

Table 12.2: Position of arthrodesis of joints.

Joint	Position
Shoulder	Flex. 25°, abd. 30°, int. rot. 45°

Elbow
  Single
  Both
	
	Flex. 75°
	One in flex. 70°, other in flex. 130°

Wrist	Dorsiflex. 20°
Hip	Flex. 15°, no add./abd. neutral rotation
Knee	Flex. 5-10°

Ankle
  Males
  Females
	
	Neutral position
	Plantar flexion for high heels

ARTHROPLASTY (SEE CHAPTER 42)

Arthroplasty is Arthro = plasty, which means making a new joint.

Indications: This is an ever-evolving field of orthopaedics. Broadly, an arthroplasty is indicated for treatment of a painful joints where the goal is to make the joint pain free while retaining the mobility. It is commonly performed for: (i) osteoarthritis of the hip, knee and shoulder; (ii) regaining movement at an ankylosed elbow; and (iii) ununited femoral neck fracture.

Types of arthroplasty (Fig. 12.4): There are three types of arthroplasty in general use.
a. *Excision arthroplasty:* In this type, one or both of the articular ends are excised so that a gap is created between them. The gap gets filled with fibrous tissue. Some mobility is maintained while this fibrous tissue is forming, and hence some range of movement is preserved at the joint. Commonly this is performed for the hip and elbow.
b. *Hemiarthroplasty or half joint replacement:* In this type, only one of the articulating surfaces is replaced by an artificial component (prosthesis) of similar type. The prosthesis is made of metal, silicon or plastic. Commonly, it is performed for fractures of

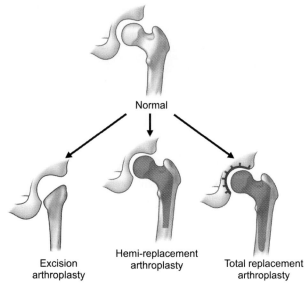

Fig. 12.4: Types of arthroplasties.

neck of the femur in elderly people (e.g., bipolar hemiarthroplasty). (Details on pages 134).
c. *Total arthroplasty or full joint replacement:* Here, both the apposing articulating surfaces are replaced by prosthetic components. There components are made us of steel or plastic or ceramic. Commonly, it is performed for hip osteoarthritis—total hip replacement (THR). (Details on page 330). Nearly all joints of the body can be replaced today.

BONE GRAFTING

Bone grafting is an operation whereby pieces of bone (bone grafts) taken from some part of a patient's body are placed at another site. Bone grafts are sometimes taken from another person or another species. Bone grafting is usually required for stimulating bone formation in a case of non-union of a fracture, or for filling bone defects. The defect may have been caused by a disease or by a surgeon trying to remove defective bone (tumour for example).

Type of bone grafts: There are three types of bone grafts (Flowchart 12.1); autograft (from the same person); allograft (from another person of the same species); xenograft (from a different species). Autografts are used most commonly.

Autogenous grafting: This is the 'gold standard' bone grafting technique. Human body has a lot of 'spare' bone for such use. Iliac crests are the *most common* site for taking bone grafts. When the graft is required for osteogenic purpose (as in non-union), cancellous bone grafts are preferred. It is available in plenty from iliac crests and upper end of tibia. When the graft is used for providing stability (as for filling bone gaps),

Flowchart 12.1: Types of bone grafts.

cortical graft is used. Fibulae are the common source of cortical bone grafts.

The grafts described above are *free grafts*. These do not survive as it is, but provide a scaffolding upon which the new bone is laid down. A bone stimulating protein called *bone morphogenetic protein* (BMP) is liberated from bone grafts, and helps in osteogenesis. Over a period of time the bone grafts are replaced by new, living bone.

Newer techniques of autogenous bone grafting are such that the vascularity of a graft is preserved while it is being placed on its receptor area. There are two ways of doing it. In one, the bone graft is taken along with a pedicle of muscle, whereby, the muscle (with its intact blood supply) continues to provide blood supply to the graft. It is called called *muscle-pedicle bone graft*. It is commonly used for treating non-union of fracture of the neck of the femur.

The other method of preserving blood supply of a bone graft is *free vascularized bone grafting*. In this, the bone (usually fibula) is taken along with the vessels supplying it. The graft thus harvested is placed at the new site, and its vessels anastomosed to the vascular bundle at host site. This way, such a graft gets its blood supply almost instantaneously. Such a graft, therefore, remains 'as it is', and gets incorporated with the parent bone much faster. Microsurgical techniques are required for free vascularized grafting.

Allogenous grafting: Allogenous bone grafts (allografts) are usually required when enough bone is not available from the host (e.g., a big defect created following a tumour resection). Such bone grafts could be obtained from another human being, living or dead. The latter is called *cadaveric graft*. Allogenous graft from live donors could be, for example, from the mother when larger amount of bone graft is required for a child. Allogenic bone graft could be from another person (amputated limb, for example). In this case, the graft needs to be preserved by different techniques. Some of the techniques of graft preservation are—deep freezing (at −70°C), freeze dried, preservation by decalcifying bone (decal bone), or by formalin preservation. Such preserved bone can be used for another patient at a later date. Hospitals performing tumour excision surgery in a big way have a regular department procuring bones from patients and cadavers, processing it and storing it. These are called *bone banks*.

Xenografting: Bone grafts from other species, usually bovine are now available off the shelf. These are available in tailor made sizes. Their use is not common yet in developing countries.

Artificial bone: This is a material derived from corals. It is hydroxyapatite with porous structure. It is supposed to have osteoconductive potential, and is being used in some countries.

Indications: Bone grafts are used mainly for three types of cases; (i) non-union of fractures—to promote union; (ii) arthrodesis of joints—to achieve fusion between joint surfaces; and (iii) filling of bone defects or cavities in a bone.

Technique: A graft may be used as a solid slab from a cortical bone (commonly a segment of the fibula), or as cancellous bone slivers or chips (commonly from the iliac crest).

SOFT-TISSUE GRAFTS

This is a whole new orthopaedic technology, where a free soft tissue graft (tendon and fascia) is taken from the body and used for bridging a soft tissue gap. Soft tissue grafts are most commonly used for ligament reconstructions (ACL reconstruction, for example). There are usually autograft (from patient's body), sometimes allografts (harvested from a donor).

TENDON TRANSFER OPERATIONS

A tendon transfer is an operation in which insertion of the tendon of a functioning muscle is moved to a new site. With this, the direction of pull of the muscle is changes and hence the muscle is used for a different function. The transfer operation is planned in such a way that loss of the transferred muscle's original function does not cause problem.

Indications: Tendon transfers have their main application in three group of conditions: (i) muscle paralysis—to restore or improve active control of a joint by utilising a healthy muscle to act in place of a paralysed one (e.g., in nerve palsy); (ii) muscle imbalance—to restore the balance between opposite groups of muscles in case one is weaker than the other (e.g., in polio); (iii) rupture of a tendon—in cases where direct suture is not practicable.

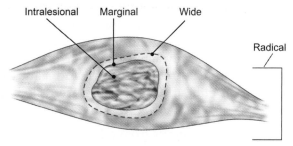

Fig. 12.5: Types of tumour excision.

The tendon transfer operation is commonly done for radial nerve palsy (Jone's transfer). Some of the

Table 12.3: Principles of tendon transfers.

Donor tendon
- Should be expandable
- Minimum power 4/5
- Amplitude of excursion to match that of the recipient muscle
- Preferably a synergistic muscle

Recipient site
- Range of movements of the joints on which the transferred muscle is expected to work should be good
- No scarring at the bed of the transferred tendon

Technical considerations
- Transferred tendon should take a straight route
- It should be placed in subcutaneous space
- Fixation must be under adequate tension

Patient considerations
- Age—minimum 5 years*
- The disease should be non-progressive

* Minimum age when a child can be trained in using the transferred muscle.

basic principles of tendon transfer procedure are as given in Table 12.3.

EXCISION OF TUMOURS

Excision of tumours (Fig. 12.5) can be of the following types: (i) *intralesional excision*: The lesion is curetted from within, as done for a simple bone cyst; (ii) *extralesional excision*: The lesion is removed along with its wall, as done for lipoma; (iii) *wide excision*: The lesion is removed with a margin of normal tissue; and (iv) *radical excision*: The tumour is removed along with the whole compartment in which it lies.

AMPUTATIONS

Amputation is the term used when a part of the limb is removed through a bone. *Disarticulation* is the corresponding term, used when a limb is removed through a joint. These operations are commonly performed for tumour ablation. This topic is discussed in detail in Chapter 40.

 What have we learnt?

- Orthopaedic treatment methods fall in two groups: Non-operative and Operative. Non-operative methods are mainly physiotherapy and medication. Operative methods are osteotomy, arthrodesis, arthroplasty, bone grafting, ligament reconstruction, tendon transfer, etc.
- Different techniques of bone grafting can be used. The most common is autografting.

Injuries Around the Shoulder, Fracture Humerus

Competencies

- ❖ **OR1.5:** Describe and discuss the aetiopathogenesis, clinical features, investigations, and principles of management of dislocation of major joints, shoulder, knee, hip.
- ❖ **OR2.1:** Describe and discuss the mechanism of injury, clinical features, investigations and plan management of fracture of clavicle.
- ❖ **OR2.2:** Describe and discuss the mechanism of injury, clinical features, investigations and plan management of fractures of proximal humerus.
- ❖ **OR2.4:** Describe and discuss the mechanism of injury, clinical features, investigations and principles of management of fracture of shaft of humerus and intercondylar fracture humerus with emphasis on neurovasular deficit.

RELEVANT ANATOMY

Shoulder girdle: It comprises of the clavicle, the scapula and the humerus. These three bones articulate with one another to give the shoulder a unique feature of freedom of movement in all directions. This maximises the reach of the hand in all directions.

The *clavicle* is the only long bone with membranous ossification. The muscles attached to its medial and lateral thirds are responsible for displacement following a fracture. Medial end of the clavicle articulates with the sternum to form the *sternoclavicular joint*, the stability of which is provided by thickened portions of the capsule. The lateral end of the clavicle articulates with the acromion process to form the *acromioclavicular joint*. The stability of this joint depends partially upon the acromioclavicular ligaments, and the more important stabilising structures, the coracoclavicular ligaments. The latter connect the conoid tubercle on the undersurface of the lateral end

of clavicle to the coracoid process. This ligament has two parts—conoid and trapezoid (Fig. 13.1). These ligaments must be torn before the acromio-clavicular joint can widely displace following an injury.

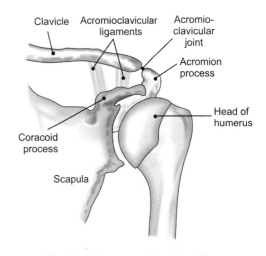

Fig. 13.1: Anatomy of the shoulder.

The *scapula* is a flat bone, thickly covered by muscles. Such thick cover do not allow displacement of fractures of this bone. Also, because of its rich vascularity, scapular fractures usually unite.

The proximal end of the humerus consists of the head articulating with glenoid cavity of the scapula (the gleno-humeral joint or the shoulder joint proper). The head is separated from the greater and lesser tuberosities by *anatomical neck.* The region below the tuberosities where the globular upper end of the bone joins the tubular shaft of the bone is called the *surgical neck.* Fractures are more common at the surgical than the anatomical neck.

Shoulder (glenohumeral) joint: This is a ball and socket joint, inherently unstable because the 'ball' is big and the 'socket' is small and shallow. Consequently, only about one-third of the humeral head is in contact with the glenoid cavity at any one time. The capsule of the shoulder joint is lax and permits freedom of movement. The strong muscles surrounding the joint contribute a great deal to the stability of this joint. The important among these are the *'rotator-cuff' muscles* (supraspinatus, infraspinatus, teres minor, sub-scapularis). The interval between subscapularis tendon and supraspinatous tendon is called *rotator interval.*

FRACTURE OF THE CLAVICLE

This is a common fracture at all age groups. It usually results from a fall on the shoulder or sometimes on an outstretched hand.

PATHOANATOMY

The junction of the middle and outer-third of the clavicle is the *most common* site; the other common site being the outer-third of the clavicle. This fracture is usually displaced. The outer fragment displaces medially and downwards because of the gravity and pull by the pectoralis major muscle attached to it (Fig. 13.2).

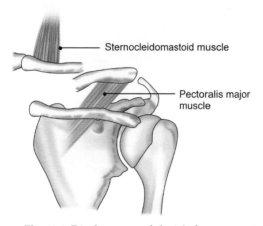

Sternocleidomastoid muscle

Pectoralis major muscle

Fig. 13.2: Displacement of clavicle fracture.

The inner fragment displaces upwards because of the pull by the sternocleidomastoid muscle attached to it.

DIAGNOSIS

Diagnosis is simple in most cases. There is a history of trauma followed by pain, swelling, crepitus, etc., at the site of fracture. One must look for any evidence of neurovascular deficit in the distal limb. The diagnosis can be confirmed on an X-ray.

TREATMENT

Fractures of the clavicle *unite readily* even if displaced, hence reduction of the fragment is not essential. A *triangular sling* is sufficient in cases with minimum displacement. Active shoulder exercises should be started as soon as the initial severe pain subsides, usually 10–14 days after the injury. A *figure-of-8 bandage* may be applied to a young adult with a displaced fracture (Fig. 13.3). It serves the purpose of immobilisation, and gives pain relief. Open reduction and internal fixation is required, either when the fracture is associated with neurovascular deficit, or in some severely displaced fractures, where it may be more of a cosmetic concern. In such cases, the fracture is fixed internally with a plate or a nail.

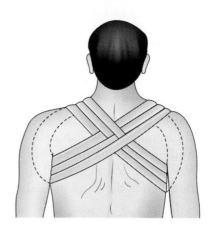

Fig. 13.3: Figure-of-8 bandage.

COMPLICATIONS

Early complications: The fractured fragment may injure the subclavian vessels or brachial plexus.

Late complications: Shoulder stiffness is a common complication, especially in elderly patients. It can be prevented by shoulder mobilisation as soon as the patient becomes pain free. Malunion and non-union (the latter being very rare) often cause no functional disability and need no treatment. Rarely, for a painful non-union of the clavicle, open reduction and internal fixation with bone grafting may be necessary.

FRACTURES OF THE SCAPULA

Fractures of the scapula are less common, and in most cases unimportant because patients recover well without much treatment. The scapula can break at four sites: (i) the body; (ii) the neck; (iii) the acromion process; and (iv) the coracoid process. Most often the fracture is undisplaced because the fragments are held in position by the surrounding muscles.

TREATMENT

The mainstay of treatment is to restore shoulder mobility by active exercises as soon as the pain subsides. A triangular sling for the period of pain and swelling (usually 1 week–10 days) is usually sufficient. In some severely displaced fractures, open reduction and internal fixation is done.

DISLOCATION OF THE STERNOCLAVICULAR JOINT

This is a rare injury. Here, the medial end of the clavicle is displaced forwards, or rarely backwards. Diagnosis is easier clinically than radiologically, because it is difficult to visualise this joint on X-ray, and hence CT scan is often required.

TREATMENT

This is by reduction using direct pressure over the dislocated end. Reduction is maintained by a figure-of-8 bandage. Recurrence is common, but causes no disability.

SUBLUXATION OR DISLOCATION OF THE ACROMIOCLAVICULAR JOINT

This is a common injury, caused by a fall on the outer prominence of the shoulder.

PATHOANATOMY

The injury may result in a partial or complete rupture of the acromioclavicular or coracoclavicular ligaments. Acromio-clavicular joint injuries are divided into three grades depending upon their severity (Table 13.1).

DIAGNOSIS

Pain and swelling localised to the acromioclavicular joint indicates an injury to this joint. In a Grade III injury the lateral end of the clavicle may be unusually prominent. X-ray with the acromioclavicular joints of both sides, for comparison, in the same film will show the subluxation or dislocation.

Table 13.1: Grades of acromioclavicular injury.

Grades	Pathoanatomy
Grade I	Minimal strain to acromioclavicular ligament and joint capsule
Grade II	Rupture of acromioclavicular ligament and joint capsule
Grade III	Rupture of acromioclavicular ligament, joint capsule and coracoclavicular ligaments

TREATMENT

Grades I and II injuries are treated by rest in a triangular sling and analgesics. Grade III injury in young athletic individuals is treated by surgical repair.

DISLOCATION OF THE SHOULDER

This is the *most common* joint in the human body to dislocate. It occurs more commonly in adults, and is rare in children. Anterior dislocation is much more common than posterior dislocation.

Shoulder instability: This is a broad term used for shoulder problems where head of the humerus is not stable in the glenoid. It has a wide, spectrum - from minor instability or a 'loose shoulder' to a frank dislocation. In the former, the patient may present with just pain in the shoulder, more so on using the shoulder. Pain occurs due to stretching of the capsule, as the head 'moves out' in some direction without actually dislocating. A patient with frank instability may present with an 'abnormal' movement of the head of the humerus. This could be partial movement (subluxation) which gets spontaneously reduced, or a dislocation. Once dislocated, it usually needs reduction by another person, with or without anaesthesia. The instability may be in one direction (unidirectional) or more (bidirectional). It may be instability in multiple directions - anterior, inferior, posterior, when it is called multi-directional instability (MDI). Isolated posterior instability is well-recognized, and presents with only pain.

MECHANISM

A fall on outstretched hand with the shoulder abducted and externally rotated, is the common mechanism of injury. Occasionally, it results from a direct force pushing the humerus head out of the glenoid cavity. A posterior dislocation may result from a direct blow on the front of the shoulder, driving the head backwards. More often, however, posterior dislocation is the consequence of an electric shock or an epileptiform convulsion.

PATHOANATOMY

Classification: Dislocations of the shoulder may be of the following types:

a. *Anterior dislocation:* In this injury, the head of the humerus comes out of the glenoid cavity and lies anteriorly. It may be further classified into three subtypes depending on the position of the dislocated head (Fig. 13.4).
   - Preglenoid: The head lies in front of the glenoid.
   - Subcoracoid: The head lies below the coracoid process. Most common type of dislocation.
   - Subclavicular: The head lies below the clavicle.

b. *Posterior dislocation:* In this injury, the head of the humerus comes to lie posteriorly, behind the glenoid.

c. *Luxatio erecta (inferior dislocation):* This is a rare type, where the head comes to lie in the subglenoid position.

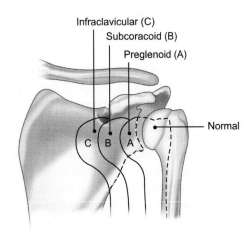

Fig. 13.4: Types of anterior dislocation of shoulder.

Pathological changes: The following pathological changes occur in the more common, anterior dislocation (Fig. 13.5):

a. *Bankart's lesion:* Dislocation causes stripping of the glenoid labrum along with the periosteum from the antero-inferior surface of the glenoid and scapular neck. The head thus comes to lie in front of the scapular neck, in the pouch thereby created. In severe injuries, it may be avulsion of a piece of bone from antero-inferior glenoid rim, called *bony Bankart lesion.*

b. *Hill-Sachs lesion:* This is a depression on the humeral head in its posterolateral quadrant, caused by impingement by the anterior edge of the glenoid on the head as it dislocates.

c. *Rounding off* of the anterior glenoid rim occurs in chronic cases as the head dislocates repeatedly over it.

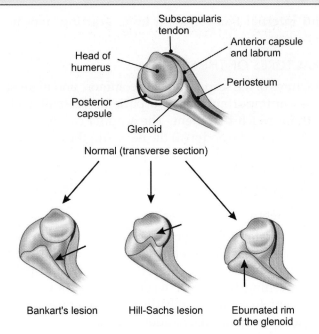

Fig. 13.5: Pathoanatomy of anterior dislocation of shoulder.

d. There may be *associated injuries:* like fracture of greater tuberosity, rotator-cuff tear, chondral damage, etc.

DIAGNOSIS

Presenting complaints: The patient enters the casualty with his shoulder abducted and the elbow supported with opposite hand. There is a history of a fall on an outstretched hand followed by pain and inability to move the shoulder. There may be a history of similar episodes in the past.

On examination: The patient keeps his arm abducted. The normal round contour of the shoulder joint is lost, and it becomes flattened. On careful inspection, one may notice fullness below the clavicle due to the displaced head. This can be felt by rotating the arm. The following are some of the signs, associated with anterior dislocation mostly of academic significance:

- *Dugas' test:* Inability to touch the opposite shoulder.
- *Hamilton ruler test:* Because of the flattening of the shoulder, it is possible to place a ruler on the lateral side of the arm. This touches the acromion and lateral condyle of the humerus simultaneously.

The diagnosis is easily confirmed on an antero-posterior X-ray of the shoulder (Fig. 13.6). An axillary view is sometimes required.

Posterior dislocation usually occurs following a convulsion. There are few symptoms and signs.

This injury is often missed on X-ray. A clinical examination eliciting loss of external rotation, and a careful look at the X-ray may help diagnose these cases. CT scan may be diagnostic.

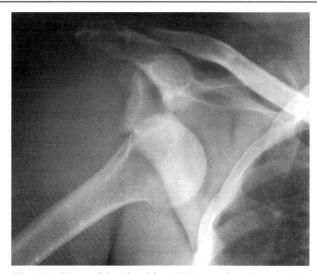

Fig. 13.6: X-ray of the shoulder, AP view, showing anterior dislocation of the shoulder.

TREATMENT

Treatment of acute dislocation is reduction under sedation or general anaesthesia, followed by immobilisation of the shoulder in a chest-arm bandage for three weeks. After the bandage is removed, shoulder exercises are begun.

TECHNIQUES OF REDUCTION OF SHOULDER DISLOCATION

Kocher's manoeuvre: This is the most commonly used method. The steps* are as follows: (i) traction - with the elbow flexed to a right angle steady traction is applied along the long axis of the humerus; (ii) external rotation - the arm is rotated externally; (iii) adduction - the externally rotated arm is adducted by carrying the elbow across the body towards the midline; and (iv) internal rotation the arm is rotated internally so that the hand falls across to the opposite shoulder.

Hippocrates manoeuvre: In this method, the surgeon applies a firm and steady pull on the semi-abducted arm. He keeps his foot in the axilla against the chest wall. The head of the humerus is levered back into position using the foot as a fulcrum.

A fracture of the greater tuberosity, often associated with an anterior dislocation usually comes back to its position as the head is reduced, and needs no special treatment.

COMPLICATIONS

Complications can be divided into early and late.

Early complications: Injury to the axillary nerve may occur resulting in paralysis of the deltoid muscle, with

a small area of anaesthesia over the lateral aspect of the shoulder. The diagnosis is confirmed by asking the patient to try to abduct the shoulder. Though shoulder abduction may not be possible because of pain, one can feel the absence of contraction of the deltoid. Treatment is conservative, and the prognosis is good.

Late complications: The shoulder is the *most common* joint to undergo recurrent dislocation. This results from the following causes: (i) anatomically unstable joint, e.g., in Marfan's syndrome; (ii) inadequate healing after the first dislocation, or (iii) an epileptic patient.

Treatment: If the disability is troublesome, operation is required. The following operations may be considered:

a. *Bankart's operation:* The glenoid labrum and capsule are re-attached to the front of the glenoid rim. This is a technically demanding procedure. Special fixation devices, called anchors are used to fix the labrum to the bone.

b. *Bristo-Latarjet operation:* In this operation, the coracoid process, along with its attached muscles, is osteotomized at its base and fixed to lower-half of the anterior margin of the glenoid. The bone part helps by augmenting bone loss form anterior glenoid, and the attached muscles (strap muscles) provide a dynamic sling support to the head of the humerus.

c. *Putti-Platt operation:* Double-breasting of the subscapularis tendon is performed in order to prevent external rotation and abduction, thereby preventing recurrences.

d. *Arthroscopic Bankart repair* (Fig. 13.7): With the development of arthroscopic techniques, it has become possible to stabilise a recurrently

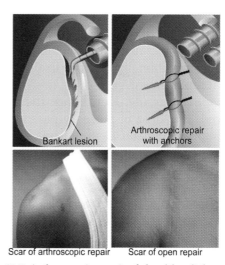

Bankart lesion

Arthroscopic repair with anchors

Scar of arthroscopic repair   Scar of open repair

Fig. 13.7: Arthroscopic repair of shoulder dislocation.

*To remember the steps of reduction, remember TEA-I (Traction, External rotation, Adduction, Internal rotation).

unstable shoulder arthroscopically. Apart from being a more cosmetic option, the rehabilitation after arthroscopic repair is faster and better. It is a technically demanding operation, and the anchor sutures used for repair are expensive. This technique is available only in select centres.

FRACTURE OF THE SURGICAL NECK OF THE HUMERUS

Fracture through the surgical neck of the humerus occurs most often in elderly women. The fracture is usually caused by a fall on the shoulder. In the majority of cases, these fractures are impacted; sometimes they are widely displaced. The possibility of this fracture should be kept in mind in all elderly persons complaining of pain in the shoulder following a fall. Often the symptoms are minimal.

It is important to properly evaluate these fractures by AP and axial X-rays. Neer has classified these fractures into 4 types depending upon the construction of the fracture. He identified 4 parts in the upper end of the humerus—shaft, head, greater tuberosity and lesser tuberosity. Depending upon in how many parts the bone has fractured, he divided them into one to four part fracture. For example, a fracture where the head, the greater tuberosity, the lesser tuberosity and the shaft, all have separated, it will be called a four-part fracture. This classification helps in deciding the treatment and prognosis.

TREATMENT

Treatment falls in the following categories:
- *Conservative treatment:* In elderly persons, even with moderate displacements, it is generally adequate to immobilise the affected shoulder in a triangular sling. As soon as the pain subsides, shoulder mobilisation is started.
- *Operative treatment:* If the fragments are widely displaced, particularly in young and active individuals, operative treatment is resorted to. It varies from minimally invasive fixation methods, to joint replacement.
- *Percutaneous wiring*: Here, once the fracture is reduced, it is held in place by passing multiple K-wires percutaneously under image intensifier control. No cut is made. It is suitable for some stable fractures, particularly in cosmetically conscious young ladies.
- *Open reduction and internal fixation*: This is used in complex fractures which are often unstable and difficult to keep in place by non-operative methods. A number of internal fixation devices

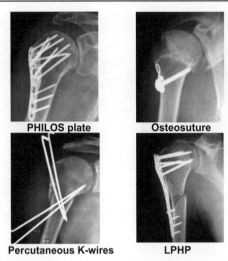

Fig. 13.8: Methods of fixation of surgical neck of the humerus.

have been in use—modern LCP based special plate (PHILOS), and Multiloc nail (Fig. 13.8).
- *Replacement arthroplasty* (Fig. 13.9): In badly comminuted fractures in an elderly, straightaway replacement arthroplasty is desirable. There are two types of replacement arthroplasty for comminuted fractures of proximal humerus – hemiarthroplasty (only head replaced), or reverse shoulder arthroplasty (a special implant where anatomy of the shoulder is reversed, as shown in Figure 13.9). Axillary nerve palsy and shoulder stiffness are common complications.

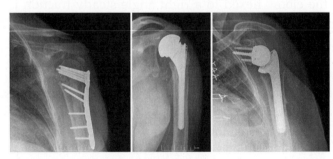

Fig. 13.9: Types of arthoplasty done for a fracture upper humerus.

FRACTURE OF THE GREATER TUBEROSITY OF THE HUMERUS

Fracture of the greater tuberosity of the humerus occurs in adults. The fracture is usually caused by a fall on the shoulder, and is undisplaced and comminuted. Sometimes, it is widely separated due to the pull by the muscle (supraspinatus) attached to it.

TREATMENT

For minimally displaced, comminuted fractures, rest in a triangular sling is enough. The shoulder is mobilised as soon as the pain subsides. For displaced fractures, open reduction and internal fixation is usually required. Painful arc syndrome (see page 304), non-union and shoulder stiffness are the usual complications.

FRACTURE OF THE SHAFT OF THE HUMERUS

This is a common fracture in patients at any age. It is usually sustained from an indirect twisting or bending force—as may be sustained in a fall on outstretched hand or by a direct injury to the arm.

RELEVANT ANATOMY

The humerus is a typical long bone (see page 8). The upper-half of the shaft is roughly cylindrical, and begins to flatten in its lower-half in the anteroposterior direction. The deltoid muscle is inserted on the deltoid tuberosity on the antero- lateral surface of the bone just proximal to its middle-third. The posterior surface is crossed obliquely by a shallow groove for the radial nerve.

The humerus is surrounded by muscles. This has the following clinical relevance: (i) the incidence of compound fractures is low; (ii) the union of fractures occurs early because a bone so well surrounded by muscles has a rich periosteal blood supply; and (iii) some degree of malunion is masked by the thick muscle cover.

PATHOANATOMY

A humerus fracture can be considered a prototype fracture because it occurs in all patterns (transverse, oblique, spiral, comminuted, segmental, etc.), may be closed or open, and may be traumatic or pathological.

Displacements are variable. It may be an undisplaced fracture, or there may be marked angulation or overlapping of fragments. Lateral angulation is common because of the abduction of the proximal fragment by the deltoid muscle (Fig. 13.10). This angulation is further increased by the tendency of the patient to keep the limb by the side of his chest, resulting in adduction of the distal fragment. Often, distraction occurs at the fracture site because of the gravity.

DIAGNOSIS

Diagnosis is simple because the patient presents with the classic signs and symptoms of a fracture. There may be wrist drop, if the radial nerve is injured. An X-ray of the whole arm including the shoulder and elbow should be done.

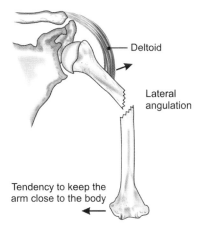

Fig. 13.10: Displacement in fracture shaft of the humerus.

TREATMENT

Most of these fractures unite easily. *Anatomical reduction is not necessary as long as the fracture is stable.* Some amount of displacement and angulation is acceptable.

This is due to the following reasons: (i) limitation of motion because of a moderate malunion in angulation or rotation goes unnoticed because of the multi-axial shoulder joint proximally; (ii) some amount of shortening goes undetected in the upper limb (unlike in the lower limb where shortening produces a limp); and (iii) the bone is covered with thick muscles so that a malunited fracture is not noticeable (unlike the tibia where malunion is easily noticeable).

Strict immobilisation is not necessary. The aim of treatment is pain relief and prevention of lateral angulation and distraction. It is possible to achieve this by conservative means in most cases.

Conservative methods: The following conservative methods are useful in most cases:

a. *U-slab* (Fig. 13.11A): This is a plaster slab extending from the base of the neck, over the shoulder onto the lateral aspect of the arm; under the elbow to the medial side of the arm. It should be moulded on the lateral side of the arm in order to prevent

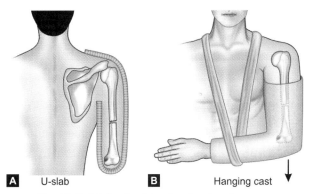

Fig. 13.11: Methods of treating fracture humerus.

lateral angulation. The U-slab is supported with a triangular sling. Once the fracture unites, the slab is removed (approximately 6-8 weeks) and shoulder exercises started.

b. *Hanging cast* (Fig. 13.11B): It is used in some cases of lower-third fractures of the humerus. The weight of the limb and the cast is supposed to provide necessary traction to keep the fracture aligned.

c. *Chest-arm bandage*: The arm is strapped to the chest. This much immobilisation is sufficient for fracture of the humerus in children less than five years of age.

In adults, early mobilisation of the limb can be begun by using a cast-brace once the fracture becomes sticky.

Operative method: In cases where a reduction is not possible by closed manipulation or if the fracture is very unstable, open reduction and internal fixation is required. Most fractures can be fixed well with plate and screws. Intramedullary nailing is another method of internal fixation. Contaminated open or infected fractures are stabilised by an external fixator.

COMPLICATIONS

Nerve injury: The radial nerve is commonly injured in a fracture of the humeral shaft. The injury to the nerve is generally a neurapraxia only. It may be sustained at the time of fracture, during manipulation of the fracture or while the fracture is healing (nerve entrapment in the callus). A special type of humerus fracture, where there is a spiral fracture at the junction of the middle and distal third, is commonly known to be associated with a radial nerve palsy. This is called *Holstein Lewis fracture*. The radial nerve injury results in paralysis of the wrist, finger and thumb extensors (wrist drop), brachioradialis and the supinator. There is a sensory change in a small area on the radial side of the back of the hand.

Treatment: For cases reporting early, treatment depends on the expected type of nerve injury (for details, refer to Chapter 10). In most closed fractures, the nerve recovers spontaneously. In open fractures, exploration is usually required. In neglected cases or when repair of a divided nerve is impractical, tendon transfers are needed. Modified Jone's transfer is most popular. Here the muscles of the forearm, supplied by median and ulnar nerves, are used for substituting wrist extension, finger extension and thumb abduction-extension. The following tendons are used:

- Pronator teres → Extensor carpi radialis brevis
- Flexor carpi ulnaris → Extensor digitorum
- Palmaris longus → Extensor pollicis longus

Delayed and non-union: Fractures of the shaft of the humerus, especially transverse fracture of the midshaft, often go into delayed or non-union. The causes of non-union are: inadequate immobilisation or distraction at the fracture site because of the gravity.

Treatment: Open reduction, internal fixation with a plate, and bone grafting is usually performed. In cases where the quality of bone is poor, an intramedullary fibular graft may be used to enhance the fixation. The limb is suitably immobilised, in addition, using a U-slab or sometimes, even a shoulder spica cast.

 What have we learnt?

- Shoulder is a group of joints—sternoclavicular, acromioclavicular, glenohumeral and scapulothoracic.
- Rotator cuff muscles are important for shoulder functions.
- Fracture of the clavicle is usually treated non-operatively.
- Anterior shoulder dislocation is a common injury. It frequently leads to recurrent dislocation.
- Treatment of humerus shaft fractures is essentially non-operative. Unstable fractures need to be operated. Non-union is treated with plating and bone grafting.

Additional information: From the entrance exams point of view

- Inferior capsule is the weakest portion of the shoulder joint.
- Tests for anterior glenohumeral instability are apprehension test, fulcrum test, crank test, Jobe's relocation test and surprise test.
- Test for posterior glenohumeral instability is jerk test.
- Sulcus test done for multi-directional and inferior instability.
- Lift off test evaluates subscapularis muscle activity.

Injuries Around the Elbow

Learning Objectives

- ❖ Discuss the classification, pathoanatomy, treatment and complications of supracondylar fracture of humerus.
- ❖ Discuss classification and treatment of olecranon fracture.

RELEVANT ANATOMY

The elbow joint is a *hinge joint*, formed by the articulation between the lower end of the humerus with the ulna (humero-ulnar joint), and with the head of the radius (humero-radial joint). The lower end of the humerus is enlarged to form the trochlea medially and capitulum laterally. Medial to the trochlea is a prominent process, i.e., medial epicondyle, and lateral to the capitulum is the lateral epicondyle. The two epicondyles are continuation of the medial and lateral supracondylar ridges respectively. The lateral epicondyle and capitulum together constitute the lateral condyle.

Three bony points relationship: The three prominent bony points around the elbow, i.e., the medial epicondyle, lateral epicondyle and tip of the olecranon are important landmarks in the diagnosis of injuries around the elbow. Normally, in an elbow flexed to 90°, these three bony points form a near isosceles triangle (Fig. 14.1), but they lie in a straight horizontal line in an extended elbow. The base of the triangle (between the two epicondyles) is the longest arm. The side between the medial epicondyle and olecranon tip

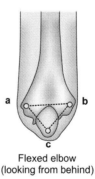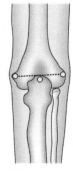

Flexed elbow
(looking from behind)

Extended elbow

Fig. 14.1: Three bony points relationship: a. Medial epicondyle, b. Lateral epicondyle, c. Tip of olecranon.

is the shortest. The head of the radius, also considered the *4th bony point*, can be palpated in a semi-flexed elbow, just distal to the lateral epicondyle. It can be better felt moving during supination-pronation of the forearm.

Carrying angle: When the elbow joint is fully extended and supinated, the forearm and the arm do not lie in a straight line, but form an angle (Fig. 14.2). This is called the carrying angle. It disappears on

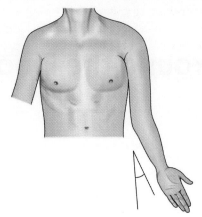

Fig. 14.2: The carrying angle.

Table 14.1: Injuries around the elbow and their mechanisms.	
Indirect	
▪ *Valgus injury*	▪ Fracture head of the radius
	▪ Fracture neck of the radius
	▪ Avulsion fracture of medial epicondyle of the humerus
▪ *Varus injury*	▪ Fracture lateral condyle of the humerus
▪ *Hyperextension injury*	▪ Supracondylar fracture of the humerus
▪ *Axial force*	▪ Fracture of the capitulum
	▪ Dislocation of the elbow
Direct	
▪ *Fall on the point of elbow*	▪ Olecranon fracture
	▪ Intercondylar fractures of humerus

flexing the elbow. The normal carrying angle is 11° in males and 14° in females. In injuries around the elbow this angle may decrease or increase.

Stability of the elbow: This mainly depends upon the inherent stability of the articulating surfaces of the elbow joint, i.e., the olecranon and the trochlea. The strong capsule and collateral ligaments add to the stability. The head of the radius rotates within an annular ligament which encircles it. In children, the head can slip out of this ligament (pulled elbow).

Ossification around the elbow: Knowledge of the appearance and fusion of different ossification centres around the elbow is necessary because these are sometimes mistaken for a fracture. Figure 14.3 shows the time of appearance of these epiphyses.

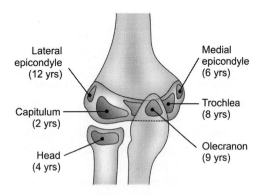

Fig. 14.3: Epiphyseal centres around the elbow and their time of appearance.

MECHANISM OF INJURY

Injuries around the elbow may result from an indirect or direct violence.

Indirect violence: This is the more common of the two mechanisms. The cause is generally a fall onto the outstretched hand. The type of force to which the elbow is subjected determines which fracture will occur. The elbow may be forced into valgus, varus, or hyperextension resulting in different injuries (Table 14.1).

Direct violence: This results either from a fall on to the point of the elbow or a direct hit on the olecranon. The result may be: (i) an olecranon fracture or (ii) an intercondylar fracture of the humerus.

SUPRACONDYLAR FRACTURE OF THE HUMERUS

This is one of the most serious fractures in childhood as it is often associated with complications.

MECHANISM

The fracture is caused by a fall on an outstretched hand. As the hand strikes the ground, the elbow is forced into *hyperextension* resulting in fracture of the humerus above the condyles.

PATHOANATOMY

The fracture line extends transversely through the distal metaphysis of humerus just above the condyles.

Types: A supracondylar fracture may be of extension or flexion type, depending upon the displacement of the distal fragment (Fig. 14.4).

The *extension type* is the more common of the two. In this, the distal fragment is extended (tilted backwards) in relation to the proximal fragment. In the *flexion type*, the distal fragment is flexed (tilted forwards) in relation to the proximal fragment. Subsequent text is limited to the more common, extension type of supracondylar fracture.

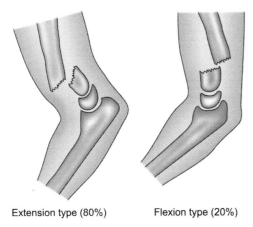

Extension type (80%)   Flexion type (20%)

Fig. 14.4: Types of supracondylar fractures.

Displacements: Commonly, a supracondylar fracture is displaced (Fig. 14.5). The distal fragment may be displaced in the following directions: (i) posterior or backward shift; (ii) posterior or backward tilt; (iii) proximal shift; (iv) medial or lateral shift; (v) medial tilt; and (vi) internal rotation.

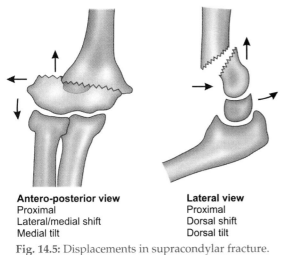

Antero-posterior view   **Lateral view**
Proximal   Proximal
Lateral/medial shift   Dorsal shift
Medial tilt   Dorsal tilt

Fig. 14.5: Displacements in supracondylar fracture.

DIAGNOSIS

Presenting complaints: The child is brought to the hospital with a history of fall, followed by pain, swelling, deformity and inability to move the affected elbow.

On examination: When presented early, before significant swelling has occurred, the following clinical signs may be observed:
• Unusual posterior prominence of the point of the elbow (tip of olecranon) because of the backward tilt of the distal fragment.
• Since the fracture is above the condyles, the three bony points relationship is maintained as in a normal elbow.

When presented late, gross swelling makes it difficult to appreciate these signs, thus making clinical diagnosis difficult. The possibility of interruption of the blood supply to the distal extremity because of an associated brachial artery injury, must be carefully looked for in all cases. Radial and ulnar pulses may be absent with or without signs of ischaemia (five P's– page 46). One must look for an injury to the median nerve (pointing index) or the radial nerve (wrist drop).

Radiological examination: Most often, it is easy to diagnose the fracture because of wide displacement.

Sometimes, the presence of ossification centres around the elbow make diagnosis of a minimally displaced fracture difficult. A comparison with an X-ray of the opposite elbow may help. The following displacements may be seen on an X-ray (Fig. 14.6).
• In an anteroposterior view, one can see the proximal shift, medial or lateral shift, medial tilt and rotation of the distal fragment.
• In a lateral view, one can see the proximal shift, posterior shift, posterior tilt and rotation of the distal fragment.

TREATMENT

Undisplaced fractures require immobilisation in an above-elbow plaster slab, with the elbow in 90° flexion. In all *displaced* fractures, the child should be admitted to a hospital because serious complications can occur within the first 48 hours. The following methods of treatment are used in displaced fractures:
a. **Closed reduction and percutaneous K-wire fixation:** Most displaced fractures are easily reduced by closed reduction, but they often slip. Hence, it is best to fix them with one or two

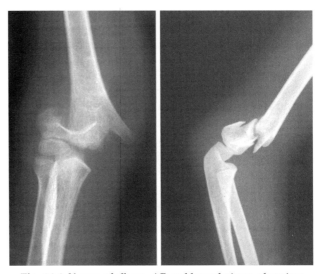

Fig. 14.6: X-rays of elbow, AP and lateral views, showing typical supracondylar fracture humerus.

K-wires, passed percutaneously under image intensifier guidance. Where facility for image intensifier is not available, a close watch on the fracture position in plaster weekly, is a must.

Technique of closed reduction of a supracondylar fracture: Closed reduction of a supracondylar fracture requires experience. It is carried out in the following steps (Fig. 14.7).

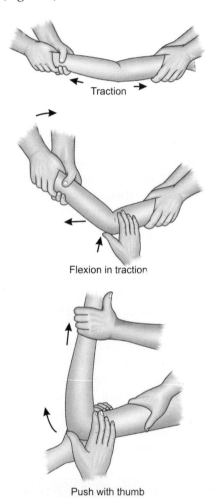

Traction

Flexion in traction

Push with thumb

Fig. 14.7: Steps in the reduction of supracondylar fracture.

Traction with the elbow in 30-40° of flexion: Traction is applied for two minutes, with an assistant giving counter-traction at the arm. While in traction, the elbow is gradually extended and the forearm fully supinated. This manoeuvre corrects proximal displacement and medial-lateral displacements. If required, the 'carrying angle' of the elbow is corrected at this stage.

Flexion in traction: With one hand maintaining traction, the upper arm is grasped with the other hand, placing the fingers over the biceps, so that the thumb rests on the olecranon. The elbow is now flexed slowly, using the hand with which traction is being applied, so as to flex the elbow

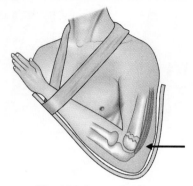

Fig. 14.8: Internal splint.

while continuous traction is maintained in the long axis of the forearm.

Pressure over the olecranon: While the above manoeuvre is continued, the thumb over the olecranon presses the olecranon (and with it the distal fragment) forward into flexion. Traction is maintained as the elbow is flexed to beyond 90°. Throughout this manoeuvre the radial pulse is felt. If it is obliterated on flexion, the elbow is extended again until the pulse returns and a posterior slab is applied in whatever position achieved. Further treatment in such cases will depend upon the acceptability of reduction. If it is possible to flex the elbow beyond 90°, the fragments become locked. The intact periosteum and triceps on the dorsal aspect of fracture act as an 'internal splint' (Fig. 14.8), thereby stabilising the reduction. A posterior slab is applied in this position for 3 weeks. It is necessary to make a check X-ray after 48 hours, and after 1 week in order to detect any redisplacement. In case no redisplacement occurs, the plaster is removed after 3 weeks.

b. **Open reduction and K-wire fixation:** In some cases, it is not possible to achieve a good position by closed methods, or the fracture gets redisplaced after reduction. In such cases, open reduction and K-wire fixation is necessary (Fig. 14.9). This is

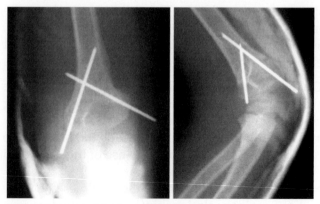

Fig. 14.9: X-rays showing a supracondylar fracture fixed with K-wires.

Flow chart 14.1: Treatment plan for supracondylar fracture.

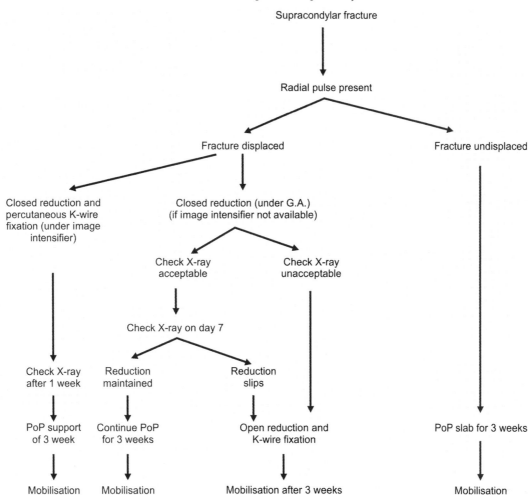

also used as a first line of treatment in some open fractures, and in those requiring exploration of the brachial artery for suspected injury.

c. **Continuous traction:** This is required in cases presenting late with excessive swelling or bad wounds around the elbow. The traction may be given with a K-wire passed through the olecranon (Smith's traction) or a below-elbow skin traction (Dunlop's traction). These methods are no longer used.

A general treatment plan for a supracondylar fracture is shown in Flowchart 14.1.

COMPLICATIONS

The supracondylar fracture is notorious for a number of serious complications. These can be:
i. Immediate—occurring at the time of fracture;
ii. Early—occurring within first 2-3 days;
iii. Late—occurring weeks to months after the fracture.

Immediate Complications

1. **Injury to the brachial artery:** This is a complication commonly associated with a displaced supracondylar fracture. The brachial artery is usually injured by the sharp edge of the *proximal* fragment (Fig. 14.10). The damage may

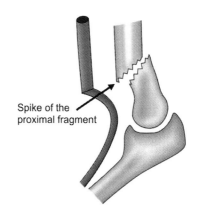

Spike of the proximal fragment

Fig. 14.10: Vascular injury in a supracondylar fracture.

Flowchart 14.2: Treatment plan for supracondylar fracture with absent pulse.

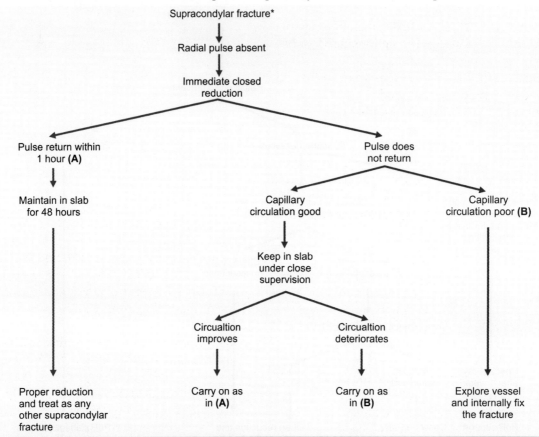

* In an open supracondylar fracture with absent pulse, wound debridement and exploration of the vessel is performed, and the fracture fixed internally as a primary procedure.

vary from just a pressure on the artery to complete disruption. The affects of arterial occlusion at the elbow differ from case to case. Most often, enough blood gets through the collaterals around the elbow to keep the hand alive, but flexor muscles of the forearm may suffer ischaemic damage leading to Volkmann's ischaemia. At times, the vascular compromise may be severe enough to result in gangrene.

The treatment plan for a supracondylar fracture with an absent pulse is shown in Flowchart 14.2.

2. **Injury to nerves:** The median nerve is the most commonly injured nerve. Radial nerve is also sometimes affected. Spontaneous recovery occurs in most cases.

Early Complications

Volkmann's ischaemia: This is an ischaemic injury to the muscles and nerves of the flexor compartment of the forearm. It is caused due to occlusion of the brachial artery by a supracondylar fracture.

Pathophysiology: Volkmann's ischaemia is the result of diminished blood supply to the flexor muscles of

the forearm. The muscles supplied by the anterior interosseous artery, a branch of brachial artery, are most susceptible to ischaemic damage because this artery is an end-artery*. Most commonly affected muscles are the flexor pollicis longus and medial half of flexor digitorum profundus. The muscle ischaemia leads to compartment syndrome (see page 47).

Diagnosis: Early diagnosis of Volkmann's ischaemia is of extreme importance. The following are some of the early signs:

- The child complains of severe pain in the *forearm.* He is unable to move the fingers fully. Ischaemic pain is more severe than the pain due to the fracture. A child needing more than usual doses of analgesics may be developing a compartment syndrome.
- *Stretch pain:* The child complains of pain in the *flexor aspect of the forearm* when the fingers are extended passively.
- Swelling and numbness over the fingers occur rather late.

---

*End artery is the one which does not have any collateral joining it.

- There is tenderness on pressing the forearm muscles.

Treatment: Volkmann's ischaemia is an emergency of the highest order. The following actions need to be taken urgently in a suspected case:
- The external splints or bandages that might be causing constriction are removed.
- The forearm is elevated and the child encouraged to move fingers.
- If no improvement occurs within 2 hours, an urgent decompression of the tight compartment is necessary. This is done by a *fasciotomy*—an operation where the deep fascia covering the flexor muscles of the forearm is slit along its entire length.

LATE COMPLICATIONS

1. **Malunion:** It is the *most common* complication of a supracondylar fracture and results in a *cubitus varus* deformity. This is because the fracture unites with the distal fragment tilted medially and in internal rotation. Malunion may occur either because of failure to achieve good reduction, or displacement of the fracture within the plaster. The cubitus varus deformity is often termed the *Gun stock deformity* (Fig. 14.11). Sometimes, the distal fragment unites with an excessive backward tilt, resulting in hyperextension at the elbow along with limitation of flexion—basically a change in the arc of movement at the elbow.

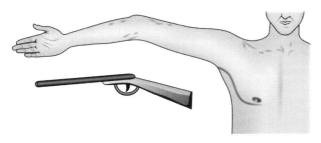

Fig. 14.11: Gun stock deformity.

Treatment: Cubitus varus deformity is a cosmetic problem, usually without much functional impairment. Mild deformity may not require treatment, but a badly deformed elbow should be corrected. Treatment is a supracondylar corrective osteotomy (French osteotomy).

2. **Myositis ossificans:** This is an ectopic new bone formation around the elbow joint, resulting in stiffness. Massage following the injury, so commonly resorted to in some places, is a major factor responsible for it.

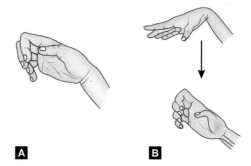

Fig. 14.12: (A) Volkmann's ischaemic contracture (VIC); (B) Volkmann's sign.

Treatment: In the early stages, the elbow is put to rest in an above-elbow slab for 3 weeks. Following this, gentle elbow mobilisation is started. In some late cases, excision of the myositic bone or excision arthroplasty of the elbow is required. Whatever treatment is undertaken, the chances of the elbow regaining full range of movement are little.

3. **Volkmann's ischaemic contracture (VIC):** This is a sequel of Volkmann's ischaemia. The ischaemic muscles are gradually replaced by fibrous tissue, which contracts and draws the wrist and fingers into flexion (Fig. 14.12A). If the peripheral nerves are also affected, there will be sensory loss and motor paralysis in the forearm and hand.

Clinical features: There is marked atrophy of the forearm, with flexion deformity of the wrist and fingers. The skin over the forearm and hand is dry and scaly. The nails also show atrophic changes. *Volkmann's sign* helps in deciding the cause of flexion deformity of the fingers. In this sign, it is possible to extend the fingers fully at the interphalangeal joints only when the wrist is flexed (Fig. 14.12B). On extending the wrist, the fingers get flexed at the interphalangeal joints. This is because when the wrist is extended, the shortened flexor muscle-tendon unit is stretched over the front of the wrist, resulting in flexion of the fingers. There may be hypoaesthesia or anaesthesia of the hand.

Treatment: Mild deformities can be corrected by passive stretching of the contracted muscles, using a turn-buckle splint (Volkmann's splint). For moderate deformities, a soft tissue sliding operation, where the flexor muscles are released from their origin at the medial epicondyle and ulna, is performed (Maxpage operation). For a severe deformity, bone operations such as shortening of the forearm bones, carpal bone excision, etc., may be required.

FRACTURE OF THE LATERAL CONDYLE OF THE HUMERUS

A common fracture in children, it results from a varus injury to the elbow.

PATHOANATOMY

The fracture fragment comprises of the capitulum and the lateral epicondyle. The fracture line runs obliquely upwards and laterally from the intercondylar area (Fig. 14.13).

In younger children, the greater part of the detached fragment may be cartilaginous, and therefore appears smaller on X-rays, than it is in reality. It is Salter and Harris *type IV* epiphyseal injury (see page 58).

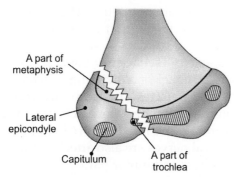

Fig. 14.13: Lateral condyle fracture.

Displacement: It is common and occurs due to the 'pull' of the common extensor muscles which take origin from the lateral epicondyle. The fragment is rotated outwards along its vertical and horizontal axis (Fig. 14.14); sometimes even as much as 90°.

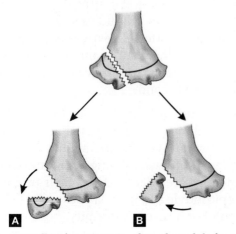

Fig. 14.14: Displacements in a lateral condyle fracture: (A) Along horizontal axis; (B) Along vertical axis.

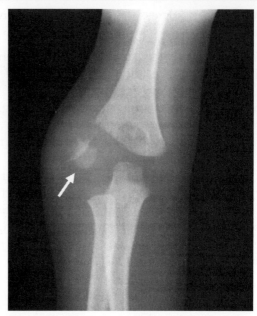

Fig. 14.15: X-ray of the elbow, AP view, showing a displaced fracture of lateral condyle of the humerus.

DIAGNOSIS

There is mild swelling and pain over the outer aspect of the elbow. This is associated with tenderness over the lateral epicondyle. The fracture is usually diagnosed on X-rays, as the symptoms are not much (Fig. 14.15).

TREATMENT

For the fracture, a type-IV epiphyseal injury, accurate reduction is important if normal growth of the elbow is to be expected. Treatment depends upon whether the fracture is displaced or not.

a. An undisplaced fracture (an uncommon situation) needs support in an above-elbow plaster slab for 2-3 weeks.
b. A displaced fracture is treated by open reduction and internal fixation using two K-wires.

COMPLICATIONS

Non-union: If unreduced, the fracture goes into non-union. This is either because of wide displacement of the fragment or a constant 'pulling' force of the extensor muscles attached to it. The result is a persistent pain or growth disturbance at the distal humeral epiphysis.

Treatment: If detected early (usually within 2 months), it is treated with open reduction and internal fixation. In late cases, it may not be possible to achieve any improvement even after open reduction. In such cases, it is better to accept the position and treat its consequences (deformity, etc.).

1. **Cubitus valgus deformity:** Diminished growth at the lateral side of distal humerus epiphysis results in a *cubitus valgus* deformity (Fig. 14.16). This may result in late ulnar nerve palsy (*tardy ulnar nerve palsy*) because of friction neuritis of the ulnar nerve as it moves over the medial epicondyle, everytime the elbow is flexed and extended.

   Treatment: No treatment is required for a mild deformity. A moderate to severe deformity may need correction by a supracondylar osteotomy. A developing tardy ulnar nerve palsy may present as tingling and numbness in the distribution of the ulnar nerve. At the earliest opportunity, the nerve should be transposed anteriorly from behind the medial epicondyle to prevent friction (anterior transposition of ulnar nerve).

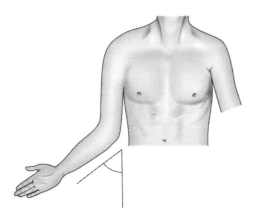

Fig. 14.16: Cubitus valgus deformity.
(Increased carrying angle).

2. **Osteoarthritis:** In cases where the articular surface is significantly disorganised, elbow osteoarthritis develops after many years. Pain and stiffness are presenting symptoms. Physiotherapy is rewarding in most cases.

INTERCONDYLAR FRACTURE OF THE HUMERUS

This is a common fracture in adults. It results from a fall on the point of the elbow so that the olecranon is driven into the distal humerus, splitting the two humeral condyles apart.

PATHOANATOMY

The fracture line may take the shape of a T or Y (Fig. 14.17). The fracture is generally badly comminuted and displaced. When displaced, the two condyles fall apart and are rotated along their horizontal axis.

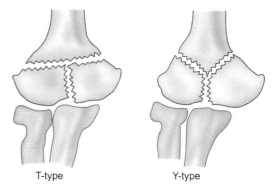

T-type   Y-type

Fig. 14.17: Types of intercondylar fractures.

DIAGNOSIS

There is generally severe pain, swelling, ecchymosis and crepitus around the elbow. The diagnosis is confirmed on X-rays.

TREATMENT

It depends upon the displacement. An undisplaced fracture needs support in an above-elbow plaster slab for 3-4 weeks, followed by exercises. A displaced fracture is treated generally by open reduction and internal fixation (Fig. 14.18). In cases with severe comminution, olecranon pin traction is given to reduce the fracture and maintain the reduction.

COMPLICATIONS

1. **Stiffness of the elbow:** This is a common complication because of the intra-articular nature of this fracture. There may be associated myositis ossificans. Treatment is by physiotherapy.
2. **Malunion:** The fracture usually unites, but may unite in a bad position. This leads to cubitus varus

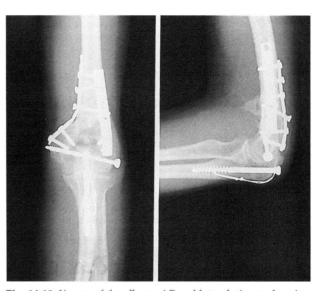

Fig. 14.18: X-rays of the elbow, AP and lateral views, showing an intercondylar fracture reconstructed with plates and screws.

or valgus deformity. A corrective osteotomy may be required for severe deformities.

3. **Osteoarthritis.**

FRACTURE OF THE MEDIAL EPICONDYLE OF THE HUMERUS

It is more commonly injured than the lateral epicondyle, because the epiphysis of the medial epicondyle appears early and fuses late with the main epiphysis of the lower humerus. Its displacement varies from minimal to displacement of the whole fragment into the elbow joint. This fracture is commonly associated with posterior dislocation of the elbow. It may be associated with an ulnar nerve injury.

Treatment is generally conservative, by immobilisation in an above-elbow slab. If displaced into the joint, it may require open reduction and internal fixation.

DISLOCATION OF THE ELBOW JOINT

Posterior dislocation is the most common type of elbow dislocation. Other dislocations are postero-medial, postero-lateral, and divergent*. It may be associated with fracture of the medial epicondyle, fracture of the head of the radius, or fracture of the coronoid process of the ulna.

Clinically, there is severe pain at the elbow. The triceps tendon stands prominent (bowstringing of triceps). The three bony points relationship is *reversed.* There is often an associated median nerve palsy. Diagnosis is easily confirmed on X-rays (Fig. 14.19).

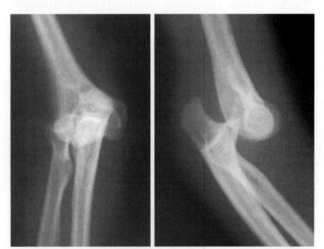

Fig. 14.19: X-rays of the elbow, AP and lateral views, showing posterior dislocation of the elbow.

---

*A dislocation of the elbow where the radius and ulna displace laterally and medially respectively (diverge).

Treatment: It is by reduction under anaesthesia followed by immobilisation in an above-elbow plaster slab for 3 weeks. Elbow stiffness and myositis are common complications.

TERRIBLE TRIAD OF ELBOW

Terrible triad of elbow is a combination injury consisting of elbow dislocation with fracture of head/neck of radius and coronoid fracture. This combination injury is very unstable and needs operative treatment.

PULLED ELBOW

This condition occurs in children between 2 and 5 years of age. The head of the radius is pulled partly out of the annular ligament when a child is lifted by the wrist. The child starts crying and is unable to move the affected limb. The forearm lies in an attitude of pronation. There may be mild swelling at the elbow. It is not possible to see the subluxated head on an X-ray because it is still cartilaginous; X-rays are taken only to rule out any other bony injury.

Treatment: The head is reduced by fully supinating the forearm and applying direct pressure over the head of the radius. A sudden click is heard or felt as the head goes back to its place. The child becomes comfortable and starts moving his elbow almost immediately.

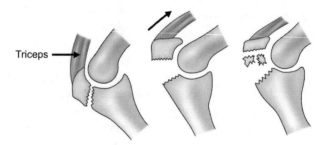

Triceps

Fig. 14.20: Types of olecranon fractures.

FRACTURE OF THE OLECRANON

This is usually seen in adults. It results from a direct injury as in a fall onto the point of the elbow.

PATHOANATOMY

The proximal fragment may be pulled proximally by the attached triceps muscle, thus creating a gap at the fracture site. The fracture may be one of the three types (Fig. 14.20).

Type I: Crack without displacement of fragments.

Type II: Clean break with separation of fragments.

Type III: Comminuted fracture.

DIAGNOSIS

Pain, swelling and tenderness are present at the point of the elbow. A crepitus or a gap between the fragments may be present. Active extension of the elbow is not possible in fractures with a gap The diagnosis is confirmed on an X-ray (Fig. 14.21).

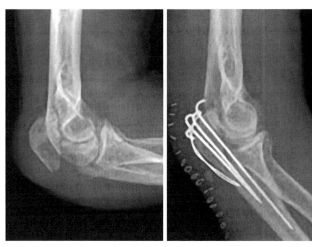

Fig. 14.21: X-ray of the elbow, lateral view, showing tension-band wiring of the olecranon.

TREATMENT

It depends upon the type of fracture:

Type I: A crack without displacement is treated by immobilising the elbow in an above-elbow plaster slab in 30 degree* of flexion. After 3 weeks the plaster is removed and elbow exercises begun.

Type II: A clean break with separation of the fragments is treated by open reduction and internal fixation using the technique of *tension-band wiring* (Fig. 14.21). It is not possible to keep the fragments together in the plaster alone because of the constant pull exerted by the triceps.

Type III: A comminuted fracture, if not separated, can be treated in a plaster slab, but if the fragments are separated, plating is required.

With improvement in methods of internal fixation, fracture of the olecranon, being an intra-articular fracture is treated by internal fixation wherever possible. This helps in early mobilisation of elbow, and hence achieving good range of movements. Recent development is use of precontoured plate specifically designed for olecranon fracture.

COMPLICATIONS

1. **Non-union** is a common complication in cases with a gap at the fracture site which prevents the fracture from uniting. Treatment is by open reduction, internal fixation and bone grafting.
2. **Elbow stiffness** occurs in some cases. Treatment is physiotherapy. In selected cases surgical release of adhesions (arthrolysis) may be required. This can be now done arthroscopically.
3. **Osteoarthritis** occurs late, often after many years in some cases, because of the irregularity of the articular surface. Treatment is physiotherapy. In selected cases, elbow replacement may be required.

FRACTURE OF THE HEAD OF THE RADIUS

This is seen *in adults,* in contrast to fractures of the neck of the radius which occurs in children. It is a valgus injury.

PATHOANATOMY

The head is deformed because of scattering of fragments. Sometimes a fragment of bone becomes loose and lies inside the elbow joint. The fracture may be of the following three types (Fig. 14.22):
1. A crack only.
2. A fragment of the head is broken off.
3. Comminuted fracture (the most common type).

DIAGNOSIS

This fracture is often missed because of minimal symptoms. There is mild pain and swelling over the lateral aspect of the elbow. A localised tenderness over the head of the radius, located immediately distal to the lateral epicondyle in a semi-flexed elbow, and *painful forearm rotation* are useful signs.

TREATMENT

It depends upon the type of fracture as discussed below:
a. **A crack only:** The fracture is treated by immobilisation in an above-elbow plaster slab for 2 weeks with the elbow at 90° of flexion and the forearm in mid-pronation.
b. **A fragment of the head broken off:** If the fragment is less than 1/3 the size of the head it can be treated as above. If it is more than 1/3 in size, or if it is lying loose inside the joint, it needs excision.

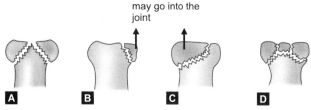

may go into the joint

Fig. 14.22: Types of fracture head of radius: (A) Undisplaced; (B) Fragment < 1/3; (C) Fragment >1/3; (D) Comminuted.

c. **Comminuted fracture with displacement:** This is treated by excision of the head.

COMPLICATIONS

1. **Joint stiffness:** Limitations of supination-pronation is a common complication associated with this injury. Treatment is persistent physiotherapy.
2. **Osteoarthritis:** It is an uncommon complication, and occurs because of joint irregularity. It usually does not cause much disability.

FRACTURE OF NECK OF THE RADIUS

This fracture occurs *in children.* It is a valgus injury of the elbow. Displacements are usually mild, and immobilisation of such fracture in an above-elbow plaster slab for 2-3 weeks is generally sufficient. In some cases with severe angulation (usually more than 60°), it may be possible to achieve acceptable reduction by closed manipulation. Sometimes, open reduction and fixation with K-wire is required. Cubitus valgus deformity may occur in a malunited fracture.

FRACTURE OF THE CAPITULUM

This is an uncommon fracture, seen in adults. The chipped off capitulum may get displaced into the joint. Due to overlap of bones, the fracture fragment may go unnoticed on X-rays. If the fragment is small or comminuted, excision is carried out. If it is a big fragment, open reduction and internal fixation is performed.

 What have we learnt?

- Three bony point relationship has a diagnostic value in elbow fractures.
- Supracondylar fracture is a common injury in children, and is fraught with complications such as malunion, Volkmann's ischaemia, etc.
- Fracture of the lateral condyle of humerus is a type IV epiphyseal injury, and needs primary internal fixation in most cases.
- A displaced olecranon fracture needs early surgery, as it commonly leads to non-union.
- Fractures around the elbow, commonly missed on X-rays are: (a) fracture capitulum; (b) fracture medial epicondyle; (c) fracture head or neck of radius; and (d) fracture lateral condyle.

Additional information: From the entrance exams point of view

- Anconeus triangle formed by radial head, lateral epicondyle and the tip of the olecranon.
- The most common cause of Volkmann's ischaemic contracture (VIC) in a child is supracondylar fracture of the humerus.
- Most common muscle involved in VIC is flexor digitorum profundus.
- Head of radius excision leads to valgus deformity at the elbow.

Injuries of the Forearm and Wrist

Competencies

- ❖ **OR2.5:** Describe and discuss the aetiopathogenesis, clinical features, mechanism of injury, investigation and principles of management of fractures of both bones forearm and Galeazzi and Monteggia injury.
- ❖ **OR2.6:** Describe and discuss the aetiopathogenesis, mechanism of injury, clinical features, investigations and principles of management of fractures of distal radius.

The radius and ulna are common sites for fracture in all age groups. These may result from direct or indirect injury. Frequently, these fractures are open, mostly from within (internal open fracture). Common combinations of injury in this region are: (i) fracture of both bones of the forearm; (ii) Monteggia fracture-dislocation and (iii) Galeazzi fracture-dislocation.

RELEVANT ANATOMY

Muscles controlling supination and pronation: Supination and pronation occur at the radio-ulnar joints. The muscles producing these movements are attached to the forearm bones, and are responsible for the rotational displacement of these fractures. The supinators of the forearm (biceps and the supinator) are attached to the radius in its proximal-third (Fig. 15.1). The pronators (pronator teres and pronator quadratus) are attached to the middle and distal-thirds of the radius respectively. This means that the supinators control the proximal half of the forearm whereas the pronators control the distal-half.

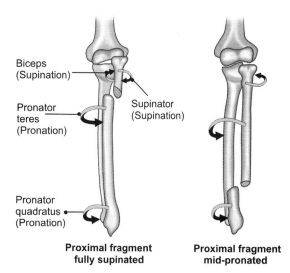

Fig. 15.1: Muscles of forearm and displacements after fracture.

Therefore, in fractures of the proximal-third of the forearm bones, the proximal half of the forearm has only supinators attached to it, and is supinated. The distal half on the other hand is pronated. In fractures of the middle-third, both the proximal and the distal halves of the forearm are in mid-pronation. This knowledge helps in predicting relative positions of the proximal and distal halves of the forearm after a fracture. Once this is known, the reduction can be obtained by realigning the distal part of the forearm in relation to the expected rotational position of the proximal part.

Radio-ulnar articulation: The radius and ulna articulate with each other by the proximal and distal radio-ulnar joints, and interosseous membrane. Hence, an injury to the forearm usually results in fractures of both the bones. In a case where there is a fracture of only one bone, and the fracture is displaced, there should be dislocation of the proximal or the distal radio-ulnar joint.

FRACTURES OF THE FOREARM BONES

The radius and ulna are commonly fractured together, hence commonly termed 'fracture of both bones of the forearm'. Sometimes, there may be an isolated fracture of either of the bone, usually without much displacement. The cause of fracture may be either an indirect force such as a fall on the hand, or a direct force such as a *'lathi'* blow to the forearm.

DISPLACEMENTS

In children, these fractures are often undisplaced or minimally displaced (greenstick fractures), but in adults they are notoriously prone to severe displacement. A combination of any of the following displacements may occur:
- Angulation - commonly medial and anterior
- Shift - in any direction
- Rotation - the proximal and distal fragments lie in different positions of rotations (e.g., the proximal fragment may be supinated and the distal pronated).

DIAGNOSIS

It is usually simple because of the obvious signs. Fractures in children are often undisplaced, may not have much signs, and are often go unnoticed.

TREATMENT

Conservative treatment has been the primary mode of treatment in the past, but recently, with availability of improved operative techniques, most of these fractures, at least in adults, are treated by operative methods. Fractures in children are even today, treated primarily by conservative methods is sufficient in most cases.

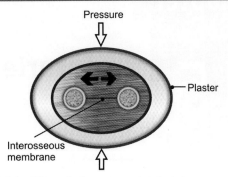

Fig. 15.2: Moulding of plaster to maintain interosseous space.

Conservative treatment: This consists of closed reduction by manipulation under general anaesthesia, and immobilisation in an above-elbow plaster cast.

Technique of closed manipulation: The elbow is flexed to 90°. The surgeon applies traction to the hand against counter-traction by an assistant grasping the upper arm. Angulation and displacement are generally corrected by traction alone. The distal part of the forearm can now be placed in the correct rotational alignment in relation to the proximal part, as judged from the site of the fracture (Refer, Fig. 15.1). Once a fracture is reduced, an above-elbow plaster cast is applied. It is important to keep the two bones apart and maintain the interosseous space, by moulding the cast while it is setting (Fig. 15.2). Weekly X-rays should be taken for 3 weeks, for early detection of redisplacement.

Open reduction and internal fixation: This is a preferred method in adults as it is difficult to obtain satisfactory reduction by closed manipulation, and also, to maintain that position in plaster. The following points have to be kept in mind while treating these fractures operatively.
- The radius and ulna should be approached through separate incisions to avoid cross union.
- Compression plating is the preferred method, the other method being intramedullary nailing.
- Additional bone grafting should be used in fractures older than three weeks.
- The limb may sometimes be immobilised post-surgery, depending upon rigidity of the fixation.
- External fixation is used in compound fracture for ease of dressing.

Deciding plan of treatment: Main point is to decide whether it is a closed or an open fracture. If it is a closed fracture, as it commonly is, the plan of treatment is as shown in Flowchart 15.1.

Flowchart 15.1: Plan of treatment of forearm bone fractures.

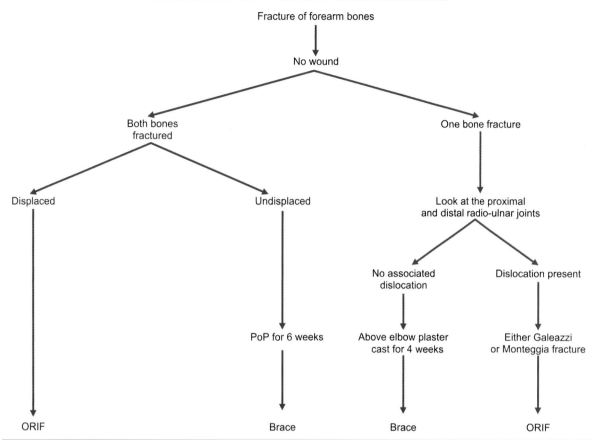

ORIF: Open reduction and internal fixation.
Brace: A plastic moulded support for the forearm with a possibility to mobilise joints, generally used after 4-6 weeks of immobilisation.

COMPLICATIONS

1. **Infection:** An open fracture of both bones of the forearm may become secondarily infected, leading to osteomyelitis.
2. **Volkmann's ischaemia:** This occurs within 8 hours of injury, as a result of ischaemic damage to the muscles of the flexor compartment of the forearm (For details, please refer to page 99).
3. **Delayed union and non-union:** Fractures of shafts of both bones of the forearm are prone to delayed union, particularly that of ulnar shaft at the junction of the middle and lower-thirds. The cause of non-union is usually inadequate immobilisation. Partial impairment of the blood supply to one of the fragments is also a contributory factor in some cases.
   Treatment: Treatment of non-union of these bones is open reduction and internal fixation using plates, and bone grafting. In a non-union involving the distal 5 cm of the ulna, good functions can be achieved by simply excising the short distal fragment.
4. **Malunion:** This results from failure to achieve and maintain a good reduction so that the bones

unite in an unacceptable position, leading to deformity and limitation of movement - especially that of rotation of the forearm. Treatment is open reduction and internal fixation using plates, and bone grafting.

5. **Cross union:** When radius and ulna fractures are joined to each other by a bridge of callus, it is called a cross union. It is likely to develop in a case where the two fractures are at the same level. It result in a complete limitation of forearm rotations.
   Treatment: If the cross union is in mid-pronation, the position most suitable for function, it is left as it is. If it occurs in excessive pronation or supination, operative treatment may be required. The cross union is undone, malalignment corrected, and the fracture internally fixed.

MONTEGGIA* FRACTURE-DISLOCATION

This is a fracture of the upper-third of the ulna with dislocation of the head of the radius. It is caused by a

---

*To remember, in Monteggia, medial side bone (i.e., ulna) is fractured.

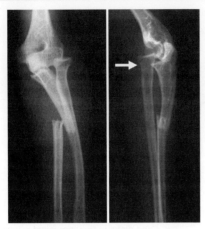

Fig. 15.3: X-rays of the forearm, AP and lateral views, showing Monteggia fracture-dislocation. Note anteriorly dislocated head of the radius (arrow).

fall on an out-stretched hand. It may also result from a direct blow on the back of the upper forearm.

TYPES

These fall into two main categories depending upon the angulation of the ulna fracture - extension and flexion type. The extension type, is the more common of the two, where the ulna fracture angulates anteriorly (extends) and the radial head dislocates anteriorly. The flexion type is where the ulna fracture angulates posteriorly (flexes) and the radial head dislocates posteriorly.

DIAGNOSIS

In a case with an isolated fracture of the ulna in its upper half, a dislocation of the head of the radius should be carefully looked for (Fig. 15.3).

TREATMENT

This is a very unstable injury, frequently redisplacing even if it has been reduced once. One attempt at reduction under general anaesthesia is justified. If reduction is successful, a close watch is kept by weekly check X-rays for the initial 3–4 weeks. In case, the reduction is not possible or if redisplacement occurs, an open reduction and internal fixation using a plate is performed. The radial head automatically falls into position, once the ulna fracture is reduced.

COMPLICATIONS

Malunion occurs commonly in cases treated conservatively, because of an undetected re-displacement within the plaster. It causes deformity of the forearm and limitation of elbow and forearm movements.

GALEAZZI FRACTURE-DISLOCATION

This injury is the counterpart of the Monteggia fracture-dislocation. Here, there is a fracture of the lower third of the radius with dislocation or subluxation of the distal radio-ulnar joint. It commonly results from a fall on an outstretched hand.

DISPLACEMENT

The radius fracture is angulated medially and anteriorly (Fig. 15.4). The distal radio-ulnar joint is disrupted, resulting in dorsal dislocation of the distal end of the ulna.

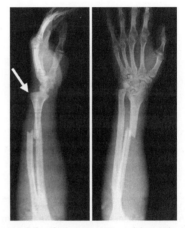

Fig. 15.4: X-rays of the forearm, AP and lateral views, showing Galeazzi fracture-dislocation. Note the dislocated distal radio-ulnar joint (arrow).

DIAGNOSIS

In an isolated fracture of the distal-half of the radius, the distal radio-ulnar joint must be carefully evaluated for subluxation or dislocation.

TREATMENT

Perfect reduction is essential for complete restoration of functions, particularly rotation of the forearm. It is difficult to achieve and maintain perfect reduction by conservative methods (except in children). Most adults require open reduction and internal fixation of the radius with a plate. The dislocated radio-ulnar joint may automatically fall back in place or may require open reduction.

COMPLICATIONS

Malunion occurs because of displacement of the fragment. It results in deformity and limitation of supination and pronation.

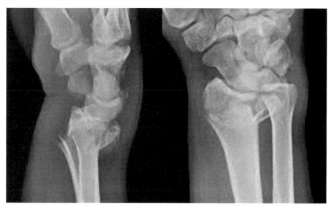

Fig. 15.5: X-ray of the wrist, AP and lateral views, showing a Colles' fracture. Note that the distal articular surface of the radius faces dorsally (tilted dorsally).

COLLES' FRACTURE

This is a fracture at the distal end of the radius, at its cortico-cancellous junction (about 2 cm from the distal articular surface), in adults, with typical displacement (Fig. 15.5). It is the most common fracture in people above forty years of age, and is particularly common in women because of post-menopausal osteoporosis. It nearly always results from a fall on an outstretched hand.

RELEVANT ANATOMY

The distal end of the radius articulates with the carpal bones (radio-carpal joint), and the distal end of the ulna (radio-ulnar joint). Normally, the distal articular surface of the radius faces ventrally and medially (Fig. 15.6). The tip of the radial styloid is about 1 cm distal to the tip of the ulnar styloid.

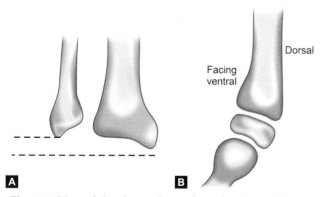

Fig. 15.6: Normal distal articular surface of radius: (A) Faces medially; (B) Faces ventrally.

PATHOANATOMY

Displacement: The fracture line runs transversely at the corticocancellous junction. In the majority of cases, one or more of the displacements described

below occur; although in a few cases it may be a crack fracture without displacement. The following are the displacements seen in Colles' fracture (Fig. 15.7):

- Impaction of fragments
- Dorsal displacement
- Dorsal tilt
- Lateral displacement
- Lateral tilt
- Supination

As the displacement occurs, some amount of comminution of the dorsal and lateral cortices, and that of the soft cancellous bone of the distal fragment occurs. Rarely, the whole of the distal fragment is broken into pieces. Some of the following injuries are commonly associated with Colles' fracture:

- Fracture of the styloid process of the ulna.
- Rupture of the ulnar collateral ligament.
- Rupture of the triangular cartilage of the ulna.
- Rupture of the interosseous radio-ulnar ligament, causing radio-ulnar subluxation.

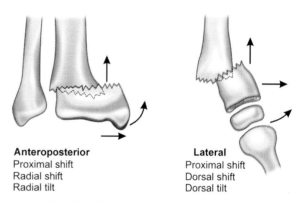

Anteroposterior
Proximal shift
Radial shift
Radial tilt

Lateral
Proximal shift
Dorsal shift
Dorsal tilt

Fig. 15.7: Displacements in Colles' fracture.

DIAGNOSIS

Clinical features: The patient presents with pain, swelling and deformity of the wrist. On examination, tenderness and irregularity of the lower end of the radius is found. There may be a typical 'dinner fork deformity' (Fig. 15.8). The radial styloid process

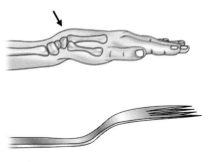

Fig. 15.8: Dinner fork deformity.

comes to lie at the same level or a little higher than the ulnar styloid process.

Radiological features: It is important to differentiate this fracture from other fractures at the same site (e.g., Smith's fracture, Barton's fracture) by looking at the displacements.

The dorsal tilt is the most characteristic displacement. It can be detected by looking at the direction of the distal articular surface of the radius on a lateral X-ray. Normally it faces ventrally*. If after fracture it faces dorsally or becomes neutral, a dorsal tilt has occurred. Similarly, a lateral tilt can be detected on an anteroposterior X-ray. Normally the distal articular surface faces medially; if it faces laterally or becomes horizontal, a lateral tilt has occurred. Most displacements can be identified on X-ray.

TREATMENT

Treatment of Colles' fracture is essentially conservative. For an undisplaced fracture, immobilisation in a below-elbow plaster cast for six weeks is sufficient. For displaced fractures, the standard method of treatment is manipulative reduction followed by immobilisation in Colles' cast (Fig. 15.9). Lately, due to improvement in surgical techniques and more functional demands of the patients, operative method is being used more and more.

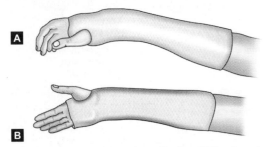

Fig. 15.9: Colles' cast: (A) In palmar flexion; (B) In ulnar deviation.

CONSERVATIVE TREATMENT

This is done by manipulation under anaesthesia and plaster cast immobilization.

Technique of closed manipulation (Fig. 15.10): The muscles of forearm must be relaxed, either by general or regional anaesthesia. The surgeon grasps the injured hand as if he was 'shaking hands'. The first step is to disimpact the fragments which have

*Normal ventral tilt of the distal articular surface can be identified on lateral X-ray of the wrist by noting that the surface faces; (i) toward the side of the thumb; and (ii) toward the thicker soft-tissues of the palm, both of which are structures on ventral side.

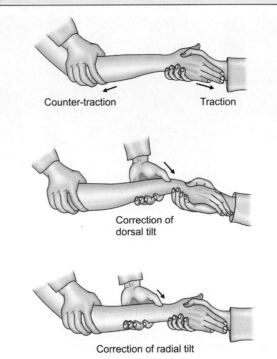

Fig. 15.10: Technique of reduction of Colles' fracture.

often been driven together. This is achieved by firm longitudinal traction to the hand against the counter-traction by an assistant who grasps the arm above the flexed elbow. Some displacements are corrected by traction alone. The surgeon now presses the distal fragment into palmar flexion and ulnar deviation using the thumb of his other hand. As this is done, the patient's hand is drawn into pronation, palmar flexion and ulnar deviation. A plaster cast is applied extending from below the elbow to the metacarpal heads, maintaining the wrist in palmar flexion and ulnar deviation. This is Colles' cast.

An X-ray is taken to check the success of the closed reduction. Besides displacements, it is important to look for correction of the dorsal tilts, i.e., the distal articular surface of the radius must face ventrally (as in a normal case).

The patient is encouraged to move his fingers as soon as the plaster dries. In addition, the shoulder and elbow joints are moved through their full range several times in a day. It is important to make check X-rays every week for the first three weeks in order to detect re-displacement. The plaster is removed after six weeks and joint mobilising and muscle strengthening exercises started for the wrist and fingers.

OPERATIVE TREATMENT

Whereas non-operative treatment remains the mainstay of treatment in elderly, where malunion is compatible with their functional requirement. In younger people more and more fractures are being treated operatively. Even in elderly people, where fracture is badly displaced or has intra-articular extension, operative treatment is preferred. The following are the common techniques of operatively treating these fractures (Fig. 15.11).

i. *Plating* (Fig. 15.11B): In this technique, the fracture is opened from the front, reduced under direct vision and fixed securely with a plate. A more recent addition to the plating technique is anatomically contoured locking compression plates.

ii. *Percutaneous pinning* (Fig. 15.11A): In this technique, the fracture is reduced under anaesthesia, under X-ray control (image intensifier). The same is fixed by passing two or more 2 mm steel wires (K-wires) percutaneously without any cutting. The fracture is thus transfixed (Fig. 15.11B). For additional support the part is immobilized in plaster for 6 weeks.

iii. *External fixation* (Fig. 15.11C): In some centres, an external fixator is used to keep the fracture 'distracted', so that the stretched ligaments and periosteum keep the comminuted fragments in place. The principle behind use of this technique is called ligamentotaxis.

COMPLICATIONS

Most patients progress rapidly to full functional recovery. Stiffness of the fingers and malunion are common complications. Other complications seen occasionally are - Sudeck's osteodystrophy, carpal tunnel syndrome, and rupture of the extensor pollicis longus tendon.

1. **Stiffness of joints:** Finger stiffness is the most common complication; the shoulder, wrist and elbow are the other joints which commonly get stiff. This occurs because of lack of exercise, and can be prevented by actively moving these joints. The joints which are out of plaster should be moved several times a day.

2. **Malunion:** A Colles' fracture always unites, but malunion occurs in a large proportion of cases. The cause of malunion is redisplacement of the fracture within the plaster so that a 'dinner fork' deformity results. There may be a limitation of wrist movement and forearm rotation.
   Treatment: Not always does a malunited Colles' fracture need treatment. Often, the only disadvantage is the ugly deformity, which does not hamper the day-to-day activities of the patient. In some active adults, the deformity and impairment of functions may be severe enough to justify correction by an osteotomy.

3. **Subluxation of the inferior radio-ulnar joint:** Shortening of the radius because of the impaction of the distal fragment leads to subluxation of the distal radio-ulnar joint. The head of the ulna becomes unduly prominent. Wrist movements, especially ulnar deviation and forearm rotations are painful and restricted.
   Treatment: A minor degree of displacement, especially in an elderly person may be accepted. In selected cases, excision of the lower end of the ulna (Darrach's resection) is worthwhile.

4. **Carpal tunnel syndrome:** This uncommon complication, occurs a long time after the fracture unites. The median nerve is compressed in the carpal tunnel, which is encroached by the fracture callus. Treatment is decompression of the carpal tunnel.

5. **Sudeck's osteodystrophy:** Colles' fracture is the most common cause of Sudeck's dystrophy in the upper limb. It is noticed after the plaster is removed. The patient complains of pain, stiffness and swelling of the hand. The overlying skin appears stretched and glossy. Treatment is by intensive physiotherapy. Full recovery takes a long time, but eventually occurs.

6. **Rupture of the extensor pollicis longus tendon:** This is an extremely rare complication and occurs a long time after the fracture has united. It is either due to loss of blood supply to the tendon at the time of fracture (a tiny vessel supplying blood to a part of the tendon is severed), or due to friction the tendon is subjected to everytime it moves over a malunited fracture. Treatment is by tendon transfer (extensor indicis to extensor pollicis longus).

SMITH'S FRACTURE (REVERSE OF COLLES' FRACTURE)

This uncommon fracture is seen in adults and in elderly people. Its importance lies in differentiating

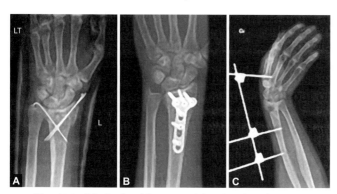

Fig. 15.11: Methods of fixation of distal radius fracture.

it from the more common Colles' fracture which occurs at the same site. It differs from Colles' fracture in that the distal fragment displaces ventrally and tilts ventrally. Treatment is by closed reduction and plaster cast immobilisation for 6 weeks. Operative treatment with plating is preferred in selected patients. Complications are similar to those in Colles' fracture.

BARTON'S FRACTURE

This is an intra-articular fracture of the distal radius. Here, the fracture extends from the articular surface of the radius to either its anterior or posterior cortices. The small distal fragment gets displaced and carries with it, the carpals (Fig. 15.12).

Depending upon the displacement, there is a volar Barton's fracture (anterior type), and a dorsal Barton's fracture (posterior type). *Treatment* is closed manipulation and a plaster cast. Open reduction and internal fixation with plate may be required in those cases where closed reduction fails. It may be considered as a primary choice in young adults with significantly displaced fractures.

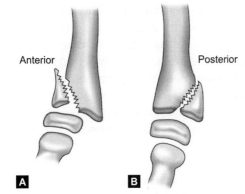

Fig. 15.12: Barton's fracture:(A) Anterior; (B) Posterior.

SCAPHOID FRACTURE

A scaphoid fracture is more common in young adults. It is rare in children and in elderly people. Commonly, the fracture occurs through the waist of the scaphoid (Fig. 15.13). Rarely, it occurs through the tuberosity. It may be either a crack fracture or a displaced fracture.

DIAGNOSIS

Clinical features: Pain and swelling over the radial aspect of the wrist following a fall on an outstretched hand, in an adult, should make one suspect strongly the possibility of a scaphoid fracture. On examination, one may be able to elicit tenderness in the scaphoid

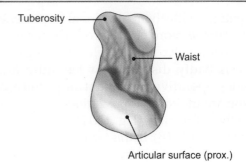

Fig. 15.13: The scaphoid bone.

fossa* (anatomical snuff box). A force transmitted along the axis of second metacarpal may produce pain in the region of the scaphoid bone.

Radiological features: Whenever suspected, an oblique view of the wrist, in addition to the antero-posterior and lateral views, is essential. Sometimes, it is just a crack fracture (Fig. 15.14) and is not visible on initial X-rays. If a fracture is strongly suspected, X-rays should be repeated after 2 weeks.

TREATMENT

Scaphoid fracture has been an apparently innocuous fracture but with high rate of non-union. The treatment used to be primarily conservative in the past, needing use of plaster for long periods. With improvement in operative techniques, this fracture is treated operatively more often than not.

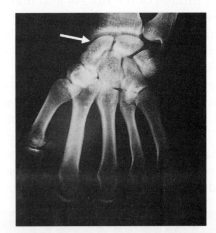

Fig. 15.14: X-ray of the wrist showing fracture of the scaphoid.

Conservative treatment: Usually reserved for undisplaced fractures. In this, the affected hand is immobilised in a scaphoid cast for 3–4 months. Sometimes, the fracture may not be visible on the

---

* It is the fossa between tendons of extensor pollicis longus and brevis, at the wrist.

initial X-ray, and becomes obvious only on X-rays done 3–4 weeks from injury. All such cases with clinical suspicion of a scaphoid fracture, are initially treated in a scaphoid cast for 2 weeks. After 2 weeks, an X-ray is taken again. Sometimes, the fracture becomes visible at this stage, because of resorption of the fracture ends. In such cases, it is treated as any other scaphoid fracture. If there is no fracture visible even after 2 weeks, the plaster is removed and patient treated as soft tissue injury to the wrist by appropriate physiotherapy.

Scaphoid cast: This is a cast extending from below the elbow to the metacarpal heads, includes the thumb, up to the interphalangeal joint. The wrist is maintained in a little dorsiflexion and radial deviation (glass holding position).

Operative treatment: There is a shift towards treatment of these fractures operatively at the very first instance due to high rate of non-union. There are two ways of treating them operatively: (i) open reduction and internal fixation using a special compression screw (Herbert screw); (ii) Percutaneous reduction and fixation under image intensifier control, using Herbert screws (Fig. 15.15).

COMPLICATIONS

Fractures of the scaphoid bone are potentially troublesome. The incidence of complications, inspite of the best treatment, is high. The most important complications are as follows:

1. **Avascular necrosis:** The blood supply of the scaphoid is precarious. In fractures through the waist, there is high probability of the proximal fragment becoming avascular. The patient

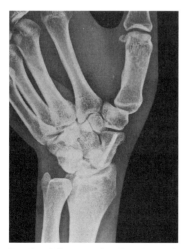

Fig. 15.15: Scaphoid fracture fixed with Herbert's screw.

complains of pain and weakness of the wrist. On the X-ray one finds non-union of the fracture with sclerosis and crushing of the proximal pole of the scaphoid.

Treatment: It is a difficult problem to treat. If the patient is symptomatic, the avascular segment of the bone is excised. In some cases, the wrist develops osteoarthritis, and is treated accordingly (as discussed later).

2. **Delayed and non-union:** A high proportion of cases of fractures of the scaphoid go into delayed or non-union. More than one factor contributes to this. It may be because of imperfect immobilisation, the synovial fluid hindering the formation of fibrinous bridge between the fragments, or impaired blood supply to one of the fragments. The diagnosis is made on the X-ray. In delayed union, the fracture, line may persist on X-ray even after 4–6 months. In non-union, distinct radiological features present are: (i) rounding of the fracture surfaces; (ii) the fracture becomes rather sharply defined; and (iii) cystic changes occur in one or both fragments. In a late case of non-union, changes of wrist osteoarthritis such as joint space reduction, osteophyte formation may also be seen.

Treatment: The treatment of delayed union and non-union depends largely on the severity of the symptoms. In a case where functions are not much impaired, nothing needs to be done. In a case where there is wrist pain and weakness of grip, operative intervention is necessary. For delayed union, bone grafting is sufficient. For non-union, the type of operation depends upon the presence of associated osteoarthritis of the radio-carpal joint. Once this happens, it is too late to expect relief by aiming at fracture union alone. An excision of part of the radio-carpal joint, or its fusion may be required.

3. **Wrist osteoarthritis:** In some cases of scaphoid fractures, osteoarthritis of the wrist develops as a result of avascular necrosis or non-union. Treatment depends upon the symptoms. Conservative treatment with hot fomentation and physiotherapy is sufficient in most cases. In some, excision of the styloid process of the radius; or in extreme cases, wrist arthrodesis may be required.

LUNATE DISLOCATIONS

These are rare dislocations of the wrist. These are of two types: lunate dislocation and peri-lunate

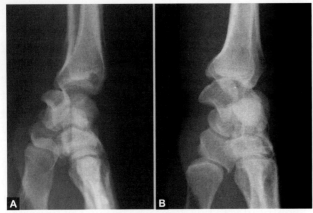

Fig. 15.16: Lateral views of the wrist X-rays showing: (A) Lunate dislocation; (B) Peri-lunate dislocation.

dislocation (Fig. 15.16). In *lunate dislocation* the lunate dislocates anteriorly but the rest of the carpals remain in position. In *peri-lunate dislocation*, the lunate remains in position and the rest of the carpal bones dislocate dorsally. The former type is more common. *Treatment* is usually by open reduction. Severe loss of wrist movements is inevitable. Avascular necrosis of the lunate is a common complication.

What have we learnt?

- Forearm fractures are common, usually displaced. Open reduction has become a method of choice in unstable, displaced fractures; and in those associated with radio-ulnar joint dislocations (Monteggia and Galeazzi).
- Colles' fracture occurs at the corticocancellous function of the distal radius. It is often comminuted and displaced. It usually malunites, but this does not cause much functional disability. Colles' fracture should be differentiated from less common Smith's fracture and Barton's fracture.

Additional information: From the entrance exams point of view

Fractures of both bones of the forearm, above the insertion of the pronator teres is immobilised in supination, below the insertion of the pronator teres is immobilised in mid-neutral position.

Learning Objectives

- ❖ Discuss evaluation and approach to treatment of a crushed hand.
- ❖ Discuss types, diagnosis and treatment of tendon injuries of the hand.

The hand is an important functional unit of the upper limb without which the whole of the upper limb becomes almost useless. This calls for adequate treatment of all hand injuries, howsoever minor they may appear. The following discussion includes only the important hand injuries.

BENNETT'S FRACTURE-DISLOCATION

It is an oblique *intra-articular* fracture of the base of the first metacarpal with subluxation or dislocation of the metacarpal [Fig. 16.1(A)]. It is sustained as a result of a longitudinal force applied to the thumb.

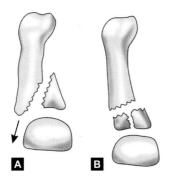

Fig. 16.1: (A) Bennett's fracture; (B) Rolando's fracture.

TREATMENT

Accurate reduction and restoration of the smooth joint surface is important. This is because, being an intra-articular fracture, if not reduced accurately, it will lead to incongruity of the articular surfaces.

This would increase the chances of developing osteoarthritis. The following methods of treatment are used:

a. **Closed reduction and percutaneous K-wire fixation** under an image intensifier, is a good technique. K-wire is used and incorporated in a plaster cast (Fig. 16.2).

b. **Open reduction and internal fixation** with a K-wire or a screw may be necessary in some cases.

COMPLICATIONS

Osteoarthritis develops if the joint surface is left irregular. It may cause persistent pain and loss of grip, so the patient is disabled when attempting heavy work. Excision of the trapezium may be required in particularly painful arthritis cases.

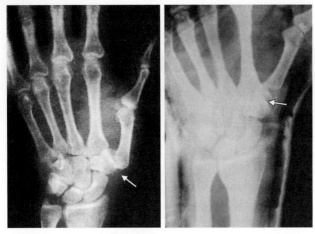

Fig. 16.2: X-rays showing Bennett's fracture-dislocation fixed with K-wire.

ROLANDO'S FRACTURE

This is a complete articular, 'T' or 'Y' shaped fracture of the first metacarpal [Fig. 16.1(B)]. Perfect reduction is not as important as in Bennett's fracture-dislocation. Treatment is by accurate reduction and fixation with 'K¹' wires (Fig. 16.2) and immobilisation in a thumb spica for 3 weeks.

FRACTURES OF THE METACARPALS

Fractures of the metacarpal shaft are common at all ages. The common causes are: (i) a fall on the hand, (ii) a blow on the knuckles (as in boxing) and (iii) crushing of the hand under a heavy object. Fracture of one or more metacarpals may occur. The fracture may be classified, according to the site, as follows:

a. Fracture through the base of the metacarpal, usually transverse and undisplaced.
b. Fracture through the shaft—transverse or oblique. These fractures are usually not much displaced because of the splinting effect of the interossei muscles and adjacent metacarpals. When more than one metacarpal shafts are fractured, this "autoimmobilisation" advantage is lost. Such fractures are unstable and require operative treatment.
c. Fracture through the neck of the metacarpal—It commonly affects the neck of the fifth metacarpal. The distal fragment is tilted forwards. It is usually sustained when a closed fist hits against a hard object [Boxer's fracture (Fig. 16.3)].

TREATMENT

Conservative treatment is sufficient in most cases. It consists of immobilisation of the hand in a light dorsal slab for 3 weeks. A minimal displacement is acceptable, but in cases with severe displacement or angulation, reduction is necessary. Reduction is achieved in most cases by closed reduction; and the same is held in place by percutaneously inserted K-wires. In some widely displaced fractures and in those with multiple metacarpal fractures, open reduction and secure internal fixation is done. It used to be using K-wires in the past, where extended period of additional immobilization was required. In present days, these fractures are fixed with mini plates and screws (Fig. 16.4). Advantage is early mobilisation and back to functions.

FRACTURES OF THE PHALANGES

These are common fractures, generally sustained by fall of a heavy object on the finger or crushing of fingers. The fractures can have various patterns, and may be displaced or undisplaced.

TREATMENT

Union is not a problem; the problem is maintaining proper alignment of the fracture. Treatment is as follows:

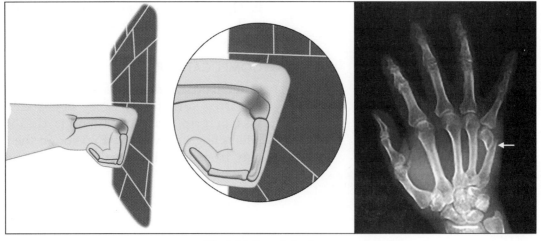

Fig. 16.3: Boxer's fracture.

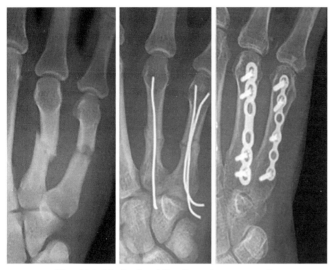

Fig. 16.4: Methods of fixation of metacarpals.

a. **Undisplaced fracture:** Treatment is basically for the relief of pain. A simple method of splintage is to strap the injured finger to an adjacent finger for 2 weeks (Fig. 16.5A). After this, finger mobilisation is started.

b. **Displaced fracture:** An attempt should be made to reduce the fracture by manipulation, and then immobilising in a simple malleable aluminium splint (Fig. 16.5B). Active exercises must be started not later than 3 weeks after the injury. If displacement cannot be controlled by the above means, a percutaneous fixation or open reduction and internal fixation using K-wire, may

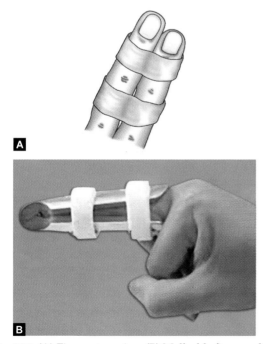

Fig. 16.5: (A) Finger strapping; (B) Malleable finger splint.

be necessary. A comminuted fracture of the tip of the distal phalanx does not need any special treatment, and attention should be directed solely to treatment of any soft tissue injury.

Mallet finger (Baseball finger) results from the sudden passive flexion of the distal interphalangeal joint so that the extensor tendon of the distal interphalangeal (DIP) joint is avulsed from its insertion at the base of the distal phalanx. Sometimes it takes a fragment of bone with it. Clinically, distal phalanx is in slight flexion. *Treatment* is by immobilising the DIP joint in hyperextension with the help of an aluminium splint or plaster cast.

DISLOCATION OF THE METACARPOPHALANGEAL JOINTS

These are uncommon injuries, resulting from hyperextension of the metacarpophalangeal (MP) joint, so that the head of the metacarpal button-holes through the volar capsule. The MP joint of the index finger is affected most commonly. Open reduction is required in most cases.

AMPUTATION OF FINGERS: PRINCIPLES OF TREATMENT

1. Every effort should be made to save as much length of the thumb as possible.
2. Amputations in children are more conservative.
3. Finger tip amputations need reconstruction in such a way that full-thickness skin covers the tip.
4. In amputations at the level of the distal phalanx, replantation is not possible.
5. Replantation is not performed in the elderly persons, or sometimes in labourers who do not need delicate functions of the hand. In such cases, rather the finger is amputated and the stump closed.
6. Thumb reconstruction is possible using microsurgical technique by: (i) replantation; (ii) pollicisation of the finger (one of the fingers is made into a thumb) and (iii) transfer of a toe with its neurovascular bundle using microsurgery.

TENDON INJURIES OF THE HAND

Flexor tendons of the fingers are commonly injured by sharp weapons. Extensor tendons are injured less commonly.

DIAGNOSIS

Often these injuries are missed. The reason is that an apparently 'small' cut wound in the hand is sutured as it is, without examining for the underlying tendon injury which goes unnoticed. Hence, whenever confronted with a wound over hand or wrist (or foot), one must visualise the tendons and nerves underlying that wound, and test for their function.

Testing for flexor tendons: For this, we must know the action of each and every flexor tendon in the hand.

Flexor carpi radialis and flexor carpi ulnaris: These are flexors of the wrist. To test for these, the patient is asked to palmar-flex the wrist. Normally, this motion occurs in the long axis of the forearm. In case tendon of one of the flexor carpi (radialis or ulnaris) is cut; the wrist while being flexed will deviate in the direction of the muscle whose tendon is intact. For example, if flexor carpi radialis is cut, on asking the patient to palmar-flex the wrist, one will see that the hand goes towards the ulnar side. The tendon of the muscle which is working can also be felt as it gets taut when the muscle contracts.

Flexor digitorum: There are two groups of these tendons, the flexor digitorum superficialis (FDS) and flexor digitorum profundus (FDP). The FDS flexes the proximal interphalangeal (PIP) joint; the FDP flexes primarily the distal interphalangeal (DIP) joint. But, since FDP runs across the PIP joint also, it causes flexion at this joint as well. To test FDP, the PIP joint of the respective finger is stabilized (Fig. 16.6A), and the patient asked to flex the DIP joint. It will not be possible if FDP of that finger is cut. FDS is tested by looking at flexion at PIP joint. But, in the presence of an intact FDP, even if FDS of that finger is cut, it will be possible to flex the PIP joint by the action of the FDP (which works on both PIP and DIP joints). This makes testing of cut FDS a little tricky. To be able to test the FDS

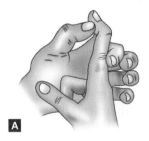

A

For testing flexor digitorum profundus.

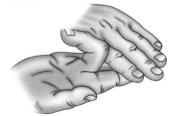

B   For testing flexor digitorum superficialis.

Fig. 16.6: Methods of testing flexor tendons of finger.

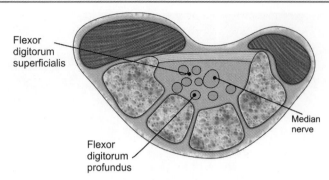

Fig. 16.7: Cut section through the wrist, showing arrangement of flexor tendons at that level.

of a finger, the action of FDP of that finger is to be eliminated. This is done by hyperextending the other fingers (Fig. 16.6B). By doing so, the FDP of the finger being tested is kept taut. This is because profundus tendons of all the fingers are interconnected by fibrous strands.

The arrangement of tendons of finger flexors is such at the wrist, that tendons of some fingers are cut more often than those of the others (Fig. 16.7). Small digital nerves and vessels run alongside flexor tendons, and are commonly cut along with flexor tendons.

Testing for extensor tendons: If extensor tendon of a finger is cut, the metacarpophalangeal (MP) joint cannot be extended. It is sometimes possible to mistake extension of the fingers at IP joints (and not at MP joints) as an indication of 'extensors working'. The finger extensors (extensor digitorum) extend only the MP joints. The IP joints are extended by slips from extensor expansion constituted by the lumbricals and interossei.

TREATMENT

Tendon injuries may be treated by the following methods:

a. **Primary repair,** end-to-end, if it is a clean cut injury. In the finger if both flexor tendons are cut, *only* the profundus tendon is repaired.

b. **Delayed repair,** reconstruction by tendon graft is performed if it is a crushed tendon. The palmaris longus is the most commonly used tendon for grafting.

c. **Tendon transfer:** If a tendon cannot be reconstructed, or sometimes as a matter of choice, another dispensable tendon can be transferred to its position, e.g., in rupture of the extensor pollicis longus, the extensor indicis can be used.

The results of tendon repair are best in injuries at the wrist, and are worst in those in the 'danger area' of the hand, i.e., the area of pulleys (between distal palmar crease and proximal interphalangeal joint). The danger area is also known as *'no man's land'*. Extensor tendon repair has better prognosis than flexor tendon repair. The main complication of tendon surgery is post-operative adhesion of the tendon to the surrounding tissues, thereby not allowing the tendon to glide properly.

CRUSH INJURY TO THE HAND

With industrialisation, the incidence of crush injury to the hand is on the rise. In developing countries, farm injuries, machine injuries and road traffic accidents constitute a majority of such injuries. The purpose of treatment in such injuries is to restore function of the hand. With advances in microsurgical techniques and powerful antibiotics, a lot of 'badly crushed hands', which were not considered salvageable in the past, can now be rehabilitated to useful function.

CONSIDERATIONS FOR AMPUTATION

The most demanding aspect of treatment of a crushed hand is the assessment of the injury. The first question faced by the treating doctor is whether the hand or its part is salvageable. The only indication for a primary amputation is an irreversible loss of blood supply to the part. In the absence of such an indication, a number of factors must be considered in deciding whether an amputation is advisable. These are discussed as follows:

a. **Age of the patient:** In children, amputation is indicated only when the part is totally non-viable. However, in persons over 50 years of age, amputation of one or two digits, except the thumb, may be indicated when both digital nerves and both flexor tendons are severed.
b. **Cause of crushing:** The severity of crushing can be judged from the history of injury. High speed, machine injuries produce more crushing than those caused by fall of a heavy object onto the hand. The causative factor also determines the extent of contamination, and thereby chances of infection; which in turn influences the decision to salvage the hand or not.
c. **Time since injury:** In developing countries, often a patient reaches the hospital after considerable delay, without proper first-aid. In such situations, there is increased risk of infection and poor tissue viability, which may tilt the balance in favour of an amputation.
d. **Severity of crushing:** A systematic examination of the hand, with a viewpoint to evaluate the five tissue areas (skin, tendon, nerve, bone and joint) helps in judging the severity of crushing. When three or more of these require special procedures such as grafting of skin, tendon suture, alignment

of bone and joint, amputation should be strongly considered.
e. **The part of the hand affected:** Every effort should be made to salvage as much of thumb and index finger as possible. One should be hesitant in amputating a finger when other fingers are also injured.
f. **Other considerations:** In some cases, the expected ultimate function of the part may not be good enough to warrant the time and effort required of the patient in not amputating the part. For example, a person engaged in manual labour may be served better by amputating a severely crushed finger, and putting him back to work, than subjecting him to a series of operations only to produce a 'cosmetic' finger.

PRINCIPLES OF TREATMENT

Hand injuries are usually neglected as they tend to occur in poor strata of the society. Even so called minor hand injuries can result in severe disability and make the whole upper limb useless. Careful evaluation, and treatment at specialized hand unit is key to good results. Once it has been decided on initial evaluation, that the crushed part of the hand can be salvaged, the purpose of treatment is to restore functions. Following basic principles guide the surgeon:

a. **Assessment of the injury:** A detailed history and thorough clinical examination is most important for accurate assessment of the injury. It is done in two stages: (i) soon after the patient is seen, preferably under sedation/GA, and (ii) again prior to the operation. The purpose of first examination is to assess whether the injury needs care in a specialised hand care unit. The basic principle guiding the assessment is that each one of the deeper structures must be considered damaged until proved otherwise. An orderly examination is helpful. Attention is first directed to the skin and then to bones, tendons and nerves. Repeated assessment over a period of time is important.
b. **Treatment priorities:** The first priority is thorough cleaning and debridement of the wound. Next is stabilisation of fractures and dislocations, and after that is wound closure with or without skin graft, skin flaps, etc. Nerves and tendons may be repaired in the primary phase of the care, but this is of secondary importance.
c. **Individual tissue considerations:** Even debridement of a crushed hand needs sufficiently experienced surgeon. The following strategy is adopted:
   i. Skin should be excised conservatively. Any enlargement of the skin wound must not cross a skin crease.

ii. Skeletal stabilisation is performed if fracture or dislocation is unstable. Joshi's fixator (JESS system) is a versatile fixator for stabilising all types of fractures of the bones of the hand, with the possibility of adequate soft tissue care. Small K-wires can also be used for this purpose. More recent is use of mini-plates, whereby the fractures can be securely fixed, and early rehabilitation.

iii. Primary repair of the extensor tendons, if ends can be visualised, is usually possible. Repair of the flexor tendons must not be attempted if the wound is grossly contaminated or if extensive dissection is required to find its ends. Cut ends of the tendons are either tagged to each other or to the surrounding tissues in order to prevent retraction. Secondary suture or grafting can be carried out 3–6 weeks later in such cases.

iv. Dead muscles, and those with doubtful viability are excised with care to avoid nerves. Digital nerves can be repaired primarily in a clean wound, or they can be repaired after 3–6 weeks.

d. **Proper splintage (Fig. 16.8):** Proper splintage of the hand during treatment is necessary, otherwise the ligaments at MP and IP joints shorten, causing stiffness. The ideal position of immobilisation is with the MP joints in 90° of flexion and IP joints in extension (Jame's position). In this position, the collateral ligaments of these joints are kept. If possible, the fingertips are left visible to evaluate circulation from time to time.

e. **Supportive care:** The following supportive care is required:

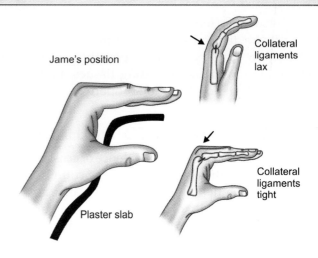

Fig. 16.8: Position of immobilisation of a hand.
(Note: MP joints in 90° flexion, IP joints in extension).

- Elevation of the hand for first 3-4 days to avoid oedema
- Finger movements to avoid oedema and stiffness
- Antibiotics, prophylaxis against tetanus and gas gangrene
- Suitable analgesics
- Dressings as necessary

Rehabilitation: In the initial period, this consists of exercises, wax bath and splintage. Later, various appliances may be designed to help the patient perform better. Once maximum benefit has been obtained by physiotherapy, secondary operations may be considered for further improvement in functions.

 What have we learnt?

- Intra-articular fracture of Ist metacarpal has to be accurately reduced, as it causes disabling arthritis.
- Minimally displaced metacarpal fractures can be treated by splintage.
- Phalangeal fractures need accurate reduction, sometimes surgically.
- Tendon injuries around the hand are often missed. A thorough clinical examination of each and every tendon is the key to diagnosis.
- Crushed hand is a serious injury. Prognosis depends upon accurate initial assessment, good first-aid and splintage, and early referral to specialised facility.

Additional information: From the entrance exams point of view

- The proximal fragment of a scaphoid fracture is more prone to avascular necrosis due to retrograde blood flow to the proximal fragment.
- Lunate dislocation can lead to median nerve injury.
- The incidence of injury in carpal bones is scaphoid > triquetral > trapezium > lunate.
- Bennett's fracture is difficult to maintain in a reduced position due to the pull of the abductor pollicis longus.
- Skier's thumb/Gamekeeper's thumb is an injury to the ulnar collateral ligament of the metacarpophalyngeal joint. It is injured during skiing, holding a catch and twisting the neck of small animals. An incomplete rupture is treated conservatively with a thumb spica or functional cast brace. A complete rupture is treated by surgical repair.
- Stener lesion occurs when the adductor pollicis aponeurosis becomes interposed between the retracted ligament, and this hinders healing.

Chapter 17

Pelvic Fractures

Topics

- ❖ Relevant anatomy
- ❖ Classification
- ❖ Pathoanatomy
- ❖ Diagnosis
- ❖ Treatment
- ❖ Complications

Competency

- ❖ **OR2.7:** Describe and discuss the aetiopathogenesis, mechanism of injury, clinical features, investigations and principles of management of pelvic injuries with emphasis on hemodynamic instability.
- ❖ **OR2.9:** Describe and discuss the mechanism of injury, clinical features, investigations and principle of management of acetabular fracture.

The incidence of pelvic fractures are on the rise following the increased number of vehicular accidents. It is commonly found as one of the fractures in a patient with multiple injuries. Often this fracture is not a serious management problem in itself, but may become so, because of the visceral complications so often associated with it. These fractures occur in all age groups but are most common in young adults.

RELEVANT ANATOMY

Pelvic ring: The pelvis is a ring-shaped structure joined in the front by the pubic symphysis and behind by the two sacroiliac joints. There are projecting iliac wings on either side, a frequent site of fractures. The pelvic ring is formed, in continuity from the front, by pubic symphysis, pubic crest, pectineal line of pubis, arcuate line of the ilium, and ala and promontory of the sacrum (Fig. 17.1). Fractures in the anterior half of the ring may have an associated injury in the posterior half. Such injuries make the pelvic ring unstable.

Stability of the pelvis: The stability of the pelvic ring depends, posteriorly on the sacroiliac joints and anteriorly on the symphysis pubis. The sacroiliac joints are bound in front and behind by the strong, band-like, sacroiliac ligaments (Fig. 17.2). The pubic symphysis is reinforced by ligamentous fibres above and below it.

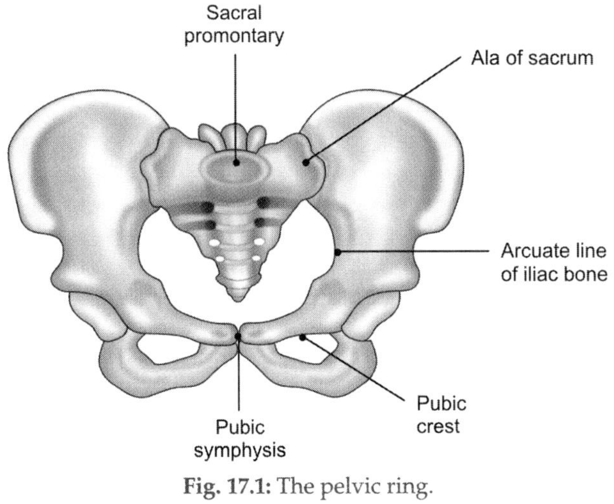

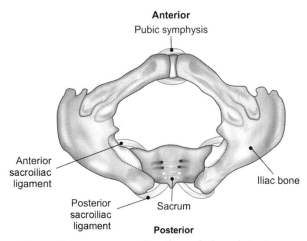

Fig. 17.1: The pelvic ring.

Fig. 17.2: Transverse section through the pelvic ring.

Accessory ligaments of the pelvis, such as iliolumbar ligament, sacrotuberous ligament and sacrospinous ligament provide additional stability to the ring.

Nerves in relation to the pelvis: The obturator nerve and the lumbo sacral trunk passes over the ala of the sacrum, and crosses the pelvic brim. These are likely to suffer injury in fractures in this region.

CLASSIFICATION

Marvin Tile (1988) classifies pelvis fractures on the basis of stability into three types: Types A, B and C (Table 17.1). Type A, the minimally displaced stable fractures, were previously known as 'isolated' fractures. Types B and C, the unstable fractures, were previously known as 'pelvic ring disruption' injuries.

Table 17.1: Classification of pelvic injuries (Tile, 1988).
Type A: Stable ▪ A1 – Fractures of the pelvis not involving the ring ▪ A2 – Stable, minimally displaced fractures of the ring **Type B: Rotationally unstable, vertically stable** ▪ B1 – Open-book type ▪ B2 – Lateral compression - ipsilateral ▪ B3 – Lateral compression - contralateral (Bucket-handle type) **Type C: Rotationally and vertically unstable** ▪ C1 – Unilateral ▪ C2 – Bilateral ▪ C3 – Associated with acetabular fracture

Type A: Stable, minimally displaced fractures: In this type, the pelvic ring is stable and the displacement is mild and insignificant. This type also involves the avulsion fractures of the parts of pelvis and fractures of the iliac wing, pubic rami fractures and undisplaced fractures of the acetabulum. These are generally treated conservatively, and have good prognosis.

Type B: Unstable fractures - rotationally unstable but vertically stable: In this type of injury, the pelvis is unstable. Rotational displacement can occur but no vertical displacement can occur. *Open-book injury* occurs when an anteroposterior force causes disruption of symphysis pubis, and thus tends to open up the pelvis (Fig. 17.3). There is no vertical displacement. The lateral injury to the pelvis is also a type of unstable pelvic fracture (type B). In this, the pelvis is hit from the side, resulting in compression injury to the posterior ring and fracture of the pubic ramus. This type of injury occurs when a pedestrian is hit from the side by a vehicle.

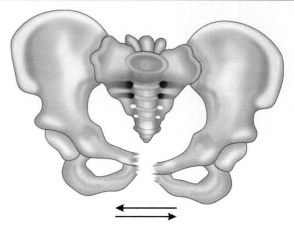

Fig. 17.3: Type B pelvis injury. Rotational displacement, no vertical displacement.

Type C: Unstable - rotationally and vertically: These are the most unstable injuries, the essential feature being vertical instability (Fig. 17.4). It usually occurs due to fall from height.

TYPE A INJURY—ISOLATED FRACTURES

This is the most common injury but the least serious of the three types. Any part of the pelvis may be affected. The essential feature being that the pelvis remains stable. Complications are uncommon in these relatively minor fractures of the pelvis. The following are some of the fractures included in this group:

Ischiopubic Rami Fracture

These are the most common of pelvic fractures. One or more rami may be fractured on one or both sides; the latter is called as *straddle fracture*. Displacement is usually minimal. The fracture of rami may extend into the acetabulum. There may be an associated injury to the urethra or bladder.

Clinically the patient presents with pain and tenderness over the fracture site. Sometimes, a

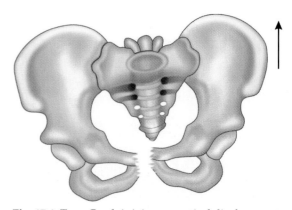

Fig. 17.4: Type C pelvis injury—vertical displacement.

patient with multiple injuries may not have any complaint referring to this fracture, and it is detected by the routine pelvic compression test (see page 124).

Radiologically, once an ischiopubic rami fracture is detected, one must carefully rule out an associated fracture in the posterior half of the pelvic ring (i.e., fracture through sacrum, sacroiliac joint or ilium). It is only after this is done that a diagnosis of 'isolated' pubic rami fracture can be made.

Treatment: These fractures pose no problems in successful union. Treatment is basically for relief of pain. Bed rest for 1–3 weeks is usually sufficient.

Iliac Wing Fracture

This is a relatively uncommon fracture resulting from direct injury to the wing of the ilium (e.g., in a road traffic accident). Sometimes, these patients may lose so much blood from 'vascular' iliac wings that they develop hypovolaemic shock. The fractures are otherwise without complications, and unite in 4–6 weeks with rest and analgesics.

AVULSION FRACTURE OF ANTERIOR INFERIOR ILIAC SPINE

The straight head of the rectus femoris muscle takes its origin from the anterior inferior iliac spine. Sometimes, due to a violent contraction of this muscle, as may occur during a jump, sprinting activity or kicking sports, the anterior inferior iliac spine may be pulled off (avulsed). The fracture unites quickly in 3–4 weeks without any complication.

ACETABULAR FRACTURES

Some of the undisplaced or minimally displaced fractures of the acetabulum can be considered in this group of relatively 'benign' fractures. These fractures usually unite without any complication. Late, secondary osteoarthritis develops in some cases because of the irregularity of the articular surface following the injury.

TRANSVERSE FRACTURES OF SACRUM AND COCCYX

Transverse fractures of the sacrum below the $S_{2,3}$ level, and that of the coccyx do not affect the stability of pelvis. Hence they are also considered Type A-type injuries.

TYPES B AND C INJURIES (RING DISRUPTION INJURIES)

These are uncommon but more important injuries because of the higher incidence of associated complications. Road traffic accidents are the most common cause of such injuries.

PATHOANATOMY

If a portion of the pelvic ring is broken, and the fragments displaced, there must be a fracture or dislocation in another portion of the ring. The following combinations of fracture and dislocation in anterior and posterior halves of the pelvis may occur:

Anterior	Posterior
■ Fracture of superior and inferior pubic rami ■ Disruption of pubic symphysis	■ Fracture through ala of sacrum ■ Dislocation through SI joint ■ Fracture through ilium

Displacements: It is generally slight. The type of displacement depends upon the force causing the fracture. The following displacements may occur:

a. *External rotation* of the hemi-pelvis (open-book type): The pelvic ring is opened up from the front like a book. There may be a pubic symphysis disruption or rami fractures in front and damage to the sacroiliac joint behind.

b. *Internal rotation of hemi-pelvis:* This may result from a lateral compression force. There may be an overlap anteriorly with or without a posterior lesion.

c. *Rotation superiorly* (bucket-handle type): The hemi-pelvis rotates superiorly along a horizontal anteroposterior axis.

d. *Vertical displacement:* This results from a vertical force causing upward displacement of half of the pelvis.

DIAGNOSIS

Clinical examination: Pelvic fractures are major injuries, often with little or no clinically obvious deformity. It may be one of the fractures in a seriously injured patient where the surgeon's attention may be diverted to other injuries with more obvious manifestations. A pelvic fracture must be carefully looked for in all cases of road accident, especially in those with multiple injuries, those associated with hypovolaemic shock, and those with major lower limb fractures (fracture of the femur, etc.). The pelvic compression test is a useful screening test in all such cases.

Pelvic compression test: The patient lies supine on the couch. The examiner compresses both iliac crests of the patient's pelvis towards each other. Any pain during this manoeuvre or a 'springy' feeling, is an indicator of pelvic fracture. A pelvic distraction test may reveal similar findings.

In displaced pelvic fractures there may be shortening of one of the lower limbs. The limb may lie in external rotation. There may be a haematoma in the region of pubic symphysis or at the back, in the region of sacroiliac joints. Palpation may reveal a localised tenderness or crepitus. A gap at the symphysis pubis is occasionally felt. There may be signs due to associated injury to the urethra, bladder or intestine, etc., as discussed on page 126. There may be anaesthesia or weakness of one leg due to injury to the sciatic plexus.

Radiological examination: Pelvis with both hips - AP is the basic X-ray required for screening purposes. In case there is a pelvic injury, special views (inlet/outlet views) are also sometimes necessary

CT scan helps in better evaluation of posterior injuries and also in cases where operative intervention is contemplated. With current CT scan machines 3-dimensional reconstruction is possible, which also helps in better evaluation of the fracture.

TREATMENT

The importance of treatment of pelvic fractures lies in identifying the possibility of life-threatening hypovolaemic shock and associated visceral injuries. The patient should be moved as little as possible, as movement at the fracture site may result in further bleeding or fat embolism.

Once the patient is stabilised, an assessment regarding the nature of the injury is made by suitable X-ray examination. Further treatment of the pelvic fracture depends on the type of fracture and presence of associated complications. In case a complication like urethral injury, etc., is present, emergency treatment for the same is executed. A pelvic fracture may fall into one of the following three categories from the treatment viewpoint:

a. **An injury with minimal or no displacement:** The patient is advised absolute bed rest for 3-4 weeks. Once the fracture becomes 'sticky' and the pain subsides, gradual mobilisation and weight bearing is permitted. It takes around 6-8 weeks for the patient to be up and about.

b. **An injury with anterior opening of the pelvis** (open-book injury): A minimal opening up (less than 2.5 cm) does not need any special treatment, and is treated on the lines of (a). Reduction is needed if the opening is more than 2.5 cm. This is done by manual pressure on the two iliac wings so as to 'close' the pelvic ring. The reduction thus

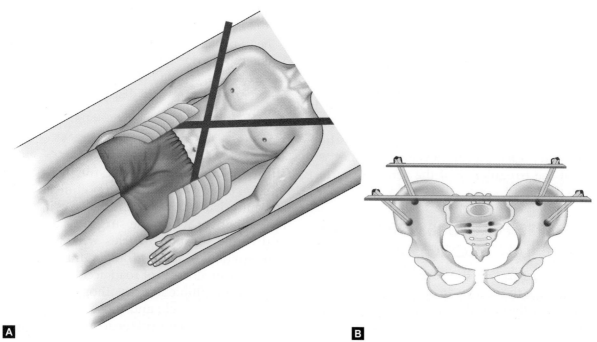

A   **B**

Fig. 17.5: Treatment of 'open-book' injury: (A) Hammock-sling; (B) External fixator.

Flowchart 17.1: Treatment plan for pelvic ring disruption injuries.

achieved is maintained by one of the following methods:

- *External fixator:* This is a reliable and comfortable method. Two or three pins threaded at the tip (Schanz pin) are inserted in the anterior part of the wing of the iliac bone on each side. After reduction of the displacement by manual pressure, the pins are clamped to a metal rod or frame placed transversely over the front of the pelvis (Fig. 17.5B).
- *Internal fixation:* The pubic symphysis disruption may be reduced and internally fixed with a plate.
- *Hammock-sling traction* (Fig.17.5A): It was a popular method in the past but poses nursing problems. The patient requires prolonged hospitalisation.

c. **Injuries with vertical displacement:** These are the most difficult pelvic injuries to treat. These are treated by bilateral upper tibial skeletal traction. A heavy weight (upto 20 kg) may be required to achieve reduction. After 3 weeks, the weight is reduced to about 10 kg to maintain the position. The traction is removed after 6-8 weeks, and the patient mobilised.

Flowchart 17.1 shows a treatment plan for pelvic ring disruption injuries.

There is now a trend towards treating these fractures by operative reduction and stabilisation. This method allows early mobility of the patient, and appealing to both the surgeon and the patient. However, it requires adequate facilities and a surgeon well-versed in operative fixation of these fractures.

COMPLICATIONS

1. **Rupture of urethra:** This is commonly associated in cases where wide disruption of symphysis pubis and pubic rami fractures is present. The urethra in males is more commonly injured—membranous urethra being the most common site. The rupture may be complete or incomplete, partial thickness

or full thickness. Diagnosis may be made by three cardinal signs of urethral injury, i.e., blood per urethra, perineal haematoma and distended bladder.

Treatment: It may be possible to pass a catheter gently in a case with partial and incomplete urethral tear. In case this fails, the help of a uro-surgeon should be sought. Principles of treatment are: (i) drainage of the bladder by suprapubic cystostomy; and (ii) micturating cystourethrogram after 6 weeks to assess the severity of urethral stricture, and treatment accordingly.

2. **Rupture of bladder:** The bladder is ruptured in pubic symphysis disruption or pubic rami fractures. In case the bladder is full at the time of injury, the rupture is usually extraperitoneal, and urine extravasates into perivesical space. Diagnosis may be suspected if a patient has not passed urine for a long time after the fracture. Catheterisation may be successful but only a few drops of blood-stained urine come out. A cystourethrogram will distinguish between a bladder and a urethral rupture.

Treatment: An urgent operation is required, preferably by a urologist. The principles of treatment are: (i) to repair the rent in the bladder; (ii) drainage of the bladder by an indwelling catheter, and (ii) to drain the urine in the prevesical space.

3. **Injury to rectum or vagina:** There may be disruption of the perineum with damage to the rectum or vagina. General surgeons and gynaecologists suitably manage these injuries.

4. **Injury to major vessels:** This is a rare but serious complication of a pelvic fracture. The common iliac artery or one of its branches may be damaged by a spike of bone. Aggressive management is crucial. If facilities are available, embolisation of the bleeding vessel under X-ray control is a good procedure. In other cases, the vessel is explored surgically and ligated or repaired.

5. **Injury to nerves:** In case of major disruption of the pelvic ring with marked vertical displacement of half of the pelvis, it is common for the nerves of the lumbo-sacral plexus to be injured. The damage may be caused by a fragment pressing on the nerves, or by stretching. *Treatment* is conservative. Recovery occurs in some cases, but in most the injury is irreversible and the consequent paralysis permanent.

6. **Rupture of the diaphragm:** A traumatic rupture of the diaphragm sometimes occurs in cases with severely displaced pelvic fractures. It is worthwhile getting an X-ray of the chest in case a patient with pelvic fracture complains of breathing trouble or pain in the upper abdomen. *Treatment* is by surgical repair.

 What have we learnt?

- Pelvic fractures are serious, potentially life-threatening injuries.
- These are often associated with visceral injuries.
- Prolonged hospitalization and in-bed immobilisation becomes necessary for treatment of these fractures.
- Operative fixation, resulting in early mobilisation has become a desired treatment now.

Additional information: From the entrance exams point of view

- In a pelvic fracture, the blood loss is 4–8 units.
- Jumper's fracture is a type of pelvic fracture.
- Kocher-Langenbeck approach is for posterior caudal exposure.
- Ilioinguinal approach is for internal or anterior approach.
- Extended iliofemoral approach is to expose both the anterior and posterior columns of acetabulum.

Injuries Around the Hip

Competencies

- ❖ **OR1.5:** Describe and discuss the aetiopathogenesis, clinical features, investigations, and principles of management of dislocation of major joints, shoulder, knee, hip.
- ❖ **OR2.10:** Describe and discuss the aetiopathogenesis, mechanism of injury, clinical features, investigations and principles of management of fractures of proximal femur.

These constitute some of the most difficult injuries of the musculoskeletal system, from treatment point of view. The following injuries will be discussed in this chapter: (i) dislocations of the hip; (ii) fractures of neck of the femur (intra-capsular); and (iii) intertrochanteric fractures (extra-capsular).

RELEVANT ANATOMY

The hip joint is a ball and socket joint with inherent stability, largely as a result of the adaptation of the articulating surfaces of the acetabulum and femoral head to each other. The capsule and ligaments of the joint provide additional stability.

The *acetabulum* faces an angle of 30° outwards and anteriorly. The normal neck-shaft angle of the femur is 125° in adults, with 15° of anteversion. The neck is made up of spongy bone with aggregation of bony trabeculae along the lines of stress. The most important of these is the *medial longitudinal trabecular stream.* These run from the lesser trochanter, along the medial cortex of the neck to the posteromedial quadrant of the head (Fig. 18.1). A thin vertical plate of bone springs from the compact medial wall of the shaft, and extends into the spongy bone of the neck. This is called the *calcar femorale.*

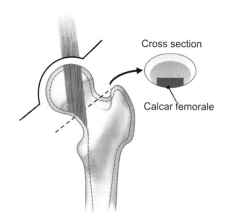

Fig. 18.1: Medial longitudinal trabeculae.

Blood supply of the femoral head: This comes from three main sources (Fig. 18.2): (i) the *medullary vessels* from the neck; (ii) the *retinacular vessels* entering from the lateral side of the head; and (iii) the *foveal vessel* from the ligamentum teres. The most important of these, (i) and (ii) are generally cut off following a fracture of the neck of the femur, and sometime result in avascular necrosis of the head.

- **Biomechanics of the hip:** The centre of gravity for a normal person, while standing, lies just in front of S$_2$ vertebra. When the person stands on one leg, the body weight tends to tilt the pelvis

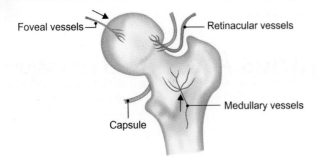

Fig. 18.2: Blood supply of head of the femur.

down to the other side. This tilt happens with the ipsilateral hip acting as a fulcrum. To counter this tilt, the abductors of the hip on the side on which one is standing, contract. It is like a lever system (Fig. 18.3). It thus helps in keeping the pelvis horizontal. This lever system (hip joint-neck of the femur – abductor muscles) is called *abductor mechanism of the hip*. It is important to understand this mechanism as this is relevant in interpreting a lot of symptoms of the hip. Quite a few treatment methods are based on understanding of this abductor mechanism.

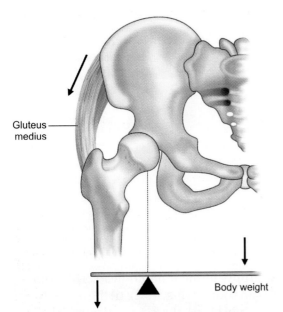

Fig. 18.3: Abductor mechanism of the hip.

DISLOCATIONS OF THE HIP

CLASSIFICATION

There are three main types of dislocations of the hip: (i) posterior dislocation (the *most common*); (ii) anterior dislocation; (iii) central fracture-dislocation. All of these may be associated with fracture of the lip of the acetabulum.

POSTERIOR DISLOCATION OF THE HIP

In this, the head of the femur is pushed out of the acetabulum posteriorly. In about 50% of cases, this is associated with fracture of the posterior lip of the acetabulum, in which case it is called a fracture-dislocation.

MECHANISM OF INJURY

The injury is sustained by violence directed along the shaft of the femur with the hip flexed. It requires a moderately severe force to dislocate a hip, as occurs in motor accidents. The occupant of the car is thrown forwards and his knee strikes against the dashboard. The force is transmitted up the femoral shaft, resulting in posterior dislocation of the hip. It is, therefore, also known as *dashboard injury*.

DIAGNOSIS

Clinical features: An isolated posterior dislocation of the hip is easy to diagnose. The patient presents with a history of severe trauma followed by pain, swelling and deformity (flexion, adduction and internal rotation). There is shortening of the leg. One may be able to feel the head of the femur in the gluteal region. The injury is sometimes missed, especially when associated with other more obvious injuries such as fracture of the shaft of the femur. It may also go unnoticed in an unconscious patient. To avoid this mistake, it is a convention to do X-ray the pelvis in *all* patients with fracture of the femur.

Radiological features: The femoral head is out of the acetabulum. The thigh is internally rotated, and hence the lesser trochanter is not visible. Shenton's line* is broken. One must look for any bony chip, either from the posterior lip of the acetabulum or from the head. A comparison from the opposite, normal side may be useful. CT scan may be necessary in cases where an associated fracture is suspected.

TREATMENT

Reduction of a dislocated hip is an *emergency.* Longer the head remains out, more the chances of it becoming avascular. In most cases it is possible to reduce the hip by *manipulation under* general anaesthesia. The chip fracture of the acetabulum, if present, usually falls in place as the head is reduced. *Open reduction* may be required in cases where: (i) closed reduction fails - usually in those presenting late; (ii) if there is intra-articular loose fragment not allowing accurate reduction; and (iii) if the acetabular fragment is large,

*It is an imaginary semi-circular line joining medial cortex of the femoral neck to lower border of the superior pubic ramus. See also Fig. 26.7 on page 217.

and is from the weight bearing part of the acetabulum. Presence of such a fragment makes the hip unstable.

Technique of closed reduction: The patient is anaesthetised and placed supine on the floor. An assistant grasps the pelvis firmly. The surgeon flexes the hip and knee at a right angle (Fig. 18.4), and exerts a pull along the long axis of the femur. Usually one hears a 'sound' of reduction, after which it becomes possible to move the hip freely in all directions. The leg is kept in light traction with the hip abducted, for 3 weeks. After this, hip mobilisation exercises are initiated.

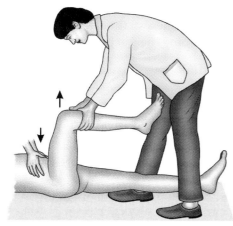

Fig. 18.4: Technique of reduction of hip dislocation.

COMPLICATIONS

1. **Injury to the sciatic nerve:** The sciatic nerve lies behind the posterior wall of the acetabulum. Therefore, it may be damaged in a posterior dislocation of the hip; more so if the dislocation is associated with a large bony fragment from the posterior lip of the acetabulum.
   Treatment: Injury is a neurapraxia in most cases and recovers spontaneously. In cases where the fragment of the posterior lip is not reduced by closed method, open reduction of the fracture, and nerve exploration may be required. If the sciatic nerve is severely damaged at this level, prognosis is poor.
2. **Avascular necrosis of the femoral head:** In some 15-20% of cases of posterior dislocation of the hip, the femoral head undergoes avascular necrosis. The changes of avascular necrosis appear on X-rays generally 1–2 years after the injury. The avascular head appears dense, and gradually collapses - wholly or in part. The patient complains of pain in the hip after a seemingly painless period following treatment for a dislocated hip. Over a period of a few years, changes of osteoarthritis

become apparent, clinically and radiologically. Such cases eventually need hip replacement.
3. **Osteoarthritis:** This is a late complication of hip dislocation, occurring a few to many years after the injury. The underlying cause may be an avascular deformed head, or an incongruous acetabulum and femoral head. The treatment is initially conservative. In some cases an operation may be necessary. Commonly, a total hip replacement is required (see also page 330).
4. **Myositis ossificans:** This occurs a few weeks to months after the injury. The patient complains of persistent pain and stiffness of the hip. X-rays shows a mass of fluffy new bone around the hip. It is particularly common in patients with head injury. Treatment is rest and analgesics (for details see page 52).

ANTERIOR DISLOCATION OF THE HIP

This is a rare injury, usually sustained when the legs are forcibly abducted and externally rotated. This may occur in a fall from a tree when the foot gets stuck and the hip abducts excessively, or in a road accident. Clinically, the limb is in an attitude of external rotation. There may be *true lengthening*, with the head palpable in the groin. Treatment is by closed manipulation. Complications are similar to that of posterior dislocation.

CENTRAL FRACTURE-DISLOCATION OF THE HIP

In this common injury, the femoral head is driven through the medial wall of the acetabulum towards the pelvic cavity (Fig. 18.5). The displacement of the head varies from the minimal to as much as the whole head

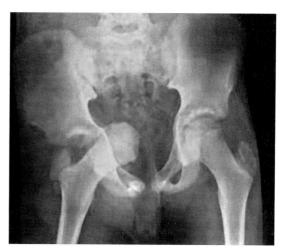

Fig. 18.5: X-ray of the hip, AP view, showing central fracture-dislocation.

lying inside the pelvis. Joint stiffness and osteoarthritis are inevitable. Therefore, the aim of treatment in these cases is to achieve as congruous an articular surface as possible. For this, skeletal traction is applied distally and laterally. If the fragments fall in place and reasonably reconstitute the articular margins, the traction is continued for 8–12 weeks. In some young individuals, in whom the fragments do not fall back in place by traction, surgical reconstruction of the acetabular floor may be necessary.

COMPLICATIONS

Hip stiffness, myositis and osteoarthritis are common complications of this injury.

FRACTURE OF NECK OF THE FEMUR

There are two fractures in the region of neck of the femur—intracapsular and extracapsular. As a matter of convention, the term 'fracture of the neck of the femur' is used for extracapsular fracture of the neck (Fig. 18.6). The extra-capsular fracture is commonly addressed as intertrochanteric fracture. The necessity to differently classify these two fractures which are otherwise in close proximity is due to the fact that *they behave differently*. Whereas, fracture of neck of the femur almost never unites, intertrochanteric fracture nearly always unites. Other differences between these two 'neighbours' are as given in Table 18.1 on page 132.

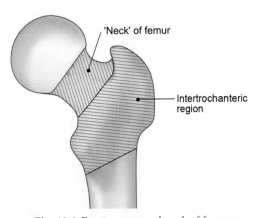

Fig. 18.6: Fracture around neck of femur.

PATHOANATOMY

Most of these fractures are displaced, with the distal fragment externally rotated and proximally migrated (Fig. 18.7). Such displacements also occur in intertro-chanteric fracture in which displacements are *more marked*. This happens because in an intracapsular frac-ture, the capsule of the hip joint is attached to the distal fragment. This capsule prevents excessive rotation and displacement of the distal fragment (and with it, the limb). On the other hand, intertrochanteric fracture is

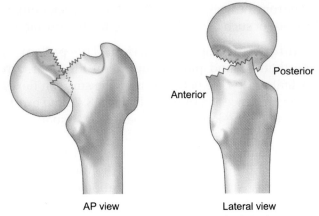

Fig. 18.7: Displacements in fracture neck of the femur.

outside the attachment of the capsule, and hence, there is nothing stopping the fracture from displacing.

CLASSIFICATION

Fractures of the neck of the femur can be classified on different basis as discussed below:

a. **Anatomical classification (Fig. 18.8):** On the basis of anatomical location of the fracture, it can be classified as: (i) subcapital—a fracture just below the head; (ii) transcervical—a fracture in the middle of the neck; or (iii) basal—a fracture at the base of the neck. The more proximally the fracture is located, the *worse* is the prognosis.

b. **Pauwel's classification:** This classification is based on the angle of inclination of the fracture in relation to the horizontal plane (Pauwel's angle, Fig. 18.9). The fractures are divided into three types (types I–III). The more the angle, the more unstable is the fracture, and *worse* the prognosis.

c. **Garden's classification:** This is based on the degree of displacement of the fracture (mainly rotational displacement). The degree of displacement is judged from change in the direction of the medial trabecular stream of the neck, in relation to the

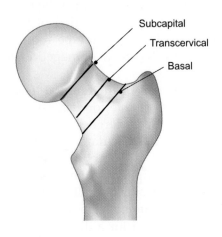

Fig. 18.8: Anatomical classification.

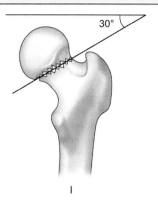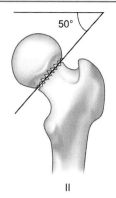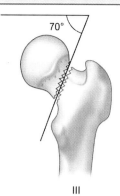

Fig. 18.9: Pauwel's classification.

bony trabeculae in the weight bearing part of the head and in the corresponding part of the acetabulum (Fig. 18.10).

- *Stage 1*: The fracture is *incomplete,* with the head tilted in posterolateral direction, so that there is an *obtuse* angle laterally at the trabecular stream. This is also called an impacted or abducted fracture.
- *Stage 2*: The fracture is *complete but undisplaced,* so that there is a break in the trabecular stream with little angulation.
- *Stage 3*: The fracture is *complete and partially displaced.* As the distal fragment rotates externally, it causes internal rotation of the head. One can make out rotation of the head and displacement of the fracture by carefully following the medial trabecular stream. The trabecular stream at the fracture site is broken and displaced. Alignment between the trabeculae of the head and the acetabulum is also lost because of the rotation of the head in relation to the acetabulum.
- *Stage 4*: The fracture is *complete and fully displaced.* As the distal fragment rotates further outwards,

it looses contact with the head, which springs back to its original position. Therefore, whereas there is a total loss of contact between the head and neck trabecular streams, those between the head and the acetabulum are normally aligned.

Though Garden's classification is scientifically more appealing, it is often difficult to decide the stage of the fracture on the basis X-rays.

MECHANISM

In elderly people, the fracture occurs with a seemingly trivial fall. Osteoporosis is considered an important contributory factor at this age. In young adults, this fracture is the result of a more severe injury. The fracture is uncommon in children.

DIAGNOSIS

Clinical features: Typically, the patient is an elderly, brought to the casualty department with complaints of pain in the groin and inability to move his limb or bear weight on the limb. Often the injury is innocuous such slipping on a wet floor, missing a step, etc. There may not be much pain, as also little swelling. It is for

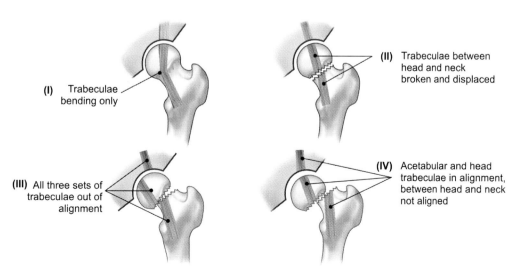

Fig. 18.10: ❖ Garden's classification.

this reason that this injury is often diagnosed late, and is misdiagnosed as 'muscle injury'. In such cases, it is only after a few days or weeks, when the patient refuses to put load on that limb, that suspicion of a fracture occurs. Occasionally, the fracture may be impacted, and in such a case, the patient may come walking, with only complaint being pain in the groin. Careful examinations reveals the following:

- *External rotation* of the leg, the patella facing outwards.
- *Shortening* of the leg, usually slight.
- *Tenderness* in the groin.
- *Attempted hip movements* painful, and associated with severe spasm.
- *Active straight leg raising* not possible.

Clinically, it is possible to differentiate this fracture from an intertrochanteric fracture which presents with similar signs. In general, signs and symptoms are more in an inter-trochanteric fracture (Table 18.1).

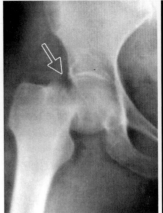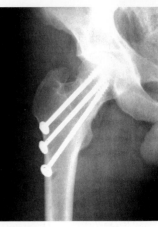

Fig. 18.11: X-rays of the hip, showing fracture neck of the femur; fixed with three cancellous screws.

Table 18.1: Differences between fracture neck of the femur and inter-trochanteric fracture.		
Point	**Fracture neck femur**	**Intertrochanteric fracture**
Age	After 50 yrs	After 60 years
Sex	F > M	M > F
Injury	Trivial	Significant
Ability to walk	May walk in impacted fracture	Not possible
Pain	Mild	Severe
Swelling	Nil	Severe
Ecchymosis	Nil	Present
Tenderness	In Scarpa's triangle	On the greater trochanter
External rotation deformity	Less than 45°	More than 45°
Shortening	Less than 1 inch	More than 1 inch
Treatment	Internal fixation always	Can be managed in traction
Complications	Non-union	Malunion

Radiological features (Fig. 18.11): While asking for X-rays, it is useful to ask for X-ray of pelvis including both hips. This helps in comparing the two sides. The following features should be noted on X-rays:

- Break in the medial cortex of the neck.
- External rotation of the femur, evident from lesser trochanter appearing more prominent*.
- Overriding of greater trochanter, so that it lies above the level of the head of the femur.

---

* The lesser trochanter is situated posteromedially on the shaft. So if the leg is externally rotated, the lesser trochanter appears more prominent on the X-ray.

- Break in the trabecular stream.
- Break in Shenton's line (page 217).

In *impacted fracture,* the only radiological finding is bending of the trabeculae. There is no clear cut fracture line. Comparison with the opposite hip may be useful.

TREATMENT

This fracture is rightly termed an *'unsolved fracture'* because of the high incidence of complications. Two factors which make the treatment of this fracture particularly difficult are: (i) the *blood supply* to the proximal fragment (the head) is cut off; and (ii) it is *difficult to achieve reduction* and maintain it. The later happens because the proximal fragment is too small. Because of these factors, the fracture invariably needs operative treatment. There are numerous controversies in the treatment of this fracture. Discussed below is a balanced approach followed in most hospitals.

Impacted fracture: Earlier, undisplaced/impacted neck femur fractures were treated non-operatively by splinting. It was noticed that large percentage would displace in due course. Hence, current trend is to treat these fractures operatively. In children, these are managed using multiple smooth pins and a hip spica. In adults, fixation with multiple cannulated cancellous screws is preferred. Though an impacted fracture can be treated by conservative methods, an accurate assessment using CT scan should be done. Often, fractures which appear impacted on X-rays are not so as per CT scan.

Unimpacted or displaced fractures: In younger patients (up to 60 years* of age), the aim is to achieve union. This is done by closed reduction and internal

---

* It is the physiological age which is considered. It means that the appearance, activities and health of the patient is that of a healthy person at 60 years of age. Often a patient may be more than 60 years, but physiologically younger, or vice versa.

fixation with cannulated cancellous screws or DHS. In some younger patients presenting late (after 3 weeks), closed reduction may be difficult, and hence open reduction is resorted to. An accurate reduction and good fixation is important for a good result. The following are some of the commonly used internal fixations devices.

- Multiple cancellous screws – most commonly used.
- Dynamic hip screw (DHS) – used sometimes.
- Multiple Knowle's pins/Moore's pins used in children.

The technique of internal fixation: The technique being described here is, use of multiple cancellous screws. The screws used are partially threaded (Fig. 18.11), the threaded part holds in the head, whereas the smooth part permits controlled collapse of the fracture, which helps in union. Facility of image intensifier is a must. Under anaesthesia, the patient is fixed to a special operating table (fracture table). The fracture is reduced by closed manipulation. The reduction is checked on image intensifier. The base of the greater trochanter is exposed and a guide-wire inserted in the centre of the femoral neck. If the position of the guide-wire is satisfactory, a cannulated screw is threaded over it. Minimum three screws, preferably parallel, are necessary. Cannulated screws make the operation simple. After the operation, no external immobilisation is required. The patient is allowed to sit up in bed,

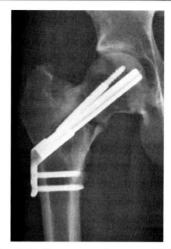

Fig. 18.12: Fracture neck system (FNS).

and be out of bed with crutches (nonweight-bearing) in the early post-operative period. Gradual weight bearing is permitted as the fracture shows evidence of union (usually 3-4 months).

Recent addition to fixation devise for fracture neck of femur is FNS (fracture neck system). This is a minimally invasive technique of providing biomechanically superior fixation (Fig. 18.12)

McMurray's osteotomy was a popular operation in the past, but is of historical value today. Flowchart 18.1 shows the treatment plan of these fractures in adults.

Flowchart 18.1: Treatment plan of fresh (< 3 weeks) fracture of neck of the femur.

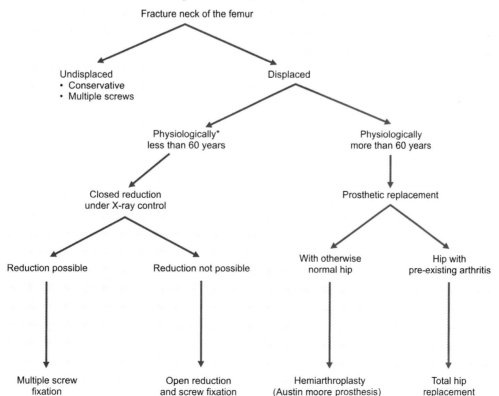

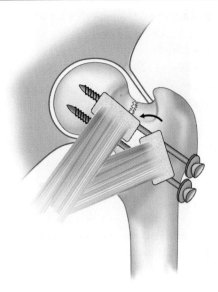

Fig. 18.13: Meyer's procedure.

Meyer's procedure (Fig. 18.13): This operation is used in treating the fractures presenting late or those with significant comminution at the fracture site. It is also used for non-union of the femoral neck fractures. In this procedure, the fracture is reduced by exposing it from behind. It is fixed with multiple screws and supplemented with a *vascularised muscle-pedicle bone graft* taken from the femoral attachment of the quadratus femoris muscle.

It is the physiological age which is considered. It means that the appearance, activities and health of the patient is that of a healthy person at 60 years of age. Often a patient may be more than 60 years, but physiologically younger, or vice versa.

Hip replacement (Fig. 18.14): In the elderly, since failure of union and AVN is reasonably high, it is

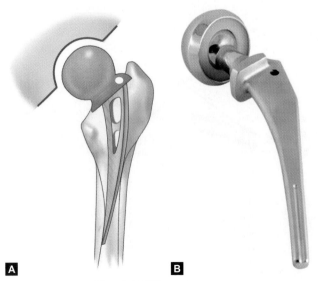

Fig. 18.14: Hip replacement.

preferable to excise the head of the femur and *replace* it by an artificial part (prosthesis). This could be a partial hip replacement (hemiarthroplasty) or total hip replacement (THR).

Hemiarthroplasty: In this, the head of the femur is excised and replaced by a prosthesis. There are two type of hemiarthroplasty - unipolar and bipolar. *Unipolar prosthesis* has one-piece 'head' with an attached stem. The stem is introduced into the medullary canal, and the head sits over the neck of the femur (Fig. 18.14A). In *bipolar prosthesis*, the head has two parts - a smaller head, and a mobile plastic cup on top of it (Fig. 18.14B). Hence, in this, movement occurs at two planes - one between the acetabulum and the plastic cup, and other between the plastic cup and the head. This is why it is called 'bipolar' It is supposed to be mechanically superior (For details see pages 329).

Total hip replacement: This has become a popular option for fracture neck of femur in active elderly. It is supposed to give better results in terms of pain relief and longevity of the prosthesis. Here both, the head of the femur and acetabulum are replaced with artificial components (see page 330).

Treatment of cases presenting late: Patient with fracture of the neck of the femur often present late, either because the fracture was not diagnosed on time or the facilities for treatment were not available. If presented later than 2-3 weeks, these are difficult problem to treat. Closed reduction is often not possible, and opening the fracture is associated with complications such as avascular necrosis. In patients above 60 years of age, replacement arthroplasty is a better option. In younger patients, it's a real challenge to treat these cases. Treatment depends upon whether the head of the femur is 'vascular' or not. This can be assessed by bone scanning or MRI. If the head is vascular, the hip is reconstructed by either osteotomy (McMurray's or Pauwel's), or reconstruction procedures such as Meyers' operation. If the head is not vascular, and the patient is young, bipolar prosthesis is preferred.

COMPLICATIONS

1. **Non-union:** It occurs in approximately 30 to 40% of intracapsular fractures. It is due to two factors working simultaneously: (a) inadequate immobilisation of the fracture even with internal fixation; and (b) poor blood supply of the head fragment. The patient presents either with a fracture not treated at all, or a fracture which has failed to unite even after treatment. The main complaint is pain and inability to bear weight on the affected limb. The limb is short and externally rotated. Active straight-leg-raising is not possible.

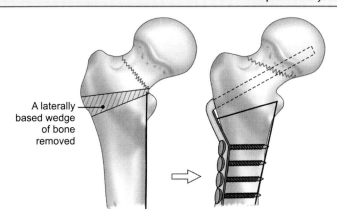

Fig. 18.15: Pauwel's osteotomy for non-union of fracture of the neck of the femur.

A laterally based wedge of bone removed

The pain may be minimal and hip movements may be *increased* because of free mobility at the fracture site (pseudarthrosis). Trendelenburg's test will be positive. Telescopy will be present. (See annexure – clinical methods, page 344–345). In a patient who has been treated by internal fixation, non-union should be suspected if there is renewed pain after seemingly normal progress. Diagnosis can be made on X-rays or CT scan. Often, there is sudden deterioration in these cases; with acute pain, external rotation of the limb, shortening, and inability to walk. This is because the implant, which was 'holding' a hitherto ununited fracture, finally gives way (implant failure).

Treatment: The treatment of non-union depends upon the age of the patient, and on whether or not there is avascular necrosis of the femoral head. In patients beyond the age of 60 years, replacement arthroplasty is performed. In younger individuals, attempt is made to preserve the head of the femur by one of the following methods:

a. *Neck reconstruction:* The fracture is exposed from behind, the ends freshened and the fracture stabilised with multiple screws and muscle-pedicle graft (Baksi's procedure). Some surgeons use free fibular graft for reconstructing the neck.

b. *Pauwel's osteotomy:* This is a valgus ostestomy at the level of the lesser trochanter (Fig. 18.15). A valgus effect so created at the fracture site results in converting the shearing forces at the fracture site into compression forces. The osteotomy is fixed with double-angle blade plate. It is a technically demanding operation.

2. **Avascular necrosis:** After a fracture through the neck, all the medullary blood supply and most of the capsular blood supply to the head are cut off. The viability of the femoral head may therefore depend almost entirely on the blood supply through the ligamentum teres. If this blood supply is insufficient, avascular necrosis of a segment or whole of the head occurs. This may, in addition, be a cause of non-union. The avascular head may collapse and become deformed. These changes may not become evident early. It is only after a few months to as long as 2 years, that one can diagnose avascular necrosis on X-rays. MRI is the best investigation for this purpose. Deformation of the head results in osteoarthritis after a few years. *Treatment:* A fracture of the neck of the femur with avascular necrosis of the head is a very difficult problem to treat. In *young* patients treatment options are between attempt at reconstruction by Meyer's procedure or replacement. In adults, total hip replacement (THR) is preferred. In *elderly* patients, a hemi-replacement arthroplasty is good enough. In cases where there is a pre-existing damage to the hip joint per se, a total hip replacement may be preferred.

3. **Osteoarthritis:** It develops a few years following fracture of the neck of femur. It may be because of: (i) avascular deformation of the head; or (ii) union in faulty alignment. The patient presents with pain and stiffness of the joint. Initially the pain is intermittent, but later it persists. *Treatment:* It depends upon the age and functional requirement of the patient. Younger patients are treated by an intertrochanteric osteotomy or partial hip replacement. For an elderly patient, total hip replacement is the best option.

INTERTROCHANTERIC FRACTURES

Fractures in the intertrochanteric region of the proximal femur, *involving either* the greater or the lesser trochanter or both, are grouped in this category (Fig. 18.16).

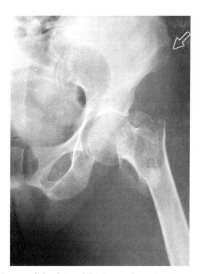

Fig. 18.16: X-ray of the hip, AP view, showing intertrochanteric fracture.

In the elderly, the fracture is normally sustained by a sideway fall or a blow over the greater trochanter. In the young, it occurs following violent trauma, as in a road traffic accident.

PATHOANATOMY

The distal fragment rides up so that the femoral neck-shaft angle is reduced (coxa vara). The fracture is generally comminuted and displaced. Rarely, it can be an undisplaced fracture.

DIAGNOSIS

Clinical features: As for fractures of the neck of the femur, the patient is brought in with a history of a fall or road accident, followed by pain in the region of the groin and an inability to move the leg. There will be swelling in the region of the hip, and the leg will be short and externally rotated. There is tenderness over the greater trochanter. The physical findings in such a case are *more marked* compared to those in a fracture of the neck of the femur.

Radiological features: Diagnosis is easy on an X-ray. Presence of comminution of the medial cortex of the neck, avulsion of the lesser trochanter and extension of the fracture to the subtrochanteric region indicate an *unstable* fracture, and a poor prognosis.

TREATMENT

Contrary to fracture of the neck of the femur, trochanteric fractures *unite readily*. The main objective of treatment is to maintain a normal femoral neck-shaft angle during the process of union. This can be done by conservative means (traction) or by internal fixation. In elderly patients, internal fixation is preferred because in them prolonged bed rest (as much as 3-4 months) in traction may cause complications related to recumbency, i.e., bed sores, pneumonia, etc.

Conservative methods: There are a number of tractions described for an intertrochanteric fracture. Those used most frequently are Russell's traction (Fig. 18.17) and skeletal traction in a Thomas splint.

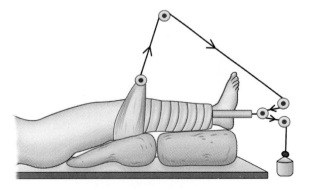

Fig. 18.17: Russell's traction.

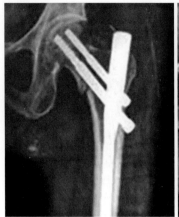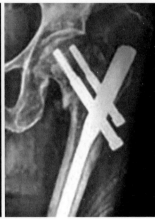

Fig. 18.18: Devices used for internal fixation of an intertrochanteric fracture.

With the success of operative methods, whereby, early mobilisation is possible, conservative methods are used less often.

Operative methods: The fracture is reduced under X-ray control and fixed with internal fixation devices. The most commonly used ones are: (i) Dynamic hip screw (DHS) (Fig. 18.18) and (ii) Proximal femoral nail (PFN). Proximal femoral nail is the implant of choice for patients with unstable fractures. External fixation and Ender's nails are useful, minimally invasive options for patients with bed sores, and for those who are unfit for a major operation. For some badly comminuted fractures with osteoporotic bones, achieving union is a difficult task, and hence, a primary replacement arthroplasty is done in such cases.

COMPLICATIONS

1. **Malunion:** As discussed earlier, intertrochanteric fractures almost always unite, but because of possible failure in keeping the fragments aligned, these often malunite. Malunion gives rise to coxa vara (decreased femoral neck-shaft angle), shortening and the leg in external rotation.
   Treatment: In elderly patients, malunion does not cause a great deal of disability, except a limp while walking, and shortening. Compensation for this shortening, by giving a suitable shoe raise, suffices in most cases. In *young people* with severe coxa vara and shortening, correction may be required. This is achieved by an intertrochanteric osteotomy whereby the neck-shaft angle is corrected and held in the proper position by internal fixation devices.

2. **Osteoarthritis:** Due to changes in the hip biomechanics following trochanteric fractures, osteoarthritis of the hip develops after a few years. The patient complains of pain and stiffness

in the hip after a reasonably symptom free period following union of the fracture. An X-ray confirms changes of osteoarthritis in the hip joint.

Treatment: In the early stages, treatment is by physiotherapy. Later, a trochanteric osteotomy (in younger patient) or a total hip replacement (in elderly patient) may be required.

 What have we learnt?

- Injury around the hip is common in elderly.
- Fracture neck of femur is notorious for complications such as non-union.
- Treatment of fracture neck of femur in younger patients is by internal fixation (head preservation), and in the elderly by replacement (head replacement).
- Intertrochanteric fractures are cousins of fracture neck femur, but very different behaviour-wise. Union usually occurs, though malunion is common. These can be treated by conservative methods, but internal fixation is preferred.

Additional information: From the entrance exams point of view

- Main blood supply to the head of the femur in adults is the lateral ascending cervical or retinacular and epiphyseal branches of the medial circumflex femoral artery.
- The most common hip injury in the elderly patient is intertrochanteric (extracapsular fractures).
- Occult fracture neck of femur is best diagnosed by MRI.
- Maximum chances of avascular necrosis in subcapital fractures.
- Fracture head of femur classified by Pipkin classification.
- Femoral head palpable on per rectal examination in central dislocation of hip.
- Paralysis of gluteus medius/minimus supplied by the superior gluteal nerve causes Trendelenburg's gait.

Competency

❖ **OR2.12:** Describe and discuss the aetiopathogenesis, clinical features, investigations and principles of management of fracture shaft of femur in all age groups and the recognition and management of fat embolism as a complication.

A fracture of the shaft of the femur is usually sustained by a severe violence as may occur in a road accident. The force causing the fracture may be indirect (twisting or bending force while landing on one leg) or direct (hit directly by an object as in a traffic accident).

PATHOANATOMY

The fracture may occur at any site, and is equally common in the upper, middle and lower third of the shaft. It may be a transverse, oblique, spiral or comminuted, depending upon the nature of the fracturing force.

Displacements: In children, the fracture does not displace a great deal; but in adults, more often than not, there is marked displacement. The proximal fragment is flexed, abducted and externally rotated by the pull of the muscles attached to it (Fig. 19.1). The distal fragment is adducted because of attachment of adductor muscles spanning the thigh on the medial side. The unsupported fracture-end of the distal fragment sags because of the gravity. There is proximal migration (overriding) of the distal fragment because of the pull by the muscles traversing across the fracture.

DIAGNOSIS

Clinical features: The patient presents with a history of severe violence followed by classic signs

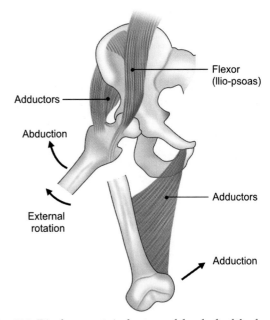

Fig. 19.1: Displacements in fracture of the shaft of the femur.

of fracture in the region of the thigh (pain, swelling, deformity, abnormal mobility, etc.). Diagnosis is not difficult. At times the violence may not be significant, and it is just that the whole body force comes on the femur and fractures it. A pathological fracture is suspected whenever the force causing fracture is not much.

Radiological examination: X-rays done for a femoral shaft fracture must include the *whole* femur. In addition, an X-ray of the pelvis should be done as, it is not uncommon that a patient with fracture of the femur has an associated injury to the pelvis.

TREATMENT

Fracture of the shaft of the femur occurs in so many different forms that practically all methods of fracture treatment discussed in Chapter 3 may be applicable. The treatment methods can be conservative or operative.

Conservative methods: This consists of the following:

a. *Traction:* A fracture of the shaft of the femur can be treated by traction, with or without a splint. Skin traction is sufficient in children, but skeletal traction is required in adults. Skeletal traction is given by a Steinmann pin passed through the upper-end of tibia. Thomas splint is used to control fragments.

b. *Hip spica:* This is a plaster cast incorporating part of the trunk and the limb. It may be a single spica (involving only the fractured limb) or *one-and-a-half* (1½) as shown in Figure 19.2. It can be safely used for immobilising these fractures in children. It has been used in the past for treating fractures in adults, but no more.

With wider availability of operative methods, more and more fractures of the shaft of femur are treated operatively, even in children. The main reason for this shift is, operative treatment being more comfortable and predictable.

Operative methods: Intramedullary nailing and plating are the two commonly used methods of

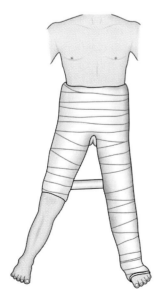

Fig. 19.2: Hip spica (1½).

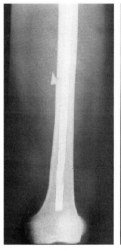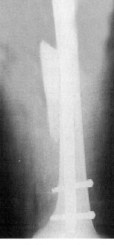

Fig. 19.3: X-rays showing intramedullary nailing done for fracture of femoral shaft.

operative treatment, though, wherever possible, intramedullary nailing is preferred. Plating is chosen where good hold is not possible by a nail. The fracture may be reduced by closed or open methods. In general, open fractures are treated with external fixators initially to avoid infections due to internal placement of implants. Once the wound heals or is granulating, one can switch to internal fixation. The following are some of the commonly used techniques of treating fracture femur operatively.

a. *Nailing:* This is a technique where the fracture is reduced and a rod (nail) inserted into the medullary canal. This can be done by open technique (open nailing)—where the fracture is opened, reduced under vision, and the rod inserted. The other method is closed nailing. In this, the fracture is reduced without opening it. This is done under X-ray control (image intensifier), by giving appropriate traction. The nail can be introduced into the medullary canal from proximal end (greater trochanter) or from distal end. All this is done under X-ray monitoring using image intensifier. Closed nailing is a minimally invasive, and modern counterpart of conventional, open nailing. The recent addition to nailing technique is interlocking. In this, the nail 'locked' at two end using bolts going from lateral cortex of the bone into a hole in the nail to the far cortex. This locks the nail in place. Apart from being minimally invasive, closed nailing has advantages over open nailing as the rate of infection is much less and healing is much quicker. Closed nailing and interlock nailing are technically demanding operations. A certain amount of surgical skills and an image intensifier is necessary for it.

b. *Plating (fixing with a thick strip of metal):* Plating may be used for fractures where good hold can not be provided by a nail. Some such situations are—medullary canal being too wide for a nail to provide hold, or the fracture is too comminuted (Fig. 19.4). Plating technique has undergone tremendous development over the years—from conventional plating, to compression plating to modern locking plate technique (discussed in Chapter 5). Special, condylar blade-plate, may be used for fractures closer to either end of the bone. Recent addition to plating for ends of the femur are pre-contoured plates (anatomical plates).

With the advent of interlock nailing, the fractures of femoral shaft, which were earlier unsuitable

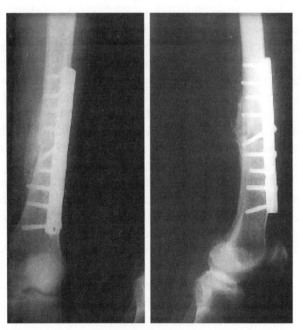

Fig. 19.4: X-rays showing plating done for fracture of distal third of the shaft of the femur.

for conventional nailing, can be satisfactorily stabilized. Therefore, there is a general trend towards nailing the fractures of the shaft of the femur rather than plating.

DECIDING TREATMENT PLAN

The treatment depends primarily upon the age of the patient, location of the fracture, type of the fracture (transverse, oblique, etc.) and presence of a wound. In general, an open fracture is treated conservatively; in bad cases an external fixator may be used.

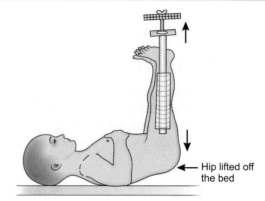

Fig. 19.5: Gallow's traction.

In children, conventionally the treatment of fracture shaft has been mostly by non-operative methods. Lately, with improvement in surgical techniques, there is a trend towards treating fractures in children, operatively. The following are some of the conventional methods of treating fracture femur in children:

a. **From birth to 2 years:** These fractures are treated by Gallow's traction (Fig. 19.5). In this, the legs of the child are tied to a overhead beam. The hips are kept a little raised from the bed so that the weight of the body provides counter-traction and the fracture is reduced. This is continued till sufficient callus forms (3–6 weeks).

b. **From 2 years to 10 years:** The treatment at this age is also essentially conservative. Different methods of traction and splintage are used to keep fragments in proper alignment. Once the fracture becomes 'sticky', further immobilisation can be provided in a hip spica.

   From 10 years to 16 years: In older children, it is more difficult to keep the fracture reduced for required period, as also it is cumbersome. It is therefore, sometimes preferred to internally fix femoral shaft fracture in this age group by thin metallic rods. These are titanium elastic nails (TENS nails). These work on the principle of 3-point fixation. Usually 2 pre-tensioned, pre-bent 'titanium elastic' nails are inserted from metaphyseal region so that no damage is done to growing regions of the bone (physis). It is a preferred method of treatment in this age group (Fig. 19.6). Sometimes, plating is preferred in children to avoid damaging the growth plate.

c. **In adults and in the elderly**, if proper facilities are available, the treatment of these fractures is done by operation. The method of fixation varies from fracture to fracture. Operative treatment allows the patient to be up and about, out of bed, with the help of crutches very early. Full weight bearing is allowed as soon as sufficient healing is seen on X-rays.

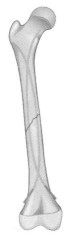

Fig. 19.6: Titanium elastic nails system (TENS).

COMPLICATIONS

The complications following a fracture of the femoral shaft can be divided into early and late.

EARLY COMPLICATIONS

1. **Shock:** In a closed fracture of the shaft of the femur, on an average, 1000–1500 mL of blood is lost. Such sudden loss of blood can result in hypovolaemic shock. Hence, all patients with this fracture should be on intravenous (IV) line, with blood arranged, in case the need arises. A close watch should be kept on pulse and blood pressure during the early post-injury period.
2. **Fat embolism:** Patient shows signs and symptoms of fat embolism after 24–48 hours of the fracture. Frequent shifting of the patient without proper splintage of the fracture should be avoided.
3. **Injury to femoral artery:** Rarely, a sharp edge of the bone may penetrate the soft tissues and damage the femoral artery. This occurs most commonly in fractures at the junction of middle and distal-third of the femoral shaft. Unless the continuity of the vessel is restored by immediate operation, the viability of the limb is in danger.
4. **Injury to sciatic nerve:** It may be damaged by a sharp bone end or by traction. The severity of damage varies from neurapraxia to complete severance of the nerve. Treatment is discussed in Chapter 10.
5. **Infection:** In cases with open fractures, wound contamination with consequent infection, can lead to osteomyelitis. The risk is maximum in fractures with extensive wounds, and those with gun-shot wounds.

LATE COMPLICATIONS

1. **Delayed union:** Although, there is no definite time period beyond which the union of a fracture is said to be delayed, but generally speaking, if union is insufficient to allow unprotected weight bearing in a fracture femur, after 5 months, union is considered delayed. X-ray may show evidence of union, but not solid enough to allow weight bearing.
   Treatment: It needs experience to decide whether continuation of conservative treatment would lead to fracture union, or an operative intervention is required. It is better to cut short the uncertainty by resorting to bone grafting, especially in an elderly person.
2. **Non-union:** It is said to have occurred when the fracture is still mobile after a few months (3 months). It may be identified on X-rays by lack of bridging callus. Sometimes, bone ends become rounded and sclerotic. A persistent micromobility at the fracture site which has been even fixed internally, may also lead to non-union. Often this comes to attention as the implant (nail or plate), used to fix the fracture, undergoes fatigue fracture of implant itself. Clinically, there may be frank mobility, pain on stressing or tenderness at the fracture site. *Treatment* is by revising the internal fixation and added bone grafting.
3. **Malunion:** If fracture of the shaft of the femur is not kept in proper position, or if it re-displaces and unites, in an unacceptable position. It is called malunion. The deformity is generally lateral angulation and external rotation. There may be significant shortening due to overlap of the fragments.
   Treatment: This depends upon the degree of malunion and age of the patient. In an elderly patient, if the disability is not much, tendency is toward accepting the deformity. Shortening may be compensated by giving a shoe raise. In younger patients, correction of the deformity is done by operative means. The deformity is corrected by re-doing the fracture or by a corrective osteotomy. The fracture is fixed again with internal fixation devices. Bone grafting is done in addition. In children, mild deformity gets corrected by the process of remodelling. Significant deformities require corrective surgery.
4. **Knee stiffness:** Some amount of temporary knee stiffness occurs in most cases of fracture of the shaft of the femur. It is possible to regain full movements with physiotherapy. At times, the stiffness persists. The following could be the reasons: (i) intra-articular and peri-articular adhesions; (ii) quadriceps adhering to the fracture site; (iii) an associated, often undetected, knee injury.

Treatment: Cases where a conscientious treatment by exercises has not been rewarding, a proper assessment of the contributing factor and its treatment is required. Intra-articular adhesions can be released by arthroscopic technique (arthrolysis), or by gentle manipulation under general anaesthesia. Quadriceps adhesion may require release, and contracted quadriceps may need to be 'lengthened' (quadriceps plasty).

 What have we learnt?

- Fracture of the femur is a major, disabling injury.
- It is treated by conservative methods in children. Most fractures in adults and elderly are treated by operation.
- Nailing and plating are the two methods of internal fixation.
- Interlock nailing is the current choice of treatment. Non-union, delayed union and malunion are common complications.

Additional information: From the entrance exams point of view

- Upper one-third shaft of femur most commonly fractured at birth.
- Maximum shortening of lower limb is seen in fracture shaft of femur and posterior dislocation of hip.

Injuries Around the Knee

Competency

❖ **OR2.11:** Describe and discuss the aetiopathogenesis, mechanism of injury, clinical features, investigations and principles of management of:
  a. Fracture patella
  b. Fracture distal femur
  c. Fracture proximal tibia with special focus on neurovascular injury and compartment syndrome.

The knee joint is the most frequently injured joint. The following injuries will be discussed in this chapter: (i) condylar fractures of the femur; (ii) fracture of the plateau; (iii) tibial plateau fractures; (iv) injuries to the ligaments of the knee; (v) injuries to the menisci of the knee; (vi) miscellaneous knee injuries.

RELEVANT ANATOMY

The knee is a hinge joint formed between the tibia and femur (tibiofemoral). The patella glides over the front of femoral condyles to form a patellofemoral joint. The stability of the knee depends primarily upon its ligaments. The functions

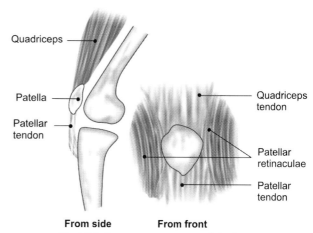

Fig. 20.1: Extensor apparatus of the knee.

of different ligaments of the knee are given in Table 20.1.

Extensor apparatus of the knee: It is constituted from proximal to distal, by quadriceps muscle, quadriceps tendon, patella with patellar retinaculae on the sides, and the patellar tendon (Fig. 20.1). Failure of any of these results in inability to actively extend the knee, called *extensor lag*.

Table 20.1: Functions of the knee ligaments.	
Ligament	**Function**
▪ Medial collateral	▪ Prevents medial opening up
▪ Lateral collateral	▪ Prevents lateral opening up
▪ Anterior cruciate	▪ Prevents anterior translation of the tibia on the femur
▪ Posterior cruciate	▪ Prevents posterior translation of the tibia on the femur

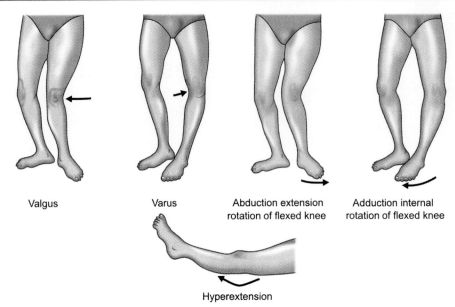

Valgus   Varus   Abduction extension   Adduction internal
                               rotation of flexed knee   rotation of flexed knee

Hyperextension

Fig. 20.2: Mechanisms of knee injuries.

MECHANISM OF KNEE INJURIES

The knee joint is subjected to a variety of forces during day-to-day activities and sports. The nature of the forces may be direct or indirect. An indirect force on the knee may be: (i) valgus; (ii) varus; (iii) hyperextension; or (iv) twisting (Fig. 20.2). Most often it is a combination of the above forces.

CONDYLAR FRACTURES OF THE FEMUR

Condylar fractures of the femur are of three types (Fig. 20.3): (i) supracondylar fractures; (ii) intercondylar

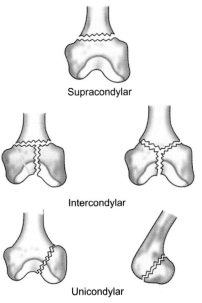

Supracondylar

Intercondylar

Unicondylar

Fig. 20.3: Condylar fractures of femur.

fractures - T or Y types; and (iii) unicondylar fractures - medial or lateral. These fractures commonly result from a direct trauma to the lower end of the femur. An indirect force more often results in unicondylar (by a varus/valgus bending force) or supracondylar fracture (by a hyperextension force). A special category of unicondylar fractures are those involving posterior femoral condyles, are called *Hoffa's fracture*.

DIAGNOSIS

Diagnosis of these fractures is suggested by pain, swelling and bruising around the knee. These fractures are often missed, when associated with more severe injuries, such as a fracture of the shaft of the femur. Diagnosis is made on X-rays. A careful assessment of the intra-articular extension of the fracture and joint incongruity must be made.

TREATMENT

Unicondylar fractures: If undisplaced, a long leg cast is given for 3-6 weeks, followed by protected weight bearing. If displaced, open reduction and internal fixation with multiple cancellous screws is performed. A buttress plate may be required in some cases.

Intercondylar fractures: The aim of treatment is to restore congruity of the articular surface as far as possible. In displaced T or Y fracture with minimal comminution, the joint is reconstructed by open reduction and internal fixation. Distal femoral anatomical LCP (locking compression plate) is the preferred option. Other options are—fixing with distal femoral nail, and condylar blade-plate.

Comminuted fractures are difficult to accurately reconstruct, but well-done open reduction and internal fixation permits early knee mobilization. In selected, badly comminuted fractures, where fixing the fracture may be nearly impossible, conservative treatment in skeletal traction may be done.

Supracondylar fractures: It is best to treat displaced supracondylar fractures with internal fixation. This could be done by closed or open techniques. Distal femoral nail or anatomical LCP may be used.

COMPLICATIONS

1. **Knee stiffness:** Residual knee stiffness sometimes remains because of dense intra- and peri-articular adhesions. A long course of physiotherapy is usually rewarding. Arthrolysis may be required in resistant cases.
2. **Osteoarthritis:** Fractures with intra-articular extension give rise to osteoarthritis a few years later.
3. **Malunion:** A malunion may result in varus or valgus deformities, sometimes requiring a corrective osteotomy.

FRACTURES OF THE PATELLA

This is a common fracture. It may result from a direct or an indirect force. In a direct injury, as may occur by a blow on the anterior aspect of the flexed knee, usually a comminuted fracture results. The comminution may be limited to a part or whole of the patella. The latter is also called a *stellate fracture* (Fig. 20.4A). Sometimes, a sudden violent contraction of the quadriceps, gives rise to a fracture with the fracture line running transversely across the patella, dividing it into two; the so-called *two-part fracture*. Most often, both of these mechanisms are at play simultaneously, so that once the fracture occurs by a direct violence, a simultaneous contraction of the quadriceps pulls the fragments apart, and results in a separated fracture of the patella with some comminution.

PATHOANATOMY

The fracture may remain undisplaced because the fragments are held in position by intact pre-patellar expansion of the quadriceps tendon in front, and by patellar retinaculae on the sides. If the force of the quadriceps contraction is strong, it will pull the fragments apart and will result in rupture of patellar retinaculae (Fig. 20.4A).

CLINICAL FEATURES

Presenting complaints: The patient complains of pain and swelling over the knee. In an undisplaced fracture the swelling and tenderness may be localised

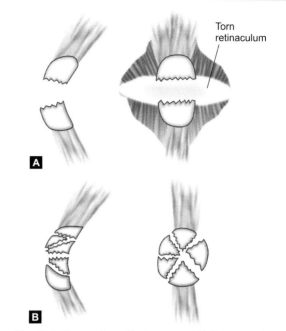

Fig. 20.4: Types of patella fractures: (A) Two-part fracture; (B) Stellate fracture.

over the patella. A crepitus is felt in a comminuted fracture. In displaced fractures, one may feel a gap between the fracture fragments. The patient will not be able to lift his leg with knee in full extension. The knee remains in a position short of full extension because of disruption of the extensor apparatus. This loss of active extension is called *extensor lag*. There may be bruises over the front of the knee—a tell-tale sign of direct trauma. The knee may be swollen because of haemarthrosis.

Radiological examination: Anteroposterior and lateral X-rays of the knee are sufficient in most cases. In some undisplaced fractures, a 'skyline view' of the patella (Fig. 20.5) may be required. A fracture with wide separation of the fragments is easy to diagnose on a lateral X-ray. Often it is not possible to visualise

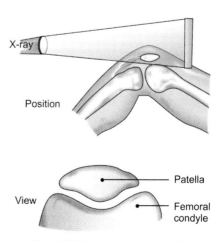

Fig. 20.5: Skyline view of patella.

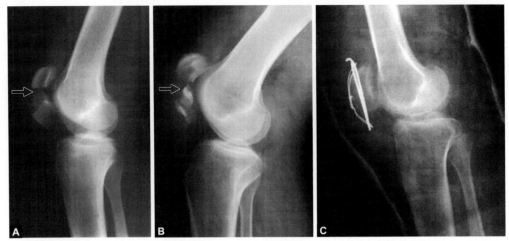

Fig. 20.6: X-rays of the knees lateral view showing: (A) Two-part fracture; (B) Comminuted fracture; (C) A fracture treated with tension-band wiring.

comminution on the X-ray; it becomes obvious only during surgery (Fig. 20.6). In a case with any doubt, as in all fractures, CT scan is done.

TREATMENT

It depends upon the type of fracture, and in some cases on the age of the patient. The following groups may be considered:

a. **Undisplaced fracture:** Treatment is aimed primarily at relief of pain. A plaster cast extending from the groin to just above the malleoli, with the knee in full extension (cylinder cast) should be given for 3 weeks. This is followed by physiotherapy. These days casts have been replaced by ready-made *long knee immobilisers.*

b. **Clean break with separation of fragments (two-part fracture):** The pull of the quadriceps muscle on the proximal fragment keeps the fragments apart, hence an operation is always necessary. The operation consists of reduction of the fragments, fixing them with *tension-band wiring (TBW)* and repair of extensor retinaculae. The knee can be mobilised early following this operation. With improvement in fixation techniques, it is possible to reconstruct even communited patella. In cases where one of the fragments constitutes only one of the poles of the patella, it is excised. The major fragment is preserved and the extensor retinaculae repaired (*partial patellectomy*). Such operations on the patella are followed by support in a cylinder cast or long knee immobilizer for 4–6 weeks.

c. **Comminuted fracture:** In comminuted fractures with displacement, it is difficult to restore a perfectly smooth articular surface, so excision of the patella (*patellectomy*) is the preferred option.

This takes care of any future risk of osteoarthritis at the patellofemoral joint. With improvement in fixation techniques, more and more comminuted fractures of the patella are being reconstructed (*patella saving operations*).

COMPLICATIONS

Knee stiffness: It is a common complication after a fracture of the patella, mostly due to intra- and peri-articular adhesions. Treatment is by physiotherapy. Sometimes, an arthroscopic release of adhesions may be required.

Extensor weakness: This results from an inadequate repair of the extensor apparatus or due to quadriceps weakness.

Osteoarthritis: Patellofemoral osteoarthritis occurs a few years after the injury due to irregularity of articulating surface of the patella.

INJURIES TO THE LIGAMENTS OF THE KNEE

With increasing sporting activities, injuries to the knee ligaments are on the rise. The type of injury depends upon the direction of force and its severity.

MECHANISM

Knee ligaments are injured most often from indirect, twisting or bending forces on the knee. The various mechanisms by which knee ligaments are injured are given below:

- **Medial collateral ligament:** This ligament is damaged if the injuring force has the effect of abducting the leg on the femur (*valgus force*). It ruptures most commonly from its femoral attachment.

- **Lateral collateral ligament:** This ligament is damaged by a mechanism just the reverse of above, i.e., adduction of the tibia on the femur *(varus force)*. Commonly, the ligament is avulsed from head of the fibula with a piece of bone. Lateral collateral ligament injuries are uncommon because the knee is not often subjected to varus force (the knee is not likely to be hit from the inside).
- **Anterior cruciate ligament:** This ligament is *most commonly* ruptured, often in association with the tears of collateral ligaments. Commonly, it occurs as a result of twisting force on a semi-flexed knee. Often it is a triad-injury to medial collateral ligament, medial meniscus and anterior cruciate ligament, called *O'Donoghue triad.*
- **Posterior cruciate ligament:** This ligament is damaged if the anterior aspect of the tibia is struck with the knee semi-flexed so as to *force the tibia backwards* on to the femur *(Dashboard injury).*

PATHOANATOMY

The ligament may tear at either of its attachment. Sometimes, taking a chip of bone from the attachment. The ligament may be torn in its substance (mid-substance tear). The severity of the tear varies from a rupture of just a few fibres to a complete tear (see classsification of ligament injury on page 5).

It may be an 'isolated' ligament injury, or more than one ligaments injured (multi-ligament injury). The combination depends upon the direction and severity of the force. Rarely, in a very severe injury, the knee may get dislocated and a number of ligaments injured.

DIAGNOSIS

Clinical examination: Pain and swelling of the knee are the usual complaints. Often, the patient is able to give a history of having sustained a particular type of deforming force at the knee (valgus, varus, etc.), followed by a sound of something tearing. The pain may be localised over the torn ligament (in cases of injury to superficial, collateral ligaments), but there is vague pain if deeper ligaments—cruciate ligaments are injured. The swelling (haemarthrosis) is variable, but appears *early* after the injury.

Damage to the medial and lateral collateral ligaments can be assessed clinically by *stress tests** (see page 6).

Pain at the site of the torn ligament and/or an abnormal 'opening up' of the joint on trying to stress the ligament,

indicate a tear. Cruciate ligaments prevent anterior–posterior gliding of the tibia. The anterior cruciate prevents anterior glide, and the posterior cruciate prevents posterior glide. This property is made use in designing tests to diagnose these injuries.

Tests for diagnosing ACL tear: These are as follows:
- Anterior drawer test: The knee is kept in 90 degree flexion. The upper end is held between two ands and a gentle pull is made in anterior direction. There is increased movement compared to the opposite side.
- Lachmann test: In this test, anterior glide of the tibia is judged with the knee in 10–15 degrees of flexion. This is a more sensitive for diagnosis of ACL tear.
- Pivot-shift test: This is a specific test for diagnosing ACL tear.

Tests for diagnosing PCL tear: These are as follows:
- Posterior sag sign: With both the knees bent to 90 degrees, one can appreciate a posterior sagging of upper tibia as noticed by loss of prominence of tibial tuberosity.
- Posterior drawer test: This is similar to anterior drawer except that here it is possible to push the upper tibial posteriorly.
- Quadriceps active test: In this test, when in 90 degree knee flexion, there is a posterior sag, when one asks the patient to try to extend the knee while the examiner stabilizes the foot on the bed, one notices correction of the sag. This sign helps in differentiating whether excessive anteroposterior mobility is due to ACL or PCL deficiency.

Essential features of common knee ligament injuries are given in Table 20.2.

Radiological examination: A plain X-ray may be normal, or a chip of bone avulsed from the ligament attachment may be visible. MRI is the investigation of choice for diagnosing ligament injuries. In doubtful cases stress X-rays are taken, generally under sedation or general anaesthesia.

Other investigation: Arthroscopic examination may be needed wherever in doubt.

Approach to a patient with knee haemarthrosis: Injury to the knee resulting in acute swelling is a common presentation. This, *knee haemarthrosis* may be due to: (i) an intra-articular fracture of bones constituting the knee—femur, tibia or patella; (ii) knee ligament injury; (iii) meniscus tear and (iv) patellar subluxation or dislocation. It is usually not possible to examine. The knee is immobilised in ready-made splints called long

---

* In an acutely injured knee, stress test is performed under anaesthesia.

Table 20.2: Essential features of knee ligament injury.

Name of the ligament	Mechanism of injury	Clinical features			
		Pain	Swelling	Tenderness	Tests
Medial collateral	Valgus force	Medial side	Medial side	Medially, on the femoral condyle	Valgus stress + at 30° knee flexion
Lateral collateral	Varus force	Lateral side	Lateral side	Laterally, on fibular head	Varus stress + at 30° knee flexion
Anterior cruciate	Twisting extension	Diffuse	Haemarthrosis	Vague	Anterior drawer test + Lachmann test + pivot-shift test
Posterior cruciate	Backward force on tibia	Diffuse	Haemarthrosis	Vague	Posterior sag sign, posterior drawer test +, quadriceps active test

knee immobiliser. An X-ray is the first investigation, where a fracture can be easily diagnosed. Of all cases where no fracture can be seen, a gentle clinical examination may indicate the diagnosis of a ligament injury or patellar subluxation. In cases, with no bony injury, initial treatment is immobilisation in a splint. Once the pain subsides and swelling reduces, it may be possible to make a more exact diagnosis. In general, the knee is rested for 3 weeks, followed by mobilisation and physiotherapy. Where one suspects a significant injury, an MRI is asked for. Once the diagnosis is confirmed, one may adopt a conservative approach or may consider surgery. In some cases, examination under anaesthesia and arthroscopy may be required to come to a diagnosis. In young females presenting with acute knee haemarthrosis following a twisting knee injury, it is a self-reduced patellar subluxation unless proved otherwise.

TREATMENT

Treatment of ligament injuries is a controversial subject. Conventionally, these injuries have been treated by non-operative methods. With availability of more accurate initial diagnosis, newer surgical techniques, and increased demands of the patient, trend is to operatively treat ligament injuries. Operative treatment is indicated in high-demand athletic individuals.

Conservative method: The haematoma is aspirated and the knee is immobilised in a cylinder cast or commercially available long-knee immobiliser. Most cases of grade I and II injuries can be successfully treated by this method. After a few weeks, the swelling subsides, and adequate range of motion and strength can be regained by physiotherapy.

Operative methods: The operation is usually performed 2-3 weeks after injury, once the acute phase subsides. It consists of the following:
a. *Repair of the ligament:* It is performed for fresh, grade III collateral ligament injuries. In cases presenting after 2-3 weeks, an additional reinforcement is provided by a fascial or tendon graft (repair with reinforcement).
b. *Reconstruction:* This is done in cases of ligament injuries with features of knee instability. A ligament is 'constructed' using patient's own tendons (autograft). One may use a tendon taken from cadaver (allograft). Synthetic ligaments were tried but have gone out of fashion.

Knee ligaments are torn more often than they are diagnosed. Unfortunately, since this injury is not detected on X-rays, it gets neglected. Patients usually present late with symptoms of knee giving way (instability). The treatment at this stage depends upon activity level of the patient.

For a patient with sedentary lifestyle, adequate stability is achieved with physiotherapy alone. In active patients, ligament reconstruction is necessary.

The ACL is the most common to be ruptured. The treatment of choice is arthroscopic ACL reconstruction. In this, the torn ligament is replaced with a tendon graft. This is done endoscopically (arthroscopic surgery), without opening the joint.

Technique: The joint is first examined by a 4 mm telescope (arthroscope). A tendon graft taken from patellar tendon or hamstring tendons is introduced into the knee through bone tunnels. The graft is fixed at both ends with screws or other devices. Bioabsorbable screws are now being used. Arthroscopic surgery has advantages of being minimally invasive, and results in quick return to function with minimal risks. A number of techniques of ligament reconstruction have come into vogue, the emphasis being essentially to do the surgery with minimum tinkering to inside of the joint (biological reconstruction).

COMPLICATIONS

1. **Knee instability:** An unhealed ligament leads to instability. The patient 'loses confidence' on his knee, and the knee often "gives-way". Persistent

instability leads to meniscus tears, and cartilage injuries. Surgery is usually required.

2. **Osteoarthritis:** A neglected ligament injury may result in further damage to the knee in the form of meniscus tear, chondral damage, etc. This eventually leads to knee osteoarthritis.

TIBIAL PLATEAU FRACTURES

These are common fractures sustained in two-wheeler accidents when one lands on the knee. Either or both condyles of tibia are fractured. The mechanism of injury is: (a) an indirect force causing varus or valgus force on the knee or (b) a direct hit on the knee.

Types of fracture: These fractures commonly occur in six patterns (Schatzker types). Type I-IV involve only one condyle, lateral or medial. Type V and VI are more complex intercondylar fractures.

Symptoms and signs: The patient complains of pain and swelling, and inability to bear weight. Often crepitus is heard or felt. Diagnosis can be made on X-rays. CT scan may be required for accurate evaluation.

Treatment: Like most fractures, both conservative and operative methods can be used. Conservative methods are used for minimally displaced fractures, and those in elderly people. There is more and more trend towards accurate reduction and early mobilisation of these fractures. Surgical treatment of these fractures is a technically demanding procedure, and needs variety of equipment and lot of experience.

MENISCAL INJURIES OF THE KNEE

These constitute a common group of injuries peculiar to the knee, frequently being reported with increasing sporting activity.

MECHANISM

The injury is sustained when a person, standing on a semi-flexed knee, *twists* his body to one side. The twisting movement, an important component of the mechanism of injury, is possible only with a flexed knee. During this movement the meniscus is 'sucked in' and nipped as rotation occurs between the condyles of femur and tibia. This results in a longitudinal tear of the meniscus. The meniscus may be torn with a minor twisting, as may occur while walking on uneven surface. A degenerated meniscus in the elderly may get torn by minimal or no injury. The medial meniscus gets torn more often because it is *less mobile* (being fixed to the medial collateral ligament).

PATHOANATOMY

The meniscus is torn *most commonly* at its posterior horn. With every subsequent injury, the tear extends anteriorly. The meniscus, being an avascular structure, once torn does not heal*. If left untreated, it undergoes many more subtears, and damages the articular cartilage, thus initiating the process of osteoarthritis.

Types of meniscal tear: The bucket-handle tears (Fig. 20.7) are the *most common* type; others are radial, anterior horn, posterior horn and complex tears. Some underlying pathological changes in the meniscus make it prone to tear. These are discoid meniscus (the meniscus, unlike the normal semilunar shape, is shaped like a disc), degenerated meniscus (in osteoarthritis), and a meniscal cyst.

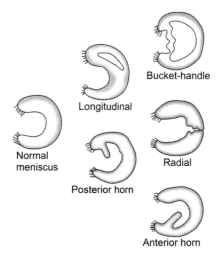

Fig. 20.7: Types of meniscus tear.

CLINICAL FEATURES

Presenting complaints: The patient is generally a young male actively engaged in sports like football, volleyball, etc. The presenting complaint is recurrent episodes of pain, and locking** of the knee. At times, the patient complains of a '*jhatka*', a sudden jerk while walking, or 'something flicking over' inside the joint. This may be followed by a swelling, appearing after a few hours and lasting for a few days. After some time, the pain becomes persistent but with little or no swelling.

---

* The peripheral meniscal tears, being in a vascular area, often heal.
** True locking is an inability to extend the knee for the last few degrees. It is different from 'pseudo-locking' where the knee catches temporarily in one position due to sudden pain. The latter may occur in cases with a loose body. It may also occur due to hamstring muscles spasm, thus not allowing the knee to get extended.

On tracing back the symptoms to their origin, one often finds a history of a classic twisting injury to the knee, followed by a swelling appearing overnight* as effusion collects. After the effusion subsides, the knee may remain in about 10 degrees of flexion, beyond which the patient is unable to extend his knee (locking). This is because the torn portion of the meniscus gets interposed between the femoral and the tibial condyles. Locking may be missed because the attention is drawn to more obvious signs of pain and swelling. The displaced fragment sometimes returns to its original position spontaneously and thus the original episode of locking may never be noticed. Every successive episode of locking may be either spontaneously corrected or may need manipulation by the patient or a physician. The history of sudden locking and unlocking, with a click located in one or other joint compartment, is *diagnostic* of a meniscus tear.

On examination: In a typical episode presenting after injury, the knee may be swollen. There may be tenderness in the region of the joint line, either anteriorly or posteriorly. The knee may be locked. Gentle attempts to force full extension produces a sensation of elastic resistance and pain, localised to the appropriate joint compartment. In between the episodes, the knee may not have any finding except wasting of the quadriceps. The manoeuvres carried out to detect a hidden meniscus tear are McMurray's and Apley's test (see Annexure I).

Often it is difficult to diagnose the cause of knee symptoms on history and clinical examination. Such non-specific symptom-complex is termed as internal derangement of the knee (IDK).

RADIOLOGICAL EXAMINATION

With meniscal tears there are no abnormal X-ray findings. X-rays are taken to rule out any associated bony pathology. MRI is an investigation of choice for detecting meniscus tears. It is a very sensitive investigation, and sometimes picks up tears which are of no clinical significance.

ARTHROSCOPY

This is a technique where a thin endoscope, about 4-5 mm in diameter—the arthroscope, is introduced into the joint through a small stab wound, and

---

* The swelling in a case of meniscus tear is due to synovial reaction, hence appears after a few hours. This is unlike the swelling in other knee injuries, where haemarthrosis results in early swelling.

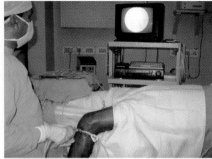
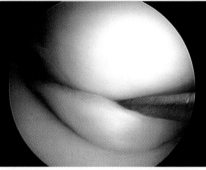

Fig. 20.8: Arthroscopic examination of the knee. The lower picture is an arthroscopic appearance of inside of the knee.

inside of the joint examined (Fig. 20.8). For details see Chapter 41.

TREATMENT

Treatment of acute meniscal tear: If the knee is locked, it is manipulated under general anaesthesia. No special manoeuvre is needed. As the knee relaxes, the torn meniscus falls into place and the knee is unlocked. The knee is immobilised for 2-3 weeks, followed by physiotherapy. In a case where locking is not present, immobilisation in a long knee immobiliser is done. With this modality, some peripheral tears will heal. Rest of the tears may continue to produce recurrent symptoms. If they do, attempt is made to repair them (meniscus suturing). If meniscus is badly damaged, excision of a part of it is done.

Treatment of a chronic meniscal tear: Treatment of meniscus tear has undergone a significant change in last few decades. Earlier, it was considered to be a vestigial structure, and excision of the torn meniscus was a routine. This was done by open surgery in olden days, and by arthroscopic surgery in recent years. Overall, arthroscopic techniques has made it possible to do the job without inflicting further damage to the knee. This technique is a significant advancement as it can be done as a day-care procedure. Since it is a minimally invasive technique, early return to work is possible.

Recent research has established that menisci are not 'useless' structures as was thought earlier. Hence, wherever possible the trend is to preserve the meniscus by suturing. The state-of-the-art in meniscus surgery is *arthroscopic meniscus suturing.*

RARE INJURIES AROUND THE KNEE

Dislocation of the knee: This rare injury results from severe violence to the knee so that all of its supporting ligaments are torn. It is a major damage to the joint, and is often associated with injury to the popliteal artery. Treatment is by reduction followed by immobilisation in a cylinder cast. Recent studies have shown superior results by operative treatment of these severe knee injuries, by multiple ligament reconstruction.

Disruption of extensor apparatus: Injury from sudden quadriceps contraction most often results in fracture of the patella. Sometimes, it may result in tearing of the quadriceps tendon from its attachment on the patella, or tearing of the attachment of the patellar tendon from the tibial tubercle. In either case, operative repair of the tendon is required.

Dislocation of the patella: The patella usually dislocates laterally. It can be one of three types: (i) acute dislocation; (ii) recurrent dislocation; and (iii) habitual dislocation.

Acute dislocation of the patella results from a sudden contraction of the quadriceps while the knee is flexed or semi-flexed. The patella dislocates laterally and lies on the outer side of the knee. The patient is unable to straighten the knee. The medial condyle of femur appears more prominent. Sometimes, the dislocation reduces spontaneously but one can elicit marked tenderness anteromedially as a result of the rupture of the tissues at that site. *Treatment* consists of reduction and immobilisation in a cylinder cast or long knee immobiliser for 3 weeks. Sometimes, a piece of bone covered with articular cartilage (osteochondral fragment), may be chipped off from the patella or the femoral condyle at the time of dislocation (Fig. 20.9). This results in repeated episodes of pain, swelling and sensation of a loose body. Arthroscopic removal of the fragment or its refixation, depending upon the size, may be required.

Recurrent dislocation of the patella: After the first episode of dislocation if it happens during adolescence, the

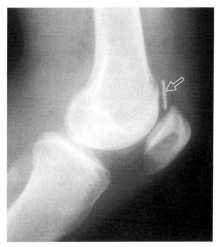

Fig. 20.9: X-ray of the knee, lateral view, showing an intra-articular osteochondral fragment.

dislocation tends to recur with more and more ease. The reason for recurrence may be for a variety of reasons. These could be due to systemic factors such as excessive generalized joint laxity, or local factors such as; (i) a small patella; (ii) a patella alta (i.e., the patella is high-lying in the shallower part of intercondylar groove); (iii) genu valgum; (iv) increased Q angle (angle between the line of quadriceps pull and line of patellar tendon and rarely and (v) due to tortional deformities in femur and tibia (intortion of femur and extortion of tibia). *Treatment* depends on the cause. A thorough evaluation by clinical examination and imaging evaluation including CT scan is required to understand the root cause of the recurrent dislocation. In vast majority, it is simply due to unhealed tissues on the medial side of the patella (medial patello-femoral ligament – MPFL), and the same is reconstructed using tendon graft. In cases where contributing factors as mentioned above are identified, an additional procedure to correct the same is done.

Habitual dislocation of the patella: It means that the patella dislocates laterally *everytime* the knee is flexed. The patient presents early in childhood. Underlying defects are very similar to those in recurrent dislocation. In addition, a shortened quadriceps (vastus lateralis component) may result in an abnormal lateral pull on the patella when the knee is flexed. *Treatment* is by release of the tight structures on the lateral side and repair of the lax structures on the medial side. An additional 'checkrein' mechanism of some sort is created to prevent re-dislocation.

What have we learnt?

- Knee injuries are commonly sustained in scooter accident and sports.
- Fractures around the knee are difficult injuries as they commonly lead to knee stiffness. Hence, open reduction and internal fixation is the more popular method of treatment.
- Internal derangement of the knee (IDK) is a term used to group all the other, non-bony injuries of the knee. These consist of ligament injuries, meniscus injury and patello femoral problems.
- MRI is an important investigation for diagnosis of ligament and meniscus injuries.
- Arthroscopic surgery has become a standard method of treating meniscus and ligament injuries of the knee.

Additional information: From the entrance exams point of view

- In 90° flexion of the knee, the tibial tuberosity is in line with the centre of the patella, on extension, it moves towards the lateral border due to the screw home mechanism.
- People with anterior cruciate deficient knees have a problem climbing downhill.
- Dial test, tests posterolateral corner and the posterior cruciate ligament.
  - Posterolateral corner deficiency positive at 30° flexion.
  - Posterior cruciate ligament positive at both 30° and 90° flexion.
- Physiological locking occurs with internal rotation of the femur over a fixed tibia by the quadriceps, unlocking refers to the lateral rotation of the femur over a stabilised tibia by the popliteus.
- Rotation force is most important in causing a meniscal injury.

Injuries to the Leg, Ankle and Foot

Competencies

- ❖ **OR2.13:** Describe and discuss the aetiopathogenesis, clinical features, investigation and principles of management of:
  - a. Fracture both bones leg
  - b. Calcaneus
  - c. Small bones of foot.
- ❖ **OR2.14:** Describe and discuss the aetiopathogenesis, clinical features, investigation and principles of management of ankle fractures.

FRACTURES OF SHAFTS OF TIBIA AND FIBULA

RELEVANT ANATOMY

The tibia is the major weight bearing bone of the leg. It is connected to the less important bone, the fibula, through the proximal and distal tibio- fibular joints. Like fractures of forearm bones, these bones frequently fracture together, and are referred to as 'fracture both bones of leg'. The following are some of the characteristics of these bones.

a. **A subcutaneous bone:** This is responsible for the large number of open tibial fractures. Also, often there is loss of bone through the wound.

b. **Fractures in this region** are often associated with massive loss of skin, necessitating care by plastic surgeons, early in the treatment.

c. **Precarious blood supply:** The distal-third of tibia is particularly prone to delayed and non-union because of its precarious blood supply. The major source of blood supply to the bone is the medullary vessels. The periosteal blood supply is poor because of few muscular attachments on the to the distal-third. The fibula, on the other hand is a bone with many muscular attachments, and thus has a rich blood supply.

Hinge joints proximally and distally: Both, the proximal and distal joints (the knee and ankle) are hinge joints. So, even a small degree of rotational mal-alignment of the leg fracture becomes noticeable. This is unlike a fracture of the femur or humerus, where some degree of rotational mal-alignment goes unnoticed because of the polyaxial ball and socket joints proximally.

MECHANISM

The tibia and fibula may be fractured by a direct or indirect injury.

Direct injury: Road traffic accidents are the most common cause of these fractures, mostly due to direct violence. The fracture occurs at about the same level in both bones. Frequently the object causing the fracture lacerates the skin over it, resulting in an open fracture.

Indirect injury: A bending or torsional force on the tibia may result in an oblique or spiral fracture respectively. The sharp edge of the fracture fragment may pierce the skin from within, resulting in an open fracture.

PATHOANATOMY

The fracture may be closed or open, and may have various patterns. It may occur at different levels (upper, middle or lower-third). Occasionally, it may be a single bone fracture i.e., only the tibia or the fibula is fractured. Displacements may be sideways, angulatory or rotational. Occasionally, the fracture may remain undisplaced.

CLINICAL FEATURES

The patient is brought to the hospital with a history of injury to the leg followed by the classic features of a fracture, i.e., pain, swelling, deformity, etc.

There may be a wound communicating with the underlying bone.

RADIOLOGICAL FEATURES

The diagnosis is usually confirmed by X-ray examination. Evaluation of the anatomical configuration of the fracture on X-ray helps in reduction.

TREATMENT

For the purpose of treatment, fractures of the tibia and fibula may be divided into two types: closed or open.

Closed fractures: Treatment of closed fractures, both in children and in adults, is by closed reduction under anaesthesia followed by an above-knee plaster cast. In children, it is possible to achieve good alignment in most cases, and the fracture unites in about 6 weeks. In adults, the fracture unites in 16–20 weeks. Sometimes, reduction is not achieved, or the fracture displaces in the plaster. In both these cases, open reduction and internal fixation is required.

The *trend is changing* with the availability of minimally invasive techniques such as of closed nailing. More and more unstable tibial fractures are being treated, right in the begining by *closed interlock nailing*.

Open fractures: The aim in the treatment of open fractures is to convert it into a closed fracture by judicious care of the wound, and simultaneously keep the fracture in good alignment. Following methods can be used for treating an open fracture, depending upon its grade.

- *Grade I:* Wound dressing through a window in an above-knee plaster cast, and antibiotics.
- *Grade II:* Wound debridement and primary closure (if less than 6 hours old), and above-knee plaster cast. The wound may need dressings through a window in the plaster cast.
- *Grade III:* Wound debridement, dressing and external fixator application. The wound is left open.

The *trend is changing*, from primarily conservative treatment to operative treatment, in care of open tibial fractures. More and more open fractures in grade I and II are being fixed internally. In a number of other cases, a delayed operation (ORIF) is done once the wound is taken care of.

Technique of closed reduction: Under anaesthesia, the patient lies supine with his knees flexed over the end of the table. The surgeon is seated on a stool, facing the injured leg. The leg is kept in traction using a halter, made of ordinary bandage, around the ankle (Fig. 21.1). The fracture ends are manipulated and good alignment achieved. Initially, a below-knee cast is applied over evenly applied cotton padding. Once this part of the plaster sets, the cast is extended to above the knee.

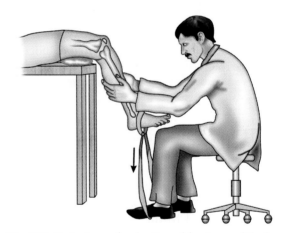

Fig. 21.1: Technique of reduction of fractures of the leg.

Wedging: Sometimes, after a fracture has been reduced and the plaster applied, check X-ray shows a little angulation at the fracture site. Instead of cutting open the plaster and reapplying it, it is better to *wedge* the plaster as shown in Figure 21.2. In this technique, the plaster is cut circumferentially at the level of the fracture, the angulation corrected by forcing open the cut on the *concave* side of the angulation, and the plaster reinforced with additional plaster bandages.

Once the fracture becomes 'sticky' (in about 6 weeks), above-knee plaster is removed and below-knee PTB (patellar tendon bearing) cast is put. Use of modern, synthetic casting tapes (made of plastic polymer) has made conservative treatment more convenient. Once the fracture has partly united, the cast can be

Flowchart 21.1: Treatment plan of tibial shaft fractures.

Fracture of both bones
of the leg

Closed

Open

Undisplaced

Displaced

Stable

Unstable

PoP cast
for 4 wks

Closed reduction

Grade I
Wound debridement + PoP
cast with dressing through
a window in the cast

Satisfactory

Not satisfactory

PoP cast
with 2-weekly
check X-ray for first
4 wks

Grade II
Wound debridement
+ external fixator

Change to PoP cast
once the wound
heals

Maintain
position
for 4 wks

Displaces

Continue PoP
for 12 wks

Grade III
External fixator +
early bone grafting

PTB cast or
brace for 6 wks

PTB for 4 wks
(if required)

Closed/open
nailing

Closed
nailing

Closed
nailing

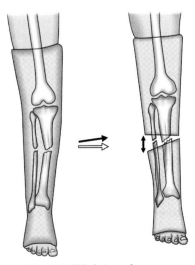

Fig. 21.2: Wedging of a cast.

replaced by removable plastic supports (braces), in which joints can be mobilized.

Role of operative treatment: Open reduction and internal fixation is necessary when it is not possible to achieve a satisfactory alignment of a fracture by non-operative methods. The internal fixation device used may be a plate or an intra-medullary nail depending upon the configuration of the fracture. Interlock nailing provides the possibility of internally fixing a wide spectrum of tibial shaft fractures. With the availability of facilities, operative treatment has now become a method of preference.

Deciding the plan of treatment: It depends on whether the fracture is closed or open. A practical plan of treatment is as shown in Flowchart 21.1.

COMPLICATIONS

1. **Delayed union and non-union:** Fractures of the tibia sometimes take unusually long to unite; more so *the ones in the lower-third.* In some cases, clear signs of non-union become apparent on X-rays. The most important factor responsible for delayed and non-union is the *precarious blood* supply of the tibia; others being frequent compounding with loss of fracture haematoma, wound infection, etc. Failure of union results in pain and inability to bear weight on the leg.

   Treatment: Treatment of delayed union and non-union is essentially by bone grafting, with or without internal fixation. Following treatment options are available:

   a. Nailing with bone grafting: This is indicated in cases of non-union, where the alignment is not acceptable, or there is free mobility at the fracture site. Some surgeons prefer plating and bone grafting.

   b. Phemister grafting: This used to be a popular method in the past, done for selected cases which fullfil the following criteria:
   - There is minimal or no mobility at the fracture site (fibrous union).
   - The fracture has an acceptable alignment.
   - The knee joint has a good range of movement.

   In this technique, grafting is performed without disturbing the sound fibrous union at the fracture site. The aim is to stimulate bone formation in the 'fibro-cartilaginous tissue' already bridging the fracture. Cancellous bone grafts are placed after raising the *osteo-periosteal* flaps around the fracture (Fig. 21.3). In addition, petalling (lifting slivers of cortical bone attached at base) is carried out around the fracture. This results in bony union in about 3–4 months.

   c. Ilizarov's method: This method is useful in treatment of difficult non-unions of tibia. These are non-unions with bone gap, infection, or those with bad overlying skin (details on page 35).

2. **Malunion:** Some amount of angulation is acceptable in children as it gets corrected by remodelling. In adults, displacements especially angulations and rotations are not acceptable. These cause problems in walking and result in early osteoarthritis of the knee and ankle. Treatment requires correction of the deformity by redoing the fracture and fixing it by plating or nailing, and bone grafting.

3. **Infection:** Because of the frequency with which tibial fractures are associated with a communicating skin wound, contamination and subsequent infection is a common complication. Most often the infection is superficial and is controlled by dressing and antibiotics. Sometimes, the underlying bone gets infected, in which case more elaborate treatment on the lines of osteomyelitis may be necessary (see page 172). The fracture in such cases often does not unite. Ilizarov's method is the treatment of choice in such infected non-unions.

4. **Compartment syndrome** (see page 47): Some cases of closed fracture of the tibia may be associated with significant crushing of soft tissues, leading to compartment syndrome. A compartment syndrome should be suspected if a fracture of the tibia is associated with excessive pain, swelling and inability to move the toes. Immediate operative decompression of the compartments is imperative.

5. **Injury to major vessels and nerves:** Occasionally a fracture of the tibia, especially in the upper-third of the shaft may be associated with injury to the popliteal artery or the common peroneal and tibial nerves. Therefore, examination of the neurovascular status of the limb in a fresh case is of vital importance to prevent serious complications like vascular gangrene, etc.

Treatment of these complications is as discussed in Chapter 7.

ACHILLES TENDON DISORDERS

Achilles tendon is largest and strongest tendon of body. It is required for locomotion. It is formed by joining together of tendons of medial and lateral heads of gastrocnemius and soleus muscles.

During life time, the tendon is subjected repetitive stress. This leads to degenerative changes within the

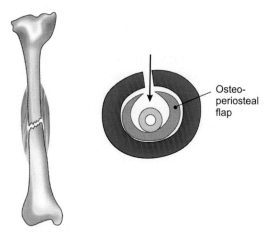

Osteo-periosteal flap

Fig. 21.3: Phemister grafting.

substance of the tendon, and can lead to spontaneous rupture. Sometime there may be history of a rather trivial injury. There are two common forms of presentations:

1. Achilles tendinosis: This is a condition due to degeneration of tendon collagen, and it results in disabling pain.
2. Achilles rupture: This may occur due to sudden contracture of the muscle. Often the background factor is degeneration.

Diagnosis is made on clinical examination, where a distinct gap can be felt in the continuity of the tendon. There may be hypertrophy of the tendon due to chronic rupture. *Thompson test* is diagnostic of a complete Achilles tendon rupture. In this, with knee bent, when calf is squeezed, the ankle normally goes into plantar flexion. This is missing if there is a complete rupture of tendo-Achilles. MRI is confirmatory.

Treatment: In acute, primarily traumatic ruptures, primary repair is done. More often, the tendon rupture has a background of degeneration. In such cases masterly neglect may produce good functional results. Some gait abnormality, acceptable with normal life, may persist.

ANKLE INJURIES

The bones forming the ankle joint are a frequent site of injury. A large variety of bending and twisting forces result in a number of fractures and fracture-dislocation at this joint. All these injuries are sometimes grouped under a general title 'Pott's fracture'.

RELEVANT ANATOMY

The ankle joint is a modified hinge joint. The 'socket' is formed by the distal articular surfaces of the tibia and fibula, the intervening tibio-fibular syndesmosis, ligament and the articular surfaces of the malleoli. These together constitute the *ankle-mortise* (Fig. 21.4). The superior articular surface of the talus (the dome) articulates with this socket.

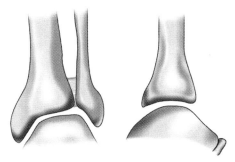

Fig. 21.4: The ankle-mortise.

The strong tibio-fibular syndesmosis, along with the medial and lateral malleoli make the ankle a strong and stable articulation. Therefore, pure dislocation of the ankle is rare. Commonly, dislocation occurs only with fractures of the malleoli or torn deltoid and syndesmotic ligaments. The elongated posterior part of the distal articular surface of the tibia, often termed as *posterior malleous* gets fractured in some ankle injuries.

Ligaments of the ankle: The ankle joint has two main ligaments; the medial and lateral collateral ligaments (Fig. 21.5).

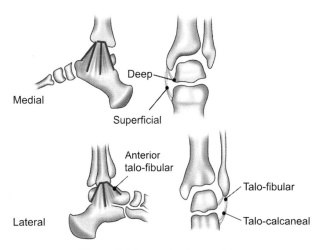

Fig. 21.5: Ligaments of the ankle.

Medial collateral ligament (deltoid ligament): This is a strong ligament on the medial side. It has a superficial (tibio-calcaneal) and a deep (tibio-talar) part.

Lateral collateral ligament: This is a weak ligament and is often injured. It has three parts: (i) anterior talo-fibular; (ii) calcaneo-fibular in the middle; and (iii) posterior talo-fibular.

Some terms used in relation to ankle injuries (Fig. 21.6): Following are some of the terms used to describe different forces the ankle may be subjected to:

a. *Inversion* (adduction): Inward twisting of the calcaneum at talo-calcaneal joint.
b. *Eversion* (abduction): Outward twisting of calcaneum at talo-calcaneal joint.
c. *Supination:* Inversion plus adduction of the foot so that the sole faces medially and is in plantar flexion.
d. *Pronation:* Eversion and abduction of the foot so that the sole faces laterally and is in dorsiflexion.
e. *Rotation* (external or internal): A rotatory movement of the foot so that the talus is subjected to a rotatory force along its vertical axis.

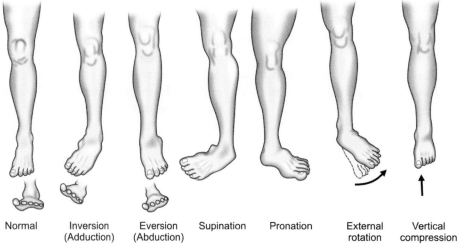

Normal　　Inversion　　Eversion　　Supination　　Pronation　　External　　Vertical
　　　　　(Adduction)　(Abduction)　　　　　　　　　　　　　rotation　compression

Fig. 21.6: Forces at the ankle.

f. *Vertical compression:* A force along the long axis of the tibia.

CLASSIFICATION

The Lauge-Hansen classification (Table 21.1) of ankle injuries is most widely used. It is based on the mechanism of injury. It is believed that a specific pattern of bending and twisting forces results in specific fracture pattern. Different types of ankle injuries have been classified on the basis of whether the foot was supinated or pronated at the time of injury, and what forces was it subjected to in that position. These following combinations are possible:
a. Supination-adduction injuries.
b. Pronation-abduction injuries.
c. Pronation-external rotation injuries.
d. Supination-external rotation injuries.

When a foot is subjected to these forces, different parts of the ankle-mortise are subjected to distraction and compression stress. The specific fracture pattern depends on the type of deforming force and its severity, as discussed below:

Supination-adduction injuries: An adduction force with the foot in *plantar-flexion* results in a sprain of the lateral ligament of the ankle. It may be either a partial or complete rupture. A partial rupture is limited to the anterior fasciculus of the lateral ligament (talo-fibular component). In a complete rupture, the tear extends backwards to involve the whole of the lateral ligament complex. As complete rupture occurs, the talus tends to subluxate out of the ankle-mortise.

The inversion force on an ankle *in neutral or dorsiflexed position* results in an avulsion fracture of lateral malleolus to begin with, usually transverse and below the joint line (low transverse). A more severe force results in additional fracture of the medial malleolus, typically, a fracture with the fracture line running *obliquely* upwards from the medial angle of the ankle-mortise (Fig. 21.7).

Table 21.1: Lauge-Hansen classification of ankle injuries.				
Type of injury	**On medial side**	**Tibio-fibular syndesmosis**	**On lateral side**	**Others**
Supination-Adduction Injury	Medial malleolus fracture with nearly vertical to oblique fracture line	Normal	Avulsion fractures of lat. malleolus or Lateral collateral ligament injury	—
Pronation-Abduction injury	Avulsion fracture of medial malleolus (low) or Medial collateral ligament	Normal or Torn	Fracture of lateral malleolus at the level of ankle mortice or proximal with *comminution* of its lateral cortex	
Pronation-external rotation injury	Transverse fracture of med. malleolus *at the level* of ankle-mortise	Torn	Spiral fracture of the fibula *above* the level of ankle-mortise	
Supination-external rotation injury	Transverse fracture of medial malleolus *at the level* of ankle-mortise	Normal or Torn	Spiral fracture of the lat. malleolus *at the level of* ankle-mortise	Fracture of the posterior malleolus

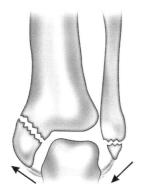

Fig. 21.7: Supination-adduction injury.

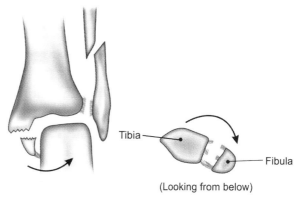

(Looking from below)

Fig. 21.9: Pronation-external rotation injury.

Pronation-Abduction injuries: In this type, the medial structures are subjected to a distracting force and the lateral structures to compressive force. This results in rupture of the deltoid ligament or a low-lying transverse fracture of the medial malleolus (avulsion fracture) on the medial side. On the lateral side, a fracture of the lateral malleolus *at the level* of the ankle-mortise or more proximal level with comminution of the outer cortex occurs (Fig. 21.8). The talus, with both malleoli fractured, subluxates laterally. This commonly produces *bimalleolar fracture.*

Supination-external rotation injuries: With the foot supinated, the talus twists externally within the mortise. As the medial structures are lax, the first structure to give way is that on the lateral side, the head of the talus striking against the lateral malleolus, producing a *spiral fracture at the level* of the ankle-mortise. The next structure to break is the posterior malleolus. As the talus rotates further, it hits against the medial malleolus resulting in a transverse fracture (Fig. 21.10). The tibio-fibular syndesmosis may remain intact or get torn depending upon level

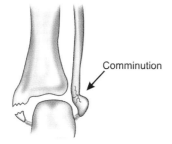

Comminution

Fig. 21.8: Abduction injury.

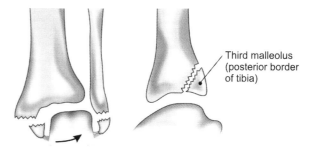

Third malleolus (posterior border of tibia)

Fig. 21.10: Supination-external rotation injury.

Pronation-external rotation injuries: When a pronated foot rotates externally, the talus also rotates outwards along its vertical axis. The first structures to give way are those on the medial side. There may occur a transverse fracture of the medial malleolus at the level of the ankle-mortise, or a rupture of the medial collateral ligament. With further rotation of the talus, the anterior tibio-fibular ligament is torn. This is followed by a spiral fracture of the lower end of the fibula. This fracture occurs above the level of ankle joint, and indirectly indicates injury to tibio-fibular syndesmosis. (Fig. 21.9). Occasionally, the fibular fracture may occur as high as the neck of the fibula (Maisonneuve's fracture). The continuing rotational force may further tear the posterior tibio-fibular ligament or may cause fracture of posterior malleolus. This makes it *trimalleolar fracture*.*

of fracture of fibula. In extreme cases, the whole foot along with the three malleoli, is displaced.

Tibial pilon fracture: This fracture at the ankle occurs as a result of primarily axial compression force, whereby the dome of the talus hit the distal articular surface of tibia. It results in variable comminuted fracture of the distal tibial articular surface with or without a fracture of the fibula (Fig. 21.11). This type

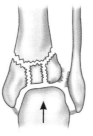

Fig. 21.11: Vertical compression injury-Pilon Fracture.

---

* It is important to recognise disruption of tibio-fibular syndesmosis on a *proper* AP X-ray of the ankle, and reconstruct it.

of fracture is often associated with severe injury to skin and soft tissue around ankle.

CLINICAL FEATURES

There is history of a twisting injury to the ankle followed by pain and swelling. Often the patient is able to describe exactly the way the ankle got twisted. On examination, the ankle is found to be swollen. Swelling and tenderness may be localised to the area of injury (bone or ligament). Crepitus may be noticed if there is a fracture. The ankle may be lying deformed (adducted or abducted, with or without rotation).

RADIOLOGICAL EXAMINATION

Antero-posterior and lateral X-rays of the ankle are sufficient in most cases (Fig. 21.12). While examining an X-ray, it is important to make note of the following features:

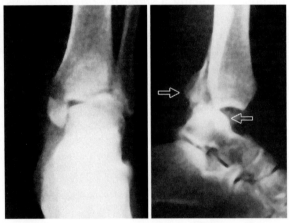

Fig. 21.12: X-rays of the ankle, AP and lateral views, showing an ankle injury. (Note, the talus is subluxated, and there is a fracture of the posterior malleolus).

Fracture line of the medial and lateral malleoli should be studied in order to evaluate the type of ankle injury (Lauge-Hansen classification). Small avulsion fractures from the malleoli are sometimes missed. These often have attached to them the whole ligament.

Tibio-fibular syndesmosis: All ankle injuries where the fibular fracture is above the mortise, the syndesmosis is bound to have been disrupted. In injuries where the fibular fracture is at the level of the syndesmosis, one must carefully look for any lateral subluxation of the talus; if it is so, width of the joint space between the medial malleolus and the talus will be more than the space between the weight bearing surfaces of tibia and talus.
- **Posterior subluxation** of the talus and fracture of posterior malleolus should be looked for, on the lateral X-ray.

- **Soft tissue swelling** on the medial or lateral side in the absence of a fracture, must arouse suspicion of a ligament injury. This should be confirmed or ruled out after thorough clinical examination and stress X-rays. CT scan and sometimes MRI.

TREATMENT

Principles of Treatment

The complexity of the forces involved produce a variety of combinations of fractures and fracture-dislocations around the ankle. The basic principle of treatment is to achieve anatomical reconstruction of the ankle-mortise. This helps in restoring good function and reducing the possibility of late onset osteoarthritis of ankle. In some undisplaced fractures, there is a role of conservative methods. In most, an operative reduction and internal fixation is required. Given below are some general principles:

Fractures without displacement: It is usually sufficient to protect the ankle in a below-knee plaster for 3-6 weeks. Good, ready-made braces can also be used in place of rather uncomfortable plaster cast.

Conservative methods: It is often possible to achieve a good reduction by manipulation under general anaesthesia. The essential feature of the reduction is to concentrate on restoring the alignment of the foot to the leg. By doing so the fragments automatically fall into place. Once reduced, a below-knee plaster cast is applied. If the check X-ray shows a satisfactory position, the plaster cast is continued for 8-10 weeks. The patient is not allowed to bear any weight on the leg during this period. Check X-rays are taken frequently to make sure the fracture does not get displaced. If everything goes well, the plaster is removed after 8-10 weeks. Physiotherapy is begun thereafter to regain movement at the ankle.

Fractures with displacement: Aim of treatment is to ensure anatomical reduction of the ankle-mortise. This means, ensuring anatomical reduction of medial, lateral and posterior malleoli, and reduction of the talus accurately within the mortise. Following modes of treatment may be useful:

Operative methods: Most surgeons are now resorting to internal fixation for all displaced fractures of ankle without attempting closed reduction. This helps to achieve perfect alignment as well as stable fixation of fragments. This subsequently, allows early motion of the ankle joint, thereby improving overall results. This approach is justified in hospitals where trained staff and all equipment necessary for such work is available.

Internal fixation: In general, operative reduction and internal fixation may be used in cases where closed reduction has not been successful, or the reduction has slipped during the course of conservative treatment. The following techniques of internal fixation are used depending upon the type of fracture.

Medial malleolus fracture
- Transverse and mildly oblique fracture - compression screw, tension-band wiring
- Vertical or highly oblique fracture - Butress plating

Lateral malleolus fracture
- Transverse fracture - tension-band wiring
- Spiral fracture - compression screws plus neutralising plate
- Comminuted fracture - bridge plating as a internal splint.

Posterior malleolus
Very small undisplaced posterior malleolus can be left alone provided syndesmosis has been well reduced and stabilized. Bigger fragment (>20%) always needs stabilization. This could be achieved by one or two compression screws with or without a buttress plate. The latter is required if size of the posterior malleolus is really huge. If left unreduced and unfixed, it leads to gradual posterior subluxation of the ankle.

Tibio-fibular syndesmosis disruption—needs to be examined in all malleolar fractures after internal fixation of medial and lateral malleolus. This is done by trying to move the fibula in AP direction. When required, it is stabilised by inserting a long screw from the fibula into the tibia-syndesmotic screw.

All major ligament injuries, e.g., that of deltoid ligament, lateral ligament should be repaired.

External fixation: This may be required in cases where closed methods cannot be used, e.g., open fractures with bad crushing of the muscles and tendons, with skin loss around the ankle.

COMPLICATIONS
Simple types of ankle injuries are almost free of complications. More serious fracture-dislocation may be complicated because of improper treatment. Sometimes, the nature of injury is such that perfect functions cannot be restored. The following complications may occur:
1. **Stiffness of the ankle:** Following immobilisation in plaster, stiffness occurs. In ankle injuries, resolution of gravitational oedema takes a long time due to sluggish venous return. It is most common in elderly persons. With persistent treatment, using limb elevation, crepe bandage and active toe movements, oedema subsides. It may be necessary to continue ankle exercises for a long period (6-8 months).
2. **Osteoarthritis:** Since most ankle fractures involve the articular surfaces, anything short of a perfect anatomical reduction with smooth and congruous joint surfaces will lead to wear and tear of the articular cartilage. This will start the process of degenerative osteoarthritis. Greater the irregularity of the articular surfaces, more rapidly will the degenerative changes progress. The patient will complain of persistent pain, swelling and joint stiffness. Once established, osteoarthritis cannot be reversed. In a case where the disability (pain, etc.) is severe, it may be required to fuse the talus to the tibia (ankle arthrodesis).

SPRAINED ANKLE
It is the term used for ligament injuries of the ankle. Commonly, it is an inversion injury, and the lateral collateral ligament is sprained. Sometimes, an eversion force may result in a sprain of the medial collateral ligament of the ankle.

Diagnosis: The patient gives history of a twisting injury to the ankle followed by pain and swelling over the injured ligament. Weight bearing gives rise to excruciating pain. In cases with complete tears, patient gives a history of feeling of 'something tearing' at the time of the injury.

There may be swelling and tenderness localised to the site of the torn ligament. If a torn ligament is subjected to stress by the following manoeuvres, the patient experiences severe pain:
- Inversion of a plantar-flexed foot for anterior talo-fibular ligament sprain.
- Inversion in neutral position for complete lateral collateral ligament sprain.
- Eversion in neutral position for medial collateral ligament sprain.

Radiological examination: X-rays of the ankle (AP and lateral) are usually normal. In some cases, *stress X-rays* may be done to judge the severity of the sprain. A tilt of the talus greater than 20° on forced inversion or eversion indicates a complete tear of the lateral or medial collateral ligament respectively.

Treatment: It depends upon the severity of sprain:
- *Grade I:* RICE=Rest, Immobilisation, Cold packs and Elevation. This is followed by weight-bearing mobilisation as and when tolerated and active exercises.
- *Grade II:* RICE with immoblisation by a removable brace. Rest of the treatment is like grade I injuries.

- *Grade III:* Weight-bearing is delayed while rest of the treatment is similar to grade II sprain. A supervised physiotherapy is required in these injuries to regain stability and strength.

Current trend is to treat ligament injuries, in general, by 'functional' method, i.e., without immobilisation. Treatment consists of RICE, for the first 2-3 days. The patient begins early protected range of motion exercises. Methods are devised by which during mobilisation, stress is avoided on 'healing' ligaments, and the muscles around the joint are built up. For this approach, a well-developed physiotherapy unit is required. For grade III ligament injury to the ankle, especially in young athletic individuals, operative repair is preferred by some surgeons.

CHRONIC ANKLE SPRAIN

Chronic recurrent sprain ankle is a disabling condition. If a course of physiotherapy and modification in shoe has not helped, a detailed evaluation with MRI and arthroscopy may be necessary. Accompanying pain in chronic ankle sprains is due to a) impingement of the scarred capsule or b) osteochondral lesion of the talus. Arthroscopic surgery is a good technique for diagnosis and treatment of such cases.

FRACTURES OF THE CALCANEUM

RELEVANT ANATOMY

The calcaneum forms the bone of the heel. Its superior surface articulates with the talus, and the anterior surface with the cuboid. Its inferior surface is prolonged backwards as the *tuber calcanei.* Normally, the angle between the superior articular surface (between talus and calcaneum) and the upper surface of the tuberosity is 35° (tuber-joint angle, Fig. 21.13). It is reduced in most fractures of the calcaneum.

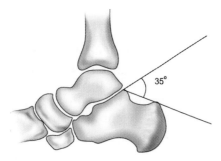

Fig. 21.13: Tuber-joint angle.

PATHOANATOMY

Fractures of the calcaneum are often caused by *fall from height onto the heels,* thus both heels may be injured at the same time. The fracture may be simple

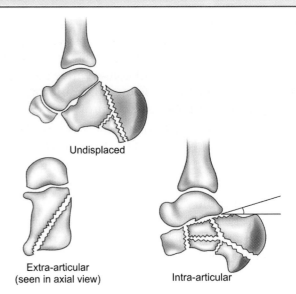

Fig. 21.14: Types of fracture calcaneum.

or comminuted. It can be restricted to (i) an isolated fracture, usually in the region of the tuberosity without involvement of articular facet, (ii) more often a compression injury where the bone is shattered like an egg shell. The degree of displacement of fragments varies according to the severity of trauma. The fracture may be of one of the following types (Fig. 21.14).

- **Undisplaced fracture** resulting from a minimal trauma.
- **Extra-articular fracture**, where the articular surfaces remain intact, and the force splits the calcaneal tuberosity vertically.
- **Intra-articular fracture**, where the articular facet of the calcaneum fails to withstand the stress. It is shattered and is driven downwards into the body of the bone, crushing the delicate trabeculae of the cancellous bone. This is the *most common* type of fracture.

DIAGNOSIS

Clinical features: The patient often gives a history of a fall from height, landing on their heels (e.g., a thief jumping from the first floor of a house). There is pain and swelling in the region of the heel. The patient is not able to bear weight on the affected foot. On examination, there is marked swelling and broadening of the heel.

Conservative methods: It is often possible to achieve a good reduction by manipulation under general anaesthesia. The essential feature of the reduction is to concentrate on restoring the alignment of the foot to the leg. By doing so the fragments automatically fall into place. Once reduced, a below-knee plaster cast is applied. If the check X-ray shows a satisfactory position, the plaster cast is continued for 8-10 weeks.

The patient is not allowed to bear any weight on the leg during this period. Check X-rays are taken frequently to make sure the fracture does not get displaced. If everything goes well, the plaster is removed after 8-10 weeks and the patient undergoes above the level of ankle joint physiotherapy to regain movement at the ankle. Usually there will be ecchymosis around the heel and on the sole. Movement at the ankle is not appreciably impaired.

Many cases of compression fractures of the calcaneum are associated with a compression fracture of a vertebral body (usually in the dorso-lumbar region), fractures of the pubic rami, or an atlanto-axial injury. One must look for these injuries in a case of a fracture of the calcaneum.

Radiological examination: It is possible to diagnose most calcaneum fractures on a lateral X-ray of the heel. In some cases, an additional axial view of the calcaneum may be required. Very often, rather than a clear fracture line extending through the calcaneum, there occurs crushing of the bone. This can be diagnosed on a lateral X-ray of the heel by reduction in the tuber-joint angle (Fig. 21.15).

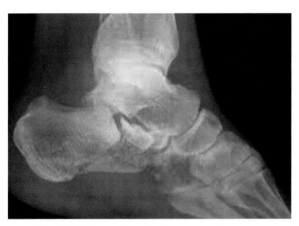

Fig. 21.15: X-ray showing fracture calcaneum.

TREATMENT

Undisplaced fracture: Below-knee plaster cast for 3 weeks followed by weight-bearing after 8 weeks, and mobilisation thereafter.

Intra-articular compression fracture: These are serious calcaneum fractures, and were treated conservatively in the past. Results were often poor, and there was onset of early talo-calcaneal arthritis in vast majority. For this, quite a few patients used to required arthrodesis of the subtalar joint.

In recent times, with improvement in surgical techniques, there is a growing trend to restore the articular surface, height and width of calcaneus by surgical intervention. The surgery is technically demanding and requires a long learning curve. A poorly performed surgery has a high complication rate whereas a well done surgery is followed by good functional recovery.

COMPLICATIONS

1. **Stiffness** of the subtalar and mid-tarsal joints: Some amount of stiffness of the subtalar joint, resulting in limitation to the inversion-eversion motion of the foot is inevitable in most compression fractures of the calcaneum. Stiffness can be kept to minimum by reduction and internal fixation and early physiotherapy.

2. **Osteoarthritis:** Because of the irreparable distortion of the subtalar joint surface, osteoarthritis is an expected complication. It results in pain and stiffness, most noticeable while walking on an uneven surface. A patient with a severe disability may require fusion of the subtalar joint (arthrodesis).

FRACTURES OF THE TALUS

Fractures of talus may range from small chip fracture of one of the articular surfaces of the talus, to more serious fracture such as fracture of the neck or body of the talus.

RELEVANT ANATOMY

Blood supply to the talus: This is the only bone of the foot without any muscle attachment. The main blood supply to the talus is from the anastomotic ring of blood vessels, the osseous vessels entering its neck and running postero-laterally within the bone to supply its body. Therefore, blood supply to the body of the talus is often cut-off following fractures occurring through the neck.

MECHANISM

Fracture of the neck of the talus results from forced dorsiflexion of the ankle (Fig. 21.16). Typically, this injury is sustained in an aircraft crash where the

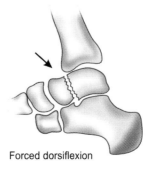

Forced dorsiflexion

Fig. 21.16: Mechanism of injury of fracture neck of the talus.

rudder bar is driven forcibly against the middle of the sole of the foot (Aviator's fracture), resulting in forced dorsiflexion of the ankle; the neck, being a weak area, gives way. This may be associated with dislocation of the body of the talus backwards, out of the ankle-mortise. Vascularity of the body of the talus may be compromised.

DIAGNOSIS

Unless carefully examined on a lateral X-ray of the ankle, this fracture is frequently missed because of the overlapping of the tarsal bones.

TREATMENT

It depends upon the displacement. If undisplaced, a below-knee plaster cast for 8-10 weeks is sufficient. In a displaced fracture, open reduction and internal fixation of the fracture with screws is required.

COMPLICATIONS

1. **Avascular necrosis and non-union:** Because of the poor blood supply, after a fracture through the neck, the body of the talus can becomes avascular. The avascular fragment fails to unite with rest of the bone and gradually collapses, leading to deformation of the bone, and eventually osteoarthritis of the ankle.
2. **Osteoarthritis:** Besides avascular necrosis of the talus, an associated injury to its articular cartilage may lead to osteoarthritis of the ankle. The patient complains of pain and stiffness. *Treatment* is mostly by physiotherapy and fomentation. In severe cases, an ankle arthrodesis may be needed.

INJURIES OF THE TARSAL BONES

Fractures and dislocations of other tarsal bones are uncommon. Most of the fractures can be treated by a below-knee plaster cast. Most dislocations at any of the tarsal joints (subtalar, talo-navicular or inter-tarsal) can be treated by manipulation and immobilisation in a plaster cast. Sometimes, an open reduction and internal fixation with K-wires or small plates may be required. Crush injury of cuboid has been named *Nutcracker fracture*. A fracture dislocation of second tarso-metatarsal and associated injuries has been termed *Lisfranc injury*. The diagnosis and adequate treatment by surgical intervention of these injuries is essential to maintain normal biomechanics of foot.

FRACTURES OF THE METATARSAL BONES

Most metatarsal fractures are caused by direct violence from a heavy object falling onto the foot. A metatarsal fracture may be caused by repeated stress without any specific injury (*March fracture*). Some of the commoner types of metatarsal fractures are discussed below.

FRACTURE OF THE BASE OF 5TH METATARSAL (JONES' FRACTURE)

This is a fracture at the base of the 5th metatarsal, caused by the pull exerted by the tendon of the peroneus brevis muscle inserted on it. Clinically, there is pain, swelling and tenderness at the outer border of the foot, most marked at the base of the 5th metatarsal. Diagnosis is easily confirmed on X-ray (Fig. 21.17). Treatment is by a below-knee walking plaster cast for 3 to 5 weeks.

FRACTURE OF THE METATARSAL SHAFTS

One or more metatarsal shafts may be fractured, mostly following a crush injury. Treatment is by below-knee plaster cast for 3-4 weeks.

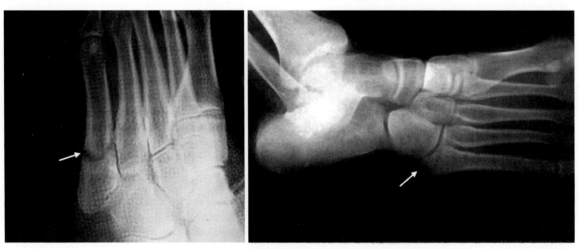

Fig. 21.17: X-ray of the foot, oblique view, showing Jone's fracture (arrow).

MARCH FRACTURE

It is a 'fatigue' fracture of neck of second or third metatarsal, resulting from long continued or often repetitive stress, particularly from prolonged walking or running in those not accustomed to it. Thus, it may occur in army recruits freshly committed to marching – hence the term 'March fracture'. The fracture heals spontaneously with rest, so treatment is purely symptomatic.

FRACTURES OF PHALANGES OF THE TOES

These are common injuries, most often resulting from fall of a heavy object, or twisting of the toes. The great toe is injured most commonly. Satisfactory general alignment is maintained in most cases and forefoot is off loaded in a special shoe. The lesser toes fracture (2nd to 5th toes) is covered with a soft woolly dressing and strapped to the toe adjacent to it (Buddy strapping).

 What have we learnt?

- Fracture both bones of leg is one of the commonest fracture of lower extremity.
- These fractures are commonly open, hence associated with complications.
- Closed interlock nailing is a usual method of treating these fractures.
- Ankle injuries are common, operative stabilisation is the treatment of choice.
- Fracture of calcaneum occurs due to fall from height, requires specialized surgical intervention.

Additional information: From the entrance exams point of view

- Tuber-joint angle (Bohler's angle), Gissane (crucial) angle and neutral triangle are measured on a lateral radiograph in a calcaneal fracture.
- Most common site for ligament injury in the body is the ankle.
- Most common mode of ankle injury is inversion and plantar flexion of the foot.
- Most common cause of insertional tendonitis and rupture is Achilles tendon overuse.

Infections of Bones and Joints

Competency

❖ **OR3.1:** Describe and discuss the aetiopathogenesis, clinical features, investigations and principles of management of bone and joint infections:
   a. Acute osteomyelitis
   b. Subacute osteomyelitis
   c. Acute suppurative arthritis
   d. Septic arthritis and HIV infection
   e. Spirochaetal infection
   f. Skeletal tuberculosis.

Infection of the bone by micro-organisms is called osteomyelitis. Conventionally, an unqualified term 'osteomyelitis' is used for infection of the bone by pyogenic organisms. Osteomyelitis can be acute or chronic.

ACUTE OSTEOMYELITIS

This can be primary (haematogenous) or secondary (following an open fracture or bone operation). Haematogenous osteomyelitis is the commonest, and is often seen in children.

RELEVANT ANATOMY

Metaphysis of the long bones (Fig. 22.1): It is a highly vascularised zone. From the diaphysis the medullary arteries reach up to the growth plate; the area of greatest activity, and branch into capillaries. The venous system begins in this area and drains toward the diaphysis. Thus, the vessels in this zone are arranged in the form of

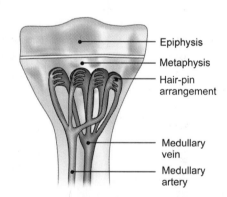

Fig. 22.1: Vascular arrangement at metaphysis of a long bone.

a loop (hair-pin arrangement). The blood stasis resulting from such an arrangement is probably responsible for the metaphysis being a favourite site for bacteria to settle, and thus a common site for osteomyelitis.

In most joints, the capsule is attached at the junction of the epiphysis with the metaphysis, i.e., the

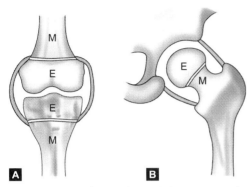

Fig. 22.2: Types of metaphysis: (A) Extra-articular, (B) Intra-articular.

metaphysis is *extra-articular* (Fig. 22.2). In some joints, part of the metaphysis is *intra-articular*, so that the infection from the metaphysis can spread to the joint, resulting in pyogenic arthritis.

ETIOPATHOGENESIS

Staphylococcus aureus is the commonest causative organism. Others are *Streptococcus* and *Pneumococcus*. These organisms reach the bone via the blood circulation. Primary focus of infection is generally not detectable.

The bacteria, as they pass through the bone, get lodged in the metaphysis. Lower femoral metaphysis is the commonest site. The other common sites are the upper tibial, upper femoral and upper humeral metaphyses.

Pathology: The host bone initiates an inflammatory reaction in response to the bacteria. This leads to bone destruction and production of an inflammatory exudate and cells (pus). Once sufficient pus forms in the medullary cavity, it spreads in the following directions (Fig. 22.3).

a. *Along the medullary cavity:* Pus trickles along the medullary cavity and causes thrombosis of the

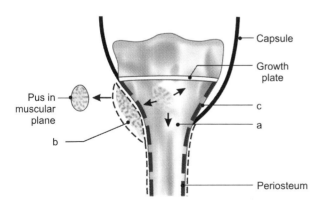

Fig. 22.3: Spread of pus from metaphysis: a. Along medullary cavity, b. Out of the cortex, c. To the joint.

venous and arterial medullary vessels. Blood supply to a segment of the bone is thus cut-off.

b. *Out of the cortex:* Pus travels along Volkmann's canals and comes to lie sub-periosteally. The periosteum is thus lifted off the underlying bone, resulting in damage to the periosteal blood supply to that part of the bone. A segment of bone is thus rendered avascular (sequestrum). Dimensions of this segment vary from a small invisible piece to the whole diaphysis of the bone (Fig. 22.4). Pus under the periosteum generates sub-periosteal new bone (periosteal reaction). Eventually the periosteum is perforated, letting the pus out into the muscle or subcutaneous plane, where it can be felt as an abscess. The abscess if unattended, bursts out of the skin, forming a discharging sinus.

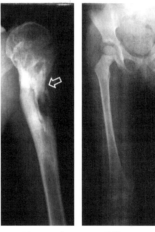

Fig. 22.4: X-rays showing different sizes of sequestra in osteomyelitis.

c. *In other directions:* The epiphyseal plate is resistant to the spread of pus. At times it may be affected by the inflammatory process. The capsular attachment at the epiphysis-metaphysis junction prevents the pus from entering the nearby joint. *In joints with an intra-articular metaphysis, pus can spread to the joint, and cause acute pyogenic arthritis,* e.g., in the hip, in the shoulder, etc.

DIAGNOSIS

The diagnosis of acute osteomyelitis is basically clinical. It is a disease of childhood, more common in boys, probably because they are more prone to injury.

Presenting complaints: The child presents with an acute onset of pain and swelling at the end of a bone, associated with systemic features of infection like fever, etc. Often the parents attribute the symptoms to an episode of injury, but the injury is usually

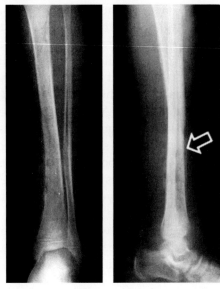

Fig. 22.5: X-ray of leg, AP and lateral views, showing acute osteomyelitis of tibia. (Note early periosteal reaction–arrow).

coincidental. One may find a primary focus of infection elsewhere in the body (tonsils, skin, etc.).

Examination: The child is febrile and dehydrated with classic signs of inflammation—redness, heat, etc., localised to the metaphyseal area of the bone. In later stages, one may find an abscess in the muscle or in the subcutaneous plane. There may be swelling of the adjacent joint, mostly because of either sympathetic effusion, but often due to concomitant arthritis.

Investigations: Investigations provide few clues in the early phase of the disease.

- **Blood:** There may be polymorphonuclear leucocytosis and an elevated ESR and CRP. A blood culture done at the peak of the fever may yield the causative organism.
- **X-rays (Fig. 22.5):** The *earliest* sign to appear on the X-ray is a periosteal new bone deposition (periosteal reaction) at the metaphysis. It takes about 7-10 days to appear.
- **MRI:** MRI is the investigation of choice in cases with doubtful diagnosis. It shows bone oedema, bone destruction, soft tissue oedema and pus collection. It also helps in deciding where to put the needle to aspirate in case it is so required.

DIFFERENTIAL DIAGNOSIS

Any acute inflammatory disease at the end (metaphysis) of a bone in a child should be taken as acute osteomyelitis unless proved otherwise. Following are some of the differential diagnoses to be considered:

a. **Acute septic arthritis:** This can be differentiated from acute osteomyelitis by the following features in arthritis:

- Tenderness and swelling localised to the joint rather than the metaphysis, in arthritis.
- Movement at the joint is painful and restricted in arthritis, whereas relatively painless in osteomyelitis.
- In case there is doubt, joint fluid may be aspirated under aseptic conditions, and the fluid examined for inflammatory cells.

b. **Acute rheumatic arthritis:** The features are similar to acute septic arthritis. The *fleeting character* of joint pains, elevated ASLO titer and high CRP values may help in diagnosis.

c. **Scurvy:** It is uncommon these days, but used to be considered in the differential diagnosis of acute osteomyelitis. Since, there is formation of sub-periosteal haematomas in scurvy, the same may mimic acute osteomyelitis radiologically. The relative absence of pain, tenderness and fever in scurvy may a pointer to it not being osteomyelitis.

d. **Acute poliomyelitis:** In the acute phase of poliomyelitis there is fever, and the muslces are tender. This often mimics acute osteomyelitis but absence of bone tenderness helps in differentiating the two.

In a child with musculo-skeletal symptoms, parents often tend to relegate symptoms to an episode of injury. Hence, often in the initial phase, a lot of non-traumatic conditions (such as osteomyelitis) are misdiagnosed as 'injury'. This may give a wrong lead, and one may proceed with treatment as one would do for a fracture or soft tissue injury (putting them in a plaster, for example). The child continues to be symptomatic, and it is only later, once the plaster is removed, that one comes to know that it was infection and not trauma. Therefore, any *readily given history of trauma, particularly in children, has to be looked at with caution.* The relevance of trauma – when, how, what type, should be established, before making a diagnosis of injury as the cause to patient's symptoms.

TREATMENT

Early, adequate treatment of acute osteomyelitis is the key to success. The child is admitted and investigated. Treatment depends upon the duration of illness after which the child is brought. Cases can be arbitrarily divided into two groups:

a. **If the child is brought within 48 hours of the onset of symptoms:** If a child is brought early, it is supposed that pus has not yet formed and the inflammatory process can be halted by systemic antibiotics. Treatment consists of rest, antibiotics and general building-up of the patient. The limb is put to rest in a splint or by traction. Choice of initial antibiotics is a cover of broad-spectrum antibiotics. The choice depends upon the age of the child. In children less than 4 months of age, a combination of Ceftriaxone and Vancomycin in appropriate dose is preferred. In older children, a combination of Ceftriaxone and Cloxacillin is given. Antibiotics are started after taking appropriate samples for culture from blood or synovial fluid. Antibiotics are changed to specific ones depending upon the culture and sensitivity report.

The child is adequately rehydrated with intravenous fluids. Response to the above treatment is evaluated by frequent assessment of the patient. A four hourly temperature chart and pulse record is maintained. It is a good idea to outline the area of local tenderness precisely, with the help of the back of a match stick over regular intervals. If the patient responds favourably, fever will start declining and local inflammatory signs will diminish. As the child improves, the limb can be mobilised. Weight bearing is restricted for 6-8 weeks. After 2 weeks, antibiotics can be administered by oral route for a total period of 6 weeks. If the patient does not respond favourably within 48 hours of starting the treatment, further investigation with MRI , and surgical intervention is required.

b. **If the child is brought after 48 hours of the onset of symptoms:** If the child is brought late or if he does not respond to conservative treatment, it is taken for granted that there is already a collection of pus within or outside the bone. Detection of pus is often difficult by clinical examination because it may lie deep to the periosteum. An ultrasound examination of the affected part may help in early detection of deep collection of pus. MRI is another comprehensive investigation.

Surgical exploration and drainage is the mainstay of treatment at this stage. The idea is to release the pus pent up inside the meduallry cavity. If not done so, the pus may travel to up and down the medullary cavity producing widespread bone necrosis and sequestrum formation. Drainage is done by a drill hole made in the bone in the region of the metaphysis. If pus wells up from the drill hole, the hole is enlarged until free drainage is obtained. A swab is taken for culture and sensitivity. The wound is closed over a sterile suction drain. Rest, antibiotics and hydration are continued post-operatively. Gradually, the inflammation is controlled and the limb is put to use. Antibiotics are continued for 6 weeks.

COMPLICATIONS

This can be divided into two types, general and local:

General complications: In the early stage, the child may develop septicaemia and pyaemia. Either complication, if left uncontrolled, may prove fatal.

Local complications: It is unfortunate that a large number of cases of acute osteomyelitis in developing countries develop serious complications. Most of these are because of delay in diagnosis, and inadequate treatment. Some of the common complications are as follows:

1. *Chronic osteomyelitis:* It is the *commonest* complication of acute osteomyelitis. There are hardly any radiological features in the early stage. Also, often such cases are wrongly treated as injury. Poor host resistance is another reason for the chronicity of the disease. These factors may to persistence of infection, sequestrum formation and pent-up pus in the cavities inside the bone (Fig. 22.6).

2. *Acute pyogenic arthritis:* This occurs in joints where the metaphysis is intra-articular, e.g., the hip (upper femoral metaphysis), the shoulder (upper humeral metaphysis), etc.

3. *Pathological fracture:* This occurs through a bone which has been weakened by the disease or by the window made during surgery. It can be avoided by adequately splinting the limb.

4. *Growth plate disturbances:* It may be damaged leading to growth disturbances. There may be complete or partial cessation of growth. This may give rise to shortening, deformity of the limb, and sometimes even lengthening (due to hyperemia around the metaphysis).

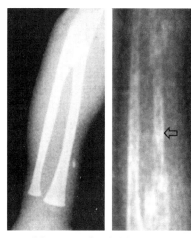

Fig. 22.6: X-rays of forearm of a child showing osteomyelitis of the radius. The X-ray on the right shows the sequestration of the whole shaft.

Secondary Osteomyelitis

This condition arises from a wound infection in open fractures or after operations on the bone. The incidence of these cases are on the rise because of increase in operative intervention in the treatment of fractures.

The constitutional symptoms are less severe than those in haematogenous osteomyelitis as the wound provides some drainage. The condition can be largely prevented by adequate initial treatment of open fractures, and adherence to sterile operating conditions for routine orthopaedic operations.

Chronic Osteomyelitis

Conventionally, the term 'chronic osteomyelitis' is used for chronic pyogenic osteomyelitis. Although, with proper initial care of acute osteomyelitis and better nutritional status of the population, its incidence is on the decline. It still continues to be an important problem in parts of developing countries. The other causes of chronic osteomyelitis are tuberculosis, fungal infections, etc. There are three types of chronic osteomyelitis:

a. Chronic osteomyelitis secondary to acute osteomyelitis.
b. Garre's osteomyelitis.
c. Brodie's abscess.

PATHOLOGY

Acute osteomyelitis commonly leads to chronic osteomyelitis because of the following reasons:

a. **Delayed and inadequate treatment:** This is the commonest cause for the persistence of an osteomyelitis. Delay causes spread of pus within the medullary cavity and sub-periosteally. This results in the death of a part of the bone (sequestrum formation). Destruction of cancellous bone leads to the formation of cavities within the bone. *Such 'non-collapsing' bone cavities and sequestra are responsible for persistent infection.*

b. **Type and virulence of organism:** Sometimes, despite early and adequate treatment, the body's defense mechanism may not be able to control the damaging influence of a virulent organism, and the infection persists.

c. **Reduced host resistance:** Malnutrition compromises the body's defense mechanisms, thus letting the infection persist.

When infection persists because of the above reasons, the host bone responds by generating more and more sub-periosteal new bone. The sub-periosteal bone

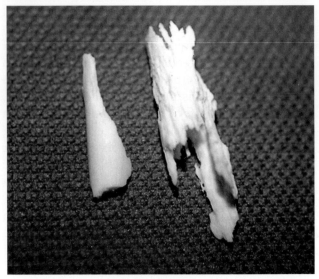

Fig. 22.7: Bone sequestra (Note the rough outer surface).

is deposited in an irregular fashion, and hence, an osteomyelitic bone has an irregular surface. Persistent laying down of new bone results in thickening of the bone. Continuing discharge of pus results in the formation of a sinus. With time, the sinus tract gets fibrosed and the sinus becomes fixed to the bone. *A persistent sinus adhered to the bone is an important clinical sign of underlying pathology being osteomyelitis.*

Sequestrum is a piece of dead bone, surrounded by infected granulation tissue trying to 'eat' the sequestrum away. It appears pale and has a smooth inner and rough outer surface (Fig. 22.7), because the latter is being constantly eroded by the surrounding granulation tissue. History of *"a piece of bone from a discharging sinus"* helps in clinching a diagnosis of osteomyelitis.

Different types of sequestra seen in different conditions as shown in Table 22.1.

Involucrum is the dense sclerotic bone overlying a sequestrum. There may be some holes in the involucrum for the pus to find way out. These holes

Table 22.1: Different types of sequestra.	
Type	**Disease**
Tubular	Pyogenic
Ring	External fixator
Black	Actinomycosis
Coralliform	Perthe's disease
Coke	Tuberculosis
Sandy	Tuberculosis
Feathery	Syphillis

are called *cloacae*. The *bony cavities* are lined by infected granulation tissue.

DIAGNOSIS

Diagnosis is suspected clinically but can be confirmed radiologically by its characteristic features. The disease begins in childhood but may present at any age. The lower-end of the femur is the *commonest* site.

Presenting complaints: A chronic discharging sinus is the *commonest* presenting symptom. The onset of sinus may be traced back to an episode of acute osteomyelitis during childhood. Often sinuses heal for varying periods, only to reappear with each acute exacerbation. Quality of discharge varies from sero-purulent to thick pus. There may be a history of extrusion of small bone fragments from the sinus. Often the only symptom in a chronic osteomyelitis is persistent pain – no fever, swelling, etc. Diagnosis in such cases is usually clinched on X-rays or MRI done as a matter of investigation.

Pain is usually minimal but may become aggravated during acute exacerbations. Generalised symptoms of infection such as fever, etc., are present only during acute exacerbations. A patient with chronic osteomyelitis may present with complications discussed subsequently (see page 173).

Examination: Some of the salient features observed on examination are as follows:
- **Chronic discharging sinus:** This is a characteristic feature of chronic infection. A *sinus fixed* to the underlying bone indicates that infection is coming from the bone. There may be sprouting granulation tissue at its opening, suggesting a sequestrum within the bone. The sequestrum may be visible at the mouth of the sinus itself. The sinus may be surrounded by healed puckered scars, indicating previous healed sinuses.
- **Thickened, irregular bone:** This can be appreciated on comparing the girth of the affected bone with that of the bone on the normal side.
- **Tenderness** on deep palpation, usually mild, is present in some cases.
- **Adjacent joint** may be stiff, either due to excessive scarring in the soft tissues around the joint, or because of associated arthritis of the joint.

INVESTIGATIONS

Radiological examination:
X-rays: X-rays are hallmark in the diagnosis of chronic osteomyelitis. The following are the salient features:
- *Thickening and irregularity* of the cortices
- *Patchy sclerosis*

- *Bone cavity:* This is seen as an area of rarefaction surrounded by sclerosis
- *Sequestrum:* This appears *denser* than the surrounding normal bone because the decalcification which occurs in normal bone, does not occur in dead bone. Granulation tissue surrounding the sequestrum gives rise to a radiolucent zone around it. A sequestrum may be visible in soft tissues
- *Involucrum* and *cloacae* may be visible.

CT scan: CT scan is a better imaging modality in better understanding an osteomyelitic bone. It is indicated in patients where (a) the diagnosis is in doubt; (b) before surgery, for better defining the cavities and sequestra. The latter may not be well appreciated on X-rays. Exact localisation of a cavity or sequestrum has bearing on surgical treatment.

Sinogram: It is indicated in situations where there is extensive involvement of the bone, and while planning surgery, one cannot decide on X- rays or even CT scan, where the pus may be coming from. Knowledge of the same helps in improving outcome of surgical treatment. In this test, a sterile thin catheter is introduced into the sinus as far as it can go. Then, a radio-opaque dye is injected and an X-rays taken. The radio-opaque dye travels to the root of the infection, and thus helps localise cavity and sequestra better.

Blood: A blood examination is usually of no help. ESR and CRP may be normal or mildly elevated. Total blood counts may be normal, but may be increased during acute exacerbation.

Pus: Pus culture may grow the causative organism. Swab should be taken from depth of the sinus after proper cleaning of the skin. This avoids contamination. If an organism is grown, it may be useful in controlling the acute on chronic stage of the disease. It may also help in selecting the pre-operative antibiotics as and when operation is planned.

DIFFERENTIAL DIAGNOSIS

A discharging sinus on a limb indicates deeper infection which could be from tissues other than the bone - skin downward. A history of bone piece discharge from a sinus is *diagnostic* of chronic osteomyelitis. Other differential diagnoses to be considered in the absence of such a conclusive history are as follows:
a. **Tubercular osteomyelitis:** The discharge is often thin and watery. A tubercular sinus may show its characteristic features such as undermined margins and bluish surrounding skin. Tubercular osteomyelitis is often multifocal. Patient may be suffering from or may have suffered from pulmonary tuberculosis.

b. **Soft tissue infection:** A longstanding soft tissue infection with a discharging sinus may mimic osteomyelitis. Absence of thickening of underlying bone, and absence of sinus fixed to the bone, may point towards the infection *not coming* from the bone. Absence of any radiological changes in the bone would help conform the diagnosis.

c. **Ewing's sarcoma:** A child with Ewing's sarcoma sometimes presents with a rather sudden onset pain fever and swelling mostly in the diaphysis, but sometimes in metaphysis. Radiological appearance (periosteal reaction, thickening of bone) often resembles that of osteomyelitis. A needle biopsy will usually settle the diagnosis. It will be disaster to treat a case of Ewings as that of osteomyelitis, with curettage, etc.

TREATMENT

Principles of treatment: Treatment of chronic osteomyelitis is primarily surgical. Antibiotics are useful only during acute exacerbations and during post-operative period. Aim of surgical intervention is: (i) removal of dead bone; (ii) elimination of dead space and cavities; and (iii) removal of infected granulation tissue and excision of sinuses.

Operative procedures: Following are some of the operative procedures commonly performed:

a. *Sequestrectomy:* This means removal of the sequestrum. If it lies within the medullary cavity, a window is made in the overlying involucrum and the sequestrum removed. One must wait for adequate involucrum formation before performing sequestrectomy. Premature removal may lead to fracture.

b. *Saucerisation:* A bone cavity is a 'non-collapsing cavity'. So, there is always some pent-up pus inside it, which is responsible for the persistence of an infection. In saucerisation, the cavity is converted into a 'saucer' by removing its wall (Fig. 22.8). This allows free drainage of the infected material.

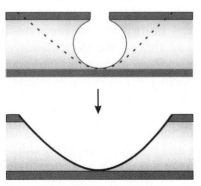

Fig. 22.8: Saucerisation.

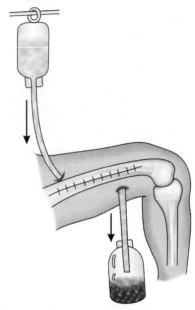

Fig. 22.9: Continuous suction irrigation.

c. *Curettage:* The wall of the cavity, lined by infected granulation and scar tissue, is curetted until the underlying normal-looking bone is seen. The cavity is sometimes obliterated by filling it with antibiotic impregnated cement beads or by mobilizing a muscle flap to obliterate dead space.

d. *Excision of an infected bone:* In a case where the affected bone can be excised *en bloc* without compromising the functions of the limb, it is a good method, e.g., osteomyelitis of a part of the fibula. With the availability of Ilizarov's technique, an aggressive approach, i.e., excising the infected bone segment and building up the gap by transporting a segment of the bone from adjacent part has shown good results (Ref. page 35).

e. *Amputation:* It may, very rarely, be preferred in a case with a long-standing discharging sinus, especially if the sinus undergoes a malignant change.

In most cases, a combination of these procedures is required. After surgery the wound is closed over a *continuous suction irrigation system* (Fig. 22.9). This system has an inlet tube going to the medullary cavity, and an outlet tube bringing the irrigation fluid out. A slow suction is applied to the outlet tube. The irrigation fluid consists of suitable antibiotics and a detergent. The medullary canal is irrigated in this way for 4 to 7 days. There are quite a few local antibiotic delivery systems are in vogue – antibiotic-laden absorbable pellets, antibiotic laden absorbable collagen, etc.

COMPLICATIONS

1. **An acute exacerbation** or 'flare up' of the infection occurs commonly. It subsides with a period of rest, and antibiotics, either broad- spectrum or based on the pus culture and sensitivity report.

2. **Growth abnormalities:** Osteomyelitis may cause growth disturbances at the adjacent growth plate, in one of the following ways:
   - *Shortening,* when the growth plate is damaged.
   - *Lengthening* because of increased vascularity of the growth plate due to the nearby osteomyelitis.
   - *Deformities* may appear if a part of the growth plate is damaged and the remaining keeps growing.

3. **Pathological fracture** may occur through a weakened area of the bone. Treatment is by conservative methods.

4. **Joint stiffness** may occur because of scarring of soft tissues around the joint or due to the joint gettting secondarily involved.

5. **Sinus tract malignancy** is a rare complication. It occurs many years after the onset of osteomyelitis. It is usually a squamous cell carcinoma. The patient may need amputation.

6. **Amyloidosis:** As with all other long standing suppurations, this is a late complication of osteomyelitis.

PROGNOSIS

To cure a bone infection is very difficult. Operative intervention may be useful if there is an obvious factor responsible for the persistence of the infection, e.g., sequestrum, cavity, etc.

GARRE'S OSTEOMYELITIS

This is a sclerosing, non-suppurative chronic osteomyelitis. It may begin with acute local pain, low-grade pyrexia and swelling. Pyrexia and pain subside about the fusiform osseous enlargement persists. There is tenderness on deep palpation. There is no discharging sinus. Shafts of the femur or tibia are the most commonly affected.

The importance of Garre's osteomyelitis lies in differentiating it from bone tumours, which commonly present with similar features, e.g., Ewing's tumour or low-grade osteosarcoma. CT scan is an important imaging modality.

Treatment is guarded. Acute symptoms subside with rest and broad-spectrum antibiotics. Sometimes, making a gutter or holes in the bone bring relief in pain.

BRODIE'S ABSCESS

It is a special type of osteomyelitis in which the body's defense mechanisms have been able to contain the infection so as to create a chronic bone abscess containing pus or jelly-like granulation tissue surrounded by a zone of sclerosis (Fig. 22.10).

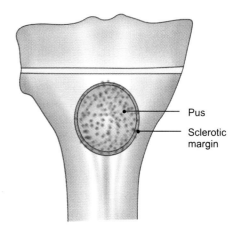

Fig. 22.10: Brodie's abscess.

CLINICAL FEATURES

The patient is usually between 11 to 20 years of age. Common sites are the upper-end of the tibia and lower-end of the femur. It is usually located at the metaphysis. A deep boring pain is the predominant symptom. It may become worse at night. In some instances, it becomes worse on walking and is relieved by rest. Occasionally, there may be a transient effusion in the adjacent joint during exacerbation of symptoms. An examination may reveal tenderness and thickening of the bone.

Radiological features: The radiological picture is diagnostic. It shows a circular or oval lucent area surrounded by a zone of sclerosis. The rest of the bone is normal. CT may be required for better evaluation.

Treatment is by operation. Surgical evacuation and curettage is performed under antibiotic cover. If the cavity is large, it is packed with antibiotic laden bone cement beads.

SALMONELLA OSTEOMYELITIS

This occurs during the convalescent phase *after an attack* of typhoid fever. It is subacute type of osteomyelitis, usually occurring in the ulna, tibia, or vertebra. Often, multiple bones are affected, sometimes *bilaterally symmetrical.* The predominant radiological feature is a diaphyseal sclerosis. The disease occurs more commonly in children with sickle-cell anaemia.

SEPTIC ARTHRITIS

This is an arthritis caused by pyogenic organisms. Typically, it presents as an acute painful arthritis, but it may present as subacute or chronic arthritis. Other terms often used to describe this condition are pyogenic arthritis, infective arthritis or suppurative arthritis.

ETIOPATHOGENESIS

It is more common in children, and males are more susceptible. Other predisposing factors are poor hygiene, poor resistance, diabetes, etc. *Staphylococcus aureus* is the commonest causative organism. Other organisms are *Streptococcus, Pneumococcus* and *Gonococcus.* The organisms reach the joint by one of the following routes:

Haematogenous: This is the commonest route. There may be a primary focus of infection in the form of pyoderma, throat infection, septicaemia, etc.

Secondary to nearby osteomyelitis: This is a particularly common route in joints with intra-articular metaphysis, e.g., the hip, shoulder, etc.
a. **Penetrating wounds:** The knee, being a superficial joint, is often affected via this route.
b. **Iatrogenic:** This may occur following intra-articular steroid injections in different arthritis, and during femoral artery punctures for blood collection.
c. **Umbilical cord sepsis** in infants can travel to joints.

As the organism reaches the joint by one of the above routes, there begins an inflammatory response in the synovium resulting in the exudation of fluid within the joint. Joint cartilage is destroyed by inflammatory granulation tissue and lysosomal enzymes in the joint exudate. Outcome varies from complete healing to total destruction of the joint. The latter may result in a complete loss of joint movement (ankylosis).

DIAGNOSIS

Diagnosis is mainly clinical. The patient is usually a child. The knee is the commonest joint affected. Other joints commonly affected are the hip, shoulder, elbow, etc.

Presenting complaints: In its typical acute form, a child with septic arthritis presents with a severe throbbing pain, swelling and redness of the affected joint. This is associated with high grade fever and malaise. The child is unable to use the affected limb. In its subacute form, the parents may notice that the child is not allowing anybody to touch the joint. He

may not be moving it properly. In the lower limbs, a painful limp may be the first thing to draw attention. It may be associated with low grade fever.

On examination: The child is generally severely toxic with high temperature and tachycardia. The affected joint is swollen and held in the position of ease (Table 22.2). Palpation reveals increased temperature, tenderness and effusion. There is severe limitation in the joint movements in all directions. Any attempt at either passive or active movements causes severe pain and muscle spasms. In subacute forms, some amount of joint movement is possible.

Table 22.2: Position of ease of common joints.	
Joint	**Position of ease**
Shoulder	Adduction, internal rotation
Elbow	Flexion, mid pronation
Wrist	Flexion
Hip	Flexion, abduction, external rotation
Knee	Flexion
Ankle	Plantar-flexion

INVESTIGATIONS

Radiological examination: Diagnosis in early stage is crucial. X-rays are usually normal. A careful look at the X-ray may reveal increased joint space and a soft tissue shadow corresponding to the distended capsule due to swelling of the joint. *Ultrasound examination* is useful in detecting collection in deep joints such as the hip and shoulder. If found, one could aspirate the fluid and send for culturing the organism responsible for infection.

In the later stage, the joint space is narrowed. There may be irregularity of the joint margins. Occasionally, there may be a subluxation or dislocation of the joint.

Blood shows neutrophilic leucocytosis. ESR is markedly elevated. A blood culture may grow the causative organism.

Joint aspiration is the quickest and the best method of diagnosing septic arthritis. The fluid may show features of acute septic inflammation (Table 22.3). Gram staining provides a clue to the type of organism, till one gets the culture report.

DIFFERENTIAL DIAGNOSIS

A case with an acute septic arthritis should be differentiated from the following conditions:
a. **Other acute inflammatory conditions:** Diseases near a joint, such as acute osteomyelitis, acute

Table 22.3: Synovial fluid examination.				
Points	**Normal**	**Non-inflammatory**	**Inflammatory**	**Septic**
Gross examination				
▪ Volume (mL)	Often < 3.5 mL	Often > 3.5 mL	Often > 3.5 mL	> 3.5 mL
▪ Viscosity	High	High	Low	Variable
▪ Colour	Colourless	Straw yellow	Yellow	Variable
▪ Clarity	Transparent	Transparent	Translucent	Opaque
Examination in lab				
▪ WBC count	< 200	200-2000	2000-7500	> 10000
▪ PMN leucocytes	< 25%	< 25%		
▪ Culture	–	–	> 50%	> 75%
▪ Mucin clot	Firm	Firm	–	+
▪ Glucose level	Equal to blood glucose	Nearly equal to blood glucose	Friable < 25 mg% of blood glucose	Friable > 25 mg% of blood glucose
▪ Crystal examination	Positive in Gout – Sodium biurate	Positive in pseudogout – Ca pyrophosphate		

lymphadenitis, acute bursitis, etc. may mimic an arthritis because in some of these conditions, the joint is kept in a deformed position. Also, there may be pain and muscle spasm with attempted movements, but these signs are basically because the body is trying to prevent any motion in the vicinity of the inflamed part. Careful examination reveals that reasonably pain free movements are present at the joint, and the movements are not limited in *every* direction. The swelling may also be localised to one side of the joint.

b. **Other causes of acute arthritis:** An acute septic arthritis should also be differentiated from other causes of arthritis as discussed below:

   ▪ *Rheumatic arthritis:* Commonly a migratory polyarthritis, but may present with only one joint affected. The subsequent fleeting character of the arthritis, high C-reactive protein levels in the serum, and joint aspiration helps in its diagnosis.

   ▪ *Haemophilia:* A past history of a bleeding disorder, especially in a boy with an acute painful joint, would suggest the diagnosis. Abnormal bleeding and clotting times are helpful for confirmation.

   ▪ *Tubercular arthritis:* It may sometimes present in a rather acute form. A past or family history of tuberculosis may be present. Joint aspiration and AFB examination may help in its diagnosis.

TREATMENT

In its early stage, before any signs of joint destruction appear on X-ray, a correct diagnosis and aggressive treatment can save a joint from permanent damage. Whenever suspected, diagnosis of septic arthritis *must be confirmed or ruled out by joint aspiration.* Broad-spectrum antibiotics should be started by parenteral route. A combination of Ceftriaxone and Cloxacillin, in appropriate doses is usually given. These are subsequently changed to specific antibiotics as per aspirate culture and sensitivity reports. The joint must be put to rest in a splint or in traction.

Whenever pus is aspirated, the joint should be opened up (arthrotomy), washed and closed with a suction drain. The same can be now done arthroscopically. As the inflammation is brought under control, general condition of the patient improves, fever and local signs of inflammation subside, the joint is then gradually mobilised. Antibiotics are continued for 6 weeks.

In late cases, with radiological destruction of the joint margins, subluxation or dislocation, it is not possible to expect joint movement. In such cases, after an arthrotomy and extensive debridement of the joint, it is immobilised in the position of optimum function, so that as the disease heals, ankylosis occurs in that position.

COMPLICATIONS

These can be divided into general and local, as for osteomyelitis. Inadequate early treatment leads to the following local complications.

1. **Deformity and stiffness:** The joint gets stiff due to intra-articular and peri-articular adhesions. In cases with advanced disease, the articular

cartilage may be completely damaged, resulting in *ankylosis.* Bony ankylosis is the usual outcome of a neglected septic arthritis.

Pathological dislocation: As the joint gets filled with inflammatory exudate, the supporting ligaments and joint capsule get stretched. Muscle spasm associated with the disease may result in pathological dislocation of the joint. Posterior dislocation of the hip and triple displacement of the knee occur (Fig. 22.11).

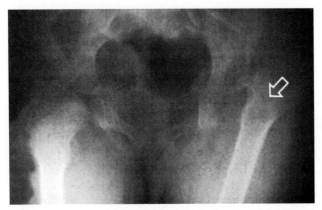

Fig. 22.11: X-ray showing pathological dislocation, as a sequelae of septic arthritis of the hip.

2. **Osteoarthritis:** Even if septic arthritis has been treated rather early, some permanent changes in the articular cartilage occur, and give rise to early osteoarthritis a few years later.

SEPTIC ARTHRITIS IN INFANCY (TOM-SMITH ARTHRITIS)

This is a septic arthritis of the hip seen in infants. At this age, the head of the femur is cartilaginous and is rapidly and completely destroyed by the pyogenic process. Onset is acute with rapid abscess formation, which may burst out or be incised and heals rapidly. Usually it is mistaken as a superficial infection and the child presents some time later with complaint of a limp without any pain. On examination, it is found that the child walks with an unstable gait. The affected leg is shorter and hip movements are *increased* in all directions. Telescopy test is positive. On X-ray, one finds complete absence of the head and neck of the femur.

Clinically, this condition closely resembles a congenital dislocation of the hip (CDH) which also sometimes presents at that age. Complete absence of the head and neck, and a normally developed round acetabulum differentiate this condition from CDH. In the latter, acetabulum is shallow.

GONOCOCCAL ARTHRITIS

Gonorrhoea may be complicated by acute arthritis which arises within two weeks of urethral discharge. As a rule the inflammation is confined to sub-synovial layers. Though the fluid in the joint may be purulent, granulation tissue does not invade the joint. Very often the inflammation subsides without pus formation.

Onset is sudden, similar to septic arthritis, but the general condition of the patient is well maintained in spite of severe local signs. This is typical of gonococcal arthritis. Knee is the commonest joint affected. Treatment is similar to that of septic arthritis. Penicillin is the drug of choice.

SYPHILIS OF THE JOINTS

CONGENITAL SYPHILIS

The joint may be affected early or late in congenital syphilis.

Early: During infancy, osteochondritis in the juxta-epiphyseal region results in breakdown of the bone and cartilage.

Late: A manifestation of congenital syphilis, 'Clutton's joints' is a painless synovitis occurring at puberty. It most commonly affects the knee and elbow, mostly bilaterally.

ACQUIRED SYPHILIS

The joints may be affected in the secondary and tertiary stages of acquired syphilis. In the secondary stage, transient polyarthritis and polyarthralgia involving the larger joints occur. In tertiary stage, gummatous arthritis occurs where the larger joints are most often involved. *Neuropathic (Charcot's) joint* is an indirect consequence of syphilis. Please refer to a Medicine textbook for tests carried out for the diagnosis of syphilis.

FUNGAL INFECTIONS

Fungal infections of the bone occur usually in patients with suppressed immunological status. The infection, particularly common in a rural population, is that of the foot, called 'Madura foot'. As the infection results in a tumour-like mass, it is also called 'Mycetoma'.

MADURA FOOT

This is caused by *Maduromycosis.* It starts as a nodular swelling over the dorsum or sole of the foot. The nodule bursts and discharges a thin pus. Gradually more nodules form and result in a swollen foot with a nodular surface and multiple discharging sinuses.

Pain is not a prominent feature, unless there is a secondary infection. The pus, characteristically contains small black granules, which on microscopic examination reveal the fungus. X-ray shows soft tissue swelling around the foot bones. There may be multiple small sieve-like erosions in the bones of the foot.

Treatment: In early stages, the lesion responds to massive doses of penicillin or dapsone. In later stages, once the foot has become disorganised and there are multiple discharging sinuses, amputation may be necessary.

LEPROSY AND ORTHOPAEDICS

Leprosy is known in the society as a disease producing ugly deformities and mutilations. Deformities are seen in all types of leprosy, but are more common in tuberculoid and polyneuritic types.

Mechanisms causing disability: Nerve involvement leading to anaesthesia, dryness of the skin, and paralysis, is primarily responsible for deformity and disability of hands and feet. These factors predispose the affected limb to misuse, resulting in ulceration, scar formation and secondary infection. These, in turn, add to disability and create a vicious cycle whereby loss of deep tissue results. Flowchart 22.1 summarises the mechanism of disability.

Clinical manifestations of leprosy relevant from viewpoint of orthopaedics are: (i) deformities; (ii) motor weakness and muscle atrophy; (iii) trophic ulcers; (iv) mutilations; and (v) neuritis.

Flowchart 22.1: Pathogenesis of disability in leprosy.

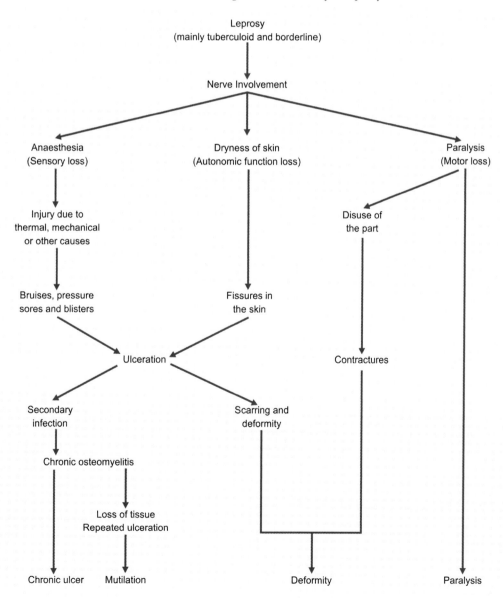

DEFORMITIES

The primary factor responsible for deformities in leprosy is involvement of peripheral nerves, but secondary factors contribute to a large percentage of deformities. The latter are totally preventable, hence important. Some such factors are malpositioning of paralysed limbs, scarring and ulceration, self inflicted injuries to an anaesthetic part, etc. Nerves commonly affected in leprosy are those in superficial locations. In order of frequency these are: ulnar nerve at the elbow, median nerve above the wrist and common peroneal nerve at the knee. Following are the common deformities seen:

- **Hand:** Common deformities in the hand are—partial claw hand in ulnar nerve palsy, total claw hand in ulnar plus median nerve palsy, ape-thumb deformity in median nerve palsy and wrist drop in radial nerve palsy.
- **Foot:** Foot drop occurs commonly due to involvement of common peroneal nerve.

Treatment: A great deal of deformities in leprosy are preventable, firstly by early detection of leprosy and adequate drug therapy; secondly by health education about hygienic care of anaesthetic foot, prevention of insect bites, proper splintage of paralysed part, and prompt and adequate care of trophic ulcers. Conservative treatment using splints, exercises and other physiotherapeutic measures are used in most cases. In some cases, surgical correction of the deformity is required. For details about methods of correction of deformities in general, please refer to Chapter 11.

MOTOR WEAKNESS AND MUSCLE ATROPHY

As a result of nerve involvement, commonly seen motor weakness are claw hand and wrist drop in the hand, and foot drop in the leg. Conservative treatment is by splints. Following reconstructive procedures may be performed in some cases.

- **For claw hand:** Paul Brand's multi-tail tendon transfer.
- **For opponens weakness:** Opponens plasty, a tendon transfer operation where tendon of flexor digitorum superficialis of the ring finger is rerouted so that it passes through a pulley created at the flexor carpi ulnaris tendon, and is attached to the thumb.
- **For wrist drop:** Jone's transfer.
- **For foot drop:** Transfer of tibialis posterior tendon on the dorsum of the foot.

TROPHIC ULCERS

These are found at anaesthetic sites, and are precipitated and perpetuated by recurrent injury or abnormal areas of pressure developing on paralysed hands and feet. Cause of injury could be mechanical, thermal, etc. Common sites of trophic ulcers are heads of first and fifth metatarsals, heels and terminal phalanges of fingers. Early manifestation may be a spontaneous blister, a nodule or an injury at the anaesthetic site. This leads to ulcer formation, which may get secondarily infected. The ulcer may extend deep and affect soft tissues and bones, and become chronic and progressive. Causes responsible for chronicity of an ulcer are: (i) impeded vascular supply; (ii) repeated trauma to the ulcer; and (iii) superadded infection.

Treatment: Prevention of ulcer is most important, because once it occurs, healing takes a long time.

Treatment of an established ulcer consists of the following:

- **Eliminating stress caused by walking**, in acute stage, by resting the foot and in later stages by application of plaster cast.
- **Eradication of infection by:** (i) debridement; (ii) sequestrectomy; (iii) securing free drainage of the wound; (iv) antibiotics; and (v) occlusive dressings.
- **Other:** Besides debridement, the role of surgery is in using *plastic surgery procedures* to cover a large ulcer. *Amputation* may sometimes be considered necessary for a big, infected ulcer with osteomyelitis.
- **Prevention of recurrences** by protecting the foot and the scar from further injuries by good care of the part, proper footwear or splints, and careful use of the part (e.g., avoiding jumping, walking in cases with foot ulcers).

MUTILATIONS

Mutilations result from recurrent trophic ulcers, sequestration of bone and decalcification of bones. These are a result of ultimate neglect of a fairly treatable condition.

NEURITIS

Leprosy may result in acute or chronic neuritis. The patient complains of pain along the course of the nerve and later, neurological symptoms. In acute stage, rest to the part and anti-leprosy chemotherapy is given. Some surgeons prefer local or systemic corticosteroids in acute stage. In chronic cases, there is diffuse thickening of the nerves. Occasionally, a nerve abscess can be palpated. Indications for surgical intervention are: (i) abscess inside the nerve – in which case it is drained; and (ii) intractable pain in a person in whom paralysis in the distribution of the nerve is already present. Neurolysis has been attempted in these cases as no further harm can be done.

What have we learnt?

- *Staphylococcus aureus* is the commonest organism to cause bone and joint infection.
- Early diagnosis is crucial in acute osteomyelitis. Bone scan may be done in suspected cases.
- Early surgical drainage may prevent an acute osteomyelitis developing into chronic.
- Treatment of chronic osteomyelitis is essentially surgical. Giving prolonged antibiotics is of no use.
- In a case of suspected septic arthritis, aspiration of the joint is the best way to confirm the diagnosis. In case of a deep joint infection, ultrasound examination can help detect increased intra-articular fluid. Ultrasound guided aspiration can be done.
- In case of septic arthritis, early surgical drainage saves the joint from permanent damage.

Additional information: From the entrance exams point of view

- The earliest sign of osteomyelitis on X-ray is loss of soft tissue planes.
- The earliest bony change on X-ray is periosteal reaction.
- Evidence of osteomyelitis on X-ray occurs after 2 weeks of onset.
- Most common cause of post-surgical, post-traumatic and osteomyelitis of the spine is *Staphylococcus aureus*.
- Most common cause of osteomyelitis in drug abusers is *Pseudomonas aeruginosa*.
- Chondrolysis is seen in septic arthritis of infancy.
- Most common cause of bone and joint infection is haematogenous.

	Septic arthritis	**Transient synovitis**
Age	0–5 yrs	6–12 yrs
ESR, WBC counts	Grossly elevated	Mild increase
Signs and Symptoms	More pronounced	Less than septic arthritis

Tuberculosis of Bones and Joints

Competency

❖ **OR4.1:** Describe and discuss the clinical features, investigation and principles of management of tuberculosis affecting major joints (Hip, Knee) including cold abscess and caries spine.

GENERAL CONSIDERATIONS

Tuberculosis (TB) is still a common infection in developing countries. After lung and lymph nodes, bone and joint is the next common site of tuberculosis in the body. It constitutes about 1–4 per cent of the total number of cases of tuberculosis.

The spine is the *most common* site of bone and joint tuberculosis, constituting about 50 per cent of the total number of cases. Next in order of frequency are the hip, the knee and the elbow. Tubercular osteomyelitis more commonly affects the ends of the long bone, unlike pyogenic osteomyelitis which affects the metaphysis. This is also the reason for early involvement of the adjacent joint in tubercular osteomyelitis. Table 23.1 shows the common musculoskeletal structures affected by tuberculosis.

ETIOPATHOGENESIS

Common causative organism is *Mycobacterium tuberculosis*. Bone and joint tuberculosis is *always* secondary to some primary focus in the lungs, lymph nodes, etc. Mode of spread from the primary focus may be either haematogenous or by direct extension from a neighbouring focus.

Table 23.1: Musculo-skeletal tuberculosis.		
Tissue	**Disease**	**Remarks**
Bone		
▪ Long bone	▪ TB osteomyelitis	▪ Tibia commonly affected
▪ Short bone (phalanges)	▪ Tuberculous dactylitis	▪ Also called *spina ventosa*
▪ Spine	▪ TB spondylitis	▪ Also called Pott's disease
Joint		
▪ Arthritis	▪ TB arthritis	▪ Hip joint commonly affected
▪ Synovium	▪ Synovial TB	▪ Knee-most common site
Others		
▪ Tendon (synovium)	▪ TB tenosynovitis of flexor tendons at wrist	▪ Compound palmar ganglion
▪ Bursae	▪ TB bursitis of trochanteric bursa	▪ Trochanteric bursitis

Pathology: Tubercular infection of the bone and synovial tissue produces similar response as it produces in the lungs, i.e., chronic granulomatous inflammation with caseation necrosis. The response may be proliferative, exudative or both:

a. *Proliferative response:* This is the more common of the two responses. It is characterised by chronic granulomatous inflammation with a lot of fibrosis.

b. *Exudative response:* In some cases, particularly in immunodeficient individuals, elderly people and people suffering from leukaemia, etc., there is extensive caseation necrosis without much cellular reaction. This results in extensive pus formation. These are also termed *non-reactive* cases.

Natural history: Inflammation results in local trabecular necrosis and caseation. Demineralisation of the bone occurs because of intense local hyperaemia. In the absence of adequate body resistance or chemotherapy, the cortices of the bone get eroded, and the infected granulation tissue and pus find their way to the subperiosteal and soft tissue planes. Here they present as *cold abscesses,* and may burst out to form sinuses. The affected bone may undergo a pathological fracture.

A tubercular osteomyelitis in the vicinity of a joint may result in the involvement of the joint.

Joint involvement is usually in the form of a low-grade synovitis, with thickening of the synovial membrane. Unlike pyogenic arthritis where proteolytic enzymes cause severe early destruction of the articular cartilage, tubercular infection causes slow destruction. Once the synovium is inflamed, it starts destroying the cartilage from the periphery. This inflammatory synovium at the periphery of the cartilage is called *Pannus.* Eventually, the articular cartilage is completely destroyed. The joint gets distended with the pus. Joint capsule and ligaments become lax, and the joint may get subluxated. Pus and tubercular debris burst out of the joint capsule to form a cold abscess, and subsequently a chronic discharging sinus.

Healing: It occurs by *fibrosis*, which results in significant limitation or near complete loss of joint movement (fibrous ankylosis). If considerable destruction of the articular cartilage has occurred, the joint space is completely lost, and is traversed by bony trabeculae between the bones forming the joint (bony ankylosis) as shown in Figure 23.1. Fibrous ankylosis is a common outcome of healed

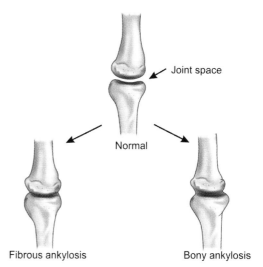

Fig. 23.1: Types of ankylosis.

tuberculosis of the joints, except in the spine where bony ankylosis follows more often.

CLINICAL FEATURES

Clinical features depend upon the site affected. Patients of all ages and both sexes are affected frequently. The onset is gradual in most cases.

Usual presenting complaints are pain, swelling, deformity and inability to use that part. Sometimes, the presentation is atypical. The following general principles will help in making a diagnosis:

a. **High index of suspicion:** Tuberculosis should be included in the differential diagnosis of any slow onset disease of the musculoskeletal system, particularly in countries where tuberculosis is still prevalent. Because of its slow onset and progress, the symptoms and signs are often minimal and non-specific. A high index of suspicion and a close watch over such symptoms in susceptible individuals, is the key to early diagnosis.

b. **Fallacious history of trauma:** Very often the patient assigns all his symptoms to an episode of injury. One should not get carried away by such information, as the injury may be coincidental. A detailed inquiry in such cases will reveal a symptom-free period between the episode of trauma and the beginning of symptoms, thus establishing the non-traumatic nature of the disease.

c. **Lack of constitutional symptoms:** Symptoms like fever, loss of appetite, weight loss, etc., are present in only about 20 per cent cases. An active primary focus is detected only in about 15 per cent of cases at the time of diagnosis; in the rest it has already healed by the time the patient presents.

Specific signs and symptoms in patients with tuberculosis at major sites will be discussed in respective sections.

INVESTIGATIONS

Radiological examination: X-ray examination of the affected part, anteroposterior and lateral views, is the single most important investigation. Findings in the early stages may be minimal and are likely to be missed. A comparison with an identical X-ray of the opposite limb or with an X-ray repeated after some period, may be helpful. Following are some of the general radiological features of tuberculosis of the bones and joints:

TB osteomyelitis: A tubercular osteomyelitis presents as a well-defined area of bone destruction, typically with minimal reactive new bone formation. This is unlike a pyogenic infection, where reactive periosteal new bone formation is an important feature.

TB arthritis: In tubercular arthritis there is reduction of the joint space, erosion of the articular surfaces and marked *peri-articular rarefaction.* This is unlike many other causes of joint space reduction such as osteoarthritis, septic arthritis, etc., where there is subchondral sclerosis instead.

X-ray features specific to different sites will be discussed in their respective sections. A chest X-ray should be done routinely to detect any tubercular lesion in the lungs.

Other investigations: Some of the following investigations may be helpful in diagnosis:

- *Blood examination:* Lymphocytic leukocytosis, high ESR.
- *Mantoux test* useful in children.
- *Serum ELISA* test for detecting anti-Mycobacterium antibodies.
- *Synovial fluid aspiration* (see Table 22.3, page 175).
- Aspiration of cold abscess and examination of pus for AFB.
- *Histopathological examination* of the granulation tissue obtained by biopsy or curettage of a lesion.

TREATMENT

Principles of treatment: Treatment of tuberculosis of bones and joints consists of control of the infection and care of the diseased part. In most cases, conservative treatment suffices; sometimes operative intervention is required.

Table 23.2: Common anti-tubercular drugs and their dosages.	
Name/Daily dose (max.)	**Side-effects**
Bactericidal	
▪ Rifampicin (RF) 10 mg/kg (600 mg)	▪ Hepatotoxicity, pink coloured urine
▪ Isoniazide (INH) 5-10 mg/kg (300)	▪ Hepatotoxicity, peripheral neuritis
▪ Streptomycin (SM) 30 mg/kg (1 gm)	▪ Vestibular damage, nephrotoxicity circumoral paraesthesia
▪ Pyrazinamide (PZ) 25 mg/kg (1.5 gm)	▪ Hepatotoxicity
Bacteriostatic	
▪ Ethambutol (ETH) 25 mg/kg for 4 weeks (1000 mg), thereafter 15 mg/kg (800 mg)	▪ Optic neuritis, colour blindness
▪ Cycloserine 10 mg/kg (500 mg)	▪ CNS toxicity - headache, tremor, dysarthria
▪ Ethionamide 25 mg/kg (750 mg)	▪ Anorexia, nausea, vomiting
▪ Para-amino salicilate (PAS) 200-400 mg/kg (12 g)	▪ Anorexia, nausea, vomiting

Control of infection: It is brought about by potent anti-tubercular drugs, rest to the affected part and the building up of patient's resistance.

a. *Anti-tubercular drugs:* Table 23.2 shows common anti-tubercular drugs, their dosage, route of administration and common side-effects. It is usual practice to start the treatment with 4 drugs - Rifampicin, INH, Pyrazinamide, Ethambutol for 3 months. In selected cases with multifocal tuberculosis, 5 drugs - RF, INH, PZ, ETH and Streptomycin, may be required for the initial period. The patient is monitored* to detect any failure to respond or for any side-effects of the drugs.

b. *Rest:* The affected part should be rested during the period of pain. In the upper extremities this can be done with a plaster slab; in the lower extremities traction can be applied. In most cases of spinal tuberculosis bed rest for a short period is sufficient; in others, support with a brace may be necessary.

c. *Building up the patient's resistance:* The patient should be given a high protein diet and exposed to fresh air and sunlight to build up his general resistance.

---

* Multi-drug resistance is a serious upcoming problem. Anti-tubercular drugs, in proper combination, in proper dosages and under close supervision is the key to its prevention.

Care of the affected part: This consists of protection of the affected part from further damage, correction of any deformities and prevention of joint contractures. Once the disease is brought under control, exercises to regain functions of the joint are carried out. Care consists of the following:

a. *Proper positioning of the joint:* The joints should be kept in proper position so that contractures do not develop.

b. *Mobilisation:* As the disease comes under control and the pain reduces, joint mobilisation is begun. This prevents contractures and helps regain movement. In cases with extreme damage to the joint, it is best to expect ankylosis of the joint in the position of most useful function.

c. *Exercises:* As the joint regains movement, muscle strength building exercises are taught.

d. *Weight bearing:* It is started gradually as osteoporosis secondary to the disease is reversed.

Operative intervention may be required in some cases. Following are some procedures commonly used:

a. *Biopsy:* For cases where the diagnosis is in doubt, a fine needle aspiration cytology (FNAC) may be performed from an enlarged lymph node or from a soft tissue swelling. An open biopsy may be necessary from a bony lesion, or in case FNAC fails to confirm the diagnosis.

b. *Treatment of cold abscess:* A small stationary abscess may be left alone as it will regress with the healing of the disease. A bigger cold abscess may need aspiration or evacuation (discussed in detail on page 189).

c. *Curettage of the lesion:* If the lesion is in the vicinity of a joint, infection is likely to spread to the joint. An early curettage of the lesion may prevent this complication.

d. *Joint debridement:* In cases with moderate joint destruction, surgical removal of infected and necrotic material from the joint may be required. This helps in the early healing of the disease, and thus promotes recovery of the joint.

e. *Synovectomy:* In cases of synovial tuberculosis, a synovectomy may be required to promote early recovery.

f. *Salvage operations:* These are procedures performed for markedly destroyed joints in order to salvage whatever useful functions are possible, e.g., Girdlestone arthroplasty of the hip (page 196).

g. *Decompression:* In cases with paraplegia secondary to spinal TB, surgical decompression may be necessary.

TUBERCULOSIS OF THE SPINE (POTT'S DISEASE)

The spine is the *most common* site of bone and joint tuberculosis; the dorso-lumbar region being the one affected most frequently.

RELEVANT ANATOMY

Development of a vertebra (Fig. 23.2): A vertebra develops from the sclerotomes which lie on either side of the notochord. The lower-half of one vertebra and upper-half of the one below it, along with the intervening disc develop from each pair of sclerotomes and have a common blood supply. Therefore, infections via the arteries involve the 'embryological' section, as in the more common paradiscal tuberculosis of the spine.

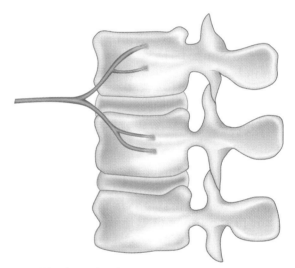

Fig. 23.2: Blood supply of vertebrae (diagrammatic, simplified).

Surface anatomy of the vertebral column: The only part of the vertebra which is accessible to palpation is its spinous process, hence this is used for localising the level of the vertebral segment. Table 23.3 shows the relationship between the vertebral spinous processes to that of some of the easily palpable anatomical landmarks. Once the affected vertebra

Table 23.3: Vertebral level – landmarks.	
▪ Most prominent spinous process at the base of the neck	T_1
▪ At the level of the spine of the scapula	D_3
▪ At the level of lower angle of the scapula	D_7
▪ Floating rib	D_{12}
▪ At the level of the iliac crests	L_4
▪ At the level of the posterior superior iliac spine	S_2

Table 23.4: Relationship between spinal and cord segments.	
Spinal segment	**Cord segment**
Cervical vertebrae	Add 1 to vertebral level
Upper dorsal vertebrae	Add 2 to vertebral level
Lower dorsal vertebrae	Add 3 to vertebral level
At D_{10}	All dorsal segments over
At D_{12}	All lumbar segments over
At L_1	All sacral segments over
Below L_1	Cauda equina

is known, the corresponding cord-segment can be found as discussed subsequently.

Cord-segment localisation: Because of the disproportionate growth of the vertebral column and spinal cord, the cord ends at the lower border of first lumbar vertebra. Beyond this, up to S2 there is only the dural sac containing a bunch of nerve roots (cauda equina). The segment of the cord which corresponds to a given vertebra is therefore above the level of that vertebra. Relationship between the spinal segment and cord segment in different regions of the spinal column is as shown in Table 23.4.

PATHOLOGY

Like tuberculosis of the bones and joints elsewhere in the body, TB of the spine is always secondary. The bacteria reach the spine via the haematogenous route, from the lungs or lymph nodes. It spreads via the paravertebral plexus of veins, i.e., Batson's plexus, which has free communication with the visceral plexus of the abdomen, a common site of tuberculosis.

Types of vertebral tuberculosis: Lesions in the vertebrae may be of the following types (Fig. 23.3):
a. *Paradiscal:* This is the *most common* type. In this, the contiguous areas of two adjacent vertebrae along with the intervening disc are affected.

b. *Central:* In this type, the body of a single vertebra is affected. This leads to early collapse of the weakened vertebra. The nearby disc may be normal. The collapse may be a 'wedging' or 'concertina' collapse (Fig. 23.4); wedging being more common.
c. *Anterior:* In this type, infection is localised to the anterior part of the vertebral body. The infection spreads up and down under the anterior longitudinal ligament.
d. *Posterior:* In this type, the posterior complex of the vertebra, i.e., the pedicle, lamina, spinous process and transverse process are affected.

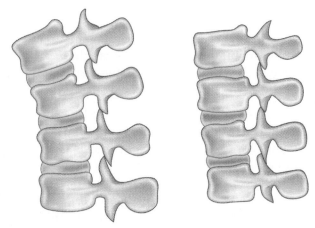

Fig. 23.4: Types of collapse of vertebrae.

Pathology: Basic pathology is the same as that in other bone and joint tuberculosis. In the more common paradiscal type, bacteria lodge in the contiguous areas of two adjacent vertebrae. Granulomatous inflammation results in erosion of the margins of these vertebrae. Nutrition of the intervening disc, which comes from the end-plates of the adjacent vertebrae is compromised. This results in disc degeneration, and as the process continues, complete *destruction*.

Weakening of the trabeculae of the vertebral body results in *collapse of the vertebra*. Type of collapse

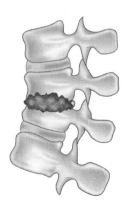 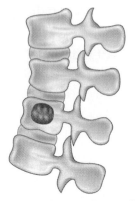 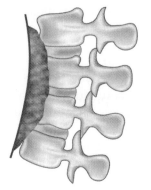 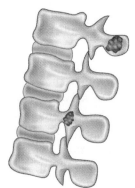

Fig. 23.3: Types of vertebral tuberculosis.

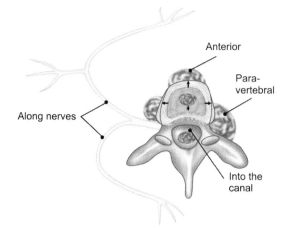

Fig. 23.5: Directions of tracking of tubercular pus from a vertebral focus.

is generally a wedging, occurs early, and is severe in lesions of the dorsal spine. This is because, in the dorsal spine the line of weight bearing passes anterior to the vertebra, so that the anterior part of the weakened vertebra is more compressed than the posterior, resulting in wedging. In the cervical and lumbar spines, because of their lordotic curvature (round forwards), wedging is less. Destruction occurs early, and is severe in children.

Cold abscess: This is a collection of pus and tubercular debris from a diseased vertebra. It is called a cold abscess because it is not associated with the usual signs of inflammation - heat, redness, etc., found with a pyogenic abscess. The tubercular pus can track in any direction from the affected vertebra (Fig. 23.5). If it travels backwards, it may press upon the important neural structures in the spinal canal. Pus may come out anteriorly (prevertebral abscess) or on the sides of the vertebral body (paravertebral abscess). Once outside the vertebra the pus may travel along the musculo-fascial planes or neurovascular bundles to appear superficially at places far away from the site of lesion.

Healing: As healing occurs, the lytic areas in the bone are replaced by new bone. The adjacent vertebrae undergo fusion by bony-bridges. Whatever changes have occurred in the shape of the vertebral body are, however, permanent.

CLINICAL FEATURES

Presenting complaints: Clinical presentations of a case of TB of the spine is very variable - from a seemingly non-specific pain in the back to complete paraplegia. Following are some of the common presenting complaints:

- **Pain:** Back pain is the most common presenting symptom. It may be diffuse; no more than a dull ache in the early stages, but later becomes localised to the affected diseased segment. It may be a 'radicular' pain i.e., a pain, radiating along a nerve root. Depending upon the nerve root affected, it may present as pain in the arm (cervical roots), girdle pain (dorsal roots), pain abdomen (dorso-lumbar roots), groin pain (lumbar roots) or 'sciatic' pain (lumbo-sacral roots).
- **Stiffness:** It is a very early symptom in TB of the spine. It is a protective mechanism of the body, wherein the para-vertebral muscles go into spasm to prevent movement at the affected vertebra.
- **Cold abscess:** The patient may present the first time with a swelling (cold abscess) or problems secondary to its compression effects on the nearby visceral structures, such as dysphagia in TB of the cervical spine. A detailed examination in such cases reveals underlying TB of the spine.
- **Paraplegia:** If neglected, which is often the case in developing countries, a case of TB of the spine presents with this serious complication. For details see Pott's paraplegia, page 189.
- **Deformity:** Attention to TB of the spine may be attracted, especially in children, by a gradually increasing prominence of the spine - a gibbus.
- **Constitutional symptoms:** Symptoms like fever, weight loss, etc., are rarely the only presenting symptoms.

EXAMINATION

The aim of examination is: (i) to pick up findings suggestive of tuberculosis of the spine; (ii) to localise the site of lesion; (iii) find skip lesions; and (iv) to detect any associated complications like cold abscesses or paraplegia. Following is the systematic way in which one should proceed to examine a case of suspected TB of the spine.

- **Gait:** A patient with TB of the spine walks with short steps in order to avoid jerking the spine. He may take time and may be very cautious while attempting to lie on the examination couch. In TB of the cervical spine, the patient often supports his head with both hands under the chin and twists his whole body in order to look sideways.
- **Attitude and deformity:** A patient with TB of the cervical spine has a stiff, straight neck. In dorsal spine TB, part of the spine becomes prominent (*gibbus or kyphus**). Significant deformity is generally absent in lumbar spine tuberculosis; there may just be loss of lumbar lordosis.

---

* There are three types of kyphotic deformities:
  i. Knuckle – prominence of one spinous process
  ii. Gibbus – prominence of two or three spinous processes
  iii. Kyphus -- diffuse rounding of the vertebral column

Table 23.5: Presentation of cold abscesses from different regions of the spine.

Region of spine	Presentation			
	Anteriorly	On the sides	Along musculo-fascial plane	Along neurovascular plane
Cervical spine	Retropharyngeal abscess	Paravertebral abscess	At the posterior border of sternocleidomastoid muscle, in the *posterior triangle* of neck	To axilla, to arm along neurovascular bundle of the arm

Thoracic spine	Mediastinal abscess	Paravertebral abscess	Trickles downward and enters either of the two lumbocostal arches:
			■ Lateral lumbocostal arch
			  - To present as *lumbar abscess*
			■ Medial lumbocostal arch
			  - To present as *psoas abscess*
				Along thoracic spinal nerves to present at
				■ Anterior chest wall
				■ Midaxillary line
				■ Posterior chest wall

Lumbar spine	Prevertebral abscess	Paravertebral abscess	Lumbar abscess or psoas abscess lower	Along neurovascular bundle of the leg to present in groin or lower down in the leg

- **Paravertebral swelling:** A superficial cold abscess may present as fullness or swelling on the back, along the chest wall or anteriorly. It is easy to diagnose because of its fluctuant nature. Sometimes, an abscess may be tense and it may not be possible to elicit fluctuation. A needle aspiration may be performed in such cases, to confirm the diagnosis. It is important to look for cold abscesses in not so obvious locations, depending upon the region of the spine affected (Table 23.5).
- **Tenderness:** It can be elicited by pressing upon the side of the spinous process in an attempt to rotate the vertebra.
- **Movement:** There is no necessity to examine for spinal movement in a patient with obviously painful spine. Spinal movement are limited in a case of TB of the spine, and can be tested, wherever considered suitable.
- **Neurological examination:** A thorough neurological examination of the limbs, upper or lower, depending on the site of tuberculosis should be performed. In addition to motor, sensory and reflexes examination, an assessment should be made of urinary or bowel functions. Aim of neurological examination is to find: (i) whether or not there is any neurological compression; (ii) level of neuro- logical compression; and (iii) severity of neurological compression.
- **General examination:** A general physical examination should be performed to detect any active or healed primary lesion. The patient may have some other systemic illness like diabetes, hypertension, jaundice, etc., which may have a bearing on further treatment.

RADIOLOGICAL INVESTIGATIONS

X-ray examination: One must *specify* the level of the suspected damage, when requisitioning an X-ray of the spine. Minimum of two views, AP and lateral, are necessary. A chest X-ray for primary focus or an X-ray of the abdomen – KUB, if a psoas abscess is suspected, may also be taken. Following are some of the important radiological features.

- *Reduction of disc space:* This is the *earliest sign* in the more common, paradiscal type of tuberculosis (Fig. 23.6A). In early stages, reduction in disc space may be minimal, and may be detectable only on comparing the height of the suspected disc with those above and below it. In advanced stages, disc space may be completely lost (Fig. 23.6B). A lateral X-ray is better for evaluation of disc space. Reduction of disc space is an important sign because in other diseases of the spine, e.g., secondaries in the spine, the disc space is well-preserved.
- *Destruction of the vertebral body:* In early stages, the contiguous margins of the affected vertebrae may be eroded. The diseased, weakened vertebra may undergo wedging. In late stages, a significant part or whole of the vertebral body may be destroyed (Fig. 23.6C), leading to angular kyphotic deformity. Severity of the deformity depends upon the extent of wedging and number of affected vertebrae (Table 23.6).
- *Evidence of cold abscess:* Radiological evidence of a cold abscess is a very useful finding in diagnosing a case of suspected spinal TB. Following abscesses may be seen on X-rays:
  - *Paravertebral abscess:* A paravertebral soft tissue shadow corresponding to the site of the affected vertebra in AP view indicates a paravertebral abscess. It may be of the following types: (i)

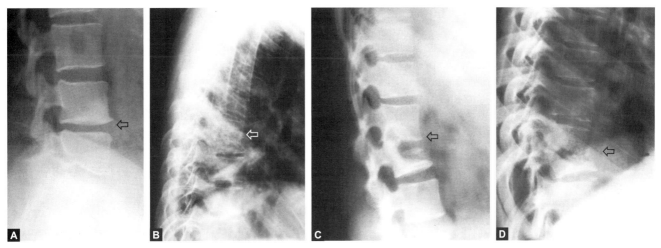

Fig. 23.6: X-ray findings in TB of the spine: (A) Early case, minimal loss of disc prolapse; (B) Complete loss of disc prolapse; (C) Destruction of vertebral bodies with loss of disc prolapse; (D) Advance destruction and wedging of vertebrae.

a fusiform paravertebral abscess (bird nest abscess - an abscess whose length is greater than its width (Fig. 23.7A); and (ii) globular or tense abscess - an abscess whose width is greater than the length (Fig. 23.7B). The latter indicates pus under pressure and is commonly associated with paraplegia.

Table 23.6: Number of affected vertebrae.

Type	No. of vertebrae involved
Knuckle	1
Gibbus	2–3
Angular kyphosis	3–4
Rounded kyphosis	>4

- *Widened mediastinum:* An abscess from the dorsal spine may present as widened mediastinum on AP X-ray.
- *Retropharyngeal abscess:* In cervical spine TB, a retropharyngeal abscess may be seen on a lateral X-ray. Normally, soft tissue shadow in front of the C3 vertebral body is 4 mm thick; an increase in its thickness indicates a retropharyngeal abscess (Fig. 23.7C).
- *Psoas abscess:* In dorso-lumbar and lumbar tuberculosis, psoas shadow on an X-ray of the abdomen may show a bulge.
- *Rarefaction:* There is diffuse rarefaction of the vertebrae above and below the lesion.
- *Unusual signs:* In tuberculosis involving the posterior complex, there may be erosion of the

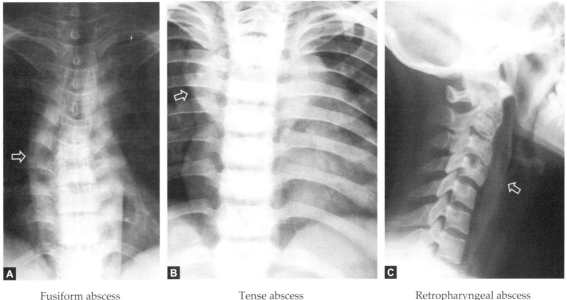

Fusiform abscess   Tense abscess   Retropharyngeal abscess

Fig. 23.7: Types of paravertebral abscesses.

posterior elements of pedicle, lamina, etc. These are better visible on oblique X-rays of the spine. Anterior type of vertebral tuberculosis may show erosion of the anterior part of the body, much the same as that possibly seen sometimes in cases with aneurysm of aorta, thus termed *aneurysmal sign.* There may be lytic lesions in the ribs in the vicinity of the affected vertebra.

- *Signs of healing:* Once the disease starts healing, the density of the affected bones gradually improves. Areas surrounding the lytic lesion show sclerosis, and over a period of time these lesions are replaced by sclerotic bone. The adjacent vertebrae undergo bony fusion.

CT scan: It may detect a small paravertebral abscess, not otherwise seen on plain X-ray; may indicate precisely the extent of destruction of the vertebral body and posterior elements; and may show a sequestrum or a bony ridge pressing on the cord (Fig. 23.8). This is a very useful investigation in cases presenting as 'spinal tumour syndrome', where there may be no signs on plain X-rays.

MRI is the investigation of choice to evaluate the type and extent of compression of the cord (Fig. 23.9). It also shows condition of the underlying neural tissues, and thus helps in predicting the prognosis in a particular case.

Biopsy: CT guided needle biopsy, or an open biopsy may be required in a case with doubtful diagnosis.

Other general investigations: Investigations like ESR, Mantoux test, ELISA test for detecting anti-tubercular antibodies, chest X-ray, etc., to support the diagnosis of tuberculosis, may be carried out whenever required.

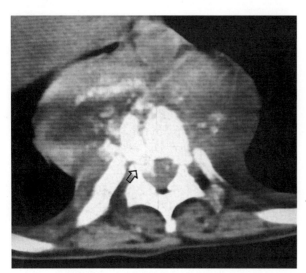

Fig. 23.8: CT scan of a case of TB spine.
(Note bony fragments in the canal).

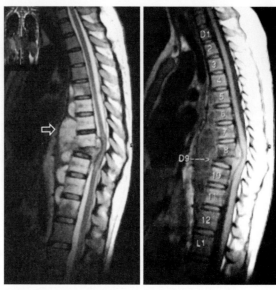

Fig. 23.9: MRI of the spine (T_1 and T_2 images), showing TB spine. (Note the compression on the cord and huge prevertebral abscess).

DIFFERENTIAL DIAGNOSIS

Cases with TB of the spine report fairly late in developing countries, so they present mostly with classic signs, symptoms and radiological features. In the early stages, and sometimes in some atypical presentations, diagnosis may be difficult. Some of the common differential diagnosis and their differentiating features are given in Table 23.7.

TREATMENT

Principles of treatment: Aim of treatment is: (i) to achieve healing of the disease and (ii) to prevent, detect early, and treat promptly any complication like paraplegia, etc. Treatment consists of anti-tubercular chemotherapy (page 182), general care (page 182), care of the spine, and treatment of the cold abscess. Only the latter two will be discussed here.

Care of the spine: This consists of providing rest to the spine during the acute phase, followed by guarded mobilisation.

- *Rest:* A short period of bed rest for pain relief may be sufficient during early stages of treatment. In cases with significant vertebral destruction, a longer period of bed rest is desirable to prevent further collapse and pathological dislocation of the diseased vertebrae. In children, a body cast is sometimes given, basically to force them to rest. Minerva jacket or a collar may be given for immobilising the cervical spine.
- *Mobilisation:* As the patient improves, he is allowed to sit and walk while the spine is supported in a collar for the cervical spine, or an ASH brace for the dorso-lumbar spine. The patient is weaned off

Table 23.7: TB of the spine: Differential diagnosis.

Symptoms	Clinical features	Investigations
Back pain		
Traumatic	History of trauma present No fever or abscess	▪ X-ray – disc height normal. ▪ Wedging of vertebrae present ▪ No paravertebral shadow seen
Secondaries/ myeloma	History of 'primary' elsewhere or myeloma	▪ Disc space normal ▪ Pedicles may be involved in secondaries ▪ Lesions in other bones present
Prolapsed disc	▪ Radiating pain ▪ SLRT – positive ▪ Localised nerve root deficit	Normal X-rays
Ankylosing spondylitis	▪ Chronic back pain, starts in lower back ▪ Diffuse morning stiffness ▪ Chest expansion reduced	▪ 'Bamboo spine' appearance on X-rays ▪ SI joints affected – hazy, fused
Neurological deficit		
Spinal tumour	▪ Present with gradually increasing neurological deficit ▪ No back pain, or other findings on spine examination	▪ X-ray – interpedicle space increased ▪ Pedicle erosion present ▪ CT myelogram confirms
Traumatic	▪ History of definite trauma present ▪ Weakness is sudden onset	X-ray suggestive of fracture-dislocation
Secondaries in the spine	▪ No history of trauma ▪ Back pain present ▪ History of 'primary' elsewhere	X-ray shows erosion of vertebrae

the brace once bony fusion occurs. He is advised to avoid sports for 2 years.

Treatment of cold abscess: A small cold abscess may subside with anti-tubercular treatment. Abscesses presenting superficially need treatment as discussed below:

- *Aspiration:* A thick needle is required because often there is thick caseous material. It should be an anti-gravity insertion with the needle entering through a zig-zag tract.
- *Evacuation:* In this procedure, the cold abscess is drained, its walls curetted, and the wound closed without a drain. This is unlike drainage of a pyogenic abscess, where a post-operative drain is always left. A psoas abscess can be drained extraperitoneally using a kidney incision.

Medical Research Council of Great Britain conducted controlled trials to study various aspects of TB spine and published findings in four reports (1973-74). Their conclusions were that: (i) Bed rest is not necessary; (ii) Streptomycin is not necessary; (iii) PoP jacket offers no benefit; and (iv) Debridement is not a good operation.

COMPLICATIONS

1. **Cold abscess:** This is the most common complication of TB of the spine. Treatment is as discussed above.

2. **Neurological compression:** At times the patient presents as a case of spinal tumour syndrome; the first clinical symptom being a neurological deficit (discussed subsequently).

POTT'S PARAPLEGIA (TB SPINE WITH NEUROLOGICAL INVOLVEMENT)

The incidence of neurological deficit has been reported to be 20 per cent. It occurs *most commonly* in tuberculosis of the dorsal spine because the spinal canal is narrowest in this part, and even a small compromise can lead to a neurological deficit.

PATHOLOGY

This consists of pressure on the neural tissues within the canal by products from the diseased vertebrae. It could occur in the following ways:

- **Inflammatory oedema:** The neural tissues become oedematous because of vascular stasis in the adjacent diseased area.
- **Extradural pus and granulation tissue:** This is the *most common* cause of compression on neural structures. The abscess formed around the diseased vertebrae may compress the neural structures from the front, much the same way as an extradural tumour.

- **Sequestra:** Devascularised bone and extruded disc material may be displaced into the canal.
- **Internal 'gibbus':** Angulation of the diseased spine may lead to formation of the bony ridge on the anterior wall of the spinal canal (Fig. 23.10). This is called the internal gibbus.

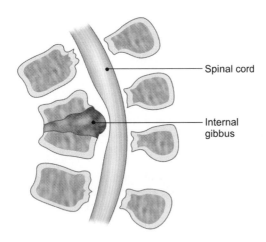

Fig. 23.10: Internal gibbus.

- **Infarction of the spinal cord:** This is an unusual but important cause of paralysis. It results from blockage of the anterior spinal artery, caused by the inflammatory reaction.
- **Extradural granuloma:** Very rarely, an extradural granuloma may form without any damage to the osseous structures. Such a patient presents with a clinical picture of a spinal tumour - the so-called *'Spinal tumour syndrome'*.

Types of Pott's paraplegia: It can be divided into two types:

a. **Early onset paraplegia,** i.e., paraplegia occurring during the active phase of the disease, usually within two years of onset of the disease.
b. **Late onset paraplegia,** i.e., paraplegia occurring several years after the disease has become quiescent, usually at least two years after the onset of disease. Pathology of the two types is different, as also is the prognosis. Table 23.8 gives the causes of neurological deficit in early and late onset paraplegia.

CLINICAL FEATURES

Neurological complications can occur in a known case of tuberculosis of the spine; or the case may present for the first time with a neurological deficit. In the latter, tuberculosis as the cause of paraplegia is detected only on examination and further investigation. Onset of paraplegia is gradual in *most* cases, but in some it is sudden. Tubercular paraplegia is usually spastic to start with. Clonus (ankle or patellar) is the most prominent early sign. Paralysis may pass with varying rapidity, through the following stages:

- **Muscle weakness**, spasticity and in-coordination due to pressure on the corticospinal tracts which are placed anteriorly in the cord and are probably more sensitive to pressure.
- **Paraplegia in extension:** Tone of the muscles is increased due to absence of normal corticospinal inhibition, resulting in paraplegia in extension.
- **Paraplegia in flexion:** Absence of paraspinal tract functions in addition to the corticospinal functions leads to paraplegia in flexion.
- **Complete flaccid paraplegia:** Paraplegia becomes completely flaccid once all transmission across the cord stops.

Grades of Pott's paraplegia: Potts' paraplegia has been graded on the basis of degree of motor involvement, into four grades (Goel, 1967):

Grade I: Patient is unaware of the neural deficit; the physician detects Babinski positive and ankle or patellar clonus on clinical examination.

Grade II: Patient presents with complaints of clumsiness, in-coordination or spasticity while walking, but manages to walk with or without support.

Grade III: Patient is not able to walk because of severe weakness. On examination, he has paraplegia in extension. There may be partial loss of sensation.

Grade IV: Patient is unable to walk, and has paraplegia in flexion with severe muscle spasm. There is near complete loss of sensation with sphincter disturbances.

Table 23.8: Causes* of paraplegia in TB of the spine.

Early onset paraplegia
- *Inflammatory causes*
  - Abscess - most common
  - Granulation tissue
  - Circumscribed tuberculous focus
  - Posterior spinal disease
  - Infective thrombosis of the spinal blood supply
- *Mechanical causes*
  - Sequestrum in the canal
  - Infected degenerated disc in the canal
  - Pathological dislocation - a ridge of bone pressing on the cord

Late onset paraplegia
- Recurrence of the disease
- Prominent anterior wall of the spinal canal in case of severe kyphosis (internal gibbus)
- Fibrous septae following healing

* Although these several mechanisms have been described as acting separately to produce paraplegia, more than one cause may be responsible in a particular patient.

INVESTIGATIONS

It is usually possible to diagnose vertebral tuberculosis as a cause of paraplegia by typical radiological signs. In some cases, a MRI scan may be done to see: (i) type of vertebral destruction; (i) presence of paravertebral soft tissue abscess; and (iii) cause of paraplegia, i.e., whether it is pus, sequestra, etc. CT scan may be required in some cases to better evaluate the vertebral canal. MRI is the investigation of choice, wherever available.

TREATMENT

Principles of treatment: Aims of treatment are as follows:

a. To *promote recovery* of the affected neural tissues, by reversing the cause responsible for compression, either by drugs or by operation.

b. To *achieve healing* of the vertebral lesion, and to support the spine till the diseased segment becomes stable.

c. To undertake *rehabilitative* measures to prevent contractures, and to regain strength in the affected part.

Treatment of Pott's paraplegia has been the topic of considerable study and discussion. Following is the treatment considered most acceptable in the author's opinion. Treatment may be divided into conservative and operative. All cases of Pott's paraplegia must be treated under supervision, after admission to a hospital.

Conservative treatment: Anti-tubercular chemotherapy forms the mainstay of treatment. All patients are started on 4-drugs anti-tubercular chemotherapy as soon as the diagnosis is made. The spine is put to absolute rest by a sling traction for the cervical spine, and bed rest for the dorso-lumbar spine. The paralysed limbs are taken care of, as discussed in the Chapter 32. During treatment, repeated neurological examination of the limbs is carried out to detect any deterioration or improvement in the neurological status.

If paraplegia improves, conservative treatment is continued. Patient is allowed to sit in the bed with the help of a brace as soon as the spine has gained sufficient strength. Bracing is continued for a period of about 6 to 12 months.

Operative treatment: If paraplegia does not improve at a satisfactory rate, or if it actually deteriorates; surgical intervention is indicated. Following are the indications for surgery considered suitable in most centres.

Absolute indications

1. Paraplegia occurring during usual conservative treatment.
2. Paraplegia *getting worse* or remaining stationary despite adequate conservative treatment.
3. Severe paraplegia with *rapid onset* may indicate severe pressure from a mechanical accident or abscess.
4. Any *severe paraplegia* such as paraplegia in flexion, motor or sensory loss for more than six months, complete loss of motor power for one month despite adequate conservative treatment.
5. Paraplegia *accompanied by uncontrolled spasticity* of such severity that reasonable rest and immobilisation are not possible.

Relative indications

1. Recurrent paraplegia, even with paralysis that would cause no concern in the first attack.
2. Paraplegia with *onset in old age:* Indications for surgery are stronger because of the hazards of recumbency.
3. *Painful paraplegia,* pain resulting from spasm or root compression.
4. *Complications* such as urinary tract infection and stones.

Rare indications

1. Paraplegia due to posterior spinal disease.
2. Spinal tumour syndrome.
3. Severe paralysis secondary to the cervical disease.
4. Severe cauda equina paralysis.

Operative procedures for Pott's paraplegia: The operative method aims at removal of the agents causing compression on the neural structures. The following operations are commonly performed:

a. **Costotransversectomy (Fig. 23.11A):** As the name suggests, this operation consists of the removal of a section of rib (about 2 inches), and transverse process. As this is done, sometimes liquid pus comes out under pressure. This is considered by some as a tense abscess relieved, and thus enough to decompress the neural tissues. It is indicated

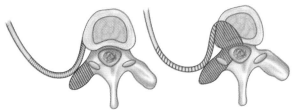

A Costotransversectomy **B** Anterolateral decompression

Fig. 23.11: Structures to be removed.

in a child with paraplegia, and when a tense abscess is visible on X-ray. In all other cases, it may not produce adequate decompression and an anterolateral decompression may be necessary.

b. **Anterolateral decompression (ALD):** This is the most commonly performed operation. In this operation, the spine is opened from its lateral side and access is made to the front and side of the cord, thus it is called anterolateral decompression. The cord is laid free of any granulation tissue, caseous material, bony spur or sequestrum pressing on it. Structures removed in order to achieve adequate exposure of the cord are; the rib, transverse process, pedicle and part of the body of the vertebra (Fig. 23.11B). Lamina or facet joints are *not* removed, otherwise stability of the spine will be seriously jeopardized.

c. **Radical debridement and arthrodesis (Hong Kong operation):** Wherever facilities are available, a radical debridement is performed by exposing the spine from front using transthoracic or transperitoneal approaches. All the dead and diseased vertebrae are excised and replaced by rib grafts. Advantage of this operation is early healing of the disease and no progress of the kyphosis.

d. **Laminectomy:** It is indicated in cases of spinal tumour syndrome, and those where paraplegia has resulted from posterior spinal disease.

Surgery for the cervical spine tuberculosis requires a separate technique; anterior decompression is preferable in this area.

PROGNOSIS

Prognosis of Pott's paraplegia depends upon the following factors:

1. **Age:** Children respond to treatment better than adults.
2. **Onset:** Acute onset paraplegia has a better prognosis.
3. **Duration:** Long-standing paraplegia has a worse prognosis.
4. **Severity:** Motor paralysis alone has a good prognosis. Sphincter involvement, i.e., urinary or bowel incontinence are bad prognostic indicators.
5. **Progress:** Sudden progress of the paraplegia has a bad prognosis.

TUBERCULOSIS OF THE HIP

After spine, the hip is affected, most commonly. It usually occurs in children and adolescents, but patients at any age can be affected.

PATHOLOGY

The basic pathology is the same as that discussed on page 181. The usual initial lesion is in the bone adjacent to the joint, i.e., either the acetabulum or the head of the femur (osseous tuberculosis). In some cases, the lesion may begin in the synovium (synovial tuberculosis), but quickly the articular cartilage and the bones are affected. A purely synovial tuberculosis, as seen in the knee joint, is uncommon in the hip. Common sites of initial bone focus in TB of the hip are as shown in Figure 23.12.

Natural history: The infected granulation tissue harbouring the bacilli, from the initial bony focus erodes the overlying cartilage or bone and reaches the joint. In early stage, this results in synovial hypertrophy and effusion. The pannus of hypertrophied synovium around the articular cartilage gradually extends over and under it. Cartilage is thus destroyed and the joint becomes full of pus and granulation tissue. Synovium gets thickened, oedematous, grey and ulcerated. Denuded of their protective cartilage, the bone ends become raw.

Multiple *cavitation* is typical of tuberculosis. Such cavities are formed in the femoral head and the acetabulum. Eventually, the head or the acetabulum gets partially absorbed. By the constant pull of the muscles acting on the hip, the remaining head of the femur may dislocate from the acetabulum onto the ilium, giving rise to the so-called *wandering acetabulum* (Fig. 23.13). In later stages, pus bursts through the capsule and spreads in the line of least resistance. It may present as cold abscess in the groin or in the region of the greater trochanter. Pus may perforate the acetabulum and appear as a pelvic abscess.

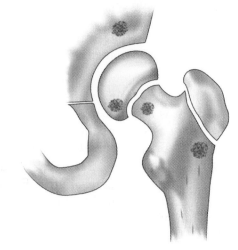

Fig. 23.12: TB hip: Common sites.

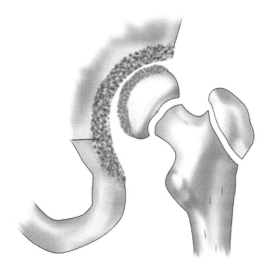

Fig. 23.13: 'Wandering' acetabulum.

Healing: If left untreated, healing may take place by fibrosis, leading to ankylosis of the hip usually in a deformed position (fibrous ankylosis).

CLINICAL FEATURES

Presenting complaints: The disease is insidious in onset and runs a chronic course. The child may be apathetic and pale with loss of appetite before definite symptoms pertaining to the hip appear. One of the first symptoms is stiffness of the hip, and it produces a limp. Initially, stiffness may occur only after rest, but later it persists all the time.

Pain may be absent in early stages, or if present, may be referred to the *knee*. The child may complain of 'night cries', the so called 'starting pain', caused by the rubbing of the two diseased surfaces, when movement occurs as a result of the muscle relaxation during sleep. Later, there may be cold abscesses around the hip or these may burst, resulting in discharging sinuses.

EXAMINATION

It should be carried out with the patient undressed. Following physical findings may be present:
- **Gait:** Lameness is one of the *first* signs. In the early stage, it is because of stiffness and deformity of the hip. Because of the flexion deformity at the hip, the child stands with compensatory exaggerated lumbar lordosis. While walking the hip is kept stiff. Forward-backward movement at the lumbar spine is used for propulsion of the lower limb. This is called the 'stiff-hip gait'. Later the limp is exaggerated by pain so the child hastens to take the weight

off the affected side. This is called the 'painful or antalgic gait'.
- **Muscle wasting:** The thigh muscles and gluteal muscles are wasted.
- **Swelling:** There may be swelling around the hip because of a cold abscess.
- **Discharging sinuses:** There may be discharging sinuses in the groin or around the greater trochanter. There may be puckered scars from healed sinuses.
- **Deformity:** Gross deformities may be obvious on inspection. Minimal deformities are compensated for by pelvic tilt and can be made obvious by tests. Commonly it is flexion, adduction and internal rotation deformity of the hip. Method of measuring deformities is as discussed in Annexure I.
- **Shortening:** There is generally a true shortening in TB of the hip, except in Stage I, in which an apparent lengthening occurs (Annexure I). Limb length discrepancy can occur at this joint not only because of actual shortening of the bones (true length) but also because of the adduction-abduction deformity, which results in pelvic tilt and thus affects the length of the limb (apparent length). The method of measuring true and apparent lengths is as discussed in Annexure I. True and apparent length, and their relation to different deformities of the hip are given in Table 23.9.
- **Movements:** Both, active and passive movements are limited in all directions. An attempted movement is associated with muscle spasm.

There may be severe limitation of movements, both active and passive, in all directions in late cases of tuberculosis. This is called ankylosis of the hip. If there is no movement at all, it is bony ankylosis.
- **Abnormal position of the head:** In a dislocated hip, the head can be felt in the gluteal region.
- **Telescopy:** This test assesses the instability of the head if it is out of the acetabulum (details in Annexure I).

	Table 23.9: Hip deformities, ASIS and limb length.	
Deformity	**ASIS level**	**Limb length**
Adduction	Higher	Apparent < true (apparent shortening)
Abduction	Lower	Apparent > true (apparent lengthening)
No adduction-abduction	Same	Apparent = true

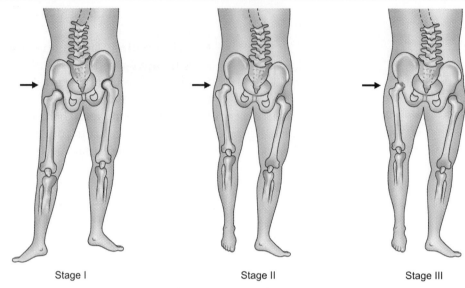

Stage I   Stage II   Stage III

Fig. 23.14: Stages of TB hip.

STAGES OF TB OF THE HIP

TB of the hip has been arbitrarily divided into three stages in its clinical course (Fig. 23.14).

Stage I (stage of synovitis): There is effusion into the joint which demands the hip to be in a position of maximum capacity. This is a position of flexion, abduction and external rotation. Since flexion and abduction deformities are only slight and are compensated for by tilting of the pelvis, these do not become obvious. The limb remains in external rotation. As the pelvis tilts downwards to compensate for the abduction deformity, the affected limb appears longer (apparent lengthening), though on measuring true limb lengths, the two limbs are found to be equal. This stage is also called the *stage of apparent lengthening*. It lasts for a very short period. Very rarely does a patient present to the hospital in such an early stage of the disease.

Stage II (stage of the arthritis): In this stage, the articular cartilage is involved. This leads to spasm of the powerful muscles around the hip. Since the flexors and adductors are stronger muscle groups than the extensors and abductors, the hip takes the attitude of flexion, adduction and internal rotation. Flexion and adduction may be concealed by compensatory tilt of the pelvis but internal rotation of the leg is obvious. As the pelvis tilts upwards to compensate for the adduction, the affected limb appears shorter (apparent shortening), although on comparing the limb lengths in similar positions, the two limbs are equal. This is also called the *stage of apparent shortening*.

Stage III (stage of erosion): In this stage, the cartilage is destroyed and the head and/or the acetabulum is eroded. There may be a pathological dislocation or subluxation of the hip. Attitude of the limb is the same as that in Stage II, i.e., flexion, adduction and internal rotation except for the fact that the deformities are exaggerated. There is *true shortening* of the limb because of the actual destruction of the bone. In addition, apparent length of the limb is further reduced because of the adduction deformity.

INVESTIGATIONS

Radiological examination: An X-ray examination of the pelvis with both hips, AP and lateral views of the affected hip are essential. Inclusion of the normal hip in the same film on the AP view helps in comparing the joint spaces on the two sides. MRI scan and bone scan may be useful in early diagnosis. Some of the radiological signs in an established case of TB of the hip are as follows:

- *Haziness:* Haziness of the bones around the hip is the *earliest* sign. To appreciate it best, the affected hip is compared with the normal hip.
- *Lytic lesion:* There may be lytic lesions in the regions specified in Figure 23.12, on page 192).
- *Reduction of joint space:* This occurs because of destruction of the cartilage. It may be uniformly or irregularly diminished, better appreciated in the early stages on comparing it with the opposite side (Fig. 23.15A).
- *Irregular outline:* The outline of the articular ends of the bone becomes irregular because of destruction by the disease process. In severe cases, a significant part of the head or acetabulum may be destroyed (Figs. 23.15B and C).

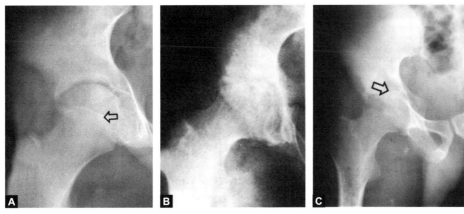

Fig. 23.15: Radiological features of TB of the hip.

- *Acetabular changes:* The head may be lying out of the acetabulum in a 'pseudo' acetabulum on the ilium - the *wandering acetabulum.* In some cases, the acetabulum simply gets enlarged and deepened with the deformed head shifted medially, giving the appearance of the *'pestle and mortar'.*
- *Signs of healing:* If the disease starts healing, there may be sclerosis around the hip.

Other investigations: The investigations that can be carried out to confirm the diagnosis are as discussed on page 171.

Biopsy: It may be needed in some doubtful cases. This is done by exposing the hip by the posterior approach and taking a piece of the synovium for histopathological examination. It is possible to do an arthroscopic biopsy.

DIFFERENTIAL DIAGNOSIS

TB of the hip is the *most common* cause of pain in the hip in children in countries where TB is still prevalent. Following differential diagnosis should be considered:

a. **Other causes of monoarthritis of the hip:** Subacute low grade monoarthritis due to low grade septic infection or rheumatoid arthritis also presents with pain and stiffness of the hip. Lack of supportive evidence for TB (like positive family history, past history) and destruction and sclerosis on X-ray, favour a diagnosis of septic arthritis. It may sometimes be difficult to differentiate the two. In rheumatoid arthritis, joint space is uniformly reduced.

b. **Inguinal lymphadenopathy or psoas abscess:** Patients with these extra-articular diseases often present with a flexion deformity of the hip because of spasm of the iliopsoas. An examination reveals that all movements of the hip *except extension* are pain free.

c. **Other diseases of the hip presenting at that age:** In a child presenting with a *limp without much pain* the following conditions should be considered:
   - *Congenital dislocation of the hip:* The limp is *painless.* It can generally be detected at birth, but is often noticed only when the child starts walking. An abnormal femoral head can be felt in the gluteal region. Telescopy test is positive. X-rays are decisive.
   - *Congenital coxa vara:* The limp is *painless.* The movements limited are abduction and internal rotation. In fact, adduction and external rotation may be increased. X-ray examination usually confirms the diagnosis.
   - *Perthes' disease:* This occurs in children in the age group of 5-10 years. The main complaint is a limp, which is generally painful. There is minimal limitation of movement, mainly that of abduction and internal rotation. Little or no shortening is present. Typically, X-ray changes are *out of proportion* to the physical findings. The joint space, unlike in TB of the hip, may even be *widened* (for details see page 309).

d. **Osteoarthritis:** This occurs in older individuals. Hip movements are limited in all directions but only terminally. There is associated pain and crepitus. Most cases are of osteoarthritis secondary to some other pathology (see Chapter 35).

TREATMENT

Principles of treatment: It is to control the disease activity, and to preserve joint movement. In early stages (Stages I and II), it is possible to achieve this by conservative treatment. In later stages (Stage II and after), significant limitation of joint functions occur despite best treatment. Treatment may be conservative or operative.

Conservative treatment: It consists of anti-tubercular chemotherapy (page 182) and care of the hip.

- *Care of the hip:* The affected hip is put to rest by immobilisation using below-knee skin traction. In addition to providing pain relief, this also corrects any deformity by counteracting the muscle spasm.
- *General care:* Same as on page 182.

Operative treatment: The following operative procedures may be indicated in TB of the hip (see plan of treatment on page 200).

- *Joint debridement:* The joint is opened using posterior approach. Pus, necrotic tissue, inflamed synovium and dead cartilage are removed from the joint. Any cavities in the head of the femur or acetabulum are curetted. The joint is washed thoroughly with saline and the wound closed. Post-operatively the joint surfaces are kept apart by traction to the leg. After the wound heals, the joint is mobilised.
- *Girdlestone arthroplasty:* The hip joint is exposed using the posterior approach. Head and neck of the femur are excised (Fig. 23.16). Dead necrotic tissues and granulation tissues are excised. Post-operatively, bilateral skeletal traction is given for 4 weeks, followed by mobilisation of the hip. It is possible to regain reasonable movement of the hip by this procedure even in severely damaged joints.
- *Arthrodesis:* In selected cases, where a stiff hip in a functional position is more suitable considering day-to-day activities of the patient, it is produced surgically by knocking the joint out.
- *Corrective osteotomy:* Cases where bony ankylosis of the hip has occurred in an unacceptable position from the functional viewpoint, a subtrochanteric

corrective osteotomy of the femur may be required.

- *Total hip replacement:* There is enough evidence now, that a total hip replacement is a useful operation in some patients with quiescent tuberculosis. But as of now in most Afro-Asian countries, where most cannot afford a total hip replacement, and where most patients want to be able to squat even at the cost of instability, an excision arthroplasty is a preferred option.

Deciding the plan of treatment: In early stages, ATT and skin traction is given. As the disease comes under control, as is evident from the relief of symptoms; joint mobilisation is begun. By physiotherapy good joint functions can be regained in most cases. In cases presenting in late stages, initial treatment is by ATT and below-knee skin traction. The traction keeps the hip in a functional position with the joint surfaces apart while healing occurs. As the disease activity comes under control and symptoms (pain, etc.) subside, a decision has to be made whether useful hip functions can be regained, depending upon the X-ray appearance of the hip. In a case, where there is no or minimal destruction of the hip joint mobilisation is begun with the hope of regaining as much movement as possible. In a case where the X-ray picture suggests significant joint damage or subluxation, one expects that normal joint functions cannot be regained. In such a situation, the options before the surgeon are essentially these:

a. To provide a *painless, mobile but unstable* joint by an excision arthroplasty (Girdlestone arthroplasty). Though the hip becomes unstable and the limb short, one can expect that patient will be able to squat on the floor.

b. To provide a *painless, stable but fixed joint* by surgically fusing the joint (arthrodesis) or by conservative means. Though the hip is stable, lack of movement, and thus an inability to squat is the major problem.

In countries, where for most of day-to-day activities squatting is required, Girdlestone arthroplasty is still considered a suitable operation. In addition to providing a mobile hip, this operation enhances healing of the disease as physical removal of the infected bone, synovium, etc., is done. In selected patients, joint debridement has resulted in a stable hip with reasonable mobility of the hip. A total hip replacement has also been advocated in some cases of healed TB.

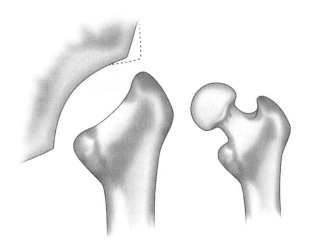

Fig. 23.16: Girdlestone arthroplasty (shaded portion excised).

Flowchart 23.1: Treatment plan for TB hip.

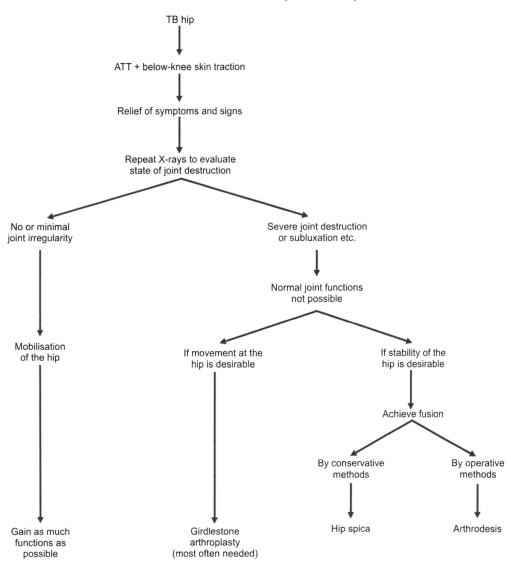

Flowchart 23.1 shows a general plan of treatment for TB of the hip.

TUBERCULOSIS OF THE KNEE

The knee is a common site of tuberculosis. Being a superficial joint, early diagnosis is usually possible. A delay in diagnosis can severely compromise joint functions.

PATHOLOGY

The basic pathology is same as that described on page 182. The disease may begin in the bone (osseous tuberculosis), usually in the femoral or tibial condyles, or more rarely in the patella. More commonly, the disease begins in the synovial membrane (synovial tuberculosis), leading to hypertrophy of the synovium. In early stages, the disease may be confined to the synovium without significant damage to the joint.

Natural history: In later stages, the articular cartilage and bone are destroyed irrespective of the site of origin. In all types, there occurs synovial hypertrophy, synovial effusion and pus formation in the joint. The hypertrophied synovium spreads under and over the cartilage and destroys it. The cartilage may become detached, leaving the bone exposed. Long-standing distension of the joint and destruction of the ligaments produces subluxation of the tibia. The tibia flexes, slips backwards and rotates externally on the femoral condyles (triple subluxation). Pus may burst out of the capsule to present as a cold abscess, and subsequently a sinus.

Healing: If untreated, nature's attempt at healing may result in fibrosis, and thereby stiffness of the joint in a deformed position. Healing is by fibrosis (fibrous ankylosis).

CLINICAL FEATURES

Presenting complaints: The patient, usually in the age group of 10-25 years, presents with complaints of pain and swelling in the knee. It is gradual in onset without any preceding history of trauma. Subsequently, pain increases and the knee takes an attitude of flexion. The patient starts limping. There is severe stiffness of the knee.

EXAMINATION

Following findings may be present on examination:

- **Swelling:** The joint is swollen, which may be due to synovial hypertrophy or effusion. The same can be detected by tests, as discussed on page 346.
- **Muscle atrophy:** Atrophy of the thigh muscles is more than what can be accounted for by disuse alone. This is an unexplained feature of joint tuberculosis.
- **Cold abscess:** There may be swelling due to a cold abscess, either around the knee or in the calf.
- **Sinus:** There may be discharging or healed sinuses.
- **Deformity:** In early stages, there is a mild flexion deformity of the knee because of effusion in the knee, and muscle spasm. Later, triple displacement (flexion, posterior subluxation and external rotation) occurs due to ligament laxity.
- **Movements:** The movements at the joint are limited. There is pain and muscle spasm on attempting movement.

INVESTIGATIONS

Radiological examination (Fig. 23.17): X-ray is essentially normal in a case of synovial tuberculosis, except for a soft tissue shadow corresponding to the distended knee. The joint space may be widened. There is diffuse osteoporosis of the bones around the joint. In osseous tuberculosis, one may see juxta-articular lytic lesions. The joint surfaces may be eroded. In later stages, joint space may be diminished or completely lost. In advanced stages, triple subluxation with cavitatory bone lesions may be present.

Other investigations along the lines already discussed on page 182 may be carried out. A biopsy is sometimes required.

DIFFERENTIAL DIAGNOSIS

Diagnosis is not difficult in a late case, but when the patient presents with synovitis, other causes of synovitis should be excluded before arriving at a diagnosis of TB of the knee. These include subacute pyogenic infection, monoarticular rheumatoid arthritis, chronic traumatic synovitis, rheumatic arthritis and haemophilic arthritis.

TREATMENT

Principles of treatment: Aim of treatment is to achieve, wherever possible, a painless mobile joint. This is possible if a patient has come early for treatment. In later stages, some amount of pain and stiffness persist in spite of treatment.

Conservative treatment: This consists of antitubercular chemotherapy, general care and local care of the part affected. It is started an all cases and decision for surgery taken if indicated, as discussed later.

Care of the knee: The knee is rested by applying below-knee skin traction or an above-knee PoP slab. This helps in the healing process, and also takes care of the associated muscle spasm which keeps the knee in a deformed position.

Operative treatment: Following operative procedures may be required in suitable cases:

- *Synovectomy:* It may be required in cases of purely synovial tuberculosis. Very often one finds 'melon seed' bodies within the joint.
- *Joint debridement:* This may be required in cases where the articular cartilage is essentially preserved. The pus is drained, the synovium excised, and all the cavities curetted.
- *Arthrodesis:* In advanced stages of the disease with triple subluxation and complete cartilage destruction, the knee is arthrodesed in functional

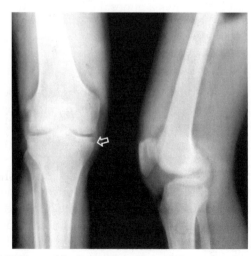

Fig. 23.17: X-ray of the knee, AP and lateral views, showing changes in tuberculosis of the knee. (Note, reduction in joint space and marginal erosions - arrow).

Flowchart 23.2: Treatment plan for TB knee.

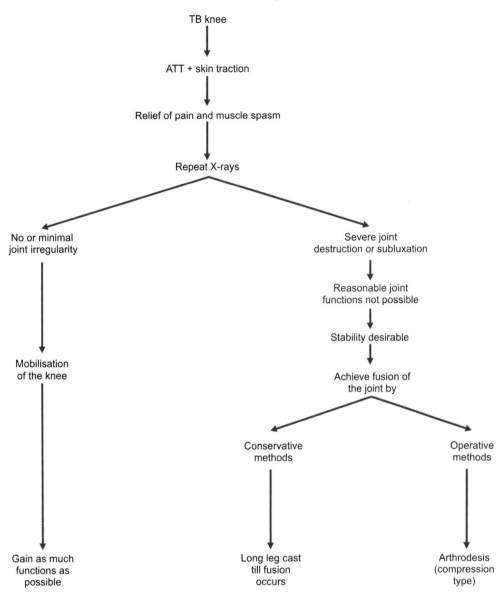

position, i.e., about 5-10° of flexion and neutral rotation. One popular method of knee arthrodesis is Charnley's compression arthrodesis.

With the current state of development of surgery, all these operations can be performed by minimally invasive arthroscopic surgery.

Plan of treatment: A plan of treatment for a case of TB of the knee is similar to that of the hip and is shown in Flowchart 23.2.

TUBERCULOSIS OF OTHER JOINTS

Other joints uncommonly affected by tuberculosis are the elbow, shoulder and ankle joints. Clinical features are similar to tuberculosis of other joints.

Diagnosis is generally possible by X-ray examination. Occasionally a biopsy may be required.

Shoulder joint tuberculosis, at times, may not produce any pus, etc., and hence is called 'caries sicca' and should always be considered in differential diagnosis of much more common shoulder problem – 'frozen shoulder'.

TB OSTEOMYELITIS

Tuberculosis of long bones: Tuberculosis rarely affect the shafts of long bones. It is usually a low grade subacute osteomyelitis of the shaft. Very often these are multifocal lesions. An important radiological feature is that the bone lysis is out of proportion to the new bone formation, unlike in pyogenic osteomyelitis. A biopsy may be necessary in some cases.

Tuberculosis of short bones: Tuberculosis of the small bones of the feet and hands is a rather common entity. These may occur as isolated lesions or as multiple ones. Diagnosis is easy with X-ray. Calcaneum is a common site (Fig. 23.18). Treatment is by rest and ATT. In cases where diagnosis is in doubt, curettage of the lesion and histopathological examination of the curetted material may be required.

Spina ventosa: This is a name given to tuberculosis of the phalanges of hand. The affected phalanx swells up like a balloon. An X-ray typically shows a lytic lesion distending the phalanx, and a lot of new bone formation.

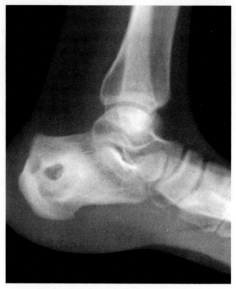

Fig. 23.18: X-ray of the calcaneum, lateral view showing tubercular cavity in the calcaneum.

 What have we learnt?

- Bone and joint tuberculosis constitute 1-4 per cent of total number of cases of tuberculosis.
- Systemic features of infection, such as fever, do not occur commonly in bone and joint tuberculosis.
- Spine is the most common site of bone and joint tuberculosis.
- Dorsolumbar spine is the most common region to get affected. Paradiscal being the most common type.
- Reduction of disc space is the earliest radiological sign of TB spine.
- It is the neurological complications associated with spine TB, which are of serious concern.
- TB hip is common cause of monoarthritis in children. Early diagnosis can save the joint from developing ankylosis.
- TB knee is of two types: Synovial and articular.
- Joints gets affected early, if there is a juxta-articular tubercular osteomyelitis.
- Treatment is focussed on (a) control of the disease, (b) functional recovery.
- Healing of tuberculous arthritis occurs by fibrous ankylosis.
- TB osteomyelitis is common in small bones.

Additional information: From the entrance exams point of view

- Tuberculosis most commonly affects the dorsolumbar region of the spine, mainly T12 L1 junction.
- The earliest feature of tuberculosis is pain.
- Tuberculosis of the spine affects the vertebral body first.
- Tuberculosis with polyarthritis is called Poncet's disease.
- Hong Kong operation is done in TB.
- Poor prognostic factors in Pott's paraplegia are acute onset, sudden progression and long-standing paraplegia.
- Most common sequelae of TB spondylitis is bony ankylosis.
- First sign of TB spine is loss of curvature of the spine followed by reduction in intervertebral space radiologically.
- Most common cause of early onset paraplegia is cold abscess.
- Triple deformity is seen in TB knee and is characterized by posterior subluxation of the knee, external or lateral rotation of the tibia and flexion of the knee. It is treated by anti-tubercular drugs with replacement or arthrodesis.

Infections of the Hand

Learning Objectives

- ❖ Describe the different types of infections in the hand and their anatomical relevance.

CLASSIFICATION

Infections of the hand can be classified into two broad categories; spreading infections and localised infections. *Spreading infections* are the ones which spread to involve a large area of the hand, e.g., lymphangitis, cellulitis, etc. *Localised infections* are those which are localised to an area of the hand because of certain anatomical factors. Infections of the hand are classified as given in Table 24.1.

ETIOPATHOLOGY

Hand infections are common in manual workers and housewives who frequently suffer small pricks or abrasions in the course of their work. *Staphylococcus aureus* is the causative organism in 80 per cent of cases; in others *Streptococcus* and other gram-negative bacteria are responsible. The organisms reach the tissue planes by direct implantation from outside or via the blood. They set up an acute inflammatory reaction, which in many cases progresses to suppuration. Without effective treatment, the infection may spread to adjacent tissue planes.

ACUTE PARONYCHIA

paronychia is an infection of the nail fold. It is the *most common* infection of the hand, and usually

Table 24.1: Hand infections.

Spreading type
- Cellulitis
- Lymphangitis

Localised type
- *On the dorsum of the hand*
  - Subcutaneous infection
  - Infection deep to the aponeurosis
- *On the palmar aspect of the hand*
  - Superficial aponeurotic infection
  - Deep aponeurotic infection
  - Thenar space infection
  - Mid-palmar space infection
- *Others*
  - Apical space of finger infection
  - Terminal pulp space infection
  - Middle volar space infection
  - Proximal volar space infection
  - Web space infection
  - Tenosynovitis
  - Space of Parona's infection

results from careless nail paring or use of unsterile manicure instruments.

Clinical features: There is pain, tenderness, redness and swelling at one or both sides of the nail fold, and at the base of the nail if suppuration has extended deep to the nail. There is a marked tenderness on pressing the nail.

Treatment: In its early stage, when no suppuration has occurred, conservative treatment may abort the infection. Once suppuration has occurred, the pus must be let out. For a mild infection, it is sufficient to raise the cuticle alone without incising, but better drainage is secured by vertical incision through the cuticle on one or both sides (Fig. 24.1). When the pus extends beneath the nail, it is necessary to remove the proximal one-third of the nail for adequate drainage.

Complications: These are: (i) extension of the infection to the pulp space and (ii) chronic paronychia.

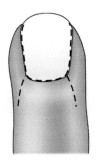

Fig. 24.1: Incision for draining acute paronychia.

APICAL SUBUNGUAL INFECTION

This is an infection of the tissues between the nail plate and the periosteum of the terminal phalanx. It results from a pin-prick or splinter beneath the nail. The lesion is excruciatingly painful with little swelling. Tenderness is maximum just beneath the free edge of the nail. The pus comes to the surface at the free edge of the nail.

Treatment: In the early stage, the infection can be aborted by conservative treatment, but once suppuration occurs, drainage is required. For drainage, a small V-shaped piece is removed from the centre of the free edge of the nail along with a little wedge of the full thickness of the skin overlying the abscess (Fig. 24.2).

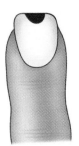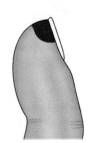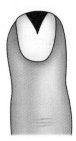

Infection   Drainage

Fig. 24.2: Apical subungual infection.

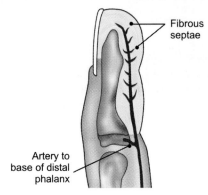

Fig. 24.3: Terminal pulp space.

Complications: Pus may spread under the nail, and may lead to a chronic sinus. Occasionally, the tip of the phalanx becomes infected.

TERMINAL PULP SPACE INFECTION (WHITLOW OR FELON)

Surgical anatomy: The terminal pulp space is the volar space of the distal digit. It is filled with compact fat, feebly partitioned by multiple fibrous septae (Fig. 24.3). At its proximal end, this space is closed by a septum of deep fascia connecting the distal flexor crease of the finger to the periosteum just distal to the insertion of the profundus flexor tendon. The digital artery, *before* it enters the space gives a branch to the epiphysis at the base of the distal phalanx. On entering the space it divides into terminal branches.

Clinical features: This is the second most common infection of the hand, commonly resulting from a pin-prick. The index finger and the thumb are affected most often. The pulp is swollen, tense and tender. A severe throbbing pain and excruciating tenderness suggest suppuration.

Treatment: In its early stage, conservative treatment may abort the infection. In the later stage, when suppuration has occurred, drainage is required. This is achieved either by incising directly over the centre of the abscess where it is pointing, or by a lateral incision just in front of the plane of the terminal phalanx.

Complications: These are: (i) osteomyelitis of the terminal phalanx, often with necrosis and sequestration of its distal half. Thromboarteritis of the terminal branches of the digital vessels accounts for this. The basal plate of the epiphysis is rarely involved; (ii) pyogenic arthritis of the distal interphalangeal joint; and (iii) very rarely, infection spreads to the flexor tendon sheath (suppurative tenosynovitis).

MIDDLE VOLAR SPACE INFECTION

Surgical anatomy: The middle volar space extends from the proximal to the distal volar creases of the finger. It is filled with loosely packed fibro-fatty tissue.

Clinical features: It commonly results from a pin-prick. Pain, swelling, and tenderness are maximally localised to this space. The finger is kept in semi-flexion. Frequently a purulent blister appears in the distal flexor crease. In early cases, it may be difficult to distinguish this infection from infection of the underlying flexor tendon sheath. However, in the former, tenderness over the *proximal end* of tendon sheath - at the base of the finger, is lacking.

Treatment: In the early stage, conservative treatment is enough. In late stage, drainage of pus via a longitudinal incision on the lateral side is performed.

Complications: Infection may spread to the distal or the proximal volar spaces, into the interphalangeal joints, or into the synovial sheath of the flexor tendons.

PROXIMAL VOLAR SPACE INFECTION

Surgical anatomy: This space is well partitioned from the middle volar space, but it communicates freely with the corresponding web space.

Clinical features: It is usually a consequence of a pin-prick. Pain, swelling and tenderness are localised to the space. Often the swelling is asymmetrical because of the concomitant involvement of the web space.

Treatment: The abscess is drained by an incision on the lateral side or at the point of maximum tenderness.

WEB SPACE INFECTION

Surgical anatomy: The web space is the triangular space between the bases of adjacent fingers; the first one being between the thumb and the index finger.

Clinical features: The infection arises: (i) from a skin crack; (ii) from a purulent blister on the forepart of the hand; or (iii) from a proximal volar space infection which communicates with the web space through the lumbrical canal (the canal that carries the lumbrical tendon from the hand into the finger). In the early stage, before localisation of infection occurs,

there is oedema over *back* of the hand. Although, the condition is strongly suspected by the location of the tenderness, a precise diagnosis is often difficult at this stage. Once localisation has occurred, signs of web space infection manifest themselves. The swelling at the base of the finger becomes obvious. In severe cases, the finger immediately adjacent to the space is 'separated' because of the mechanical effect of the abscess. Maximum tenderness is found in the web and on the volar surface of the base of the finger.

Treatment: In the early stage, conservative treatment may abort the infection. In late stage, drainage of the pus is required. The web space abscess is drained by a transverse incision on the palmar surface over the affected web space. Care needs to be taken to deepen the incision cautiously until the subcutaneous fat is reached. Only a few strands of palmar fascia need to be divided, and if pus does not flow, it is sought with a probe or a dissector. The edges of the wound are cut away so as to leave a diamond-shaped opening. When the abscess communicates with a dorsal pocket, a counter-incision is advisable on the dorsum of the hand.

Complications: Spread of the infection to the nearby spaces and tendon sheaths is a common complication.

DEEP PALMAR ABSCESS

An abscess beneath the palmar fascia is a serious but rare infection of the hand. It may be an infection in the thenar* or mid-palmar space.

Surgical anatomy: The deep palmar spaces of the hand lie in the hollow of the palm, deep to the flexor tendons and their synovial sheaths. The space is divided into two halves - a medial half (the mid-palmar space), and a lateral half (the thenar space). The posterior relation of the space is formed by the fascia covering the interossei and metacarpal bones on the medial side, and the adductor pollicis muscle on the lateral side. On the two sides of the space are the thenar and hypothenar muscles (Fig. 24.4, next on page).

Clinical features: The infection can arise from a penetrating wound, via the bloodstream, or as a complication of suppurative tenosynovitis. At an early stage, there is an intense throbbing pain, and deep tenderness in the palm. There is only little swelling on the volar aspect of the palm; rather it is severe on the dorsum of the hand, sometimes so great as to give

---

* Thenar space is not same as the space containing thenar muscles (See Fig. 26.4)

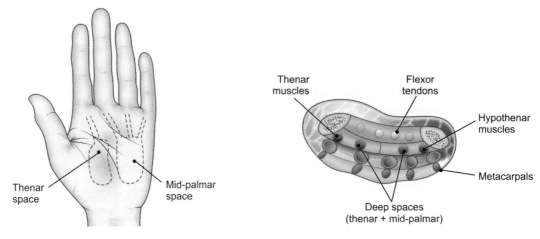

Fig. 24.4: Deep palmar spaces.

rise to what is called 'frog hand'. The fingers are kept flexed. Extension at the metacarpophalangeal joints is very painful, but painless at the interphalangeal joints. This distinguishes this condition from suppurative tenosynovitis where there is pain on extending the metacarpophalangeal as well as interphalangeal joints. Regional lymphadenopathy is commonly present.

As tension within the space mounts, the normal concavity of the palm becomes flattened. Subsequently, the pus erodes through the palmar fascia and the intense pain eases off. The palm now becomes slightly convex, and it may be possible to elicit fluctuation only at this stage of the infection.

Treatment: It is often difficult to diagnose deep palmar space infection in its early stages because of its deep location. In some cases, treatment by conservative methods may abort the infection, but more often suppuration follows. The pus, being in a deeper plane, is difficult to detect because of the lack of fluctuation. A strong suspicion and a throbbing pain are indications of deep seated pus requiring drainage. A needle aspiration may be helpful in confirming the presence of pus.

A central transverse incision is made in the line of the flexor crease, passing across the middle of the palm at the site of maximum tenderness. If pus is encountered beneath the aponeurosis, the floor of the abscess must be probed systematically for a sinus leading to a deeper plane. In order to ensure free drainage of the pus, the skin edges as well as those of the palmar fascia are trimmed.

Complications: Spread of infection to nearby spaces and tendon sheaths may occur. A chronic infection may result in a discharging sinus and stiffness of the hand.

ACUTE SUPPURATIVE TENOSYNOVITIS

This is a rare but important infection because prompt treatment is essential if the function of the finger is to be preserved.

Surgical anatomy: The flexor tendons of the hand are covered with fibrous and synovial flexor sheaths (Fig. 24.5). The fibrous sheaths exist only up to the bases of the digits. A synovial sheath lines the fibrous sheaths. In the thumb and little finger, the synovial lining extends proximally through the palm and ends 2–3 cm above the wrist. The synovial sheaths of the index, middle and ring fingers end proximally at the level of the transverse palmar skin crease. The proximal part of the sheath of the flexor tendon of the thumb is known as the *radial bursa*. The sheath of the little finger tendons open proximally into the *ulnar bursa*, which encloses the grouped tendons of the flexor digitorum superficialis and flexor digitorum profundus.

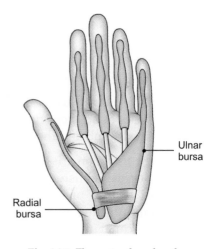

Fig. 24.5: Flexor tendon sheaths.

It should be noted that there is normal but great anatomical variation in the arrangement of the synovial tendon sheaths. The ulnar and radial bursae may communicate. The tendon sheaths of the index, middle and ring fingers may communicate with the ulnar bursa.

Clinical features: The bacteria enter the tendon sheath with the point of a needle or other sharp objects penetrating the tendon sheath. *Exceptionally,* the sheath is infected by extension from the terminal pulp space infection.

The finger is swollen throughout its length, and is acutely tender over the flexor tendon sheath.

It is held semi-flexed, and active or passive extension at the interphalangeal joint is very painful. In tenosynovitis of the little finger, the ulnar bursa also becomes involved, giving rise to swelling of the palm and sometimes fullness immediately above the flexor retinaculum. The area of maximum tenderness in an ulnar bursa infection can be elicited over that part of the bursa lying between the transverse palmar creases. This is *Kanavel's sign* (Fig. 24.6). In infections of the radial bursa, there is more swelling over the thenar eminence and thumb. The other findings are similar to other tendon sheath infections.

Treatment: An aggressive conservative treatment is started at an early stage. Clinical re-examinations

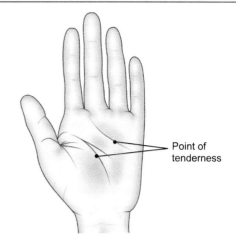

Point of tenderness

Fig. 24.6: Kanavel's sign.

are carried out every 6 hours to assess improvement. Conservative treatment is continued only so long as there is good local and general response. Any delay in decompression leads to a spread of the infection proximally into the forearm.

Complications: These are: (i) permanent stiffness of the finger in semi-flexion because of necrosis of the tendons and adhesions between the tendon and the sheath; and (ii) spread of the infection to nearby structures such as the ulnar and radial bursae.

What have we learnt?

- ▪ Hand infections are of two types: Superficial and deep.
- ▪ Early surgical intervention is preferred.
- ▪ Stiffness is a common complication.

Additional information: From the entrance exams point of view

- ▪ Felon most commonly affects the thumb.
- ▪ Kanavel's sign is seen in tenosynovitis, it consists of eliciting tenderness on percussion over the flexor tendon sheath of the finger, flexion posture of fingers with pain on hyprextension and uniform swelling involving the entire finger.

Congenital Talipes Equino Varus (CTEV)

Competency

- ❖ **OR12.1:** Describe and discuss the clinical features, investigations and principles of management of congenital and acquired malformations and deformities of:
  - a. Limbs and spine - scoliosis and spinal bifida
  - b. Congenital dislocation of hip, torticollis
  - c. Congenital talipes equino varus.

'Clubfoot' is a rather vague term which has been used to describe a number of different abnormalities in the shape of the foot, but over the years it has come to be synonymous with the most common congenital foot deformity, i.e., Congenital Talipes Equino Varus (CTEV). It occurs once in every 1000 live births.

RELEVANT ANATOMY

The joints of the foot relevant to understanding of this chapter are: (i) the ankle joint between the tibia and the talus; (ii) the subtalar joint between the talus and the calcaneum; (iii) the talonavicular joint; and (iv) the calcaneocuboid joint (Fig. 25.1).

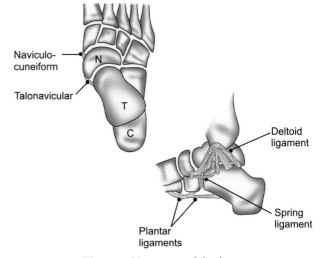

Fig. 25.2: Ligaments of the foot.

For the purpose of description, the foot is often divided into hindfoot, midfoot and forefoot. The *hindfoot* is the part comprising of talocalcaneal (subtalar) joint. *Midfoot* comprises of talonavicular, calcaneocubooid and naviculo-cuneiform joints. The *forefoot* is cuneiform-metatarsal and other joints beyond it.

The ligaments related to the etiology of clubfoot are as follows (Fig. 25.2):

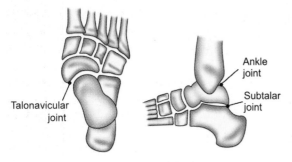

Fig. 25.1: Joints of the foot.

- *Deltoid ligament:* This is the medial collateral ligament of the ankle. It has a superficial and a deep component.
- *Spring ligament:* This is a ligament which joins the anterior end of the calcaneum to the navicular.
- *Interosseous ligament:* This ligament is between the talus and calcaneum, joining their apposing surfaces.
- *Capsular ligaments:* The thickened portions of the capsule of the talonavicular, naviculo-cuneiform, and cuneiform-metatarsal joints, termed as the capsular ligaments, are important structures in pathology of CTEV.
- *Plantar ligaments:* These are ligaments extending from the plantar surface of the calcaneum to the foot, giving rise to the longitudinal arch of the foot.

Tendons related to the pathology of clubfoot are those on the medial side of the foot (Fig. 25.3). The tendon immediately behind the medial malleolus is that of the tibialis posterior. More posteriorly are the flexor digitorum longus tendon, posterior tibial artery and nerve, and flexor hallucis longus tendon. The tibialis posterior tendon has its main insertion on the navicular. This is the *most important* muscle related to pathology of clubfoot.

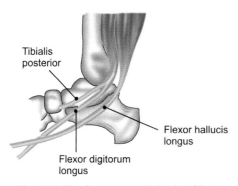

Fig. 25.3: *Tendons on medial side of foot.*

NOMENCLATURE

Before discussing this topic further, it is wise to understand the meaning of the various terms used to describe foot deformities (Fig. 25.4). The following are some such terms:

- **Equinus** (derived from 'equine', i.e., a horse who walks on toes): This is a deformity where the foot is fixed in plantar-flexion.
- **Calcaneus** (reverse of equinus)**:** This is a deformity where the foot is fixed in dorsiflexion.
- **Varus:** The foot is inverted and adducted at the mid-tarsal joints so that the sole 'faces' inwards.

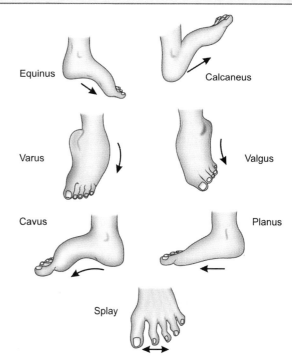

Fig. 25.4: Types of foot deformities.

- **Valgus:** The foot is everted and abducted at the mid-tarsal joints so that the sole 'faces' outwards.
- **Cavus:** The longitudinal arch of the foot is exaggerated.
- **Planus:** The longitudinal arch is flattened.
- **Splay:** The transverse arch is flattened.

Invariably, the foot has a combination of above mentioned deformities; the most common being equino-varus. The next most common congenital foot deformity is calcaneo-valgus.

ETIOLOGY

In the vast majority of cases, etiology is not known, hence it is termed idiopathic. In others, the so called secondary clubfoot, some underlying cause such as arthrogryposis multiplex congenita (AMC) can be found.

Idiopathic clubfoot: Following are some of the theories proposed for the etiology of idiopathic clubfoot:

a. **Mechanical theory:** The raised intrauterine pressure forces the foot against the wall of the uterus in the position of the deformity.

b. **Ischaemic theory:** Ischaemia of the calf muscles during intrauterine life, due to some unknown factor, results in contractures, leading to foot deformities.

c. **Genetic theory:** Some genetically related disturbances in the development of the foot have been held responsible for the deformity.

Secondary clubfoot: Following are some of the causes of secondary clubfoot:

a. **Neurogenic disorders:** In a case where there is a muscle imbalance, i.e., the invertors and plantar flexors are stronger than the evertors and dorsiflexors, an equino-varus deformity develops. This occurs in paralytic disorders such as cerebral palsy, polio, spina bifida, myelodysplasia and Freidreich's ataxia.

b. **Arthrogryposis multiplex congenita (AMC):** This is a disorder of defective development of the muscles. The muscles are fibrotic and result in foot deformities, and deformities at other joints.

PATHOANATOMY

All the tissues of the foot, i.e., the bones, joints, ligaments and muscles have developmental abnormality.

Bones: Bones of the foot are smaller than normal. Neck of the talus is angulated so that the head of the talus faces downwards and medially. Calcaneum is small, and concave medially.

Joints: Deformities occur from the malpositioning of different joints:

- **Equinus** deformity occurs primarily at the ankle joint. Other tarsal joints also contribute to it.
- **Inversion** deformity occurs primarily at the subtalar joint. The inverted calcaneum takes the whole foot with it so that the sole faces medially.
- **Forefoot adduction** deformity occurs at the mid-tarsal joints, mainly at talonavicular joint.
- **Forefoot cavus** deformity is the result of excessive arching of the foot at the mid-tarsal joints.

Muscles and tendons: Muscles of the calf are under-developed. As a result, the following muscles–tendon units are contracted:

- **Posteriorly -** Tendoachilles
- **Medially -** Tibialis posterior
  (3 muscles) - Flexor digitorum longus
                - Flexor hallucis longus

Capsule and ligaments: All the ligamentous structures on the postero-medial side of the foot are shortened. Following are some of these structures:

- **Posterior**   Posterior capsule of the ankle joint
  (3 structures) Posterior capsule of the subtalar joint
                      Posterior talofibular and calcaneo-fibular ligaments
- **Medial**   Talonavicular ligament
  (3 ligaments)   Spring ligament
                      Deltoid ligament

- **Plantar**   Plantar fascia
                      Plantar ligaments
- **Others**   Interosseous ligament between the talus and calcaneum

Skin: The skin develops adaptive shortening on the medial side of the sole. There are deep creases on the medial and posterior side. There are dimples on the lateral aspect of the ankle and midfoot.

Secondary changes: These changes occur in the foot if the child starts walking on the deformed feet. Weight, bearing exaggerates the deformity. Callosities and bursae develop over the bony prominences on the lateral side of the foot.

CLINICAL FEATURES

Presenting complaints: Though, the history dates back to birth, a child with CTEV may present some time after birth, often as late as adulthood. Following are some of the common presentations:

a. **Detected at birth:** At places where delivery is conducted by trained medical personnel, CTEV is detected at the time of routine screening of newborns for congenital mal-formations. At times, the deformity is very mild, the so-called postural equino-varus.

b. **Brought during early infancy:** At places where delivery is conducted at primary health centres, the child is generally brought to the hospital around the age of 3-6 weeks.

c. **Brought during late infancy and early childhood:** In these cases, the child has received treatment elsewhere, or the deformity has recurred, or it has never been corrected. Unfortunately, in developing countries, a large number of cases report to the hospital late.

d. **Brought during late childhood:** It is not uncommon in developing countries to have a grown up child, or sometimes an adult with clubfoot, reporting to the hospital for the first time. Ignorance, poverty and illiteracy are generally the reasons for such late presentations.

EXAMINATION

In addition to foot examination, a general examination should be carried out to detect associated malformations in other parts of the body.

Foot examination: Normally, the foot of a newborn child can be dorsiflexed until the dorsum touches the anterior aspect of the shin of the tibia (Fig. 25.5). This is a good screening test for detecting the milder variety of clubfoot. The more classic one will have the following findings:

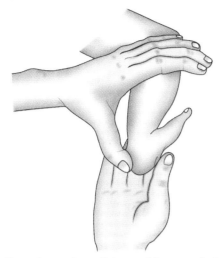

Fig. 25.5: Foot of a newborn. It is possible to touch the dorsum of the foot to the shin.

- *Bilateral* foot deformity in 60 per cent cases.
- *Size of the foot* smaller (in unilateral cases).
- Foot is in *equinus, varus and adduction*. This can be judged by the inability to bring the foot in the opposite direction. In late cases, in addition, cavus of the foot may also be present.
- *Heel is small* in size; the calcaneum may be felt with great difficulty.
- *Deep skin creases* on the back of the heel and on the medial side of the sole.
- *Bony prominences* felt on the lateral side of the foot, the head of the talus and lateral malleolus.
- *Outer side of the foot* is gently convex. There are dimples on the outer aspect of the ankle.

On attempted correction, one can feel the tight structures posteriorly (tendoachilles) and plantar warts (plantar fascia).

A child presenting late may have callosities over the lateral aspect of the foot. The calf muscles are wasted.

Terminology to describe clubfoot in different presentations is as shown in Table 25.1.

General examination: It is aimed at finding an underlying cause of the deformity as discussed on pages 207–208. A patient of residual polio may

TABLE 25.1: Terminology to describe clubfoot.

Type	Description
Supple	Foot can be brought to normal position
Rigid	Foot deformities not correctable
Resistant	Foot deformities not responding to manipulation and POP casting
Neglected	Not treated for 1 year
Relapsed	Got corrected but recurred

Table 25.2: Differences between primary and secondary clubfeet.

Differentiating features	Primary clubfoot	Secondary clubfoot
Present since birth	Yes	Sometimes
Side affected	Bilateral common (60%)	Unilateral common
Foot size	Much smaller	Normal or small
Heel size	Small with fat++	Normal with fat
Skin	Chubby, creases present	Atrophic, creases absent
Neurological examination	Essentially normal	Motor and sensory loss present
Prognosis	Good	Poor

present with equino-varus deformity, which may mimic clubfoot, but there will be paralysis of some other part of the limb. Presence of sensory deficit points to an underlying neurological cause. The presence of deformities at other joints indicate possible arthrogryposis multiplex congenita (AMC).

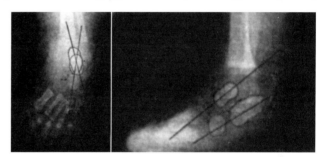

Fig. 25.6: X-rays showing reduced talocalcaneal angles in clubfoot (normal 35°).

DIAGNOSIS

This is easy in cases presenting soon after birth. In those presenting late, secondary causes of talipes equino-varus deformity must be excluded (Table 25.2). *X-rays* of the foot are done (antero-posterior and lateral) with the foot in whatever corrected position possible. The talocalcaneal angles*, in both, AP and lateral views, in a normal foot are more than 35o, but in CTEV these are reduced (Fig. 25.6). X-rays are used by some as a method of baseline documentation of the deformities and a method for assessment of correction after treatment.

TREATMENT

Principles of treatment: In principle, treatment consists of *correction* of the deformity, and its maintenance. Correction can be achieved by non-operative or

---

* This is an angle between long axis of talus and calcaneum – also called as Kite's angle.

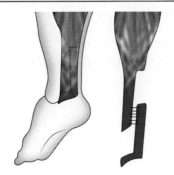

Fig. 25.7: Z-plasty of tendoachilles.

operative methods. Maintenance is continued until the foot (and its bones) grows to a reasonable size, so that the deformity does not recur.

METHODS OF CORRECTION OF DEFORMITY

A deformity can be corrected by non-operative or operative methods.

Non-operative methods: Following are the non-operative methods of correcting deformities:

a. *Manipulation alone:* In a newborn, the mother is taught to manipulate the foot after every feed. The foot is dorsiflexed and everted. While manipulating, sufficient pressure should be applied by the person so as to blanch her own fingers. This pressure should be maintained for about 5 seconds, and this is repeated several times, over a period of roughly 5 minutes. Minor deformities are usually corrected by this method alone. For major deformities, further treatment by corrective plaster casts is required.

b. *Manipulation and PoP:* In this method, the surgeon manipulates the foot after sedating the child. The foot is then held in the corrected position with plaster casts. Presently Ponsetti philosophy as discussed below, in popular. Earlier it was Kite's philosophy.

Ponsetti's philosophy: This philosophy is based on better understanding of the pathoanatomy of the deformed foot. According to Ponsetti, the calcaneo-cuboid-navicular complex is internally rotated (adducted) under the plantarflexed talus. Hence, the deformity can be corrected by bringing the complex back under the talus by gradually stretching the tight structures. This is done by putting thumb pressure *over the talus head* (and not over calcaneo-cuboid joint as in Kite's method). By doing this, the calcaneo-cuboid-navicular complex is externally rotated under the talar head.

Treatment is started within *1st week* of life. The cavus aspect of the deformity is corrected first, followed by the adduction, then varus and lastly equinus.

After every manipulation, an above-knee PoP cast is applied, which is changed every 5-7 days. It is usually possible to correct all components of the deformity within 6 weeks. The equinus deformity component often remains undercorrected, and is treated by percutaneous tenotomy of tendoachilles.

Operative methods: With the remarkable success with Ponseti method of casting, there is little role of surgical treatment even in late cases and in relapsed cases. Serial casting should be considered, as a first step, even in severe cases. Though surgery may still be required, the extent of surgery becomes much less.

In more severe deformities, which are not corrected by conservative methods, or in those that recur, operative treatment is required. Soft tissue release operations may be sufficient in younger children (younger than 3 years), but bony operations are required in older children. The following operations are performed:

a. *Postero-medial soft tissue release (PMSTR):* This operation consists of releasing the tight soft tissue structures (tendons, ligaments, capsule, etc.) on the posterior and medial side of the foot. This can be performed in younger children. In older children, an additional bony procedure is required. The following structures are generally released:

On the Posterior Side
- Lengthening of the tendoachilles by Z-plasty (Fig. 25.7).
- Release of posterior capsules of the ankle and subtalar joints.
- Release of posterior talofibular and calcaneofibular ligaments.

On the Medial Side
- Lengthening of 3 tendons*, i.e., tibialis posterior, flexor digitorum longus and flexor hallucis longus. In addition, their contracted thickened sheaths are excised.
- Release of 3 ligaments, i.e., talonavicular ligament, superficial part of the deltoid ligament and the spring ligament.
- Release of 3 more structures is needed in severe cases. These are the interosseous talocalcaneal ligament, capsules of the naviculo-cuneiform and cuneiform-first metatarsal joints.

On the Plantar Side
- Plantar fascia release.
- Release of the short flexors of the toes (flexor digitorum brevis) and abductor hallucis from their origin on the calcaneum.

---
* For ease of remembering, a 'rule of 3' makes it simple – 3 tendons, 3 ligaments and 3 more structures are released.

b. *Limited soft tissue release:* In some cases, the foot remains partially corrected after conservative treatment, and only limited soft tissue release may be sufficient as shown below:

- For equinus alone — a posterior release
- For adduction alone — a medial release
- For cavus alone — a plantar release

c. *Tendon transfers:* In some cases, the tibialis anterior and tibialis posterior (both invertors of the foot) may exert a deforming force against the weak peronei (evertors) producing a dynamic supination deformity. This muscle imbalance may be corrected by transfering the tibialis anterior to the outer side of the foot, where it acts as an everter. Minimum age for tendon transfers is 3 years.

d. *Dwyer's osteotomy:* This is an open-wedge osteotomy of the calcaneum, performed in order to correct varus of the heel (Fig. 25.8). Minimum age at which this operation can be performed is 3 years, as prior to this the calcaneum is mainly cartilaginous. Some prefer a closed-wedge osteotomy on the lateral side.

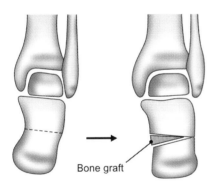

Fig. 25.8: Dwyer's osteotomy (open wedge).

e. *Dilwyn Evan's procedure:* This consists of a thorough soft tissue release postero-medial soft tissue release (PMSTR) with calcaneocuboid wedge resection and fusion (Fig. 25.9). It is used for a neglected or relapsed clubfoot, in children between 4–8 years. With wedge resection, the

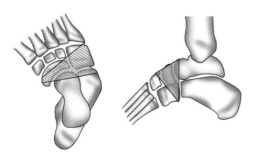

Fig. 25.9: Dilwyn Evan's operation.

lateral column is shortened, and with fusion of the calcaneocuboid joint the lateral side of the foot does not grow as much as the medial side. This results in gradual correction of the deformity.

f. *Wedge tarsectomy:* This consists of removing a wedge of bones from the mid-tarsal area (Fig. 25.10). The wedge is cut with its base on the dorsolateral side. Once the wedge is removed the foot can be brought to normal (plantigrade) position. This operation is performed for neglected clubfeet between the age of 8-11 years.

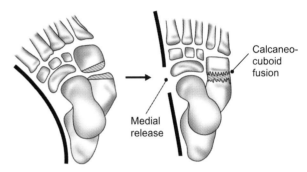

Fig. 25.10: Wedge tarsectomy (dorsolateral wedge).

g. *Triple arthrodesis:* This consists of the fusion of three joints of the foot (subtalar, calcaneocuboid and talonavicular), after taking suitable wedges to correct the deformity (Fig. 25.11). It is performed after the age of 12 years, because before this the bones are cartilaginous and it is difficult to achieve fusion. Of the three, talo-navicular joint fusion is most difficult to achieve.

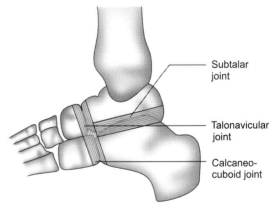

Fig. 25.11: Triple arthrodesis.

g. *Ilizarov's technique:* Using the principles of Ilizarov's technique, different components of the deformity are corrected by gradual stretching, using an external fixator. Once correction is achieved, it is maintained by plaster casts. Ilizarov's technique

Flowchart 25.1: Treatment plan for CTEV.

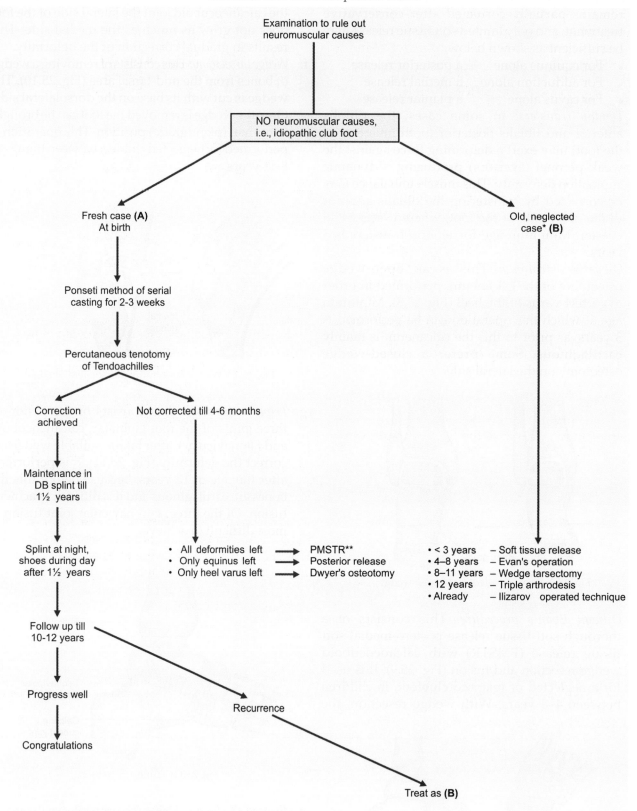

** PMSTR – Postero-medial soft tissue release

is indicated in neglected clubfeet, and in those in which it has recurred after previous operation. A simpler technique based on above principles has been popularized by Dr BB Joshi from Mumbai (JESS fixation).

METHODS OF MAINTENANCE OF THE CORRECTION

Correction once achieved, is maintained by the following methods:

a. **CTEV splints:** These are splints made of plastic, moulded in such a way that when tied with straps, it keeps the foot in corrected position.

b. **Denis-Brown splint (DB splint)/foot abduction orthosis:** This is a splint to hold the foot in the corrected position (Fig. 25.12). It is used throughout the day before the child starts walking. Once he starts walking, a DB splint is used at night and CTEV shoes during the day.

c. **CTEV shoes:** These are modified shoes, used once a child starts walking. The following modifications are made in the shoe (Fig. 25.13):
   ▪ Straight inner border to prevent forefoot adduction.
   ▪ Outer shoe raise to prevent foot inversion.
   ▪ No heel to prevent equinus.

These shoes are used until the child is 5 years old.

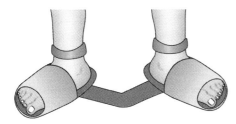

Fig. 25.12: Denis-Brown splint.

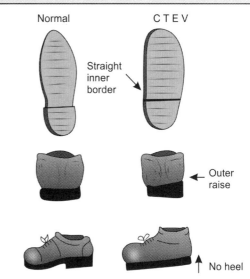

Fig. 25.13: CTEV shoes.

PLAN OF TREATMENT

Most cases which are treated early, respond well to non-operative methods. Operative methods may be indicated in the following cases:

a. A child who does not respond to non-operative treatment *(resistant clubfeet)*: These feet are generally severely deformed, 'chubby' (atypical clubfoot) or associated with underlying arthrogryposis multiplex congenita (AMC).

b. A child whose deformities have recurred *(recurrent clubfeet)*: This usually happens if correction is not maintained. The *first* deformity to recur is the equinus.

c. A child who has presented late or has not been adequately treated *(neglected clubfeet)*.

Once corrected a clubfoot has to be maintained in the corrected position by the methods described earlier. A comprehensive plan of treatment for CTEV is shown in Flowchart 25.1.

 What have we learnt?

- Idiopathic clubfoot is to be differentiated from secondary clubfoot, as the prognosis of the two is different.
- Treatment consists of manipulation and PoP, followed by maintenance in splints. Conservative treatment is successful in most cases.
- Different surgical procedures are indicated at different stages.

Congenital Dislocation of the Hip and Other Malformations

Competency

❖ **OR12.1:** Describe and discuss the clinical features, investigations and principles of management of congenital and acquired malformations and deformities of:
a. Limbs and spine - scoliosis and spinal bifida
b. Congenital dislocation of hip, torticollis
c. Congenital talipes equino varus.

CONGENITAL DISLOCATION OF THE HIP (CDH)

This is a spontaneous dislocation of the hip occurring before, during or shortly after birth. In western countries, it is one of the most common congenital disorder. It is *uncommon in India* and some other Asian countries, probably because of the culture of mother carrying the child on the side of her waist with the hips of the child abducted (Fig. 26.1). This position helps in reduction of an unstable hip, which otherwise would have dislocated. The general term "dysplastic hip" is sometimes used for these congenital malformations of the hip.

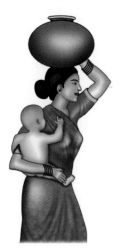

Fig. 26.1: Mother carrying a child by her side.

ETIOLOGY

Etiology is not well-understood, but the following factors appear to be important:

a. **Hereditary predisposition to joint laxity:** Heredity related lax joints are predisposed to hip dislocation in some positions.

b. **Hormone induced joint laxity:** CDH is 3-5 times more common in females. This may be due to the fact that the maternal relaxin (a ligament relaxing hormone in the mother during pregnancy) crosses the placental barrier to enter the foetus. If the hormonal environment of the foetus is a female, relaxin acts on the foetus's joints in the same way as it does on those of the mother. This produces joint laxity, and thus dislocation.

c. **Breech malposition:** The incidence of an unstable hip is about 10 times more in newborns with breech presentation than those with vertex presentation. It is possible that in breech presentation the foetal legs are pressed inside the uterus in such a way that if the hip ligaments are lax, dislocation may occur.

PATHOLOGY

Present evidence suggests that there are two distinct types of dysplastic hips: (i) those *dislocated* at birth (classic CDH); and (ii) those *dislocatable* after birth. The first are primarily due to a hereditary faulty development of the acetabulum, and are difficult to treat. The second

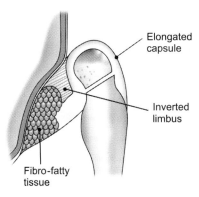

Fig. 26.2: Pathology of CDH.

are due to underlying joint laxity, with a precipitating factor causing the dislocation. Following changes are seen in a dislocated joint (Fig. 26.2):

- Femoral *head is dislocated upwards* and laterally; its epiphysis is small and ossifies late.
- Femoral neck is excessively *anteverted.*
- *Acetabulum is shallow,* with a steep sloping roof.
- Ligamentum teres is hypertrophied.
- Fibrocartilaginous labrum of the acetabulum (limbus) may be folded into the cavity of the acetabulum *(inverted limbus).*
- Capsule of the hip joint is stretched.
- *Muscles* around the hip, especially the adductors, undergo adaptive shortening.

DIAGNOSIS

Diagnosis is easy in an older child; but may be very difficult in younger children, especially during infancy. This is because of subtle clinical findings and difficulties in interpreting X-rays of these children.

CLINICAL FEATURES

CDH is more common in first born babies, more on the left, more common in females (M:F=1:5), bilateral in 20% cases. CDH may be detected at birth or soon after; sometimes not noticed until the child starts walking. Following are the salient clinical features at different ages:

- **At birth:** Routine screening of all newborns is necessary. The examining paediatrician may notice signs suggestive of a dislocated or a dislocatable hip, as discussed subsequently.
- **Early childhood:** Sometimes, the child is brought because the parents have noticed an asymmetry of creases of the groin, limitation of movements of the affected hip, or a click everytime the hip is moved.
- **Older child:** CDH may become apparent once the child starts walking. Parents notice that the child walks with a 'peculiar gait' though there is

no pain. On examination a CDH may be found to be the underlying cause.

EXAMINATION

A meticulous examination is the key to the early diagnosis of CDH. There may be limitation of hip abduction, asymmetry of groin creases or an audible click. Physical findings in a younger child may be little, and diagnosis may only be possible by special tests designed to elicit instability. These are as follows:

Barlow's test: The test has two parts. In the first part, the surgeon faces the child's perineum. He grasps the upper part of each thigh, with his fingers behind on the greater trochanter and thumb in front. The child's knees are fully flexed and the hips flexed to a right angle (Fig. 26.3). The hip is now gently *adducted.* As this is being done, gentle pressure is exerted by the examining hand in a proximal direction while the thumb tries to 'push out' the hip. As the femoral head rolls over the posterior lip of the acetabulum, it may, if dislocatable (but not, if dislocated) slip out of the acetabulum. One feels an abnormal posterior movement, appreciated by the fingers behind the greater trochanter. There may be a distinct 'clunk'. If nothing happens, the hip may be normal or may already be dislocated; in the latter, second part of the test would be more relevant.

In the second part of the test, with the hips in 90° flexion and fully adducted, held as described above, thighs are gently abducted. The examiner's hand tries to pull the hips while the fingers on the greater trochanter exert pressure in a forward direction, as if one is trying to put back a dislocated hip. If the hip is dislocated, either because of the first part of the test or if it was dislocated to start with, a 'clunk' will be

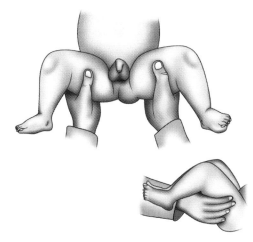

Fig. 26.3: Barlow's test.

heard and felt, indicating reduction of the dislocated hip. If nothing happens, the hip may be normal or it is an irreducible dislocation. In the latter case, there will be limitation of hip abduction. In a normal hip, it is possible to abduct the hips till the knee touches the couch.

Ortolani's test: This test is similar to the second part of Barlow's test. The hips and knees are held in a flexed position and gradually abducted. A 'click of entrance' will be felt as the femoral head slips into the acetabulum from the position of dislocation.

In an older child, the following findings may be present:
- Limitation of abduction of the hip.
- Asymmetrical thigh folds (Fig. 26.4).

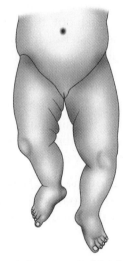

Fig. 26.4: Asymmetrical thigh folds.

- Higher buttock fold on the affected side.
- *Galeazzi's sign:* The level of the knees are compared in a child lying with hip flexed to 70° and knees flexed. There is a lowering of the knee on the affected side (Fig. 26.5).

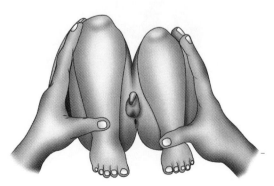

Fig. 26.5: Galeazzi sign.

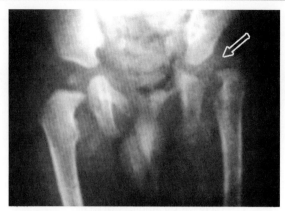

Fig. 26.6: X-ray of the pelvis of an infant with CDH on the left. (Note that the epiphysis on the affected side has not appeared yet).

- *Ortolani's test* may be positive.
- *Trendelenburg's test is positive:* This test is performed in an older child. The child is asked to stand on the affected side. The opposite ASIS (that of the normal side) dips down (details in Annexure I).
- The limb is short and slightly externally rotated. There is lordosis of the lumbar spine.
- *Telescopy positive:* In a case of a dislocated hip, it will be possible to produce an up and down piston-like movement at the hip. This can be appreciated by feeling the movement of the greater trochanter under the fingers (details in Annexure I).
- A child with unilateral dislocation exhibits a typical gait in which the body lurches to the affected side as the child bears weight on it *(Trendelenburg's gait)*. In a child with bilateral dislocation, there is alternate lurching on both sides *(waddling gait)*.
- Some hip pathologies mimicking CDH are: Coxa vara, posterior hip dislocation and paralytic hip dislocation and paralytic hip dislocation.

RADIOLOGICAL FEATURES

In a child below the age of 1 year, since the epiphysis of the femoral head is not ossified, it is difficult to diagnose a dislocated hip on plain X-rays (Fig. 26.6). Von Rosen's view may help.

Ultrasound examination is useful in early diagnosis at birth.

In an older child, the following are the important X-ray findings:
- Delayed appearance* of the ossification centre of the head of the femur.

---

* Normally, epiphysis of the head of the femur appears at 1 year of age.

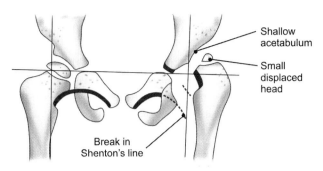

Fig. 26.7: Diagrammatic representation of the X-ray, showing break in Shenton's line.

- Retarded development of the ossification centre of the head of the femur.
- Sloping acetabulum.
- Lateral and upward displacement of the ossification centre of the femoral head.
- A break in Shenton's line (Fig. 26.7).

TREATMENT

Principles of treatment: Aim is to achieve reduction of the head into the acetabulum, and maintain it until the hip becomes clinically stable and a 'round' acetabulum covers the head. In most cases, it is possible to reduce the hip by closed means; in some an open reduction is required. Once the head is inside the acetabulum, in younger children, under the mould-like effect of the head, it develops into a round acetabulum. If reduction has been delayed for more than 2 years, acetabular remodelling may not occur even after the head is reduced for a long time. Hence, in such cases, surgical reconstruction of the acetabulum may be required.

Methods of reduction: Following methods of reduction may be used:
a. *Closed manipulation:* It is sometimes possible in younger children to reduce the hip by gentle closed manipulation under general anaesthesia.
b. In unilateral cases, reduction can be attempted till 10 years of age and till 8 years in bilateral cases
c. *Traction followed by closed manipulation:* In cases where the manipulative reduction requires a great deal of force or if it fails, the hip is kept in traction for some time, and is progressively abducted. As this is done, it may be possible to reduce the femoral head easily under general anaesthesia. An adductor tenotomy is often necessary in some cases to allow the hip to be fully abducted.
d. *Open reduction:* This is indicated if closed reduction fails. Reasons of failure of closed reduction could be the presence of fibro-fatty tissue in the acetabulum or a fold of capsule and acetabular

labrum (inverted limbus) between the femoral head and the superior part of the acetabulum. In such situations, the hip is exposed, the soft tissues obstructing the head excised or released, and the head repositioned in the acetabulum.

Maintenance of reduction: Once the hip has been reduced by closed or open methods, following methods may be used for maintaining the head inside the acetabulum.
a. *Plaster cast:* A frog leg or Bachelor's cast (Fig. 26.8).

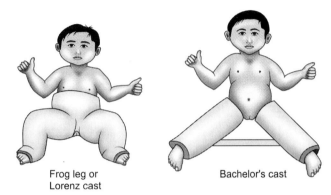

Fig. 26.8: Casts for CDH.

b. *Splint:* Some form of splint such as Von Rosen's splint (Fig. 26.9).

External splints can be removed once the acetabulum develops to a round shape. The hip is now mobilised, and kept under observation for a period of 2-3 years for any recurrence.

Acetabular reconstruction procedures: The available procedures are:
a. *Salter's osteotomy:* This is an osteotomy of the iliac bone, above the acetabulum. The roof of the acetabulum is rotated with the fulcrum at the pubic symphysis, so that the acetabulum becomes

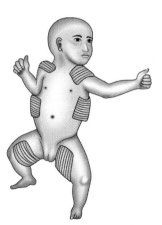

Fig. 26.9: Von Rosen's splint.

more horizontal, and thus covers the head (Fig. 26.10A).

b. *Chiari's pelvic displacement osteotomy:* The iliac bone is divided almost transversely immediately above the acetabulum, and the lower fragment (bearing the acetabulum) is displaced medially. The margin of the upper fragment provides additional depth to the acetabulum (Fig. 26.10B).

c. *Pemberton's pericapsular osteotomy:* A curved osteotomy (Fig. 26.10C) is made. The roof of the acetabulum is deflected downwards over the femoral head, with the fulcrum at the triradiate cartilage of the acetabulum.

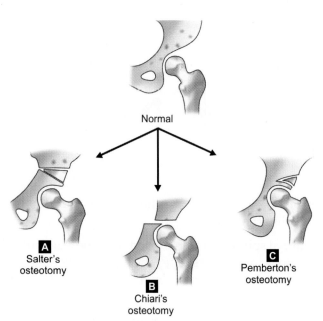

Fig. 26.10: Acetabular reconstruction procedures.

In some cases, reduction of the hip may be possible only in extreme abduction or internal rotation of the thigh. In such cases a *varus derotation osteotomy* is done at the sub-trochanteric region. The distal fragment is realigned and the osteotomy fixed with a plate.

Treatment plan: Treatment varies according to the age at which the patient presents. For convenience of discussion, this has been divided into four groups on the basis of age of the patient:

- *Birth to 6 months:* The femoral head is reduced into the acetabulum by closed manipulation, and maintained with plaster cast or splint.
- *6 months to 6 years:* It may be possible up to 2 years to reduce the head into the acetabulum by closed methods. After 2 years, it is difficult and also unwise to attempt closed reduction. This is because, when the head has been out for some time, the soft

tissues around the hip become tight. Such a hip, if reduced forcibly into the acetabulum, develops avascular necrosis of the femoral head. In these cases, reduction is achieved by open methods, and an additional femoral shortening may be required. In older children, an acetabular reconstruction may be performed at the same time or later. Salter's osteotomy is preferred by most surgeons.

- *6–10 years:* The first point to be decided in children at this age is whether or not to treat the dislocation at all. No treatment may be indicated for children with bilateral dislocations because of the following reasons:
  - The limp is less noticeable.
  - Although having some posture and gait abnormalities, these patients tend to live normal lives until their 40's or 50's.
  - Results of treatment are unpredictable and a series of operations may be required.
  - In unilateral cases, an attempt at open reduction with reconstruction of the acetabulum may be made. A derotation osteotomy is needed in most cases.
- *11 years onwards:* Indication for treatment in these patients is pain. If only one hip is affected, a total hip replacement may be practical once adulthood is reached. Sometimes, arthrodesis of the hip may be a reasonable choice.

A general plan of treatment of a child with CDH is as shown in Flowchart 26.1.

OTHER CONGENITAL MALFORMATIONS

TRUNK AND SPINE

1. **Klippel-Feil syndrome:** Congenital short and stiff neck due to fused or deformed cervical vertebrae.
2. **Sprengel's shoulder:** Failure of descent of the scapula, which is developmentally a cervical appendage, i.e., congenital high scapula.
3. **Hemivertebra:** Growth of only one half of a vertebra resulting in congenital scoliosis. This is common in the dorsal spine.
4. **Block vertebra:** The bodies of two vertebrae are joined together with no intervening disc space. This is common in the cervical spine.
5. **Spondylolysis:** A break in the pars interarticularis of one of the lumbar vertebra, commonly L_5 (see page 277).
6. **Spondylolisthesis:** Displacement of one vertebra over the one below it, because of defective development, commonly L_5 over S_1 (see page 276).

Flowchart 26.1: Treatment plan for congenital dislocation of hip (CDH).

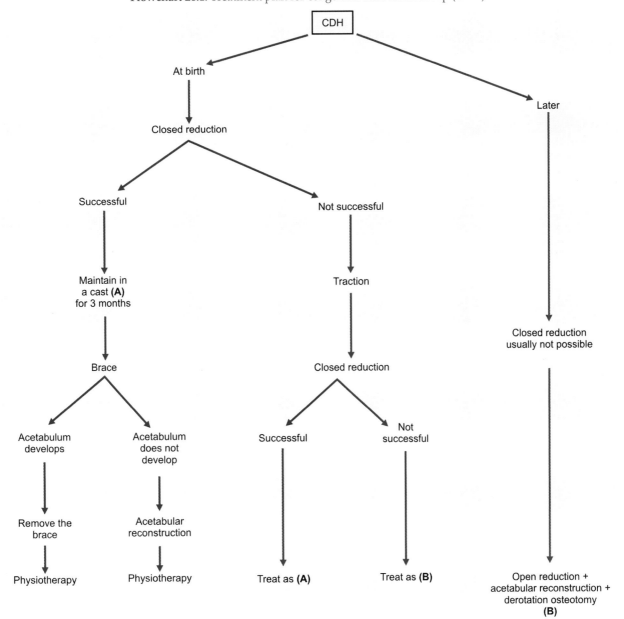

7. **Diastematomyelia:** A longitudinal fibrous or bony septum dividing the spinal canal.

UPPER LIMB

8. **Phocomelia:** Lack of development of proximal part of the limb, the distal part being present (seal limb).
9. **Absence of radius:** The hand deviates to lateral side because of lack of normal support by the radius (radial club hand or manus valgus).
10. **Congenital radio-ulnar synostosis:** The forearm bones are joined together at the proximal end, thus preventing forearm rotation.
11. **Madelung's deformity:** Defective growth of the distal radial epiphysis resulting in deformity of the distal end of the radius, and dislocation of the head of the ulna, dorsally.
12. **Syndactyly:** Webbing of two or more digits; the commonest being middle and ring fingers.
13. **Polydactyly:** More than five fingers; commonly an extra thumb.

LOWER LIMB

14. **Congenital dislocation of the hip.**
15. **Congenital coxa vara:** Reduced femoral neck-shaft angle due to a developmental defect in the growth of the proximal femur (see page 323).
16. **Congenital short femur:** Failure of development of the proximal half of the femur resulting in severe shortening.

17. **Congenital pseudarthrosis of the tibia:** A birth defect in the lower third of the tibia in children, whereby a fracture in this region fails to unite.

18. **CTEV or 'clubfoot':** Congenital deformed foot (see Chapter 25).

19. **Congenital vertical talus or 'Rocker bottom foot':** A vertically placed talus due to defective development (see page 317).

 What have we learnt?

- Congenital dislocation of the hip is uncommon in developing countries.
- Early diagnosis by ultrasound at birth, is useful.
- Aim of treatment is to put the dislocated head back in place, as soon as possible.
- Late cases need surgery, which essentially consists of reducing the head into acetabulum, and doing something to keep it there by reconstructing the acetabulum and/or femur.

Additional information: From the entrance exams point of view

- The best diagnostic modality for DDH is MRI.
- Screening for DDH done by ultrasound.
- Ultrasound-guided aspiration is the best way of differentiating septic arthritis and transient synovitis.
- Investigation of choice to diagnose early Perthes' disease is MRI.

Poliomyelitis and Other Neuromuscular Disorders

Competencies

- ❖ **OR8.1:** Describe and discuss the aetiopathogenesis, clinical features, assessment and principles of management a patient with post polio residual paralysis.
- ❖ **OR9.1:** Describe and discuss the aetiopathogenesis, clinical features, assessment and principles of management of cerebral palsy patient.

POLIOMYELITIS

Poliomyelitis, commonly called polio, is an acute infectious disease caused by the *poliovirus*. In the majority of cases, the infection may manifest merely as an episode of diarrhoea; in others the virus may affect the anterior horn cells of the spinal cord and lead to extensive paralysis of the muscles. In extreme forms, the paralysis may involve the respiratory muscles, and may lead to death.

ETIOPATHOLOGY

The poliovirus enters the body either through the *faeco-oral* route or by inhalation of droplets. The infection occurs commonly in summer. Paralysis may be precipitated after strenuous physical activity, by an intramuscular injection or in a child on cortisone therapy. A tonsillectomy, adenoidectomy or tooth extraction predisposes to paralysis during polio epidemics.

Pathogenesis: The virus multiplies in the intestine. From here it travels to the regional lymph nodes and reticuloendothelial structures, from where it enters the blood circulation. If the defense mechanism of the body is poor, the virus reaches the nervous system (mainly the anterior horn cells) via the blood

or peripheral nerves. The neurons undergo varying degree of damage—some may permanently die, others may be only temporarily damaged, still others may undergo only functional impairment due to tissue oedema. The neurons, which are permanently damaged, lead to permanent paralysis. Those which have undergone only partial damage may regenerate, and hence, partial recovery of the paralysis may occur. It is this residual paralysis called postpolio residual paralysis (PPRP) which is responsible for the host of problems associated with a paralytic limb (deformities, weakness, etc.).

CLINICAL FEATURES

Presenting complaints: Often, the patient is a child around the age of 9 months. The mother gives a history that the child developed mild pyrexia associated with diarrhoea, followed by inability to move a part or whole of the limb. The lower limbs are affected most commonly. Paralysis is of varying severity and *asymmetrical* in distribution. In extreme cases, the respiratory muscles may also be paralysed.

Often, the child is seen by a paediatrician in the early stages. When he is referred to an orthopaedic surgeon, the paralysis may already be on its way

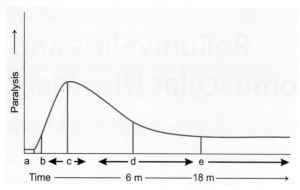

Fig. 27.1: Stages of poliomyelitis: a. Incubation period, b. Preparalysis stage, c. Stage of maximum paralysis, d. Stage of recovery, e. Postpolio residual paralysis.

to recovery. Recovery of power, if it occurs, may continue for a period of *2 years*. Most of the recovery occurs within the first *6 months*. Any residual weakness persisting after 2 years is permanent, and will not recover. For descriptive purposes, the disease is conveniently divided into five stages (Fig. 27.1).

EXAMINATION

A patient of the paralytic polio may have the following features, on examination:

a. **In the early stage**, the child is febrile, often with rigidity of the neck and tender muscles. This may be associated with diffuse muscle paralysis. The following are some of the typical features of a paralysis resulting from polio:

- It is *asymmetric*, i.e., the involvement of the affected muscles is haphazard.
- It occurs commonly in the lower limbs because the anterior horn cells of the lumbar enlargement of the spinal cord are affected most often.
- The muscle affected *most commonly* is the quadriceps, although in most cases it is only partially paralysed.
- The muscle which most often undergoes *complete paralysis* is the tibialis anterior.
- The muscle in the hand affected *most commonly is the opponens pollicis.*
- The motor paralysis is not associated with any sensory loss.
- *Bulbar or bulbospinal polio*: This is a rare but life-threatening polio, where the motor neurons of the medulla are affected. This results in involvement of respiratory and cardiovascular centres, and may cause death.

b. **In late stage (PPRP)**, the paralysis may result in wasting, weakness, and deformities of the limbs. The deformities result from imbalance between muscles of opposite groups at a joint, or due to the action of the gravity on the paralysed limb. The common deformity at the hip is flexion-abduction-external rotation. At the knee, flexion deformity is common; in severe cases *triple deformity* comprising of flexion, posterior subluxation and external rotation occurs. At the foot, equinovarus deformity is the most common; others being equinovalgus, calcaneo-valgus and calcaneocarus, in that order. In the upper limbs, polio affects shoulder and elbow muscles. Muscles of the hand are usually spared. The limb may become short. With time, the deformities become permanent due to contracture of the soft tissues and maldevelopment of the bones in the deformed position.

DIAGNOSIS

A diagnosis of poliomyelitis should be considered in an endemic area if a child presents with pyrexia and acutely tender muscles. At this stage, the poliomyelitis is usually confused with influenza, osteomyelitis, septic arthritis, scurvy, etc. Once the paralysis sets in, other common conditions producing flaccid paralysis must be excluded. Some of these are as follows:

- Pyogenic meningitis: A lumbar puncture may reveal the diagnosis.
- Post-diphtheritic paralysis.
- Guillain-Barré syndrome: This is to be considered if flaccid paralysis occurs later in life. In this syndrome, paralysis is symmetrical, and facial nerve involvement occurs early. Complete recovery usually occurs within 6 months.

In a patient presenting in the stage of residual paralysis, polio should be differentiated from other causes of flaccid paralysis. Some of these are myopathy, spina bifida, other spinal disorders producing paralysis, and peripheral neuropathy (Table 27.1).

PROGNOSIS

Of the total number of cases infected with the poliovirus, 50 per cent do not develop paralysis at all (non-paralytic polio). 40 per cent develop paralysis of a varying degree (mild, moderate, or severe). 10 per cent patients die because of respiratory muscle paralysis. Of the patients with paralytic polio, 33 per cent recover fully, 33 per cent continue to have moderate paralysis, while another 33 per cent remain with severe paralysis.

TREATMENT

Principles of treatment: Polio can be prevented by immunisation. It is important to immunise patients

Table 27.1: Differential diagnosis of residual paralysis.

Poliomyelitis	▪ Asymmetrical ▪ Lower motor neuron type ▪ No sensory loss ▪ Improves with time or is static
Myopathy	▪ Usually symmetrical, follows a pattern ▪ Lower motor neuron type ▪ No sensory loss ▪ Deteriorates with time
Spina bifida and other spinal disorders	▪ Usually symmetrical ▪ Motor + sensory loss ▪ Deteriorates with growth
Neuropathy	▪ Usually bilateral, 'glove and stocking' pattern ▪ Motor + sensory loss ▪ May improve with treatment

even after an attack of acute poliomyelitis. This is because there are three strains of the virus, and the patient could still get paralytic polio by another strain. Once polio infection occurs, there is no specific treatment for it, and there is no way of preventing the paralysis or limiting its severity. Whatever recovery from paralysis occurs is spontaneous, and there is very little a doctor can do to enhance the recovery. The role of a doctor is: (i) to provide supportive treatment during the stage of paralysis or recovery; (ii) to prevent the development of deformities during this period; and (iii) to use, in a more efficient way, whatever muscles are functioning. The treatment appropriate to each stage of the disease is best considered stage by stage.

a. **Stage of onset:** It is generally not possible to diagnose polio at this stage. In an endemic area, if a child is suspected of having polio, intramuscular injections and excessive physical activity should be avoided.

b. **Stage of maximum paralysis:** In this stage, the child needs mainly supportive treatment. A close watch is kept for signs suggestive of bulbar polio. These are signs of paralysis of the vagus nerve, causing weakness of the soft palate, pharynx and the vocal cords—hence problem in deglutition, and speech. A respirator may be necessary to save life if the respiratory muscles are paralysed. Paralytic limbs may have to be supported by splints to prevent the development of contractures. All the joints should be moved through the full range of motion several times a day. Muscle pain may be eased by applying hot packs.

c. **Stage of recovery:** The patient should be kept under close supervision of a skilled physiotherapist. The principles of treatment during this stage are as follows:

▪ *Prevention of deformity* by proper splintage, and joint mobilising exercises.

▪ *Correction of the deformity* that may have already occurred (discussed in Chapter 11).

▪ *Retraining of muscles* that are recovering by exercises. Progress is judged by repeated examination of the motor power of the paralysed limb (muscle charting).

▪ *Encourage walking* with the help of appliances, wherever possible (Fig. 27.2).

d. **Stage of residual paralysis:** It is the stage where more active orthopaedic treatment is required. It consists of the following:

▪ Detailed *evaluation of the patient:* Most patients with residual polio (PPRP) walk with a limp, with or without calipers. An assessment is made whether functional status of the patient can be improved. For this, an evaluation of the deformities and muscle weakness is made. Gait can be improved by the use of a caliper or by operations.

▪ *Prevention or correction of deformities:* The main emphasis is on prevention of deformity. This is done by splinting the paralysed part in such a way that the effect of muscle imbalance and gravity is negated (details in Chapter 11). An operation may sometimes be required to prevent the deformity. For example, in a foot with severe muscle imbalance between opposite group of muscles, a tendon transfer operation is done. This produces a more 'balanced' foot, hence less possibility of deformity. Commonly performed operation for correction of deformities are as follows:

  ◦ For hip deformity (flexion-abduction-external rotation): Soutters' release.

  ◦ For knee flexion deformity: Wilson's release.

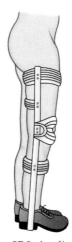

Fig. 27.2: A caliper.

- For equinus deformity of the ankle: Tendoachilles lengthening.
- For cavus deformity of the foot: Steindler's release.

- *Tendon transfers:* The available muscle power is redistributed either to equalise an unbalanced paralysis, or to use the motor power for a more useful function (see page 84). It is not done before 5 years of age, as the child has to be manageable enough to be taught proper exercises. More commonly performed tendon transfers are as follows:
  - Transfer of extensor hallucis longus (EHL) from the distal phalanx of great toe to the neck of the first metatarsal (modified Jone's operation). This is done to correct first metatarsal drop in case of tibialis anterior muscle weakness.
  - Transfer of peroneus tertius and brevis muscles (evertors of the foot) to the dorsum of the foot. The transfer is required in a foot with dorsiflexion weakness. Evertors can be spared for more useful function of dorsiflexion of the foot.
  - Hamstring (knee flexors) transfer to the quadriceps muscle to support a weak knee extensor.
- *Stabilisation of flail joints:* Joints with such severe muscle paralysis that the body loses control over them are called *flail joints.* Stabilisation of these joints is necessary for walking. This can be achieved by operative or non-operative methods. Non-operative methods consist of calipers, shoes, etc. Operative methods consist of fusion of the joints (e.g., triple arthrodesis for stabilisation of the foot).
- *Leg length equalisation:* In cases where a leg is short by more than 4 cm, a leg lengthening procedure may be required.

CEREBRAL PALSY (CP)

This is defined as a *non-progressive* neuromuscular disorder of cerebral origin. It includes a number of clinical disorders, mostly arising in childhood. The essential features of all these disorders is a varying degree of upper motor neuron type of limb paralysis (spasticity), together with difficulty in coordination (ataxia) and purposeless movements (athetosis).

ETIOPATHOLOGY

Birth anoxia and injuries are the *most common* cause of CP in developing countries. Causes can be divided into prenatal, natal and postnatal (Table 27.2).

Table 27.2: Causes of cerebral palsy.

Prenatal causes	■ Defective development ■ Kernicterus
Natal causes	■ Birth anoxia* ■ Birth injury
Postnatal causes	■ Encephalitis ■ Meningitis ■ Head injury

* Most common

Pathology: The pathology of this disorder is the degeneration of the cerebral cortex or basal ganglion, either because of their faulty development or because of damage caused by the various factors given in Table 27.2.

CLINICAL FEATURES

Presenting complaints: The clinical features vary according to the severity of the lesion, the site of the neurological deficit and the associated defects.

- *Severity of lesion:* The lesion may be mild in 20 per cent of cases, in which case the child may remain ambulatory without any help and may never require consultation. In the majority (almost 50 per cent of cases), the child requires help with ambulation. The usual presentation is a child less than one year old, in whom the parents have noticed a lack of control on the affected limb. There is a delay in the developmental milestones such as sitting up, standing or walking. In about 30 per cent of cases, the involvement is severe, and the child is bed-ridden.
- *Pattern of involvement:* The pyramidal tracts are involved in 65 per cent of cases, and they present with spasticity, exaggerated reflexes, etc. One or all the limbs may be involved. The most common pattern is a symmetrical spastic paresis of the lower limbs, resulting in a tendency to flex and adduct the hips (scissoring), to keep the knees flexed and the feet in equinus. Less commonly, it may present as monoplegia, hemiplegia or quadriplegia. In the upper limb, there is typical flexion of the wrist and fingers with adduction of the thumb and pronation of the forearm. In 35 per cent of cases, extrapyramidal symptoms such as ataxia, athetoid movements, dystonia predominate.
- *Associated defects:* These consist of speech defect, sensory defect, epilepsy, occular defects and mental retardation. About 50 per cent of the patients are severely mentally retarded, 25 per cent have moderate mental retardation and 25 per cent have borderline mental retardation.

EXAMINATION

On examination, there may be weakness of muscles, the distribution of which is variable. This leads to marked muscle imbalance, resulting in deformities. The joints are stiff because of spasticity; hence when a steady pressure is applied, the muscle relaxes and the deformity is partially corrected. As the pressure is released, the spasm returns immediately. The tendon reflexes are exaggerated, and clonus may be present.

The patient exhibits a lack of voluntary control when asked to hold an object. As the patient tries to move a single group of muscles, other groups contract at the same time (athetoid movements). Mental deficiency may be present. There may also be defective vision and impaired hearing.

TREATMENT

Principles of treatment: The aim of treatment is to maintain and develop whatever physical and mental capabilities the child has. It consists of: (i) orthopaedic treatment; and (ii) speech and occupational therapy.

Orthopaedic treatment consists of the prevention and correction of deformities, and keeping the spasticity under check. Methods of controlling the spasticity are: (i) drugs— e.g., Diazepam, Beclofen; (ii) phenol nerve block; and (iii) neurectomy. Neurectomy may be required to control severe muscle spasm interfering with optimal rehabilitation. Obturator neurectomy is performed for spasm of adductors of the thigh. A number of other operative procedures may be necessary for improving selective functions.

Speech therapy and occupational therapy constitutes an important adjunct to the overall treatment of the child. Mild cases can be looked after at home, but specialised residential schools are required for severely handicapped children.

PROGNOSIS

Complete cure is impossible since an essential part of the brain is destroyed and cannot be repaired or replaced. All that can be hoped for is improvement. Depending upon the severity of the underlying damage, a child can be made independent enough to earn his own living in due course. A child formerly dependent on others for many daily activities may often become independent. This needs a great amount of patience and perseverance on the part of the parents and attendants of the child. In spite of all the treatment, there are a few in whom worthwhile improvement cannot be gained.

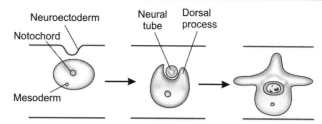

Fig. 27.3: Development of vertebral column.

SPINA BIFIDA

RELEVANT ANATOMY

The vertebral bodies develop from the mesoderm around the notochord. From the centre of each body extend two projections which grow around the neural canal to form the vertebral arch (Fig. 27.3). The two halves of the arch fuse in the thoracic region, from where the fusion extends up and down. Failure of fusion of these arches gives rise to spina bifida. It is often associated with maldevelopment of the spinal cord and the membranes.

TYPES

The defect varies in severity from a mere failure of fusion of the spinous processes, to a bony defect with a major aberration in the development of the neural elements. Accordingly, there are two main types of spina bifida: (i) spina bifida occulta; and (ii) spina bifida aperta.

Spina bifida occulta: This is the mildest and the *most common*. In this, the failure of the vertebral arches to fuse results in bifid spinous processes of vertebrae. The following are some of the important features:
- *Most common site:* This is common in the lumbosacral spine; S_1 being the most common site.
- *Externally,* the skin may be normal or there may be tell-tale signs in the form of a dimple in the skin, a lipomatous mass, a dermal sinus or a tuft of hair.
- *Neurological impairment* is not related to the severity of the bone defect. The most common manifestation of neurological involvement is a muscle imbalance in the lower limbs with selective muscle wasting. This leads to foot deformities because of muscle imbalance; common ones being equinovarus or cavus. The cause of neural impairment may be: (i) tethering of the cord to the undersurface of the skin by a fibrous membrane (*membrana reuniens);* (ii) tethering of the cord to the filum terminale; (iii) bifid cord, transfixed with an antero-posterior bone bar (diastematomyelia); or (iv) defective neural development (myelodysplasia).

Treatment: A symptomless patient, where the lesion is detected on an X-ray taken for some other problem, needs no treatment. Cases presenting with backache respond to physiotherapy. Cases presenting with a neurological deficit need to be evaluated regarding the cause and likelihood of worsening of the neurological deficit. MRI is the imaging modality of choice. Surgical treatment may be required in some cases. *Orthopaedic treatment* is the same as for a paralytic limb, i.e., (i) prevention and correction of deformities; (ii) using residual muscle power for more useful functions by tendon transfers and joint stabilisation; (iii) giving support for walking.

Spina bifida aperta: This developmental defect involves not only the vertebral arches but also the overlying soft tissues, skin, and often the meninges. In severe cases, the nerve tube itself may be exposed. The following are some of the important features:

Most common site: The dorsolumbar spine is affected most commonly. There is a variable structural defect of closure of the embryonal neural tube giving rise to the following (Fig. 27.4):

a. *Meningocele,* i.e., protrusion of meninges through a defect in the neural arch. This contains only CSF.
b. *Meningomyelocele,* i.e., the protrusion of the meninges along with some neural elements (normally developed spinal cord or cauda equina).
c. *Syringomyelocele,* i.e., the central canal of the cord is dilated (syringomyelia), and the cord lies within

the protruded meningeal sac together with the nerves arising from it.
d. *Myelocele:* This results from an arrest in the development at the time of closure of the neural groove. An elliptical raw surface, representing the ununited groove is seen. At the upper end of this surface opens the central canal through which CSF may be seen leaking.

With the exception of spina bifida occulta, myelocele is the *most common* type of spina bifida; though many of these cases are stillborn. If the child is born alive, death ensues within a few days from infection of the cord and meninges. The other types of spina bifida with neural development defects where the patient often survives is meningocele and meningomyelocele. There may be mild to severe paralysis of the lower limbs. These children are often born with deformities, particularly flexion-adduction contracture of the hip, and deformities of the foot. These deformities are the direct result of muscle imbalance due to paralysis. There may be urinary and bowel incontinence.

Treatment: Treatment of this condition consists of: (i) treatment of the basic defect, i.e., spina bifida; (ii) orthopaedic treatment to prevent and correct the deformities, and to use the residual motor power in the best possible way; and (iii) urological treatment for bladder incontinence.

DISORDERS OF THE MUSCLES

These diseases are still incurable. Accurate diagnosis is important: (i) to rule out other treatable disorders; (ii) to act as a guide to optimal rehabilitation efforts; and (iii) to permit genetic counselling.

DEFINITIONS

Myopathy is a *generic term* for somatic motor dysfunctions due to diseases of the skeletal muscles, i.e., dysfunctions not otherwise attributable to lesions of the central nervous system, the lower motor neuron (LMN) or the neuro-muscular junction (NMJ).

Myopathy may be inherited or acquired. The underlying pathological process may be restricted to the muscles or may affect other organ systems as well. In an inherited myopathy, the defect may be: (i) abnormal cellular enzymes; (ii) abnormal structural proteins; or (iii) both. It is the inherited myopathy with structural protein as its underlying defect, which is designated *muscular dystrophy* (Flowchart 27.1). It comprises of a group

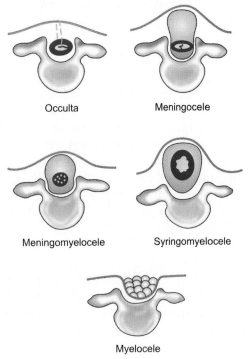

Occulta   Meningocele

Meningomyelocele   Syringomyelocele

Myelocele

Fig. 27.4: Types of spina bifida.

Flowchart 27.1: Approach to a patient with motor dysfunction.

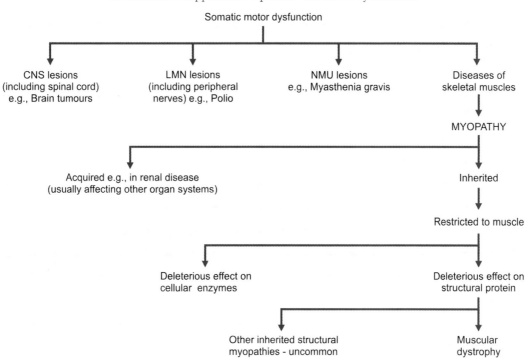

of heterogenous disorders that share in common: (i) bilateral, usually symmetrical, topographically patterned loss of strength and muscle wasting; (ii) progression over several years; and (iii) largely non-specific laboratory and histologic evidence of myofibril necrosis. One type of dystrophy is distinguishable from another type by the following criteria:

- Age at clinical onset.
- Type of inheritance.
- Distribution of physical findings.
- Presence or absence of myotonia.
- Progression of illness (temporal profile).
- Evidence of any additional genetically determined medical problem.

There are no proven pathognomonic clinical or laboratory tests to diagnose a muscular dystrophy. A confirmed family history is a very strong indicator of diagnosis. Classic syndromes present few diagnostic problems, but unfortunately incomplete or atypical forms are common. Diagnostic accuracy is directly proportional to the reliability of the neurologic data (the history, physical examination, and ancillary laboratory findings), and the care with which it is analysed (Flowchart 27.2, next page). A systematic approach as suggested below helps in arriving at the correct diagnosis.

a. First localise the neuroanatomic site of the lesion. (Is it in the CNS, LMN, NMJ, or muscle?).
b. Establish its most likely pathogenetic mechanism (is it an inherited or acquired, myopathy?). If inherited, is it metabolic or structural? If acquired, is it infectious, metabolic, toxic drug induced, or dysimmunologic?
c. Identify a particular disease consistent with the site of the lesion and presumed pathogenesis.

Treatment: It is difficult. Most of the common types pursue a gradual course leading to severe muscular weakness. In selected cases, treatment along the lines of a paralytic limb may be used (refer to page 228).

PERIPHERAL NEUROPATHIES

This topic is discussed in detail in Medicine textbooks, and is discussed here since a paralysis secondary to neuropathy may present to an orthopaedic surgeon. Peripheral neuropathies are of two types—mononeuropathy, and poly- neuropathy. Mononeuropathy is commonly due to trauma and other causes as discussed in Chapter 10. The causes of polyneuropathy are as given in Table 27.3, next page.

Nutritional deficiency, diabetes and infections constitute majority of the cases of polyneuropathy.

Flowchart 27.2: Muscular dystrophy — How to distinguish various types?

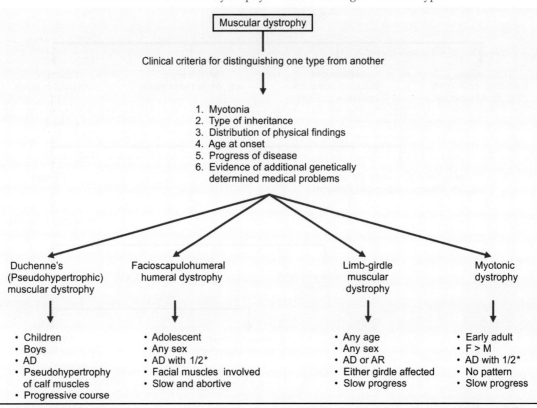

Guillain–Barré syndrome is an important treatable cause. The cause of neuropathy can be found in about 50-60 per cent of cases by clinical examination and investigations. The patient presents with bilateral involvement, complains of weakness of most distal group of muscles and paraesthesias in the distal parts of the extremities. There is loss of deep jerks in the affected extremities, and glove and stocking type of hypoaesthesia. A detailed neurological examination should be performed in all cases.

TREATMENT

It consists of the following:
- Treatment of the underlying cause, if possible.
- Prevention of contractures by splintage and physiotherapy.
- Care of the anaesthetic limb by protecting it from injury.
- Treatment of neuropathic pain with analgesics and nerve blocks.

Table 27.3: Common causes of peripheral polyneuropathies.	
Toxic	*Infections*
■ Alcoholism	■ Leprosy, Diphtheria
■ Drugs: Nitrofurantoin, INH, Diphenylhydantoin	■ Guillain-Barre syndrome
■ Metals: Pb, As, Hg	
	Genetic causes
Deficiency states	■ Peroneal muscular atrophy
■ Vitamin B_1 deficiency	■ Progressive hypertrophic polyneuropathy
■ Vitamin B_{12} deficiency	
■ Multiple deficiencies	*Inflammatory causes*
■ Malnutrition	■ Polyarteritis nodosa (PAN)
■ Malabsorption	■ Rheumatoid arthritis
	■ Systemic lupus erythematosus (SLE)
Metabolic diseases	
■ Diabetes mellitus	*Malignancy*
■ Uraemia	■ Carcinoma bronchus
■ Acute intermittent porphyria	■ Lymphoma
■ Hepatic failure	■ Multiple myeloma

What have we learnt?

- It is the residue of polio, which needs treatment by orthopaedic surgery.
- In the initial stage, aim is to prevent occurrence of deformity. In late stages, reconstructive surgery is required to improve the functional capability of the affected part.

Additional information: From the entrance exams point of view

- Progression of congenital scoliosis is maximum in unilateral unsegmented bar with a hemivertebra.
- Progression of congenital scoliosis is least with a block vertebra.

Bone Tumours

Competency

- ❖ **OR10.1:** Describe and discuss the aetiopathogenesis, clinical features, investigations and principles of management of benign and malignant bone tumours and pathological fractures.

The term 'bone tumour' is a broad term used for benign and malignant neoplasms, as well as 'tumour-like conditions' of the bone (e.g., osteochondroma). Metastatic deposits in the bone are more common than primary bone tumours. Of the primary bone malignancies, multiple myeloma is the *most common*. Osteochondroma is the most common benign tumour* of the bone. Most primary malignant bone tumours occur in children and young adults; in whom these constitute one of the common malignant tumours. The nature of a bone tumour can be suspected based on the type of destruction seen on an X-ray (Table 28.1).

Classification and nomeclature of bone tumours is given in Table 28.2.

Table 28.1: Types of lesions radiographically.

Type of Lesion	Aggression	Examples
Geographic lesion: Well-defined lesion	Least aggressive	Simple bone cyst
Moth eaten: Less well-defined with a moth eaten appearance	More aggressive	Low grade osteosarcoma Giant cell tumour
Permeative lesion: Least defined	Most aggressive	Telengiectatic osteosarcoma

BENIGN TUMOURS

OSTEOMA

This is a benign tumour composed of sclerotic, well-formed bone protruding from the cortical surface of a bone. The bones involved most often are the skull and facial bones. Generally, the tumour is of no clinical significance except that it may produce visible swelling. Sometimes, it may bulge into one of the air sinuses (frontal, ethmoidal or others), and cause obstruction to the sinus cavity, leading to pain.

Treatment: No treatment is generally required except for cosmetic reasons, where a simple excision is sufficient. It is not a pre-malignant lesion.

OSTEOID OSTEOMA

It is the *most common* true benign tumour of the bone. Pathologically, it consists of a nidus of tangled arrays of partially mineralised osteoid trabeculae surrounded by dense sclerotic bone.

Clinical presentation: The tumour is seen commonly between the ages of 5–25 years. The bones of the lower extremity are more commonly affected; *tibia*

---

* Though it is not a true neoplasm.

Table 28.2: Nomenclature and classfication of bone tumours (WHO classification simplified).

a. Bone forming tumours

- Benign — Osteoid osteoma, osteoma Osteoblastoma
- Indeterminate — Aggressive osteoblastoma
- Malignant — Osteosarcoma conventional, variants

b. Cartilage forming tumours

- Benign: — Osteochondroma (exostosis) Enchondroma (chondroma) Chondromyxoid fibroma Chondroblastoma
- Malignant — Chondrosarcoma

c. Giant cell tumour (GCT)

- A benign aggressive tumor

d. Hematopoietic neoplasms

- Malignant — Solitary plasmacytoma Multiple myeloma Lymphoma

e. Ewing sarcoma/primitive neuroectodermal tumor

f. Vascular tumours

- Benign — Haemangioma Glomangioma
- Malignant — Angiosarcoma

g. Others

- Benign — Neurilemmoma Neurofibroma
- Malignant — Malignant fibrous histiocytoma Liposarcoma Undifferentiated sarcoma Adamantinoma

h. Tumour-like lesions

- Bone cysts – simple or aneurysmal
- Fibrous dysplasia – mono or polyostotic
- Reparative giant cell granuloma (e.g., epulis)
- Fibrous cortical defect
- Eosinophilic granuloma

located in the diaphysis of long bones. Posterior elements of the vertebrae are a common site. The presenting complaint is a nagging pain, worst at night, and is relieved by *salicylates.* There are minimal or no clinical signs, except for mild tenderness at the site of the lesion, and a palpable swelling if it is a superficial lesion.

Diagnosis: It is generally confirmed on X-ray. The tumour is visible as a zone of sclerosis surrounding a radiolucent nidus usually less than 1 cm in size (Fig. 28.1A). In some cases, the nidus may not be seen on a plain X-ray because of the extensive surrounding sclerosis. It may only be detected on a CT scan. CT scan is the imaging modality of choice to confirm osteoid osteoma.

Treatment: Radiofrequency (RF) ablation is the treatment of choice. Complete excision of the nidus along with the sclerotic bone is done where facility for radiofrequency ablation is not available. Prognosis is good. It is not a pre-malignant condition.

UNCOMMON BENIGN TUMOURS OF THE BONE

Osteoblastoma: This is a benign tumour consisting of vascular osteoid and new bone. It occurs in the jaw and the spine. If in long bones, it occurs in the diaphysis or metaphysis, but *never* in the epiphysis. It occurs in patients in their 2nd decade of life. The patient presents with an aching pain. Radiologically, it is a well-defined radiolucent expansile bone lesion 2-12 cm in size. There is minimal reactive new bone formation. *Treatment* is by curettage.

Chondroblastoma: This is a cartilaginous tumour containing characteristic multiple calcium deposits.

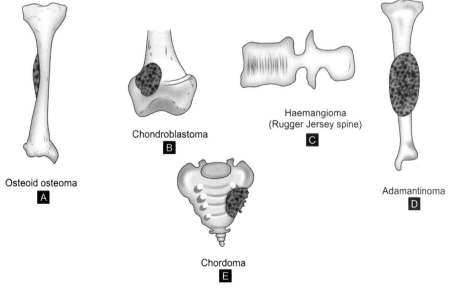

Osteoid osteoma A
Chondroblastoma B
Haemangioma (Rugger Jersey spine) C
Adamantinoma D
Chordoma E

Fig. 28.1: Benign tumours of the bone.

It typcally occurs before skeletal maturity, and is located in the epiphysis. Bones around the knee are commonly affected. Radiologically, there is a well-defined lytic lesion surrounded by a zone of sclerosis. Areas of *calcification within the tumour* substance give rise to a mottled appearance (Fig. 28.1B). *Treatment* is by curettage and bone grafting. In deep seated, small lesions, radiofrequency (RF) ablation is an option.

Haemangioma of the bone: This is a benign tumour of angiomatous origin, commonly affecting the vertebrae and the skull. It occurs in young adults. Common presenting symptoms are persistent pain and features of cord compression. At times the lesion is asymptomatic. Typically, one of the lumbar vertebrae is affected. Radiologically, it appears as *loss of horizontal striations* and prominence of vertical striations of the affected vertebral body (Fig. 28.1C). The importance of this tumour lies in differentiating it from more common diseases like TB spine or metastatic bone disease of the spine. *Treatment* depends upon the symptoms. Often it is an incidental finding, and can be left alone. If causing symptoms, depending upon the situation, angioembolisation, surgery (decompression with or without stabilisation) can be considered. Radiotherapy is indicated for inaccessible lesions.

Adamantinoma: This tumour affects primarily the jaw bone or the tibial diaphysis. It occurs between 10-35 years of age. The swelling is associated with only minimal pain, and it increases in size gradually. Typically, it appears as an eccentric *multi* loculated lesion on X-ray. It is centred over the anterior cortex of the tibia, with lytic areas interrupted by sclerotic margins (Fig. 28.1D). Local recurrence is common. Treatment is by wide resection.

Chordoma: This is a malignant tumour supposedly originating from the remnants of notochord. *Sacrum* and upper cervical spine are common sites. It presents with a persistent pain and swelling, sometimes with a neurological deficit. Bone destruction is the only hallmark feature of this tumour (Fig. 28.1E). Treatment, wherever possible, is complete excision. If complete excision is not possible, radiotherapy is done.

OSTEOCLASTOMA (Giant Cell Tumour)

Giant cell tumour (GCT) is a common bone tumour with variable growth potential. It is a benign aggressive tumor with a tendency for local recurrence.

PATHOLOGY

The cell of origin is uncertain. Microscopically, the tumour consists of undifferentiated spindle cells, profusely interspersed with multinucleate giant cells. The tumour stroma is highly vascular. These giant cells were mistaken as osteoclasts, hence in the past it was called 'osteoclastoma', a term not used anymore.

CLINICAL FEATURES

The tumour is seen commonly in the age group of 20–40 years, i.e., after skeletal maturity. *The bones affected* commonly are those around the knee, i.e., lower-end of the femur and upper-end of the tibia. Lower-end of the radius is another common site. The tumour is located at the epiphysis*. It often reaches almost up to the joint surface. Common *presenting complaints* are swelling and vague pain. Sometimes, the patient, unaware of the lesion, presents for the first time with a pathological fracture through the lesion.

EXAMINATION

Examination reveals a bony swelling, eccentrically located at the end of the bone. Surface of the swelling is smooth. There may be tenderness on firm palpation. The characteristic 'egg-shell crackling' may or may not be elicited. The limb may be deformed if a pathological fracture has occurred.

DIAGNOSIS

GCT is one of the common cause of a solitary lytic lesion of the bone, and must be differentiated from other such lesions (Table 28.3). Following are some of the characteristic radiological features of this tumour:

- A solitary, may be loculated, lytic lesion.
- *Eccentric* location, often subchondral (Fig. 28.2A).
- Expansion of the overlying cortex (expansile lesion).
- *'Soap-bubble' appearance* - the tumour is homogeneously lytic with trabeculae of the remnants of bone traversing it, giving rise to a loculated appearance.
- *No calcification* within the tumour (Fig. 28.2B).
- None or minimal reactive sclerosis around the tumour.
- Cortex may be thinned out, or perforated at places.
- Tumour usually does not enter the adjacent joint.

TREATMENT

Treatment of choice for GCT is surgery. The choice of surgery is a tricky balance between doing too little or too much. On the too little side is, conservative

---

* It is the area which *was* epiphysis before its fusion with the metaphysis.

Table 28.3: Differential diagnosis of a solitary bone lesion.

Features	Giant cell tumour	Simple bone cyst	Aneurysmal bone cyst	Fibrous dysplasia
Age	20–40 years	< 20 years	10–40 years	20–30 years
Common bones	Lower femur Upper tibia Lower radius	Upper humerus Upper femur	Tibia Humerus	Neck of the femur Tibia
Location	Epiphysis	Metaphysis	Metaphysis	Metaphysis
X-ray	Soap-bubble appearance, eccentrically placed	Maximum width less than width of the growth plate	Distending lesion, 'ballooning' the bone	Multi-loculated Ground-glass appearance Trabeculations++
Treatment	Extended curettage/resection	Aspiration and steroid injection/curettage	Sclerotherapy/curettage	Observation/curettage/fixation

removal of just the tumour (curettage) and thus retaining the patient's anatomy. One does run the risk of local tumour recurrence in this approach. On the other hand, on the too much side is wide resection of the tumour, thus reducing the chances of recurrence. This approach may compromise joint functions, may sometimes mean even amputation. It all depends upon how early or late the patient presents, and also on expertise of the surgeon. More often than not, one would like to remove the tumour in toto, by what is called 'extended curettage', a good midway between just curettage and wide resection.

- **Extended curettage**: This is the most acceptable method. This involves two steps. First step is, *thorough removal of tumour tissue* while retaining the native bone and the adjoining joint. For this a high speed burr is ideal, and is used to extend the cavities. An adjuvant such as phenol, liquid nitriogen or bone cement is used for 'completeting' the removal. The second step is to *fill the cavity* so created. This may be done using bone cement/bone graft/both. Some sort of external support is required to prevent fracture.

- **Excision:** This is the treatment of choice when the tumour affects a bone whose removal does not hamper with functions, e.g., the fibula, lower-end of the ulna, etc.

- **Excision with reconstruction:** In patients where curettage is not possible because the lesion is too big, and those with multiple recurrences, a wide excision of the tumor is needed. Here, a block of bone with tumour is removed. The gap thus created is made up by some reconstructive procedure. Just for an example, in tumours affecting the lower-end of femur, the affected part is excised *en bloc,* and the defect created made up by one of the following methods:
  - *Arthrodesis by the Turn-o-Plasty procedure* (Fig. 28.3A): In this technique, the required length of the tibia is split into two halves. One half is turned upside down and fixed with the stump of the femur left after excising the tumour. A similar procedure can be used for a tibial lesion by taking half of the femur.
  - *Arthrodesis by bridging the gap* by double fibulae (Fig. 28.3B), one taken from same extremity and the other from the opposite leg (Yadav, 1990).

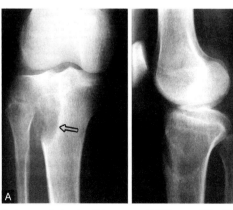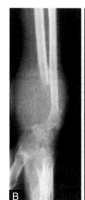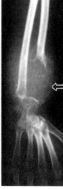

Fig. 28.2: Radiological features of giant cell tumour: (A) X-ray of the tibia, AP and lateral views, showing GCT of upper end of the tibia. (Note that the tumour is eccentrically placed); (B) X-ray of the radius, AP and lateral views, showing GCT of the lower end of the radius. (A lytic tumour, with no new bone formation).

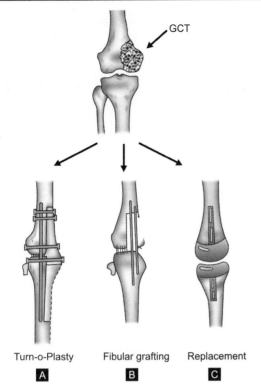

Turn-o-Plasty   Fibular grafting   Replacement

A   **B**   **C**

Fig. 28.3: Methods of treating GCT around the knee.

- *Arthroplasty:* In this procedure, the tumour is excised, and an attempt is made to reconstruct the joint in some way (Fig. 28.3C). This can be carried out using an autograft (patella to substitute the articular defect), allograft (replacing the defect with the preserved bone of a cadaver), or an artificial joint (prosthesis).
- **Amputation:** For more aggressive tumours or following recurrence, amputation may be necessary.
- **Others:** Wherever surgical removal is not feasible (e.g, sacral/vertebral locations), non-operative methods like radiotherapy may be used. It is the preferred treatment method for GCT affecting the vertebrae.
- Treatment for GCT at more common sites is as given in Table 28.4.

Table 28.4: Wide excision treatment of GCT (where extended curettage is not possible).

Site	Treatment of choice
Lower end of femur	Excision with Turn-o-Plasty
Upper end of tibia	Excision with Turn-o-Plasty
Lower end of radius	Excision with fibular* grafting
Lower end of ulna	Excision
Upper end of fibula	Excision

* Proximal end of the *opposite* fibula is preferred, since it matches the lower end of radius in shape.

PROGNOSIS

Recurrence following treatment is a serious problem. With every subsequent recurrence, the tumour becomes more aggressive.

PRIMARY MALIGNANT TUMOURS

OSTEOSARCOMA (OSTEOGENIC SARCOMA)

Osteosarcoma is the second most common, and a highly malignant primary bone tumour.

Pathology: An osteosarcoma can be defined as a malignant tumour of the mesenchymal cells, characterised by formation of osteoid or bone by the tumour cells.

Classification: This tumour has been subclassified on the basis of: (i) the clinical setting where it occurs; and (ii) its dominant histomorphology.

a. On the basis of *clinical setting,* this tumour can be divided into primary and secondary. *Primary* osteosarcoma, the more common, occurs in the age group of 15-25 years. There are no known pre-malignant conditions related to it. It is very much more malignant than the secondary one. The *secondary* osteosarcoma occurs in older age (45 years onwards). Some of the pre-malignant conditions often associated with it are Paget's disease, bone island, fibrous dysplasia, irradiation to bones, etc.

b. On the basis of *dominant histomorphology,* an osteosarcoma may be: (i) osteoblastic, i.e., with a lot of new bone formation; (ii) chondroblastic, i.e., with basic cell being a cartilage cell; (iii) fibroblastic, i.e., the basic cell being a fibroblast; and (iv) telangiectatic type, a predominantly lytic tumour.

Whatever be the histomorphologic characteristics and the site of origin, all osteosarcomas are aggressive lesions and metastasize widely through the blood stream. Lung is the most common site of metastasis. Lymph node involvement is unusual. Osteolytic type is more malignant than the osteoblastic type. Despite its aggressiveness, osteosarcoma rarely penetrates an open physeal plate. Most osteosarcomas fall into the primary conventional category, and have the following important features.

- **Age at onset:** This tumour occur between the ages of 15–25 years, constituting the most common musculoskeletal tumour at that age.
- **Common sites of origin:** In decreasing order of frequency these are: the lower-end of the femur; upper-end of the tibia; and upper-end of the humerus. However, any bone of the body may be affected.

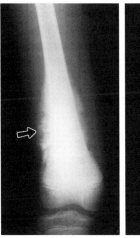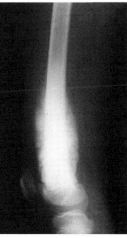

Fig. 28.4: X-ray of the femur, AP and lateral views showing osteosarcoma of lower end of the femur. (Note the metaphyseal origin and lot of new bone formation).

- **Gross appearance** of the tumour depends upon its dominant histomorphology. An *osteoblastic* tumour is greyish white, hard, and has a gritty feeling when cut. A *chondroblastic* type may appear opalescent and bluish grey. A *fibroblastic* type has a more typical fish flesh sarcomatous appearance. The highly malignant, *telangiectatic* type may have large areas of tumour necrosis and blood-filled spaces within the tumour mass. Most tumours have mixed areas.

- **Histologically,** these tumours vary in the richness of the osteoid, cartilaginous, or vascular components; but common to all is a basically anaplastic mesenchymal parenchyma with osteoid produced and lined by malignant cells.

Clinical features: Pain is usually the first symptom, soon followed by swelling. Pain is constant and boring, and becomes worse as the swelling increases in size. There may be a history of trauma, but more often it is incidental and just draws the attention of the patient to the swelling. Sometimes, the patient presents with a pathological fracture.

Examination: The swelling is in the region of the metaphysis. Skin over the swelling is shiny with prominent veins. The swelling is warm and tender. Margins of the swelling are not well- defined. Movement at the adjacent joint may be limited mainly because of the mechanical block by the swelling. The tumour may compress the neurovascular structures of the limb, and produce symptoms due to that. Regional lymph nodes may be enlarged, but are usually reactive.

Investigations: Following investigations may be carried out to confirm the diagnosis:
- **Radiological examination:** X-ray shows the following features (Fig. 28.4):

- An area of *irregular destruction* in the metaphysis, sometimes overshadowed by the new bone formation. The cortex overlying the lesion is *eroded.* There is *new bone formation* in the matrix of the tumour. The lesion is typically permeative with a wide zone of transition from normal to abnormal bone.
- *Periosteal reaction:* As the tumour lifts the peri-osteum, it incites an intense periosteal reaction. The periosteal reaction in an osteosarcoma is irregular, unlike in osteomyelitis where it is smooth and in layers.
- *Codman's triangle:* A triangular area of subperiosteal new bone is seen at the tumour-host cortex junction at the ends of the tumour.
- *Sun-ray appearance:* As the periosteum is unable to contain the tumour, the tumour grows into the overlying soft tissues. New bone is laid down along the blood vessels within the tumour growing centrifugally. This gives rise to 'sun-ray appearance' on the X-ray.

- **Serum alkaline phosphatase (SAP):** It is generally elevated, but is of no diagnostic significance. It has been considered a useful parameter for follow up of a case of osteosarcoma. A rise of SAP after an initial fall after tumour removal is taken as an indicator of recurrence or metastasis.

- **Biopsy:** An open biopsy is a standard method of confirming the diagnosis. Fine needle aspiration cytology (FNAC), otherwise a popular method of tissue diagnosis in soft tissue tumours, is not useful in diagnosis of osteosarcoma. In some advanced centres, with expert histopathologists, a core biopsy is equally effective.

Treatment: The aim is to confirm the diagnosis, to evaluate spread of the tumour (staging), and to execute adequate treatment.

a. **Confirmation of the diagnosis:** Histologically, tumour new-bone formation is pathognomonic of osteosarcoma. The appearance on histology should always be correlated with the clinical and radiological picture before making the final diagnosis.

b. **Staging:** This consists of evaluation of: (i) the extent of involvement of the affected bone and (ii) that of spread of the tumour to other sites. As complete removal of tumour is of vital importance in surgery - whether it is amputation or limb-salvage, the assessment of involvement of the local part is critical. It is done by X-ray and MRI. Make sure that the whole bone is included in the images. A detailed analysis of the extent of bone involvement, soft-tissue involvement, and that of the neurovascular bundle is made. The tumour may have skip areas in the medullary cavities, and those will need to be included in the surgical removal. Soft tissue involvement and that of neurovasular bundle can be very well made with an MRI.

c. **Treatment:** Treatment consists of local control of the tumour, and control of the micro- or macro-metastases.

- *Local control:* This is achieved by surgical ablation. There are two methods of surgical ablation - limb-sparing and amputation. Amputation used to be a standard method of surgical ablation in the past but lately, with better imaging techniques, advances in chemotherapy and possibility of surgical reconstruction, limb-sparing surgery is the preferred option. In this, a 'wide excision' of the tumour with a cuff of normal tissue all around, is done. After wide excision for limb-salvage surgery, the defect has to be reconstructed by a prosthesis, allograft, or autograft.

  As osteosarcoma is not sensitive to radiotherapy, this modality is reserved for patients having inoperable disease.

- *Control of distant macro- or micro-metastasis:* In the majority of cases, micro-metastasis has already occurred by the time diagnosis is made. These are effectively controlled by adjuvant chemotherapy, immunotherapy, etc. A solitary lung metastasis may sometimes be considered suitable for excision.

  Role of chemotherapy: Chemotherapy has revolutionised the treatment of osteosarcoma. It is usually started as a 'neo-adjuvant' chemotherapy (chemotherapy before surgery), and continued after surgery as adjuvant chemotherapy. The basic principle is that the micro-metastases which are supposed to have occurred by the time the diagnosis is made, are controlled effectively. A multi-drug combination of two or three of these drugs is used. High dose methotrexate, as a complete removal of tumour is of vital importance in surgery (whether it is amputation or limb salvage). Ifosfamide, Cisplatin and Adriamycin are the main drugs. These drugs are highly toxic and should be given in centres where their side effects can be effectively managed.

d. **Follow up:** The patient is checked up every 6–8 weeks. Any evidence of recurrence of the primary tumour, or appearance of the secondary (usually in the chest) is diagnosed early and treated. A practical plan for treatment management of a case of osteosarcoma is shown in Flowchart 28.1.

Prognosis: Without treatment, death occurs within 2 years, usually within 6 months of detection of metastasis. 5-year survival with surgery alone is 20 per cent. With surgery and adjuvant chemotherapy, a 5-year disease free period is reported to be as high as 70 per cent.

SECONDARY OSTEOSARCOMA

This is an osteosarcoma developing in a bone affected by a pre-malignant disease. Some such diseases are as given in Table 28.5. It is seen in the older age group (after 40 years). Treatment is along the lines of the conventional osteosarcoma.

PAROSTEAL OSTEOSARCOMA

This is a type of osteosarcoma, arising in the region of the periosteum. It is a slower growing tumour, seen in adults. The common site is lower-end of the femur. It is a low garde osteosarcoma, and chemotherapy is not indicated. Prognosis is much better.

EWING'S SARCOMA

This is highly malignant tumour occurring between the age of 10-20 years, sometimes up to 30 years.

Pathology: Following are some of the important pathological features:

- **Bones affected:** It commonly occurs in long bones (in two-third cases), mainly in the femur and tibia. About one-third of cases occur in flat bones, usually in the pelvis and ribs. Occasionally, it is known to have a *multicentric* origin.

- **Site:** The tumour may begin anywhere, but diaphysis of the long bone is the most common site.

- **Gross pathology:** The tumour characteristically involves a large area, or even the entire medullary cavity. The tumour tissue is grey white. It is soft and may be thin, almost like pus. The bone may be expanded, and the periosteum elevated, with subperiosteal new bone formation, often in layers. The tumour ruptures through the cortex early, and extends into the soft tissues.

- **Histopathology:** The tumour comprises of sheets of quite uniform, small cells, resembling lymphocytes. Often, the tumour cells surround a central clear area, forming a *pseudo-rosette*. The tumour grows fast and metastasises through the blood-stream to the lungs and to other bones.

Clinical features: The patient presents with pain and swelling. There may be a history of trauma preceding onset, but it is usually incidental. Often there is an associated fever and malaise in which case it may be confused with osteomyelitis.

Flowchart 28.1: Treatment plan for osteosarcoma.

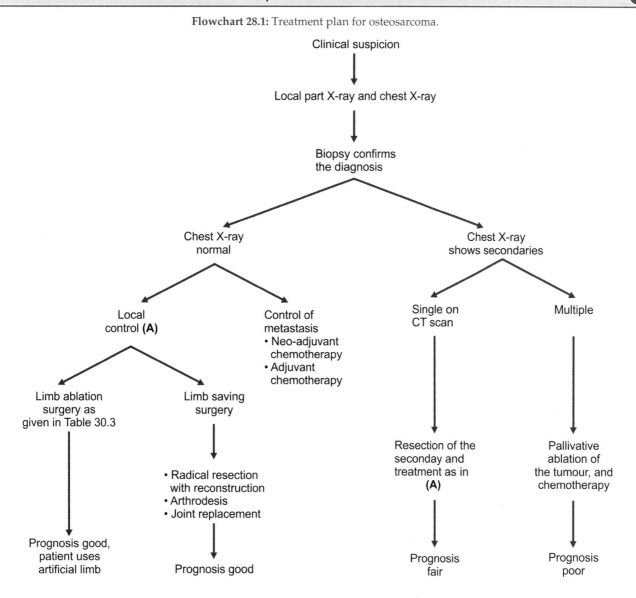

Clinical suspicion

↓

Local part X-ray and chest X-ray

↓

Biopsy confirms the diagnosis

- Chest X-ray normal
  - Local control **(A)**
    - Limb ablation surgery as given in Table 30.3
      - Prognosis good, patient uses artificial limb
    - Limb saving surgery
      - • Radical resection with reconstruction
      - • Arthrodesis
      - • Joint replacement
        - Prognosis good
  - Control of metastasis
    - • Neo-adjuvant chemotherapy
    - • Adjuvant chemotherapy
- Chest X-ray shows secondaries
  - Single on CT scan
    - Resection of the seconday and treatment as in **(A)**
      - Prognosis fair
  - Multiple
    - Pallivative ablation of the tumour, and chemotherapy
      - Prognosis poor

Examination: On examination, the swelling is usually located in the diaphysis and has features suggesting a malignant swelling.

Radiological features: In a typical case, there is a lytic lesion in the medullary zone of the midshaft of a long bone, with cortical destruction and new bone formation in layers - *onion-peel appearance* (Fig. 28.5). In atypical presentations, the tumour may be located in the metaphysis, and may be confused with osteomyelitis. It may have a predominant soft tissue component with little cortical destruction, and

Table 28.5: Pre-malignant bone lesions.

- Paget's disease
- Diaphyseal aclasis
- Enchondromatosis
- Post-radiation

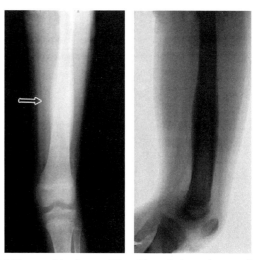

Fig. 28.5: X-rays of the femur, AP and lateral views showing Ewing's sarcoma of the femur complete removal of tumour is of vital importance in surgery (whether it is amputation or limb salvage). (Note the onion-peel appearance.)

Table 28.6: Essential features of common bone tumours.

Tumour	Age (Years)	Common sites	Common Location	Clinical features	X-ray picture	Differential diagnosis	Pathology	Treatment
Osteosarcoma	15–25	Lower end of femur, upper end of tibia	Metaphysis	Pain ++ Swelling ++ Duration is weeks–months	Sun-ray appearance, Codman's triangle, tumour new bone +	Ewing's tumour	Tumour cells with osteoid or bone formation Alkaline phosphatase increased in 50% cases	Local ablation+ Chemotherapy
Ewing's tumour*	10–20	Femur, tibia flat bones*, multi-centric**	Diaphysis	Pain ++ Swelling+ Often fever+ Duration is weeks–months	Onion-peel appearance	Osteosarcoma Osteomyelitis	Sheaths of round cells	Radiotherapy + Chemotherapy
Osteoclastoma	20–40	Lower femur Upper tibia Lower radius	Epiphysis region	Pain + Swelling + Duration–mths	Soap bubble appearance No tumour new bone	Aneurysmal bone cyst, rarely ostesarcoma	Multinucleate giant cells in fibrous stroma	Excision of tumour + Reconstruction
Chondrosarcoma	30–60	Flat bones, upper end of femur	Anywhere in the bone	Pain + Swelling +++ Duration is months–Years	Mottled calcification within the tumour with lytic areas	Osteosarcoma	Chondroblasts and cartilaginous matrix	Local ablation + Radiotherapy

* Ewing's tumour is the most common malignant tumour of flat bones.
** Ewing's tumour is the most common sarcoma of bone tumour which has multicentric origin.

may resemble a soft tissue sarcoma. In flat bones, it is primarily a lytic lesion with hardly any new bone formation.

Differential diagnosis: Ewing's sarcoma can be differentiated from other bone tumours by features given in Table 28.6. From chronic osteomyelitis, it can be differentiated by the following features in the former:

• Sequestrum
• Well-defined cloacae and a rather smooth periosteal reaction
• Located at metaphysis

Treatment: Treatment consists of multi-agent chemotherapy and local control. Chemotherapy consists of a combination of Vincristine, Adriamycin, Cisplatin alternating with Ifosfamide and Etoposide, in 14 cycles spread over 9- 10 months. Local control is done about 3 months after starting chemotherapy, and consists of limb salvage surgery (preferred), or radiotherapy or both. Ewing's sarcoma differs from osteosarcoma in that it is a highly *radio-sensitive* tumour.

Prognosis: With the available treatment, the five-year survival (and cure) is to the tune of 70 per cent, in cases where metastases have not happened.

MULTIPLE MYELOMA

It is a malignant neoplasm derived from plasma cells.

Pathology: The neoplasm characteristically affects flat bones, i.e., the pelvis, vertebrae, skull, and ribs. It may occur as a solitary lesion (plasmacytoma), multiple lesion (multiple myeloma), extramedullary myelomatosis or diffuse myelomatosis. The lesions are mostly small and circumscribed. The bone is simply replaced by tumour tissue and there is *no reactive new bone formation.*

Grossly, the tumour is soft, grey and friable. Microscopically, it consists of sheets of closely packed cells. Typically, the tumour cells have an eccentric nucleus with clumped chromatin.

Clinical features: The tumour usually affects adults above 40 years of age. Men are affected more often than women. Usual presentation is that of multiple site involvement. Common presenting complaint is increasingly severe pain in the lumbar and thoracic spine. *Pathological fractures,* especially of the vertebrae and ribs may result in acute symptoms. The patient is weak, and will have loss of weight. *Neurological symptoms* may result if the tumour presses on the spinal cord or the nerves in the spinal canal. There is local tenderness over the affected bones. There may be no swelling or deformity unless a pathological fracture occurs.

Investigations: Following investigations prove helpful:
• **Radiological examination:** Characteristic radiological features are as follows (Fig. 28.6):
  ▪ Multiple *punched out lesions* in the skull and other flat bones.
  ▪ Pathological *wedge collapse* of the vertebra, usually more than one, commonly in the thoracic spine. The pedicles are usually spared.
  ▪ Diffuse, severe rarefaction of bones (hence commonly confused with postmenopasual or senile ostepororsis).
  ▪ Erosions of the borders of the ribs.
• **Other investigations** carried out to support the diagnosis of multiple myeloma are as follows:
  ▪ *Blood:* Low haemoglobin, high ESR (usually very high), increased total protein, albumin/

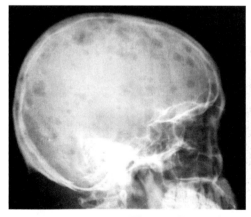
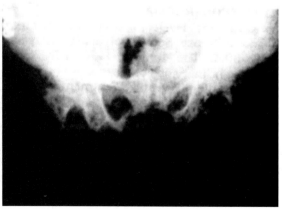

Fig. 28.6: X-rays showing features of multiple myeloma.

globulin (A/G) ratio reversed, increased serum calcium, normal alkaline phosphatase.

- *Urine:* Bence Jones proteins are found in 30 per cent of cases.
- *Serum electrophoresis:* Abnormal spike in the region of gamma globulin (myeloma spike) is present in 90 per cent of cases.
- *Sternal puncture:* Myeloma cells may be seen.
- *Bone biopsy* from the iliac crest, or a CT guided needle biopsy from the vertebral lesion may show features suggestive of multiple myeloma.
- *Skeletal survey*: A skeletal survey is a good modality to determine muticentricity.
- *Bone scan/PET Scan:* One of these may be required in cases presenting as solitary bone lesion, where lesions at other sites may be detected. There may be false-negative lesions on bone scan.
- *Biopsy:* A core needle or open biopsy from the lesion may sometimes be required to confirm the diagnosis.

Treatment: It consists of control of the tumour by chemotherapy, and splintage to the diseased part by PoP, brace, etc. Radiotherapy plays a useful role in cases with neurological compression, localised painful lesions, fractures and soft tissue masses. Complications like pathological fractures must be prevented by splinting the affected part. Treatment of a pathological fracture can be done by conservative or operative methods as discussed in Chapter 1.

Chemotherapy: The mainstay of treatment of myeloma is medical management, consisting of triple-drug regimen of Bortezomib (a targeted therapy, first line therapy), steroids, Lenalidomide, or Cyclophosphamide. Many a time, a bone marrow transplant may be required.

SOME UNCOMMON MALIGNANT TUMOURS

CHONDROSARCOMA

This is a malignant bone tumour arising from cartilage cells. It may arise in hitherto normal bone (primary chondrosarcoma), or in a pre-existing cartilaginous tumour such as enchondroma (secondary chondrosarcoma). It may arise in any bone but is common in flat bones such as scapula, pelvis and ribs.

Diagnosis: It occurs commonly in adults between 30-60 years of age, and is rare in children. The tumour has a wide spectrum of aggressiveness; from low-grade malignant to highly malignant. Metastasis occurs through the blood vessels, commonly to the

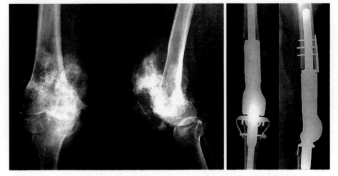

Fig. 28.7: X-ray showing chondrosarcoma of the femur (Note mottled calcification).

lungs. Presenting symptoms are pain and swelling, often of long duration. X-ray shows erosion of the cortex and bone destruction. The tumour matrix may have mottled calcification (as rings, arcs or 'popcorn' calcification) typical of a cartilaginous tumour (Fig. 28.7). This is much different to 'cloudy' or 'cotton wool' osteoid seen in osteosarcoma). Diagnosis is confirmed by a biopsy.

Treatment: Conventional chondrosarcoma are chemo and radio resistant tumours. Wide surgical removal is the only treatment. This is usually achievable by a limb-salvage surgery. An amputation is only rarely required, depending upon the behavior of the tumour. Prognosis depends upon the grade of chondrosarcoma. Role of chemotherapy and radiation therapy is only in the mesenchymal and de-differentiated types of chondrosarcoma.

SYNOVIAL SARCOMA

This is a malignant tumour, histologically a combination of synovial cells and fibroblasts. It occurs *most commonly* around the knee. It may not necessarily originate from the synovial membrane. More often than not, it is extra-articular in origin. The tumour spreads via the blood vessels, lymphatics, and along the soft tissue planes.

Treatment is by amputation, as for other bone malignancies. Prognosis is poor.

RETICULUM CELL SARCOMA

This is a tumour arising from the marrow reticulum cells. It has a clinical and pathological resemblance to Ewing's tumour, but different behaviour. It has a more favourable prognosis. Long bones are commonly affected, but it also occurs in flat bones. The most common age group affected is 20-50 years, and males are affected more commonly. Overall, it has a slow rate of growth and metastasises late. Pathological fractures occur commonly.

METASTASIS IN BONE

Metastatic tumours in the bone are *more common* than the primary bone tumours. The tumours most commonly metastatising to bone are carcinoma of the lung in the male and carcinoma of the breast in the female. Other malignancies metastasising to the bone are carcinoma of prostrate, carcinoma of thyroid, etc.

CLINICAL FEATURES

A patient with secondaries in the bone may present in the following ways:

a. It may be a patient with *known primary* malignancy, who presents with symptoms suggestive of secondaries in the bone. These symptoms are: (i) bone pain – in the spine (most common site), ribs or extremities; and (i) pathological fracture – commonly in the spine, proximal femur and humerus..

b. It may be a patient, *not a known case of primary* malignancy, who presents with: (i) bone pain, which on subsequent investigations is found to be due to a destructive lesion in the bone; or (ii) a pathological fracture through an area of bone weakened by such a lesion. On further investigations the lesion is found to be a secondary from somewhere else. All patients above 40 years of age presenting with a new bony lesion are much more likely to have metastasis or myeloma than a primary bone tumor.

Malignancies which are known to present first time with secondaries (with silent primary) are carcinoma of thyroid, renal cell carcinoma, carcinoma of the bladder, etc.

INVESTIGATIONS

A case of secondaries in the bone can be investigated as follows:

a. In a case *with known primary,* a complaint of bone pain may be due to metastatic lesion of the bone. On plain X-rays, 20-25 per cent or more of metastatic deposits are missed. Hence, in a case where bone secondaries are suspected, a bone scan should be performed (Fig. 28.8). This also helps in evaluating the extent of spread of metastasis in bones. PET scan is the most recent imaging modality for early detection of metastasis, with the advantage of picking up the primary malignancy (breast/lung, etc.) as well as extra-skeletal metastases (lung/liver, etc).

b. In a *case presenting first time* with bony secondaries, a systematic investigation programme is required to detect the primary. In spite of the best efforts, it is not possible to detect the primary in 10 per

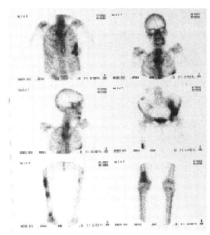

Fig. 28.8: Bone scan of a patient suspected of secondaries in the bone.

cent of cases. After a detailed history and systemic examination, the following investigations may be carried out:

- **Radiological examination:** Majority of bone secondaries are osteolytic, but a few are osteoblastic. Carcinoma of the prostate in males and carcinoma of the breast in females are the most common tumours to give rise to sclerotic secondaries in the bone. Vertebral bodies are affected most frequently. Other common sites are the ribs, pelvis, humerus and femur. Secondaries in bone are uncommon distal to the elbow and knee.

- **Blood:** A high ESR, and an elevated serum calcium are indications of bony secondaries in a suspected case. Other tests may be positive, depending upon the nature of the primary, e.g., elevated serum acid phosphatase in prostatic malignancy.

- **Other investigations:** These depend upon the site suspected on clinical examination. In a secondary without a known primary, useful investigations are an abdominal ultrasound, Barium studies, IVP, thyroid scan, etc. In patients with unknown primary, relevant imaging which may include a mammogram/X-ray or CT of chest/USG or CT of abdomen or a whole body PET CT, may be done, as the case may be.

Treatment: It consists of symptomatic relief of pain, prevention of any pathological fracture, and control of secondaries by chemotherapy or radiotherapy, depending upon the nature of the primary tumour. Role of surgery is limited, mostly to the management of pathological fractures. The aim of treatment is providing pain relief and mobility to enable the pateint to have a dignified life.

TUMOUR-LIKE CONDITIONS OF THE BONE

OSTEOCHONDROMA

This is the most common benign 'tumour' of the bone. It is not a true neoplasm since its growth stops with cessation of growth at the epiphyseal plate. It is a result of an aberration at the growth plate, where a few cells from the plate grow centrifugally as a separate lump of bone. Though the tumour originates at the growth plate, it gets 'left behind' as the bone grows in length, and thus comes to lie at the metaphysis. The stalk and part of the head of the tumour are made up of mature bone, but the tip is covered with cartilage.

Clinical presentation: The patient, usually around adolescence, presents with a painless swelling around a joint, usually around the knee. There may be similar swellings in other parts of the body in case of multiple exostosis (see page 308).

Examination: The swelling has all the features of a benign bony swelling. Usual location is metaphyseal, but often it comes to lie as far as the diaphysis. It may be a sessile or pedunculated swelling. There may be signs suggestive of complications secondary to the swelling. These are: (i) pain due to bursitis at the tip of the swelling or due to fracture of the exostosis; (ii) signs due to compression of the neurovascular bundle of the limb; (iii) limitation of joint movements due to mechanical block by the swelling and (iv) a fracture of the ostoechondroma. Occasionally, the tumour undergoes malignant transformation (chondrosarcoma). A rapid increase in the size of the tumour (particularly after skeletal maturity) and appearance of pain in a hitherto painless swelling may be suggestive of malignant transformation. *Diagnosis* is made on X-ray where one can see a bony growth made up of mature cortical bone and marrow, with a continuity between the medullary canals of the long bone and the bony growth (Fig. 28.9). The cartilage cap is not visible on the X-ray.

Treatment: When necessary because of symptoms, the tumour should be excised. The excision includes the periosteum over the exostosis; since leaving it may result in leaving a few cartilage cells, which will grow again and cause recurrence of the swelling. It is preferable to delay this excision till skeletal maturity.

ENCHONDROMA

This is a benign tumour consisting of a lobulated mass of cartilage encapsulated by fibrous tissue. Frequently the fibrous septae dividing the lobules are calcified. The tumour is seen commonly between the ages of 20–30 years. Small bones of the hands and feet are

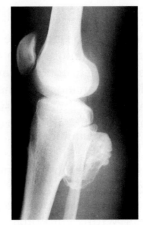

Fig. 28.9: X-ray of knee, lateral view, showing osteochondroma from upper end of tibia.

commonly affected. The presenting complaint is a long-standing swelling from one or more phalanges or metacarpals, without much pain. The swelling increases in size very slowly, often totally replacing the bone. An X-ray shows expanding lytic lesions in one or more bones (Fig. 28.10). Overlying cortices are thinned out. The tumour matrix has stippled calcification.

Treatment: An unsightly appearance or a fracture through the lesion is generally the indication for treatment. The lesion is curetted thoroughly, and the cavity, if it is big, is filled with bone grafts. Prognosis is good. Although, chondromas in small bones are not known to undergo malignant change, those in the long bones should be carefully evaluated and differentiated from a low-grade chondrosarcoma.

Uncommon presentations of enchondromas (Ollier's disease): This is a non-hereditary disorder seen in childhood. In this, masses of unossified cartilage persist within the metaphysis of some long bones, usually multiple. Growth at the adjacent epiphyseal plates may be affected, leading to shortening and deformities.

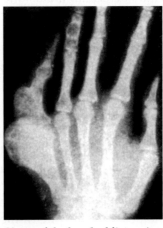

Fig. 28.10: X-ray of the hand, oblique view, showing enchondromas of the hand bones.

Maffucci syndrome: This is a hereditary disorder where multiple enchondromas and cavernous haemangiomas occur together.

SIMPLE BONE CYST

This is the only *true cyst* of the bone, different from other lesions, which though appear clear 'cyst-like' on X-ray, are actually osteolytic, sometimes solid lesions. Its etiology is not known. Pathologically, it is a cavity in the bone lined by thin membrane, and contains serous or serosanguinous yellow-coloured fluid.

Diagnosis: It occurs in children and adolescents. The ends of the long bones are the favourite sites; the *most common* being the upper-end of the humerus. The cyst itself may not produce many symptoms, and attention is brought to it by a pathological fracture through it. X-rays show a well-defined, lobulated, radiolucent zone in the metaphysis or diaphysis of a bone (Fig. 28.11A). Maximum width of the lesion is less than the width of the epiphyseal plate. The characteristic 'fallen leaf sign' may be seen on the X-ray after a fracture. A lesion close to the epiphyseal plate is considered *'active'*, as against the one away from it - say in the diaphysis.

The other common cyst of the bone with which this lesion often needs to be differentiated is the aneurysmal bone cyst (Fig. 28.11B). It also needs to be differentiated from other causes of a solitary cystic lesion in a bone as discussed in Table 28.2.

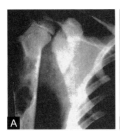 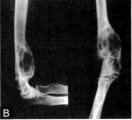

Simple bone cyst　　Aneurysmal bone cyst
Fig. 28.11: X-rays showing bone cysts.

Treatment: The cyst is known to undergo spontaneous healing, particularly after a fracture. One or two injections of methylprednisolone into the cyst results in healing. In some cases, particularly when the cyst is in weight-bearing bones or in cases where recurrence has occurred, curettage and bone grafting may be required.

ANEURYSMAL BONE CYST

This is a benign bone lesion occurring in wide age group, and affects almost any bone. It consists of a blood-filled space enclosed in a shell, ballooning up the overlying cortex – hence its name.

Diagnosis: It is common between 10-40 years of age. Common sites are the long bones, usually at their ends. A gradually increasing swelling is the predominant presentation. There is little pain. Often it presents with a pathological fracture. Typical radiological features are as follows (Fig. 28.11B):
* Eccentric well-defined radiolucent area.
* Expansion of the overlying cortex.
* Trabeculation within the substance of the tumour.

Treatment is by intralesional sclerotherapy or curettage and bone grafting. Recurrence occurs in 25 per cent cases.

FIBROUS DYSPLASIA (FIG. 28.12)

This is a disorder in which the normal bone is replaced by fibrous tissue – hence its name. The mass of fibrous tissue thus formed grows inside the bone and erodes the cortices of the bone from within. A thin layer of subperiosteal bone forms around the mass, so that the bone appears expanded.

CLINICAL FEATURES

It may affect only one bone (monostotic), or many bones (polyostotic). Often in the polyostotic variety, the bones of a single limb are affected. A polyostotic fibrous dysplasia in girls may have precocious puberty and cutaneous pigmentation (Albright's syndrome). The disease commonly occurs in children and adolescents. Pain, deformity and pathological fracture are the common presenting symptoms. The bones commonly affected are the upper-ends of femur and tibia, and ribs.

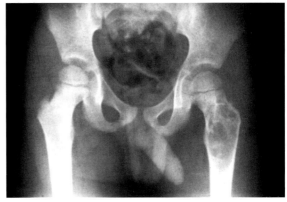

Fig. 28.12: X-rays of the pelvis showing fibrous dysplasia of upper end of the femur. (Note multiloculated lesion).

Radiologically, the affected bone shows translucent to 'ground-glass' appearance. The lesion is usually multi-loculated, expanding the cortex of the bone. Serum alkaline phosphatase is often elevated. Diagnosis is confirmed by biopsy.

Treatment depends upon the location of the lesion. In most weight-bearing bones, due to risk of pathological fracture, it is advisable to do curettage and bone grafting. In other, not so approachable locations and also in non-weight bearing bones, they can be left.

Common sites of primary bone tumours is as depicted in Figure 28.13.

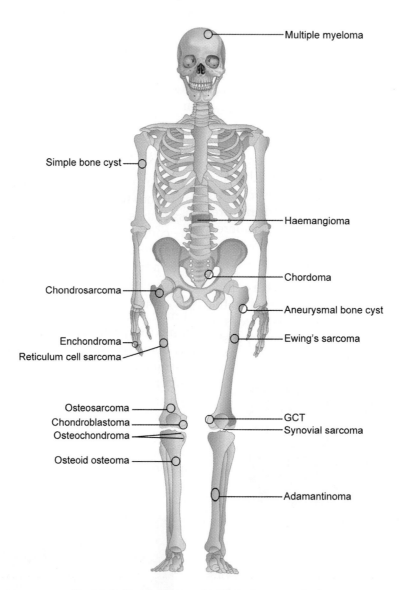

Fig. 28.13: Common sites of indiviual tumours in the human skeleton.

What have we learnt?

- Primary malignant bone tumours occur in children.
- Knee is the most common site of primary bone tumours.
- GCT is a locally agressive tumour, sometimes metastatising.
- Secondaries in the bone is a common cause of pathological fractures.
- Limb salvage, rather than amputation is the aim of modern bone tumour surgery.

Additional information: From the entrance exams point of view

Most common sites of primary bone tumours

Tumour	Site
Chondroblastoma	Epiphyseal (most common tumour in this region before puberty)
Gaint-cell tumour	Epiphyseal (most common tumour in this region after puberty)
Chondrosarcoma, osteochondroma,	Metaphyseal bone cyst, enchondroma, osteosarcoma
Gaint-cell tumour	
Ewing's tumour, lymphoma, multiple myleloma, adamantinoma, osteoid osteoma diaphyseal	

Most common sites of tumour and tumour-like lesions

Lesion	Site
Solitary bone cyst	Upper end of humerus
Aneurysmal bone cyst	Lower limb metaphysis
Osteochondroma	Distal femur
Osteoid osteoma	Neck of femur
Osteoblastoma	Vertebrae
Osteoma	Skull, facial bones
Enchondroma	Short bones of hand
Chordoma	Sacrum
Adamantinoma	Tibia
Ameloblastoma	Mandible
Fibrous dysplasia	Polyostotic—craniofacial
	Monostotic—upper femur
Multiple myeloma	Lumbar vertebrae
Osteosarcoma	Lower end femur
Ewing's sarcoma	Femur
Chondrosarcoma	Pelvis
Secondary tumours	Dorsal vertebrae

Tumour type and appearance

Tumour	Appearance
Fibrous dysplasia	Ground glass
Chondrogenic tumours	Patchy calcification
Osteogenic tumours	Homogenous calcification
Unicameral bone cyst	Fallen leaf sign

Prolapsed Intervertebral Disc

Learning Objectives

❖ Discuss the etiology, pathoanatomy clinical features and management of a case of prolapsed inter-vertebral disc.

RELEVANT ANATOMY

The intervertebral disc consists of three distinct components—the cartilage end-plates, nucleus pulposus and annulus fibrosus. The cartilage plates are thin layers of hyaline cartilage between adjacent vertebral bodies and the disc proper (Fig. 29.1). The disc receives its nutrition from the vertebral bodies via these end-plates, by diffusion.

The *nucleus pulposus* is a gelatinous material which lies a little posterior to the central axis of the vertebrae. It is enclosed in *annulus fibrosus*, a structure composed of concentric rings of fibro-cartilaginous tissue. The nucleus pulposus is normally under considerable pressure and is restrained by the crucible-like annulus. The posterior longitudinal ligament is a strap-like ligament at the back of the vertebral bodies and discs.

PATHOLOGY

The term 'prolapsed disc' means the protrusion or extrusion of the nucleus pulposus through a rent in the annulus fibrosus. It is not one-time phenomenon;

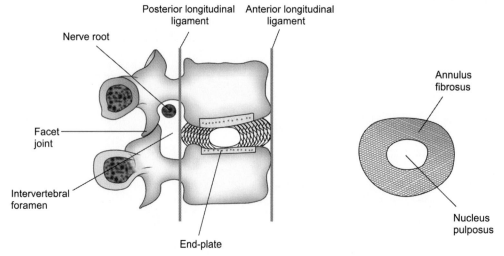

Fig. 29.1: Intervertebral disc and related structures.

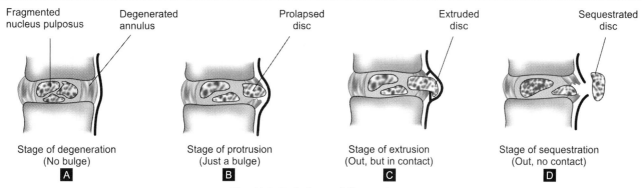

Fig. 29.2: Pathology of disc prolapse.

rather it is a sequence of changes in the disc, which ultimately lead to its prolapse. These changes consist of the following:

a. **Nucleus degeneration:** Degenerative changes occur in the disc before displacement of the nuclear material. These changes are: (i) softening of the nucleus and its fragmentation; and (ii) weakening and disintegration of the posterior part of the annulus (Fig. 29.2A).

b. **Nucleus displacement:** The nucleus is under positive pressure at all times. When the annulus becomes weak, either because a small area of its entire thickness has disintegrated spontaneously or because of injury, the nucleus tends to bulge through the defect (Fig. 29.2B). This is called *disc protrusion.* This tendency is greatly increased if the nucleus is degenerated and fragmented. Finally, the nucleus comes out of the annulus and lies under the posterior longitudinal ligament; though it has not lost contact with the parent disc. This is called *disc extrusion* (Fig. 29.2C). Once extruded, the disc does not go back. The posterior longitudinal ligament is not strong enough to prevent the nucleus from protruding further. The extruded disc may loose its contact with the parent disc, when it is called *sequestrated disc* (Fig. 29.2D). The sequestrated disc may come to lie behind the posterior longitudinal ligament or may become free fragment in the canal.

c. **Stage of fibrosis:** This is the stage of repair. This begins alongside of degeneration. The residual nucleus pulposus becomes fibrosed. The extruded nucleus pulposus becomes flattened, fibrosed and finally undergoes calcification. At the same time, new bone formation occurs at the points where the posterior longitudinal ligament has been stripped from the vertebral body and spur formation occurs.

The *site of exit* of the nucleus is usually posterolateral (Fig. 29.3) on one or the other side. Occasionally, it can be central (posterior-midline) disc prolapse. The *type* of nuclear protrusion may be—a protrusion, an extrusion or a sequestration. A dissecting extrusion (an extrusion with disc material between the body of the vertebra and posterior longitudinal ligament, stripping the latter off the body), may occur. The *most common level* of disc prolapse is between L_4-L_5 in the lumbar spine and C_5-C_6 in the cervical spine. In the lumbar spine, it is uncommon above L_3–L_4 level.

Secondary changes associated with disc prolapse: As a consequence of disc prolapse, changes occur in the structures occupying the spinal canal and in the intervertebral joints. These are as follows:

a. **Changes in structures occupying spinal canal:**
   - Commonly, the unilateral protrusion is in contact with the spinal theca and *compresses one or more roots* in their extra-thecal course. Usually, a single root is affected. Sometimes, two roots on the same or opposite sides are affected. The nerve root affected is usually the one which leaves the spinal canal below the *next* vertebra. This is because the root at the level of the prolapsed disc leaves the canal in the upper-half of the foramen (Fig. 29.1). Thus, the nerve root affected in a disc prolapse between L_4-L_5 vertebrae is L_5, although it is the L_4 root which exits the canal at this level.

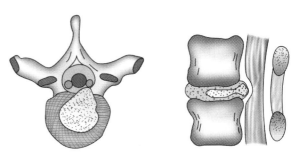

Fig. 29.3: Posterolateral disc prolapse.

■ *Pressure effects on the intra-thecal roots of* the cauda equina may occur by a sudden large disc protrusion in the spinal canal and may present as cauda equina syndrome. This is uncommon.

b. **Changes in the intervertebral joints:** With the loss of a part of the nucleus pulposus and its subsequent fibrosis, the height of the disc is reduced. This affects the articulation of the posterior facet joints. The incongruity of the facet articulation leads to degenerative arthritis.

DIAGNOSIS

The diagnosis is mainly clinical. Investigations like CT scan and MRI scan may be done to confirm the diagnosis, especially if surgery is being considered.

CLINICAL FEATURES

The patient is usually an adult between 20–40 years of age, with a sedentary lifestyle. The *most common* presenting symptom is low back pain with or without the pain radiating down the back of the leg (sciatica). A preceding history of trauma is present in some cases. In a few cases, there is a history of exertion such as having lifted something heavy or pushed something immediately preceding a sudden onset backache. The following symptoms are common:

- **Low backache:** The onset of backache may be acute or chronic. An acute backache is severe with the spine held rigid by muscle spasm, and any movement at the spine painful. The patient may be able to go about with difficulty. In extreme cases, he is completely incapacitated, any attempted movement producing severe pain and spasm. In chronic backache, the pain is dull and diffuse, usually made worse by exertion, forward bending, sitting or standing in one position for a long time. It is relieved by rest.

- **Sciatic pain:** This is usually associated with low back pain, but may be the sole presenting symptom. The pain radiates to the gluteal region, the back of the thigh and leg. The pattern of radiation depends upon the root compressed. In S_1 root compression, the pain radiates to the postero-lateral calf and heel. In L_5 root compression the pain radiates to the anterolateral aspect of the leg and ankle. In a disc prolapse at a higher level (L_2-L_3, etc.), the pain may radiate to the front of the thigh. Often the radiation may begin on walking, and is relieved on rest (neurological claudication).

- **Neurological symptoms:** Sometimes, the patient complains of paraesthesias, most often described as 'pins and needles' corresponding to the dermatome of the affected nerve root. There may be numbness in the leg or foot and weakness of the muscles. In cases with large disc material compressing the theca and roots, a cauda equina syndrome results, where the patient has irregular LMN type paralysis in the lower limbs, bilateral absent ankle jerks, with hypoaesthesia in the region of L_5 to S_4 dermatomes and urinary and bowel incontinence.

EXAMINATION

The back and limbs are examined with the patient undressed. The following observations are made:

- **Posture:** The patient stands with a rigid, flattened lumbar spine. The whole trunk is shifted forwards on the hips (Fig. 29.4). The trunk is tilted to one side (sciatic tilt or scoliosis). The sideways tilt tends to exaggerate on attempted bending forwards.

- **Movements:** The patient is unable to bend forwards; any such attempt initiates severe muscle spasm in the paraspinal muscles.

- **Tenderness:** There is diffuse tenderness in the lumbo-sacral region. A localised tenderness in the midline or lateral to the spinous process is found in some cases.

- **Straight leg raising test (SLRT):** This test indicates nerve root compression (details in Annexure I). A positive SLRT at 40° or less is suggestive of root compression. More important is a positive contralateral SLRT.

- **Lasegue test:** This is a modification of SLRT where first the hip is lifted to 90° with the knee bent. The knee is then gradually extended by the examiner. If nerve stretch is present, it will not be possible to

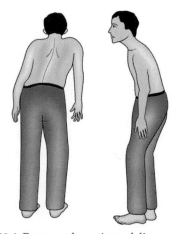

Fig. 29.4: Posture of a patient of disc prolapse.

Table 29.1: Neurological deficit in disc prolapse

Level	Nerve root affected	Motor weakness	Sensory loss	Reflexes
L_5-S_1	S_1 root	Weakness of plantar-flexors of the foot	Over lateral side of the foot	Ankle jerk sluggish or absent
L_4-L_5	L_5 root	Weakness of EHL* and dorsiflexors of the foot	Over dorsum of the foot and lateral side of the leg	Ankle jerk normal
L_3-L_4	L_4 root	Weakness of extensors of the knee	Over great toe and medial side of the leg	Knee jerk sluggish or absent

*EHL: Extensor hallucis longus

do so and the patient will experience pain in the back of the thigh or leg.

- **Neurological examination:** A careful neurological examination would reveal a motor weakness, sensory loss or loss of reflex corresponding to the affected nerve root. Of special importance is the examination of the muscles of the foot supplied by L_4, L_5 and S_1 roots, as these are the roots affected more commonly. The extensor hallucis longus muscle is *exclusively* supplied by L_5 root and its weakness is easily detected by asking the patient to dorsiflex the big toe against resistance. Sensory loss may merely be the blunting of sensation or hypoaesthesia in the dermatome of the affected root. Table 29.1 gives the neurological findings as a result of compression of different roots.

INVESTIGATIONS

Plain X-ray: It does not show any positive signs in a case of acute disc prolapse. X-rays are done basically to rule out bony pathology such as infection, etc. In a case of chronic disc prolapse, the affected disc space may be narrowed and there may be lipping of the vertebral margins posteriorly.

MRI scan: This is the investigation of choice. It shows the prolapsed disc, theca, nerve roots, etc., very clearly (Fig. 29.5). Normally, in an axial cut-section, the posterior border of a disc appears concave. In a case where there is disc prolapse, it will appear flat or convex. In the sagittal section upward and downward displacement of a prolapsed disc can be made out.

CT scan: This is done where facility for MRI is not there. The herniated disc material can be seen within the spinal canal, pressing on the nerve roots or theca.

Electromyography (EMG): Findings of denervation, localised to the distribution of a particular nerve root, helps in localising the offending disc in cases with multiple disc prolapse. This test is rarely required.

DIFFERENTIAL DIAGNOSIS

A prolapsed disc is a common cause of low backache, especially the backache associated with sciatic pain. One must be extremely cautious and avoid misdiagnosing other diseases that may mimic a disc prolapse. These include ankylosing spondylitis, vascular insufficiency, extra-dural tumour, spinal tuberculosis, etc. (see page 183).

TREATMENT

PRINCIPLES OF TREATMENT

Aim of treatment is to achieve remission of symptoms, mostly possible by conservative means. Cases who do not respond to conservative treatment for 3-6 weeks, and those presenting with cauda equina syndrome may require operative intervention.

CONSERVATIVE TREATMENT

This consists of the following:
- **Rest:** It is most important in the treatment of a prolapsed disc. Rest on a hard bed is necessary for not more than 2–4 days.
- **Drugs:** These consist mainly of analgesics and muscle relaxants.

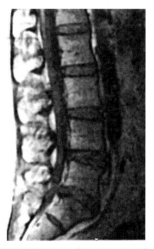

Fig. 29.5: MRI scan showing a L_5–S_1 disc.

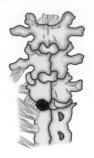
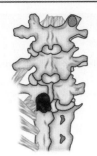
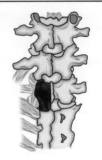
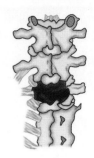

| Fenestration (ligamentum flavum excised) | Laminotomy (a border of lamina excised) | Hemilaminectomy (half of lamina excised) | Laminectomy (both laminae with spinous process excised) |

Fig. 29.6: Surgery for disc prolapse. (The shaded portion only is removed).

- **Physiotherapy:** This consists of hot fomentation, gentle arching exercises, etc.
- **Others:** These consist of lumbar traction, transcutaneous electrical nerve stimulation (TENS), etc.

OPERATIVE TREATMENT

Indications for operative treatment are: (i) failure of conservative treatment; (ii) cauda equina syndrome; and (iii) severe sciatic tilt. It consists of the following techniques:

- The **disc excision (Fig. 29.6):** Here the prolapsed or extruded part of the disc is removed by open surgery. Following are the techniques:
  - *Fenestration:* The ligamentum flavum bridging the two adjacent laminae is excised and the spinal canal at the affected level exposed.
  - *Laminotomy:* In addition to fenestration, a hole is made in the lamina for wider exposure.
  - *Hemilaminectomy:* The whole of the lamina on one side is removed.
  - *Laminectomy:* The laminae on both sides, with the spinous process, are removed. Such a wide exposure is required for a big, central disc producing cauda equina syndrome.
  - *Endoscopic discectomy:* This is a technique of disc excision where the disc is removed by using an endoscope. Fine endoscopic instruments or laser probes are inserted percutaneously through small stab wounds. It is a minimally invasive technique, and is gaining popularity. One requires adequate instrumentation and training to perform it.
- **Disc excision with spinal fusion:** In cases where the spine segment is already unstable, or is likely to become unstable with time, fusion of the affected segment is done at the same time as disc excision.
- **Disc replacement:** This is the latest technique in disc surgery, offered as an alternative to traditional surgery of disc excision. It is still not an established technique.

CERVICAL DISC PROLAPSE

Prolapse of the intervertebral disc in the cervical spine is much less common than it is in the lumbar spine. The disc between C_5-C_6 is the one affected most frequently. Postero-lateral protrusion is the most common. A typical patient presents with a vague history of injury to the neck, often a jerk or a twisting strain. Symptoms may begin hours after the episode of injury. The neck becomes stiff and the pain radiates down the shoulder to the outer aspect of the limb, up to the thumb. Paraesthesias may be felt in the hand. On examination, it may be possible to localise the neurological deficit to a particular nerve root, usually C_5. In some cases, there may be signs of cord compression from the front (UMN signs). X-rays do not show any abnormality. MRI scan is the imaging modality of choice but should be done if operative intervention is contemplated.

TREATMENT

There is a strong tendency to spontaneous recovery. Cases may present with signs of cord compression or root compression in the upper limb. Such cases may require surgery. The disc is exposed from the front and the material removed. Simultaneously, the affected segment is fused using bone graft and anterior plate.

What have we learnt?

- Disc prolapse is common at L_5–S_1.
- SLRT, particularly contralateral positive SLRT, is highly suggestive of disc prolapse.
- Treatment depends upon the stage of the disease.

Approach to a Patient with Back Pain

Learning Objectives

❖ Discuss approach to clinical diagnosis of a patient with low backache and its investigations.

LOW BACK PAIN

Back pain is an extremely common human phenomenon, a price mankind has to pay for their upright posture. According to one study, almost 80 per cent of persons in modern society will experience back pain at some time during their life. Fortunately, in 70 per cent of these, it subsides within a month. But, in as many as 70 per cent of these (in whom pain had subsided), the pain recurs.

CAUSES

Causes of back pain can be divided into: (a) specific, where the cause can be detected (Table 30.1); (b) non-specific, where no specific cause can be detected. Postural and non-specific work-related trauma, is the common reason. Amongst the whole list of specific causes of back pain, the most sinister are—tumour (metastasis), infection (tuberculosis) and trauma. Once these sinister causes are ruled out, rest are of less clinical significance. Back pain could be a feature of an extraspinal disease such as lumbar back pain due to kidney disease, low back pain due to gynaecological disease. A simple approach to a case with back pain is *to first focus on ruling out sinister causes*. For the rest,

a systematic approach to diagnosis and treatment can be adopted.

HISTORY

Age: Some diseases are more common at a particular age. *Back pain is uncommon in children, but if present, it is often due to some organic disease.* In adolescents, postural and traumatic (ligament and muscle injury) dominate the scene. In adults, spondyloarthropathy (SpA) and disc prolapse are common. SpA related back pain occurs across age group—from adolescent to early adulthood. In elderly persons, degenerative arthritis, osteoporosis and metastatic bone disease are usually the cause.

Sex: Back pain is more common in women, particularly after they have had pregnancy. This is due to excessive weight, lack of exercise leading to poor muscle tone, and nutritional deficiency (osteomalacia). In men, back pain, more often than not, is due to obesity and bad posture at work.

Occupation: A history regarding the patient's occupation may provide valuable clues to risk factors responsible for back pain. These are often not apparent to the patient, and could be a part

Table 30.1: Causes of low back pain.

Congenital causes
- Spina bifida
- Lumbar scoliosis
- Spondylolysis
- Spondylolisthesis
- Transitional vertebra
- Facet tropism

Traumatic causes
- Sprain, strain
- Vertebral fractures
- Prolapsed disc

Inflammatory causes
- Tuberculosis
- Ankylosing spondylitis
- Spondyloarthropathy (SpA)

Degenerative
- Osteoarthritis

Neoplastic
- Benign
  - Osteoid osteoma
  - Eosinophilic granuloma
- Malignant
  - Primary: Multiple myeloma, Lymphoma
  - Secondaries from other sites

Metabolic causes
- Osteoporosis
- Osteomalacia

Pain referred from viscera
- Genitourinary diseases
- Gynaecological diseases

Miscellaneous causes
- Functional back pain
- Postural back pain
  - Protuberant abdomen
  - Occupational bad posture
  - Habitual bad posture

infection and trauma occur in the dorso-lumbar spine. Postural back pain is often in the upper back.

- **Onset:** Often, there is a history of significant trauma immediately preceding an episode of back pain, and may indicate a traumatic pathology. At times the trauma happens to be a precipitating factor, and there may be underlying non-traumatic pathology. History of trauma may be there in about 40 per cent cases of disc prolapse. In most, it may be subtle trauma, resulting from a routine activity such as bending to pull something out of a drawer. Careful questioning regarding leisure activities and exercise is important because inconsistency in activity levels during work and leisure time can precipitate back pain.
- **Localisation of pain:** Pain arising from a tendon or muscle injury is localised, whereas that originating from deeper structure is diffuse. Often, pain is referred to the lower limb (*sciatica*), with associated neurological signs (numbness tingling) pertaining to a particular dermatome. This is a pointer to nerve root entrapment.
- **Progress of the pain (Fig. 30.1):** In traumatic conditions, or in acute disc prolapse, pain is maximum at the onset, and then gradually subsides over days or weeks. Back pain due to disc prolapse often has periods of remissions and exacerbations. Pain due to infection or tumour takes a progressive course, with nothing causing relief.
- **Relieving and aggravating factors:** Most back pains are worsened by activity and relieved by

of his 'routine'. People in sedentary jobs are more vulnerable to back pain than those whose work involves varied activities. Back pain is common in surgeons, dentists, computer professionals, manual workers, truck drivers, etc.

Past history: A past history of having suffered from a spinal disease such as a traumatic or inflammatory disease may point to that as the possible cause of back pain.

Features of pain: The following features are to be noted:
- **Location:** Pain may be located in the lower, middle or upper back. Disc prolapse and degenerative spondylitis occur in the lower lumbar spine;

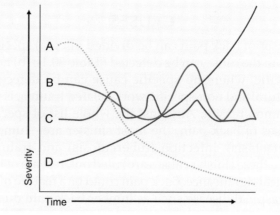

Fig. 30.1: Progression of back pain due to different etiologies: A. Traumatic, B. Disc prolapse, C. Osteoarthritis. D. Tumour/Inflammation.

rest. All back pains which have inflammatory component are worse in the morning and get better with activities (SpA, for example), and those of mechanical nature, become worse after a period of activity and get better with rest (postural, for example). Severe back pain at night that responds to a tablet of aspirin may typically be due to a benign bone tumour. Back pain with radiation, initiated on walking or standing for long, and relieved by rest, is a feature of spinal stenosis. An increase in pain during menstruation may indicate a gynaecological pathology.

Associated symptoms: The following associated symptoms may point to the cause of back pain:
- **Stiffness:** It is associated with most painful backs, but it is a prominent symptom in pain due to spondarthritis, more so early in the morning. There may be an associated limitation of chest expansion.
- **Pain in other joints:** In some rheumatic diseases (SpA), back pain may be the presenting feature, but on detailed questioning one may get a history of pain and swelling of a few more joints or pain at attachment of tendons to bone (enthesopathy). These points towards systemic disease as cause of back pain.
- **Neurological symptoms:** Symptoms such as paraesthesias, numbness or weakness may point to a lesion of the nervous tissue, or a lesion in close proximity to it (e.g., a disc prolapse).
- **Extra-skeletal symptoms:** A history suggestive of abdominal complaints, urogenital complaints, or gynaecological complaints may indicate an extra-skeletal cause of back pain.

- **Mental status** of the patient must be judged to rule out any psychological cause of back pain (hysteria, malingering, etc.). A patient suffering from an organic disease may have an significant overlay of psychological factors.

PHYSICAL EXAMINATION

The patient should be stripped except undergarments, and examined in the standing and lying down positions:

Standing position: The following observations are made in the standing position:
- **Position:** Normally a person stands erect with the centre of the occiput in the line with the natal cleft (Fig. 30.2), the two shoulders are at the same level, the lumbar hollows are symmetrical and the pelvis is 'square'. In a case with back pain, look for scoliosis, kyphosis, lordosis, pelvic tilt and forward flexion of the torso on the lower limbs. A minor scoliosis is often picked up like this.
- **Spasm:** Muscle spasm may be present in acute back pain and can be discerned by the prominence of the para-vertebral muscles at rest, which stand out on slightest movement.
- **Tenderness:** Localised tenderness may indicate ligament or muscle tear. There may be trigger points or tender nodules in cases of fibrositis. Pain originating from the sacro-iliac joint may have tenderness localised to the posterior superior iliac spine. Tenderness localized to dorso-lumbar spine is an important physical finding as that is the common site of sinister etiologies.

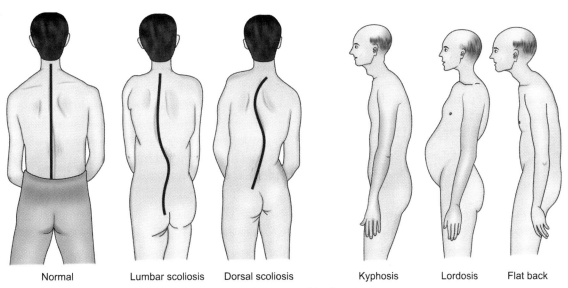

| Normal | Lumbar scoliosis | Dorsal scoliosis | Kyphosis | Lordosis | Flat back |

Fig. 30.2: Posture and back pain.

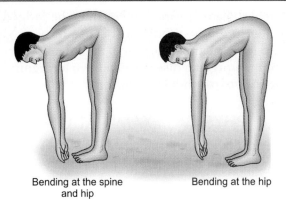

Bending at the spine
and hip

Bending at the hip

Fig. 30.3: Bending forwards.

- **Swelling:** A cold abscess may be present, indicating tuberculosis as the cause.
- **Range of movement:** There is limitation of movement in organic diseases of the spine. One must carefully differentiate spinal movements from the patient's ability to bend at the hips (Fig. 30.3).

Lying down position: In the supine position the following observations are made:
- **Straight leg raising test (SLRT):** This is a test to detect nerve root compression (Annexure I).
- **Neurological examination:** Sensation, motor power and reflexes of the lower limb are examined. This helps in localising the site of spine pathology.
- **Peripheral pulses:** The peripheral pulses should be palpated to detect a vascular cause of low back pain, which may be due to vascular claudication. The skin temperature in the affected leg may be lower.
- **Adjacent joints:** Often, the pain originates from the hip joints or the sacro-iliac joints, hence these should be examined routinely.
- **Abdominal, rectal or per vaginal examination** may be done wherever necessary. Chest expansion should be measured in young adults with back pain.

INVESTIGATIONS

The diagnosis of back pain is essentially clinical. It is conventional, not to get X-rays done in an acute back pain of less than 3 weeks duration. This is because 70% of these subside with rest, as getting X-rays done does not affect decision. On the contrary, X-ray examination is a must for back pain lasting more than 3 weeks; it being almost an extension of the clinical examination. There are a number of other investigations such as MRI scan and some blood investigations.

Radiological examination: Routine X-rays of the lumbo-sacral spine (AP and lateral) and pelvis (AP) should be done in all cases. These are useful in diagnosing metabolic, inflammatory and neoplastic conditions. Though, X-rays are usually normal in non-specific back pain, these provide a baseline.

MRI scan has become a go to modality for evaluation of a backache. It delineates soft tissues extremely well.

Blood investigations: These should be carried out if one suspects malignancy, metabolic disorders, or chronic infection (please refer to their respective Chapters for details).

Electromyography: If nerve root compression is a possibility, electromyography (EMG) may be appropriate (please refer to page 69).

TREATMENT

Principles of treatment: For specific pathologies, treatment is discussed in respective chapters. Most back pains falling in the 'non-specific' category have a set programme of treatment, mostly conservative. It consists of rest, drugs, hot packs, spinal exercises, traction, corset and education regarding the prevention of back pain.
- **Rest:** In the acute phase, absolute bed rest on a hard bed (a mattress is allowed) is advised. Bed rest for more than 2-3 weeks is of no use; rather, a gradual mobilisation using aids like brace is preferred.
- **Drugs:** Mainly analgesic—anti-inflammatory drugs are required. In cases with a stiff spine, muscle relaxants are advised.
- **Physiotherapy:** This consists of heat therapy (hot packs, short-wave diathermy, ultrasonic wave, etc.). Gradually, a spinal exercises programme is started.
- **Traction:** It is given to a patient with back pain with lot of muscle spasm. It also sometimes help in 'forcing' the patient to rest in the bed.
- **Use of corset:** This is used as a temporary measure in treating acute back pain, in back pain due to lumbar spondylosis, etc.
- **Education:** Patients must be taught what they can do to alleviate the pain and to avoid injury or re-injury to the back. This includes education to avoid straining the back in activities of daily living such as sitting, standing, lifting weight, etc. 'Back Schools' are formalised approach to this education.

MAJOR CAUSES OF LOW BACK PAIN
CONGENITAL DISORDERS

Spina bifida (see page 230 also): This and other minor congenital anomalies of the spine are present in about half the population, but are not necessarily the cause of back pain. Therefore, other pathological conditions should be ruled out before diagnosing this as the cause of symptoms. Treatment is as for non-specific back pain.

Transitional vertebrae: A transitional vertebra is the one at the junction of two segments of the spine, so that the characteristics of both segments is present in one vertebra. It is common in the lumbo-sacral region, either as lumbarisation (S_1 becoming L_6) or sacralisation (L_5 fused with the sacrum, either completely or partially).

TRAUMATIC DISORDERS

Back strain (acute or chronic): The terms back strain and back sprain are often used interchangeably. Most often this arises from a 'trauma' sustained in daily routine activities rather than from a definite injury. People prone to back strain are athletes, tall and thin people, those in a job requiring standing for long hours and those working in bad postures. Sedentary workers and women after pregnancy are also frequent candidates for back strain. Acute ligament sprain may occur while lifting a heavy weight, sudden straightening from bent position, pushing, etc. Treatment is 'non-specific' as discussed earlier.

Compression fractures: These fractures occur commonly in the thoraco-lumbar region (see page 260–261). Treatment depends upon the severity of compression. It is important to be suspicious of any underlying pathology. Diseases such as early secondary deposits in an elderly, may produce a fracture spontaneously, in one or multiple vertebrae.

INFLAMMATORY DISORDERS

Tuberculosis: Spinal tuberculosis is a common cause of persistent back pain, especially in undernourished people living in unhygienic conditions. Early diagnosis and treatment is crucial for complete recovery (details on page 183).

Ankylosing spondylitis: This should be suspected in a *young male* presenting with back pain and stiffness. Symptoms are *worst in the morning* and are relieved on walking about. Spinal movements may be markedly limited along with limitation of chest expansion.

DEGENERATIVE DISORDERS

Osteoarthritis: See page 290–292.

Prolapsed disc: See Chapter 29.

Spinal stenosis: Narrowing of the spinal canal may occur in the whole of the lumbar spine (e.g., achondroplasia), or more often, in a segment of the

Table 30.2: Differentiating between vascular and neurological claudication.

Features	Vascular claudication	Neurogenic claudication
Peripheral pulses	Absent	Present
Standing	No effect	Patient has to rest
Walking	No effect	Patient has to rest
Cycling	Reproduces pain	No effect
Pain at rest	Present	Absent
Pain relieved by	Stopping activity	Stooping forwards

spine (commonly in the lumbo-sacral region). Stenosis may be in all parts of the canal or only in the lateral part; the latter is called as root canal stenosis. It may give rise to pressure or tension on the nerves of the cauda equina or lumbar nerve roots. Typically, the patient complains of pain radiating down the lower limbs on walking some distance. The same is relieved on taking rest for a few minutes. The other reason for claudication is vascular compromise to the limb. Table 30.2 shows differentiating features between neurogenic and vascular claudication. Diagnosis of canal stenosis is confirmed on MRI. Treatment is by decompression of the spinal canal or root canal, as the case may be.

TUMOURS

Both benign and malignant tumours occur in the spine and the spinal canal. Tumours of the spinal canal, usually benign, are classified as extradural or intradural; the latter can be either intra-medullary or extra-medullary. These tumours are usually diagnosed on myelogram or CT scan. Tumours of the spine are mostly malignant, usually secondaries from some other primary tumours (details on page 241). Some more common tumours of the spine are as discussed below.

Benign tumours: These are uncommon. Osteoid osteoma is the *most common* benign tumour of the spine. It causes severe back pain, especially at night. Typically the pain is relieved by aspirin. The tumour, usually the size of a pea, is found in the pedicle or lamina. Haemangioma also occurs in the vertebral body. Meningioma is a common intradural, extra-medullary tumour which presents with back pain or radiating pain.

Malignant tumours: Multiple myeloma is the *most common* primary malignancy of the spine. Metastatic deposits are extremely common in the spine because of its rich venous connections, especially with the vertebral venous plexus. Pain often precedes X-ray evidence of a metastatic deposit. By the time a deposit is visible on X-ray, the tumour has replaced about 30 per cent of the bony content of the vertebra. A bone scan can detect the lesion earlier.

OTHER CAUSES

Metabolic disorders: Osteoporosis and osteomalacia are common causes of back pain (see page 299–301).

Spondylolysis and spondylolisthesis discussed on page 276–277.

Facet arthropathy and subtle arthritis of the facet joints can result from a degenerative disease and maldevelopment of the facets (facet tropism).

Functional back pain: At times, on detailed evaluation and investigations, no pliable cause of back pain is detected. In such cases, one must think that it could be of functional origin. Such patients are anxious personalities, have myriads of aches and pain all over the body. They have usually visited quite a few doctors and also taken multiple sittings of physiotherapy, but of no use. Some of the typical features of a patient with functional backache are as follows:

- Tenderness that is inappropriate in the clinical setting.
- Over-reaction by the patient during the physical examination
- Nondermatomal pain—physical signs inconsistent with specific roots
- Manson's test: This is a test to detect functional back pain. The patient is asked to pin-point the location of their back pain. The same is marked. After this, rest of the examination is carried out to divert patient's attention away from the back. He is then asked again to point to the painful site. In patients with functional pain, the site of pain this time will not correspond to that on first instance as the patient would have forgotten it.

APPROACH TO A PATIENT WITH BACK PAIN

The source of back pain is difficult to find because of variable factors. The aim is to identify the pathology that needs immediate treatment, such as an infection, neoplasm, disc prolapse, etc. All other back pains are treated as 'non-specific back pain' with more or less common treatment programme. While the patient is on this treatment programme, he is reviewed at regular intervals for any additional signs suggesting an organic illness. First establish whether the problem is acute (3 to 6 months) or chronic (longer than 6 months). If it is an acute pain, whether it is related to a definite episode of trauma or is spontaneous in onset. The causes are accordingly worked out (Flowchart 30.1). In cases with chronic back pain, it is helpful to judge whether it is mechanical or inflammatory by asking the patient whether rest brings relief or makes the pain worse. Accordingly, further signs and symptoms help in diagnosis (Flowchart 30.1).

INVESTIGATIONS

Plain X-rays: Plain X-rays are always done in two planes—AP and lateral. One must mention which part of the spine (upper, middle or power) needs to be X-rayed. The plain X-rays give information about congenital malformations such as fused vertebra, hemivertebra, spondylolysis and spondylolisthesis, scoliosis and degenerative spine disease (osteophytes, disc space narrowing). soft tissue shadows in relation to spine indicate infection.

MRI: MRI is the investigation of choice in diagnosis of spinal disorders. MRI helps in imaging the spinal canal, spinal cord and nerve roots. It is ideal imaging for evaluation of the disc (degeneration, protrusion, extrusion). All soft tissue pathologies such as abscess, synovial tumours and neural tumours are best diagnosed on MRI. There is no fixed rule for doing MRI. It is a go to investigation where one suspects a sinister back pathology, or when the symptoms are not settling with conservative treatment.

Blood tests: These are required based on what is being suspected in as particular case.

SCIATICA

Sciatica is a symptom and not a diagnosis. It means a pain radiating down the back of the thigh and calf. Degenerative arthritis and disc prolapse are the common causes. Some other causes are given in Table 30.3. Broadly, sciatica can either be because of inflammation of the sciatic nerve or because of compression of one of the roots constituting the sciatic nerve.

Table 30.3: Causes of sciatica.

Inflammatory
- Sciatic neuritis
- Arachnoiditis

Nerve root compression
- Compression in the vertebral canal by disc, tumour, tuberculosis
- Compression in the intervertebral foramen due to root canal stenosis because of OA, spondylolisthesis, facet arthropathy or tumours
- Compression in the buttock or pelvis by abscess, tumour, haematoma

Flowchart 30.1: Approach to a patient with low back pain.

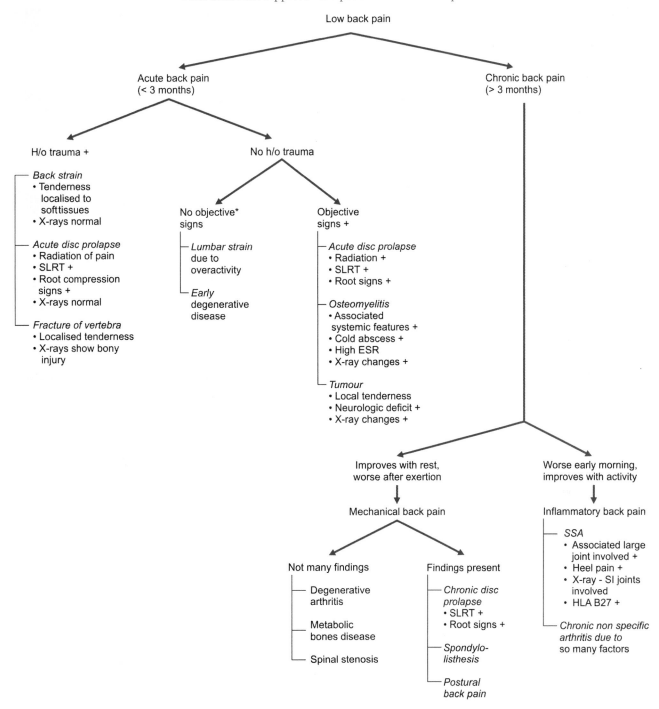

* Always keep in mind the visceral causes of back pain, if there are no findings on clinical examination of the spine.

What have we learnt?

- 70 per cent of acute back pains recover with rest.
- There are two types of back pain: (a) Inflammatory, which are worst in the morning (after rest) and (b) Mechanical, which come up after exertion.
- Treatment depends upon the cause.

Competency

❖ **OR2.8:** Describe and discuss the aetiopathogenesis, mechanism of injury, clinical features, investigations and principles of management of spine injuries with emphasis on mobilisation of the patient.

Fractures and dislocations of the spine are serious injuries because they may be associated with damage to the spinal cord or cauda equina. Thoraco-lumbar segment is the *most common* site of injury; lower cervical being the next common.

About 20 per cent of all spinal injuries result in a neurological deficit in the form of paraplegia in thoraco-lumbar spine injuries or quadriplegia in cervical spine injuries. Often, the patient does not recover from the deficit, resulting in prolonged invalidism or death.

RELEVANT ANATOMY

STRUCTURE

The vertebral column consists of 33 vertebrae (7 cervical, 12 dorsal, 5 lumbar, 5 sacral and 4 coccygeal) joined together by ligaments and muscles. Each vertebra consists of an anterior body and a posterior neural arch (Fig. 31.1). Each vertebral body

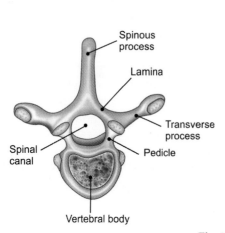

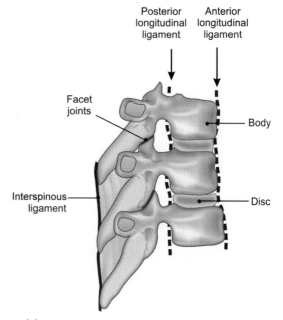

Fig. 31.1: Anatomy of the spine.

has a central part of cancellous bone and a peripheral cortex of compact bone. The margins of the upper and the lower surfaces of the vertebral body are thickened to form vertebral rings. The *neural arch* is constituted by pedicles, laminae, spinous process and articulating facets.

Between any two vertebrae is a strong 'cushion'– the intervertebral disc. It consists of two portions, a central nucleus pulposus and a peripheral annulus fibrosus. The *nucleus pulposus* is a remnant of the notochord and is made up of muco-gelatinous material. The *annulus fibrosus* is made up of fibrous tissue and surrounds the nucleus pulposus.

ARTICULATION

The entire vertebral column has similar articulation (except atlanto-axial joint). The vertebral bodies are primarily joined by intervertebral discs. Anteriorly, the vertebral bodies are connected to one another by a long, strap-like, anterior longitudinal ligament and posteriorly by a similar posterior longitudinal ligament.

The neural arches of adjacent vertebrae articulate through *facet joints.* These are synovial joints with a thick capsule. The adjacent laminae are joined together by a thick elastic ligament, the *ligamentum flavum.* Interspinous ligaments connect the adjacent spinous processes. The supraspinous ligament connects the tips of the adjacent spinous processes. Intertransverse ligaments connect the adjacent transverse processes. These ligaments are together often termed the *posterior ligament complex.*

The direction and size of the articular facets forming the facet joints is different in different parts of the spine (Fig. 31.2). In the cervical spine, they are short and more horizontally placed, becoming stouter and more vertical lower down the vertebral column. The facets of the lumbar spine are stout and vertically placed, hence *pure* dislocation (without associated fracture) does not occur in this region.

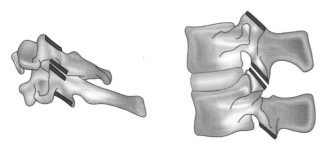

Cervical spine   Lumbar spine

Fig. 31.2: Direction of facet joints.

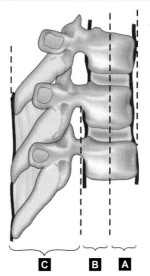

Fig. 31.3: Three column concept: (A) Anterior column; (B) Middle column; (C) Posterior column.

BIOMECHANICS OF INJURY

MODE OF INJURY

A fall from height, e.g., a fall from a tree, is the *most common* mode of sustaining a spinal injury in developing countries. In developed countries, road traffic accidents account for the maximum number. Other modes are: fall of a heavy object on the back, e.g., fall of a rock onto the back of a miner, sports injuries, etc.

STABLE AND UNSTABLE INJURIES

For purpose of treatment, it is crucial to assess the stability of an injured spine. A *stable injury* is one where further displacement between two vertebral bodies does not occur because of the intact 'mechanical linkages'. An *unstable injury* is one where further displacement can occur because of serious disruption of the structures responsible for stability. Often, it is difficult to decide with some surety whether the spine is stable; in all such cases it is safer to treat them as unstable injuries.

Three-column concept: Recent biomechanic studies show that from viewpoint of stability, the spine can be divided into three columns: anterior, middle and posterior (Fig. 31.3). The *anterior* column consists of the anterior longitudinal ligament and the anterior part of annulus fibrosus along with the anterior half of the vertebral body. The *middle* column consists of the posterior longitudinal ligament and the posterior part of the annulus fibrosus along with the posterior half of the vertebral body. The *posterior* column consists of the posterior bony arches along with the posterior ligament complex.

In different spinal injuries, the integrity of one or more of these columns may be disrupted, resulting in threat to the stability of the spine. When only one column is disrupted (e.g., a wedge compression fracture of the vertebra) the spine is stable. When two columns are disrupted (e.g., a burst fracture of the body of the vertebra) the spine is considered unstable. When all the three columns are disrupted, the spine is always unstable (e.g., dislocation of one vertebra over other).

CLASSIFICATION

Spinal injuries are best classified on the basis of mechanism of injury into the following types:

- Flexion injury
- Flexion-rotation injury
- Vertical compression injury
- Extension injury
- Flexion-distraction injury
- Direct injury
- Indirect injury due to violent muscle contraction

FLEXION INJURY

This is the *most common* spinal injury.

Examples: (i) heavy blow across the shoulder by a heavy object; (ii) fall from height on the heels or the buttocks (Fig. 31.4).

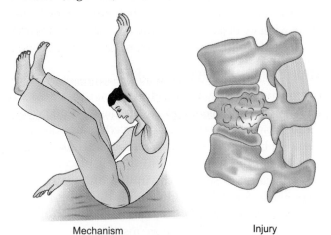

Fig. 31.4: Flexion injury.

Results: In the cervical spine, a flexion force can result in: (i) a sprain of the ligaments and muscles of the back of the neck: (ii) compression fracture of the vertebral body, C_5 to C_7; and (iii) dislocation of one vertebra over another (most common C_5 over C_6). In the dorso-lumbar spine, this force can result in the wedge compression of a vertebra (L_1 most common, followed by L_2 and D_{12}). It is a *stable* injury if compression of the vertebra is less than 50 per cent of its posterior height.

FLEXION-ROTATION INJURY

This is the *worst* type of spinal injury because it leaves a highly *unstable* spine, and is associated with a high incidence of neurological damage.

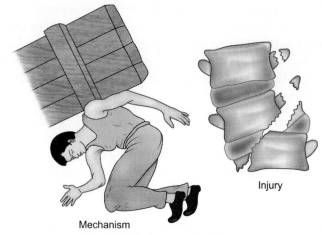

Fig. 31.5: Flexion-rotation injury.

Examples: (i) heavy blow onto one shoulder causing the trunk to be in flexion and rotation to the opposite side (Fig. 31.5); (ii) a blow or fall on posterolateral aspect of the head.

Results: In the cervical spine this force can result in: (i) dislocation of the facet joints on one or both sides; and (ii) fracture-dislocation of the cervical vertebra. In the dorso-lumbar spine, this force can result in a fracture-dislocation of the spine. Here one vertebra is twisted off in front of the one below it. While dislocating, the upper vertebra takes a slice of the body of the lower vertebra with it. There is extensive damage to the neural arch and posterior ligament complex. It is a *highly unstable* injury.

VERTICAL COMPRESSION INJURY

It is a common spinal injury.

Examples: (i) a blow on the top of the head by some object falling on the head; (ii) a fall from height in erect position (Fig. 31.6).

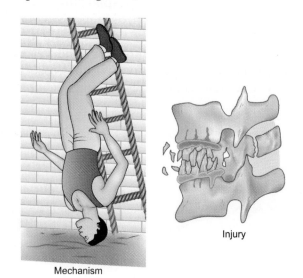

Fig. 31.6: Vertical compression injury.

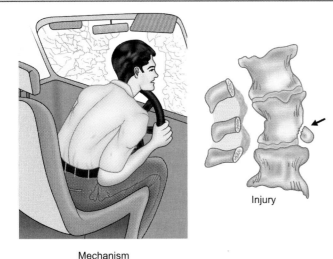

Mechanism

Fig. 31.7: Hyperextension injury.

Results: In the cervical spine, this force results in a burst fracture, i.e., the vertebral body is crushed throughout its vertical dimensions. A piece of bone or disc may get displaced into the spinal canal, causing pressure on the cord. In the dorso-lumbar spine, this force results in a fracture similar to that in the cervical spine, but due to a wide canal at this level, neurological deficit rarely occurs. It is an *unstable* injury.

EXTENSION INJURY

This injury is commonly seen in the cervical spine.

Examples: (i) motor vehicle accident—the forehead striking against the windscreen forcing the neck into hyperextension; (ii) shallow water diving—the head hitting the ground, extending the neck (Fig. 31.7).

Results: This injury results in a chip fracture of the anterior rim of a vertebra. Sometimes, these injuries *may be unstable.*

FLEXION-DISTRACTION INJURY

This is a recently described spinal injury, being recognised in western countries where use of a seat belt is compulsory while driving a car.

Example: With the sudden stopping of a car, the upper part of the body is forced forward by inertia, while the lower part is tied to the seat by the seat belt. The flexion force thus generated has a component of 'distraction' with it (Fig. 31.8).

Results: It commonly results in a horizontal fracture extending into the posterior elements and involving a part of the body. It is termed a 'Chance fracture'. It is an *unstable* injury.

DIRECT INJURY

This is a rare type of spinal injury.

Examples: (i) bullet injury; (ii) a *lathi* blow hitting the spinous processes of the cervical vertebrae.

Results: Any part of the vertebra may be smashed by a bullet, but, a *lathi* blow generally causes a fracture of the spinous processes only.

VIOLENT MUSCLE CONTRACTION

This is a rare injury.

Example: Sudden violent contraction of the psoas.

Results: It results in fractures of the transverse processes of multiple lumbar vertebrae. It may be associated with a huge retroperitoneal haematoma.

CLINICAL FEATURES

Presenting complaints: A patient with a spinal injury may present in the following ways:

- **Pain in the back** following a severe violence to the spine: The history is often so classic that one can predict the type of injury likely to have been sustained. At times the pain is slight, and one may not even suspect a spinal injury. Sometimes, a mild compression fracture of a vertebra may occur from a little jerk in the osteoporotic spine of an elderly person.
- **Neurological deficit:** Sometimes, a patient is brought to the hospital with complaints of inability to move the limbs and loss of sensation. Mostly there is a history of violence to the spine immediately preceding the onset of these

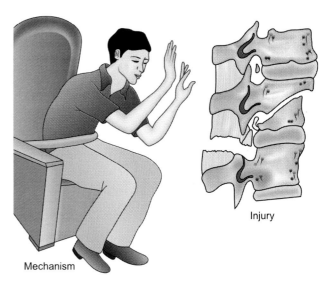

Mechanism

Fig. 31.8: The Chance fracture.

complaints. Sometimes, the paralysis may ensue late, or may extend proximally due to traumatic intraspinal haemorrhage.

EXAMINATION

A patient with suspected spinal injury should be treated as if it were certain unless proved otherwise on further clinical examination and investigation. Utmost care is required during examination and moving such a patient. Examination consists of the following:

- **General examination:** A quick general examination should be carried out to evaluate any hypovolaemic shock and associated injuries to the head, chest or abdomen.
- **Neurological examination:** It is carried out before examining the spine *per se*. By doing so, it will be possible to find the expected segment of vertebral damage. The level of motor paralysis, loss of sensation and the absence of reflexes are a guide to the neurological level of injury. It is easy to calculate the expected vertebral level from the neurological level (Table 23.4 on page 184).
- **Examination of the spine:** In a patient with a suspected spinal injury, utmost care must be observed during examination of the spinal column. If such care is not observed, in an unstable spine, movement at the fracture site may cause damage to the spinal cord. The patient should be tilted by an assistant just enough to permit the surgeon's hand to be introduced under the injured segment. One may be able to feel the prominence of one or more of the spinous processes, tenderness, crepitus or haematoma at the site of injury.

INVESTIGATIONS

Good antero-posterior and lateral X-rays *centering* on the involved segment provide reasonable information about the injury. Sometimes, special imaging techniques are required, e.g., CT scan, MRI, etc.

Plain X-rays: This is helpful in: (i) confirmation of diagnosis; (ii) assessment of mechanism of injury; and (iii) assessment of the stability of the spine. Following features may be noted on plain X-rays (Fig. 31.9).

- Change in the general alignment of the spine, i.e., antero-posterior bending (kyphosis) or sideways bending (scoliosis).
- Reduction in the height of a vertebra.

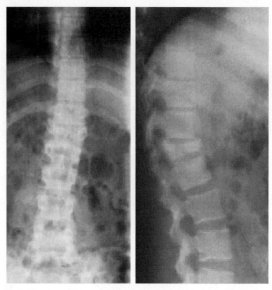

Fig. 31.9: X-rays showing compression fracture of D_{12} vertebra .

- Antero-posterior or sideways displacement of one vertebra over another.
- Fracture of a vertebral body.
- Fracture of the posterior elements, i.e., pedicle, lamina, transverse process, etc.

Occasionally, plain X-rays may appear normal in the presence of a highly unstable spinal injury. This is commonly seen in *'whiplash' injury* to the cervical spine where all the three columns of the spine are disrupted in a sudden hyperflexion followed by sudden hyperextension of the neck, e.g., after the sudden stopping of a car. Sometimes, a dislocation of the cervical spine may be spontaneously reduced so that there are only minimal findings on X-ray. Following are some of the radiological features suggestive of an unstable injury:

- Wedging of the body with the anterior height of the vertebra reduced more than half of the posterior height.
- A fracture-dislocation on X-ray.
- Rotational displacement of the spine.
- Injury to the facet joints, pedicle or lamina.
- An increase in the space between the adjacent spinous processes as seen on a lateral X-ray.

MRI: It is the best modality of imaging an injured spine. In addition to showing better the details of injured bones and soft tissues, it shows very well the anatomy of the cord.

CT scan: This can be done, where facility for MRI is not available. One can see the damaged structures more clearly, and make note of any bony fragment in the canal.

Table 31.1: Essential features of different types of spinal injuries.

Mechanism	Type of injury	Common site	Column failure	X-ray features	Stability
Flexion injury e.g., Fall on buttock/ head, heavy object falling on flexed spine	Compression fracture	$L_1 > L_2 > D_{12}$ $C_5 - C_7$	Only anterior column failure	Diminished anterior height of vertebra, posterior part remains intact	Stable
Flexion-rotation injury e.g., Fall on one side, blow on the side	Fracture-dislocation	L_1, D_{12} $C_5 - C_7$	All the three columns failure	*Direct evidence* (subluxation/dislocation) <ul><li>Posterior arch fracture</li><li>Broken facets</li><li>Vertebral body offset anteriorly</li></ul> *Indirect evidence* <ul><li>Broken ribs</li><li>Broken transverse processes</li><li>Increased disc height</li><li>Increased interspinous distance</li></ul>	Unstable
Vertical compression injury e.g., Object falling on head	Burst fracture	$C_5 - C_6$	Anterior and middle columns failure	Diminished anterior and posterior heights of vertebra CT scan may be of help in demonstrating compromise of the spinal canal by bony fragments	May be unstable
Extension injury e.g., Motor vehicle accident, shallow water diving	Avulsion fracture of anterior lip of vertebra	$C_5 - C_6$, lumbar spine	Only anterior column failure	Small chip from margin of vertebra, CT scan of no help	Stable
Flexion-distraction injury e.g., Car seat belt injury	Chance fracture	Dorsal spine	Middle and posterior column failure	Horizontal fracture line through posterior arch and posterior part of body of the vertebra	May be unstable
Direct injury e.g., Bullet injury, muscle contraction	Fracture of spinous or transverse processes	Any region	Any/All columns failure	Variable	Variable

Essential features of different types of spinal injuries is given in Table 31.1.

TREATMENT

The treatment of spinal injuries can be divided into three phases, as in other injuries:

Phase I Emergency care at the scene of accident or in emergency department.

Phase II Definitive care in emergency department, or in the ward.

Phase III Rehabilitation.

PHASE I - EMERGENCY CARE

At the site of accident: An acute pain in the back following an injury is to be considered a spinal injury unless proved otherwise. Also, all suspected spinal injuries are to be considered unstable unless their stability is confirmed on subsequent investigation. Based on this, a patient with a spinal injury has to be given utmost care right at the site of accident; the basic principle being to avoid any movement at the injured segment.

While moving a person with a suspected cervical spine injury, one person should hold the neck in traction by keeping the head pulled. The rest of the body is supported at the shoulder, pelvis and legs by three other people. Whenever required, the whole body is to be moved in one piece so that no movement occurs at the spine. The same precaution is observed in a case with suspected dorso-lumbar injury.

In the emergency department: The patient should not be moved from the trolley on which he is first received until stability of the spine is confirmed. In cases with cervical spine injury, two sandbags should be used on either side of the neck in order to avoid any movement of the neck. A quick general examination of the patient is carried out in order to detect any other associated injuries to the chest, abdomen, pelvis, limbs, etc. A thorough neurological examination of the limbs is performed. The spine is examined for any tenderness, crepitus, haematoma, etc. X-ray examination, as desired, is requisitioned.

Medical management of spinal cord injury: If the patient presents within 8 hours of injury, IV methylprednisolone is administered as a bolus dose followed by maintenance dose. Naloxone, thyrotropin-releasing hormone and GM1 gangliosides have been used.

PHASE II - DEFINITIVE CARE

Definitive care of a patient with spinal injury depends upon the stability of the spine and the presence of a neurological deficit. The aim of treatment is: (i) to avoid any deterioration of the neurological status; (ii) to achieve stability of the spine by conservative or operative methods; and (iii) to rehabilitate the paralysed patient to the best possible extent. Treatment of the various type of spinal injuries, as practiced most widely is as discussed below:

Treatment of cervical spine injuries: Cervical spine injuries are often associated with head injury, the effect of which may mask the spinal lesion. Therefore, it is necessary to get an X-ray of the cervical spine in any case of serious head injury.

Aim of treatment of cervical spine injury is to achieve proper alignment of vertebrae, and maintain it in that position till the vertebral column stabilises. Operative stabilisation of the fractured spine has become the treatment of choice, as it enhances rehabilitation. Where facilities are not available, reduction and stabilisation can be done by non-operative methods as discussed below:

Non-operative method: Reduction is achieved by skull traction applied through skull calipers—Crutchfield tongs (Fig. 31.10). A weight of up to 10 kg is applied

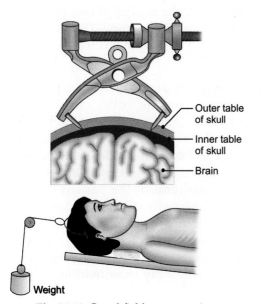

Fig. 31.10: Crutchfield tongs traction.

Outer table of skull

Inner table of skull

Brain

Weight

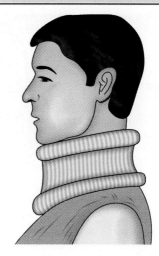

Fig. 31.11: Cervical collar.

and check X-rays taken every 12 hours. Also a close watch is kept on the patient's neurological status, because it is possible to damage the spinal cord or the medulla by injudicious traction. When it is confirmed on X-rays that reduction has been achieved, light traction is continued for 6 weeks. By this time, the soft tissues around the injured segment get sufficiently fibrosed, and further immobilisation can be done by immobilisation in a moulded PoP cast or a plastic collar. In about 3–4 months, a bony bridge forms between the subluxed vertebrae, and the spine stabilises. The collar can then be discarded.

Operation: This is a treatment method of choice wherever facilities are available. It is particularly required for: (i) irreducible subluxation because of 'locking' of the articular processes or (ii) persistent instability following conservative treatment. The operation consists of inter-body fusion (anterior fusion) or fusion of the spinous processes and laminae (posterior fusion). Internal fixation may be required.

Common cervical spine injuries:

- **Wedge compression fracture** of the vertebral body: This results from a flexion force. The posterior elements are usually intact so that the injury is *stable.*
  Treatment: Reduction is not required. The neck is kept immobilised with the help of skull traction/ sling traction. Once pain and muscle spasm subside, the neck is supported in a cervical collar, PoP cast or a brace (Fig. 31.11). Exercises of the neck are started after 8–12 weeks.
- **Burst fracture** of the vertebral body: This results from a vertical compression force. The posterior elements are usually intact but because of the severity of crushing of the vertebra, fracture is

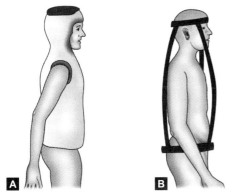

Fig. 31.12: (A) Minerva jacket; (B) Halo-pelvic traction.

considered *unstable*. It may be associated with a neurological deficit if a broken fragment from the body gets displaced inside the spinal canal.

Treatment: Where there is no neurological deficit, the injury can be treated on the same lines as for wedge compression fractures mentioned above. Management of a patient with neurological involvement is discussed later.

- **Subluxation or dislocation** of the cervical spine: A flexion rotation force or a severe flexion force may result in the forward displacement of one vertebra over the other (commonly C_5 over C_6). The displacement may be partial or complete. Sometimes, the displacement may be spontaneously reduced*, leaving a well aligned spine but significantly devoid of supporting ligament; these are *unstable injuries*. For proper assessment, in addition to antero-posterior and lateral views, oblique X-ray views may be taken. MRI gives critical information about extent of injury.

  Treatment: Surgical stabilisation is the treatment of choice. Some cases can be treated conservatively. The aim of treatment is to achieve reduction of the subluxed vertebra and maintain it in a reduced position until the spine becomes stable.

Uncommon cervical spine injuries: Included in this group are the following injuries:

- **Fracture of the atlas:** A 'burst' fracture where both, anterior and posterior arches of the atlas, are fractured by a vertical force acting through the skull is a common atlas fracture (Jefferson's fracture). Displacement is seldom severe, and more often than not, the spinal cord escapes injury. Treatment consists of traction, followed by immobilisation in Minerva jacket or halo-pelvic support (Fig. 31.12).

---

* Even with an apparently good looking alignment on the X-ray, the spine may be highly unstable.

- **Atlanto-axial fracture-dislocation:** A fracture-dislocation of the atlanto-axial joint is more common than pure dislocation (Fig. 31.13). A pure dislocation is more often associated with a neurological deficit. The displacement is commonly anterior. Treatment consists of skull traction, followed by immobilisation in a Minerva jacket. In due course, the fracture unites and a bridge of bone joins C_1 to C_2 anteriorly, thereby stabilising the spine.
- **Clay shoveller's fracture:** This is a fracture of the spinous process of D_1 vertebra. It is caused by muscular action as occurs in shovelling by labourers, hence its name.
- **Displacement of intervertebral disc:** A violent flexion-compression force can sometimes result in sudden prolapse of the nucleus pulposus of a cervical disc into the vertebral canal resulting in quadriplegia. An early decompression may give good results.

Treatment of thoracic and lumbar spine injuries: Definitive treatment of a thoracic spine injury depends upon the presence of neurological deficit and on whether it is stable or an unstable injury. In general, conservative treatment is sufficient for stable injuries.

Stable injuries: Most of these need a period of bed rest and analgesics followed by mobilisation. Initial mobilisation may be by some external support, like a brace, etc., but gradually these are discarded and an active programme of rehabilitation continued till full functions are achieved. During the period of bed rest, one must take special care of possible complications such as bed sores, chest infection, urinary tract infection, etc.

Unstable injuries: These are either associated with a neurological deficit or are likely to develop it during treatment. Open reduction and surgical stabilisation gives the best choice of recovery but conventionally, these cases have been treated non-operatively with: (i) bed rest for 6 weeks; (ii) bracing till spine stabilises; and (iii) care of the back.

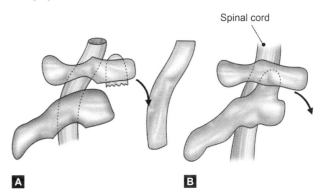

Fig. 31.13: Atlanto-axial injuries: (A) Fracture-dislocation; (B) Only dislocation.

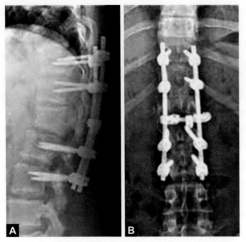

Fig. 31.14: X-rays of the spine showing methods of internal fixation of the spine by pedicular screws and rod.

Operative intervention in dorso-lumbar injuries: There are clear indications for surgery in these injuries. The goal of surgery is to restore the normal sagittal and coronal plane alignment of the spine. The spinal canal should be decompressed, and the fixation should be so secure that supplementary bracing is not needed. The indications are:

- Loss of 50% of vertebral height
- The spinal canal is compromised 50%
- There exists a 30 degree kyphosis deformity
- There is a neurologic deficit.

Operative methods: The method of fixation currently in use is pedicle screw with rod posteriorly and supported sometimes by anterior fixation (Fig. 31.14).

Flowchart 31.2 shows a practical plan of treatment of injuries to dorso-lumbar spine.

Flowchart 31.2: Treatment plan of dorso-lumbar spine injury.

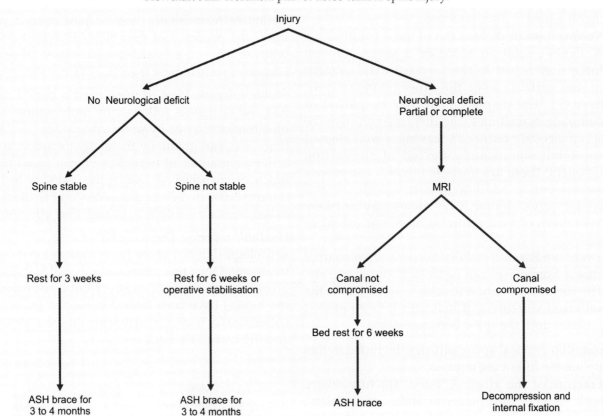

What have we learnt?

- Spinal injuries are a complex combination of bony and neural injuries.
- Meticulous care, right from the scene of injury, till final rehabilitation is necessary to prevent neurological damage.
- Stability of the injured spine is the most important parameter in deciding whether to go for operative or non-operative treatment.
- The trend is towards operative stabilisation of the spinal injuries, and their treatment in specialised centres.

Additional information: From the entrance exams point of view

- Motorcyclist's fracture is a ring fracture of the skull base.
- Most common cause of spinal cord injury in India (developing countries) is fall from height whereas in developed countries, it is road traffic accidents.
- Dislocation without fracture can be seen in the cervical spine.
- Vertebroplasty: Polymethylmethacrylate is injected into fractured (compressed) vertebral bodies to decrease pain and strengthen the bone. This does not restore the height of the vertebrae or prevent deformity.
- Baloon kyphoplasty: A small balloon is inflated in the compressed vertebral body to restore its height and alignment.
- Both procedures are absolutely contraindicated in infection, untreated coagulopathy and healed osteoporotic fractures.

Competency

❖ **OR2.8:** Describe and discuss the aetiopathogenesis, mechanism of injury, clinical features, investigations and principles of management of spine injuries with emphasis on mobilisation of the patient.

Only a small proportion of cases of spinal injuries are complicated by injury to the neural structures within the vertebral column. In the cervical spine, it may lead to paralysis of all four limbs (quadriplegia). In thoracic and thoraco-lumbar spine, it may result in paralysis of the trunk and both lower limbs (paraplegia). The terms quadriparesis and paraparesis are sometimes used for *incomplete* paralysis of all four limbs or the lower limbs respectively.

The *most common* spinal injury to be associated with paraplegia is a fracture-dislocation (flexion-rotation injury) of the dorso-lumbar spine. Quadriplegia most commonly results from fracture-dislocation (flexion-rotation injuries) at the C_5-C_6 junction. Only severely displaced lumbar spine injuries below L_1 level, produce cauda equina type of paralysis.

PATHOLOGY

The displaced vertebra may either damage the cord (very unlikely), the cord along with the nerve roots lying by its side or the roots alone. Pathologically, damage to neural structures may be a cord concussion, cord transection or root transection (Fig. 32.1).

Cord concussion: In this type, the disturbance is one of *functional loss* without a demonstrable anatomical lesion. Motor paralysis (flaccid), sensory loss and

visceral paralysis occur below the level of the affected cord segment. Recovery begins within 8 hours, and eventually the patient recovers fully.

Cord transection: In this type, the cord and its surrounding tissues are transected. The injury is anatomical and irreparable. Initially, the motor paralysis is flaccid because the cord below the level of injury is in a state of 'spinal shock'. After some time, however, the cord recovers from shock and acts as an independent structure, without any control from the higher centres. In this state, though the cord manifests reflex activity at spinal level, there is no voluntary control over body parts below the level of injury. There is total loss of sensation and autonomic functions below the level of injury.

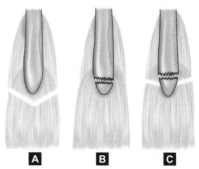

Fig. 32.1: Pathology of neural injury: (A) Only roots affected; (B) Only the cord affected; (C) Roots + cord affected.

The appearance of signs suggestive of reflex cord activity, i.e., bulbocavernosus reflex, anal reflex and plantar reflex, *without* recovery of motor power or sensations is an indicator of cord transection. These reflexes usually appear within 24 hours of the injury. In a few days or weeks, the flaccid paralysis (due to spinal shock) becomes spastic, with exaggerated tendon reflexes and clonus. Involuntary flexor spasms at different joints and spasticity leads to contractures. Sensation and autonomic functions never return.

Root transection: Spinal nerve roots may be damaged alone in injuries of the lumbar spine, or in addition to cord injury, in injuries of the dorso-lumbar spine. Neurological damage in nerve root injury is similar to that in cord transection except that in the former residual motor paralysis remains permanently flaccid and regeneration is *theoretically** possible. A discrepancy between the neurological and skeletal levels may occur in spinal injuries below D_{10} level because the roots descending from the segments higher than the affected cord level may also be transected, thereby producing a higher neurological level than expected.

Incomplete lesions: Occasionally, the neurological lesion may be incomplete, i.e., affecting only a portion of the cord. In these cases, there is evidence of *neurological sparing* distal to the injury (perianal sensation sparing is common). Such sparing is an indication of a favourable prognosis. Incomplete lesions may be of the following types. There are some classical forms of incomplete spinal cord injury:

a. *Central cord syndrome:* The central part of the spinal cord is injured due to ischemia. It is common after a hyperextension injury and is common where the vertebral canal is stenotic, usually in cervical spine. It produces sacral sensory sparing and greater motor weakness in the upper limbs than in the lower limbs. In the upper limbs the motor weakness is more distally than proximally. Painful paresthesias occur in the extremities. Upper limbs are more affected than lower limbs. Radiographs of the cervical spine are normal.

b. *Brown-Sequard syndrome:* The syndrome is hemisection of the cord, seen after a penetrating injury due to a knife stab or a gunshot. It is characterised by ipsilateral loss of proprioception, vibration sense, two point discrimination, motor loss below the level of the lesion with contralateral loss of sensitivity to pain and temperature. A patient with the Brown-Sequard syndrome would typically say that he can feel the water in a bath tub but he cannot tell its temperature. The Brown-Sequard syndrome carries the *best prognosis* amongst all the incomplete spinal cord injury syndromes.

c. *Anterior spinal cord syndrome:* This is seen when the anterior spinal artery is infarcted or when there is damage to the anterior spinal cord by a disc prolapse or a retropulsed bony fragment as in a burst fracture or in flexion injuries; there is damage to the anterior and the lateral spinothalamic tracts. The dorsal columns are intact. The injury produces bilateral loss of motor function and loss of sensitivity to pain and temperature while preserving proprioception, crude touch, vibration and position sense (because posterior columns are intact). The prognosis is poor.

d. *Posterior cord syndrome:* It is an uncommon incomplete spinal cord injury where there is injury to only the posterior columns. It is a rare injury. Clinically the patient presents with normal motor power, but has pain and burning sensation, loss of proprioception and loss of vibration distal to the lesion. Romberg's sign is positive.

e. *Conus medullaris syndrome:* This is due to an injury of the sacral cord and lumbar nerve roots within the spine canal at vertebral level T_{12} and L_1. This is a region more prone to injury as it is the junction between a mobile lumbar segment and a fixed thoracic segment. An acute injury causes an areflexic bladder and bowel and flaccid paralysis of the lower limbs, with saddle anaesthesia. In a pure conus lesion the bulbocavernosus reflex may be lost.

f. *Cauda equina syndrome:* It is marked by injury to the lumbosacral nerve roots within the neural canal from L_2 vertebral level or below, resulting in an areflexic bladder, bowel and lower limb flaccid paralysis. Saddle anaesthesia, bilateral radicular pain, numbness, areflexia or hyporeflexia may exist. There will be urinary retention and bowel incontinence. Symptoms are of the lower motor neuron type and can be asymmetrical. Cauda equina syndrome can be due to a burst fracture, or a massive disc prolapse. Decompression should be done early for better bladder and bowel recovery.

NEUROLOGICAL DEFICIT AND SPINAL INJURIES

Cervical spine: In these injuries, the segmental level of the cord transection nearly always corresponds

---

*The root, being made up of myelinated fibres, behaves like any other nerve as far as recovery is concerned. But, because the distance between the level of injury and the neuromuscular junction is big, motor recovery is only a theoretical possibility.

to the level of bony damage. A high cervical cord transection (above C_5) is *fatal* because all the respiratory muscles (thoracic and diaphragmatic) are paralysed. Transection at the C_5 segment results in paralysis of the muscles of the upper limbs, thorax, trunk, and lower limbs, with loss of sensation and visceral functions. With transection at level below the C_5 segment, some muscles of the upper limbs are spared, resulting in characteristic deformities, depending upon the level.

Thoracic lesion (between T_1 and T_{10}): In cord transection from T_1 to T_{10}, trunk limb muscles and that of lower limb are paralysed. At the tenth thoracic vertebra, the corresponding cord segment is L_1, so in injuries at this level, only the lower limbs are affected.

Dorso-lumbar lesions (between D_{11} and L_1): Between 11th dorsal and 1st lumbar vertebrae lie all the lumbar and sacral segments along with their nerve roots.

Hence, injuries at this level cause cord transection with or without involvement of nerve roots. This is the cause of difference in neurological deficit in fractures and fracture-dislocations with apparently similar X-ray appearances. In injuries of the cord with nerve root transection, paralysis in the lower limbs is mixed (UMN+LMN type). It is important to differentiate it from a lesion of cord transection with *root escape*, as the latter has a better prognosis.

Lesions below L_1: This area of the canal has only bunch of nerve roots, which subsequently emerge at successive levels of the lumbo-sacral spine. Thus, injury in this area results in root damage, resulting in flaccid paralysis, sensory loss and autonomic disturbances in the distribution of the affected roots.

CLINICAL EXAMINATION

A neurological deficit following trauma to the spine is difficult to miss. More important is to perform a thorough neurological examination to evaluate the following: (i) the level of neurological deficit; (ii) any evidence of an incomplete lesion; and (iii) any indication of complete cord transection.

INVESTIGATIONS

Radiological examination: Often there is no correlation between the severity of the injury on the X-rays and the degree of neurological deficit.

CT and MRI scan: This may be indicated in cases with incomplete paralysis, particularly if it is increasing. It

is also indicated in cases where no bony lesions are visible on plain X-rays. MRI has become the imaging modality of choice for these cases.

TREATMENT

A patient with traumatic paraplegia, wherever possible, should be admitted to specialised units, where necessary facilities for management of these cases are available. In developing countries, these cases are still managed in general hospitals. Treatment can be discussed in 3 phases:

Phase I   Emergency care at the scene of accident and in the emergency department

Phase II   Definitive care on in-patient basis

Phase III Rehabilitation

PHASE I – EMERGENCY CARE

The care in phase I is along the lines already discussed in 'treatment of spinal injuries' on page 263–264.

PHASE II – DEFINITIVE CARE

Care in phase II consists of: (i) clinical assessment of the neurological deficit; (ii) radiological and special investigations to understand the type of vertebral lesion, and to detect the possibility of persistent cord compression by a bone fragment in the vertebral canal; and (iii) care of paraplegic in the ward. (i) and (ii) are discussed in Chapter 31; (iii) is being discussed here.

Ward care of a paraplegic: Ward care of a traumatic paraplegic or quadriplegic consists of: (i) management of the fracture; (ii) nursing care; (iii) care of the bladder and bowel; and (iv) physiotherapy.

Management of the fracture: Treatment of the fracture or fracture-dislocation *per se* is the same as that for spinal injury at that level without neurological lesion. This is as discussed on page 265–266. Role of operative treatment is controversial. It consists of stabilisation of the spine by internally fixing it. This ensures better nursing care of the patient but offers no security about the recovery of neurological function. The generally accepted indications for surgery in developing countries, with limited expertise, can be considered as follows:

a. *Incomplete paralysis*, particularly if it is increasing, and a CT scan shows fragments of bone encroaching upon the spinal canal.

b. *Patient with multiple injuries*, in whom it is desirable to stabilise the spine for overall optimum care of the patient.

Nursing care: Specialised nursing care has dramatically changed the prognosis of a traumatic

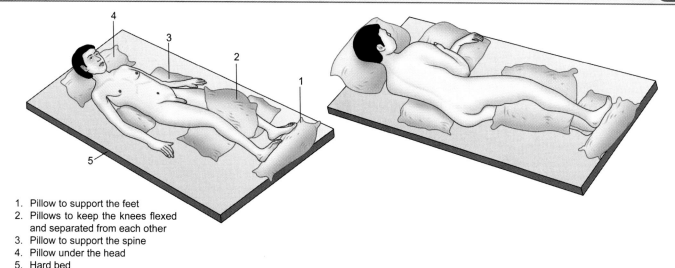

1. Pillow to support the feet
2. Pillows to keep the knees flexed and separated from each other
3. Pillow to support the spine
4. Pillow under the head
5. Hard bed

Fig. 32.2: Care of paraplegic—positioning in bed.

paraplegic. It can be considered under the following heads:

a. *Positioning in bed:* The patient is nursed flat on a hard bed with a mattress. The limbs are positioned with pillows so that contractures do not develop; also pressure points are adequately padded (Fig. 32.2).

b. *Care of the back:* Frequent turning in bed is vital so that the patient lies for equal periods on his back and on either side. The bed is kept dry and free of wrinkles. Special beds are available which provide an ease of turning the patient periodically (Stryker frame), and constantly changing pressure-point (water-bed, alpha- bed).

c. *Personal hygiene:* All personal hygiene of the patient from top to toe, is to be looked after. This includes combing hair, cleaning teeth, mouth wash, care of the skin and nails, etc.

Care of the bladder: Intermittent catheterisation is the *best* but for convenience an indwelling catheter is used. Catheter is changed once a week, and the patient is kept on prophylactic antiseptic drugs. A urine culture is done once every two weeks. As the patient becomes haemodynamically stable, catheter is periodically clamped so that the bladder capacity is maintained.

In most cases of cord transection, satisfactory automatic emptying is established within one to three months of the injury (*automatic bladder*). In a case, where the sacral segments are irrecoverably damaged, as in a cauda equina lesion, reflex emptying does not occur. In such cases, micturition will have to be started or aided by other mechanisms like abdominal straining or manual compression, etc. (*autonomous bladder*).

Care of the bowel: The patient develops bowel incontinence and constipation. The latter may result in periodic bloating up of the abdomen. A frequent soap water enema or manual evacuation of the bowel may be required.

Physiotherapy: Aim of physiotherapy in the initial few weeks is to maintain mobility of the paralysed limbs by moving all the joints through the full range gently, several times a day. Later, in cases where partial recovery occurs, exercises specifically for building up the muscle groups are taught.

PHASE III – REHABILITATION

In most cases with traumatic paraplegia and quadriplegia, the deficit is permanent. With concentrated efforts at rehabilitation, a majority of these cases can be made reasonably independent and enabled to lead a useful life within the constraints of their disability. Rehabilitation can be considered under the following headings: (i) physical rehabilitation; (ii) psychological and social rehabilitation; and (iii) economic rehabilitation.

Physical rehabilitation: It consists of making the patient as independent in his activities of daily living (ADL) as possible. The patient may be given special appliances like calipers, wheelchair, etc., for this.

Psychological and social rehabilitation: Keeping the morale of a paraplegic high is a great challenge. The doctor, nursing staff, family, friends and social organisations have a great role to play in this.

Economic rehabilitation: This is an important aspect of rehabilitation of a paraplegic. As soon as the patient is able to do a worthwhile job, efforts should be made to procure some form of remunerative employment for him.

In developed countries, these patients are managed in special *spinal injury centres*. There are now more and more surgeons in these centres who believe in the operative treatment of most cases of paraplegia and quadriplegia. According to them, stabilisation of the spine after reduction of the displacement gives the patient: (a) best chance of relieving compression on the cord, if at all and (b) helps in better nursing care of the patient.

What have we learnt?

- Traumatic paraplegia is one of the most common spinal injury.
- Recovery depends upon the nature of neural damage, and whether it is a complete or incomplete cord damage.
- Nursing care during recovery phase is crucial.
- Prolonged rehabilitation is required.

SCOLIOSIS

CLASSIFICATION

It is of two types: non-structural (transient) and structural (permanent). In structural scoliosis, the vertebrae, in addition to sideways tilt, are rotated along their long axis; in non-structural scoliosis they are not.

Non-structural scoliosis: This is a mobile or transient scoliosis. It has three subtypes, as discussed below:
1. *Postural scoliosis:* It is the *most common overall* type, often seen in adolescent girls. The curve is mild and convex, usually to the left. The main diagnostic feature is that the curve straightens completely when the patient bends forwards.
2. *Compensatory scoliosis:* In this type, the scoliosis is a compensatory phenomenon, occurring in order to compensate for the tilt of the pelvis (e.g., in a hip disease or for a short leg). The scoliosis disappears when the patient is examined in a sitting position (in case the leg is short) or when the causative factor is removed.
3. *Sciatic scoliosis:* This is as a result of unilateral painful spasm of the paraspinal muscles, as may occur in a case of prolapsed intervertebral disc.

Structural scoliosis: It is a scoliosis with a component of permanent deformity. The following are the different subtypes:

- *Idiopathic:* It is the *most common* type of structural scoliosis. It may begin during infancy, childhood or adolescence. *Infantile scoliosis* begins in the first year of life, and is different from the other in that, it can be a *resolving or progressive* type. Scoliosis beginning later in life progresses at a variable rate, and leads to an ugly deformity. The deformity is most obvious in thoracic scoliosis because of the formation of a rib hump. In the lumbar region, even a moderate curve goes unnoticed because it gets masked by the compensatory curvature of the adjacent part of the spine. Idiopathic curves progress until the cessation of skeletal growth.
- *Congenital scoliosis:* This type is always associated with some form of radiologically demonstrable anomaly of the vertebral bodies (Fig. 33.1). These are: (i) hemivertebrae (only one-half of the vertebra grows); (ii) block vertebrae (two vertebral bodies fused); or (iii) an unsegmented bar (a bar of bone joining two adjacent vertebrae on one side, thereby preventing growth on that side). These curves grow, often at a very fast rate. Sometimes, there are associated anomalies in the growth of the neural structures, leading to a neurological deficit in the lower limbs.
- *Paralytic scoliosis:* An unbalanced paralysis of the trunk muscles results in paralytic scoliosis of the

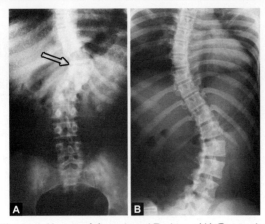

Fig. 33.1: X-rays of the spine, AP views; (A) Congenital scoliosis; (B) Idiopathic scoliosis.

spine. Poliomyelitis is the most common cause in developing countries. Other common causes are cerebral palsy and muscular dystrophies.

• *Other pathologies:* There are other causes of structural scoliosis such as neurofibromatosis which produces a *sharp* kyphoscoliosis.

PATHOLOGY

The main pathology is lateral curvature of a part of the spine. This is called the *primary curve*. The spine above or below the primary curve undergoes compensatory curvature in the opposite direction. These are called the *compensatory or secondary curves* (Fig. 33.2A). The lateral curvature is associated with rotation of the vertebrae. In curves of the thoracic spine, rotation of the vertebrae leads to prominence of the rib cage on the *convex* side, giving rise to a rib hump (Fig. 33.2B).

Any part of the thoraco-lumbar spine may be affected. The pattern of the curve and its natural evolution are fairly constant for each site. The following types are recognised: (i) dorsal scoliosis; (ii) dorso-lumbar scoliosis; and (iii) lumbar scoliosis.

DIAGNOSIS

Clinical features: In most cases, visible deformity is the only symptom. Pain is occasionally a feature in adults with a long-standing deformity. In exceptional cases of severe long-standing scoliosis, sharp angulation of the spinal cord over the apex of the curve may result in interference with cord functions, leading to a neurological deficit.

Radiological features: For proper assessment of scoliosis, a *full* antero-posterior X-ray of the spine in supine and erect positions, plus a lateral view are necessary. Severity of the curve is measured by *Cobb's angle*—an angle between the line passing through the margins of the vertebrae at the ends of the curve (Fig. 33.3A). Radiological assessment regarding the likelihood of progress of the curve can be made by looking at the iliac apophysis (Fig. 33.3B). It fuses with the iliac bone at maturity and indicates the completion of growth, and thus no possibility of the curve worsening. This is called *Reisser's sign*.

Rotation of a vertebra can be appreciated by looking at the position of the spinous processes and pedicles on AP view. Normally, a spinous process is in the centre of the vertebral body. In a case where there is a rotation of a vertebra, the spinous process is shifted

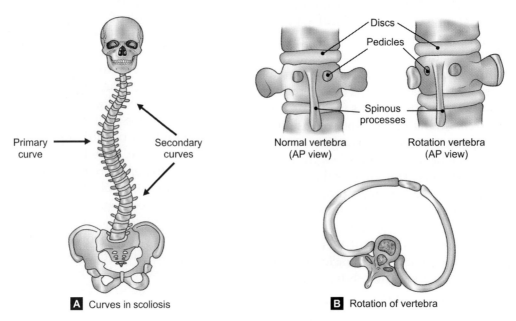

Fig. 33.2: Pathology of scoliosis.

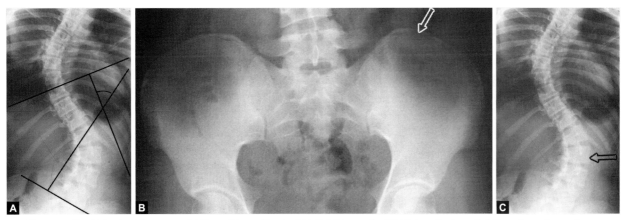

Fig. 33.3: Radiological features of idiopathic scoliosis: (A) Cobb's angle; (B) Reisser's sign; (C) Rotation of vertebrae.

to one side (Fig. 33.3C). Also, there will be asymmetry in the position of the pedicles on the two sides.

In congenital scoliosis, one may find wedging, hemivertebrae, an unsegmented bone bar between the vertebrae, fused ribs, etc. In scoliosis associated with neurofibromatosis an erosion of the vertebral bodies may be seen. Intervertebral foramina may be widened in a dumbell-shaped neurofibroma producing scoliosis.

TREATMENT

Principles of treatment: Aim of treatment is to assess the prognosis of the curve in terms of the visible deformity it is likely to produce. This depends upon: (i) the type of the curve; (ii) age at onset; and (iii) the site of the curve. Congenital curves progress at variable rates depending upon the type of vertebral malformation, but overall they grow faster than idiopathic curves. Neurofibromatotic curves progress faster. In general, younger the patient, the worse the prognosis. Thoracic curves produce the worst deformities.

As soon as it is realised that a curve is likely to progress and result in an ugly deformity, the affected part of the spine is fused. The *basic guiding principle* is that a straight, stiff spine is better than a curved, flexible one. Treatment of postural curves is non-operative. Proper training and exercises form the mainstay of treatment. Structural curves of less than 30°, and well-balanced double-curves can also be successfully treated by non-operative methods. The following are the indications for surgical intervention:
- Congenital scoliosis, where the radiological signs suggest the possibility of fast progression of the curve, especially those in the thoracic spine.
- Curves showing deterioration radiologically, and are in the region where they are likely to produce ugly deformities at pubertal growth spurt.
- Scoliosis associated with backache.

For all other curves, the patient is started on a non-operative regimen consisting of exercises and a brace. The progress of the curve is monitored clinically and radiologically every 6 months. Following are the non-operative and operative methods of treatment:

Non-operative methods: These consist of exercises to tone up the spinal muscles and give support to the spine. Following supports are commonly used:
- *Milwaukee brace:* This is named after the city of Milwaukee where it was designed (Fig. 33.4).
- *Boston brace:* It is cosmetically more acceptable.
- *Reisser's turn-buckle cast:* This is a body cast with a turn-buckle in between. Tightening of the turn-buckle stretches the concave side of the curve, thus correcting the deformity.
- *Localiser cast:* This is a body cast applied with the spine in traction. A special localiser table is required for this.

Operative methods: Operative methods comprise of fusion of the spine. In congenital scoliosis, simple

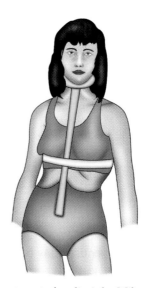

Fig. 33.4: Treatment of scoliosis by Milwaukee brace.

fusion is sufficient. In idiopathic scoliosis, the spine is fused after achieving some correction by stretching the spine. Stretching could be done pre-operatively by traction (Cotrel traction), localiser cast, or halo-pelvic distraction system. It could be achieved per-operatively by pedicle screw and rod fixation.

KYPHOSIS

This is a general term used for excessive backward convexity of the spine. It is of two types; round or angular.

Round kyphosis means a gentle backward curvature of the spinal column. It is caused by diseases affecting a number of vertebrae (e.g., senile kyphosis). Such a kyphosis may be localised to a segment of the spine, or it may be diffuse.

Angular kyphosis means a sharp backward promi-nence of the spinal column. It may be prominence of only one spinous process because of the collapse of only one vertebral body—as may occur in a compres-sion fracture of a vertebra. This is called as *knuckle*. There may be a kyphosis localised to a few vertebrae, and is called as *gibbus*.

It is seen commonly in tuberculosis where usually two or more vertebrae are affected.

CAUSES

The following are the common causes of diffuse kyphosis:
a. **Postural:** This is the *most common* type, seen in tall individuals, especially in some tall women, because of their tendency to stand with a forward stoop. It occurs in the upper dorsal spine, and can be corrected by postural training and physiotherapy.
b. **Compensatory:** If there is an exaggerated lumbar lordosis due to some disease, the thoracic spine develops compensatory kyphosis.
c. **Scheuermann's disease:** It is a common type. There is a gentle round kyphosis in the *lower thoracic spine*. It is due to osteochondritis affecting the ring-epiphyses of the vertebral bodies. On X-rays, the vertebral bodies appear wedge-shaped, narrower in front. There may be a dull constant pain during early stages of the disease, but later, only kyphosis remains. Conservative treatment is adequate for most patients with pain as the complaint. If the deformity is severe, especially if it is compromising the activities in any way, surgical intervention may be required.
d. **Ankylosing spondylitis:** The disease produces a stiff and kyphotic spine. It begins in young men as

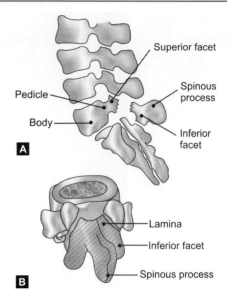

The shaded portion remains with the lower vertebra

Fig. 33.5: Spondylolisthesis.

low backache, which gradually spreads to affect the whole spine. Chest expansion is reduced because of the limitation of movements at the costo-vertebral joints. In a few cases, hips and shoulders are also affected.

SPONDYLOLISTHESIS

Spondylolisthesis is forward displacement of a vertebra over the one below it (Fig. 33.5A). It commonly occurs between L_5-S_1, and between L_4-L_5. Occasionally, the displacement is backwards (retrolisthesis).

PATHOLOGY

Normally, forward displacement of a vertebral body is prevented primarily by the engagement of its articular processes with that of the vertebra below it. The attachments of the intervertebral disc and ligaments between vertebrae also check this displacement, but to a small extent. Thus, any defect in this 'check' mechanism leads to spondylolisthesis. Accordingly, spondylolisthesis has been divided into the following types:
a. **Isthmic:** This is the *most common* type overall. The lesion is in the pars interarticularis*. Three sub-types are recognised:
  - Lytic: Fatigue fracture of the pars inter articularis
  - Intact but elongated pars interarticularis

---

*Pars interarticularis: As the name suggests, it is the part of the vertebra bridging the superior and inferior articular facets.

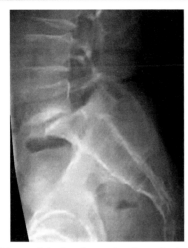

Fig. 33.6: X-ray of the lumbar spine, lateral view, showing spondylolisthesis of L₄ over L₅ vertebra.

- Acute fracture of the pars interarticularis. The defect allows the separation of the two halves of the vertebra. The anterior half (i.e., the body with the pedicles and superior articular facet) along with the whole of the spinal column above it, slips forwards over the vertebra below. The posterior half of the affected vertebra (i.e., laminae and inferior articular facets), remain with the lower vertebrae (Fig. 33.5B).

b. **Dysplastic:** In this, the *least* common type, there is a congenital abnormality in the development of the vertebrae, so that one vertebra slips over the other.

c. **Degenerative:** This is seen fairly commonly in elderly people. The posterior facet joints becomes unstable because of osteoarthritis, and subluxate. Vertebral displacement is occasionally backwards rather than forwards (retrolisthesis). Displacement is usually not severe, and neurological disturbance is unusual.

d. **Pathological:** This type results from a genera-lised or localised bone disease weakening the articulation between the vertebrae.

e. **Traumatic:** This is a very rare type, where one vertebra slips over other following an injury.

DIAGNOSIS

Clinical features: The isthmic type of spondy-lolisthesis presents in adolescents and young adults. The degenerative type occurs in old age. The presenting symptom is usually backache, with or without sciatica. Symptoms become worse on standing or walking. Sometimes, there may be neurological symptoms in the lower limbs. In a large number of cases, the abnormality is symptomless, and is detected on a routine X-ray taken during screening for a health checkup.

On examination, there is often a visible or palpable 'step' above the sacral crest due to the forward displacement of the spinal column. There may be increased lumbar lordosis. There may be evidence of stretching of the sciatic nerve, as found by the straight leg raising test (SLRT).

X-ray examination: Anterior displacement of one vertebra over other can be seen on a lateral view of the spine (Fig. 33.6). The displacement can be graded into four categories depending upon the severity of slip. Grade I spondylolisthesis means vertebral displacement up to 25 per cent of the antero-posterior width of the lower vertebral body, whereas grade IV means the complete forward displacement of the affected vertebra. An *oblique view* of the spine may show defect in the pars interarticularis. In this view, in a normal vertebra, the pars interarticularis looks like a 'scottish dog' (Fig. 33.7). If the appearance is that of a scottish dog 'wearing a collar', the defect is in the isthmus (pars interarticularis), and the patient has a *spondylolysis* (a defect without slipping of the vertebra). If the head of the 'scottish dog' is separated from the neck, the patient has *spondylolisthesis* (a defect with slip of the vertebra).

TREATMENT

Principles of treatment: For a mild symptomless spondylolisthesis, no treatment is required. When symptoms are mild, they are adequately relieved by conservative methods, such as a brace and spinal exercises. When symptoms are moderately severe or more, especially if these hamper the activity of the patient, an operation may be required.

Methods of treatment: These consist of conservative and operative methods.

Conservative methods consist of rest and external support to the affected segment followed by flexion

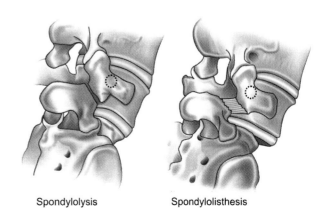

Spondylolysis   Spondylolisthesis

Fig. 33.7: Scottish dog sign (seen in oblique views of the spine).

exercises. The patient is advised to change his job to a physically less demanding one.

Operative methods consist of decompression of the compressed nerves if any, followed by fusion of the affected segments of the spine. This is commonly achieved by fusion between the transverse processes of adjacent vertebrae (intertransverse fusion). Use of internal fixation devices like pedicular screws and rods has helped in early mobilisation of the patient.

 What have we learnt?

- Scoliosis is sideways curvature of spine, different from kyphosis and lordosis, which are antero-posterior curves.
- Non-structural scoliosis is transient, whereas structural is permanent.
- Treatment depends upon severity of the scoliotic curve, its location and how it is likely to affect cosmesis and functions.

Competency

❖ **OR2.3:** Select, prescribe and communicate appropriate medications for relief of joint pain.
❖ **OR5.1:** Describe and discuss the aetiopathogenesis, clinical features, investigations and principles of management of various inflammatory disorder of joints.

DEFINITIONS

Arthritis is an inflammation of a joint. It is characterised by pain, swelling and limitation of joint movement. The cause may be purely a local pathology such as pyogenic arthritis, or a more generalised illness such as rheumatoid arthritis.

Arthralgia is a term used for pain in a joint, *without* any other signs of inflammation.

CLASSIFICATION

From the clinical viewpoint, arthritis can be divided into two types: (i) monoarthritis; and (ii) polyarthritis. Monoarthritis will usually mean that it is a disease affecting just one joint. The causes of that are as shown in Table 34.1. Sometimes monoarthritis may be early presentation of a developing systemic inflammatory disorder such seronegative spondyloarthritis. In such cases, over

Table 34.1: Types of arthritis.

- **Monoarthritis**
  Pyogenic arthritis, Tubercular arthritis, Haemophilic arthritis, Secondary osteoarthritis, Gout - sometimes
- **Polyarthritis**
  Rheumatoid arthritis, Rheumatic fever, Juvenile chronic polyarthritis Primary osteoarthritis, seronegative, spondarthritis

Table 34.2: New diagnostic criteria for rheumatoid arthritis (1987).

- Morning stiffness
- Swelling of three or more specified joints
- Swelling of joint(s) in the hands and wrist
- Symmetrical swellings
- Rheumatoid nodule
- Rheumatoid factor positive
- X-ray changes—erosion or unequivocal peri-articular osteopenia

If four or more of these are present, it is rheumatoid arthritis

Sensitivity of these criteria 93 per cent
Specificity of these criteria 90 per cent

a period of time, monoarthritis may blow up into a full-fledged polyarthritis. It is impostant to search for features of polyarthritis (involvement of other joints, and enthesopathy) by direct questioning. Wheres monoarthritis is primarily the domain of orthopaedic surgeons, polyarthritis is treated by rheumatologists. Some common causes of the two types of arthritis are given in Table 34.1.

RHEUMATOID ARTHRITIS

Rheumatoid arthritis is a chronic systemic inflammatory disease primarily affecting synovial joints. It is diagnosed as per the criteria laid down by American Rheumatism Association in 1987 (Table 34.2).

ETIOPATHOLOGY

Etiology: The exact etiology is not known. Following factors have been thought to play a role in causation of the disease:

- *A genetic* predisposition is strongly suspected because of certain histocompatibility markers associated with it (HLA-drw4/HLA-DR1).
- *Agents* such as mycoplasma, clostridium and some viruses (EB virus) have been implicated in its etiology.

It is now believed that rheumatoid arthritis results from exposure of a genetically predisposed individual to some infectious agent. This leads to autoimmunity and formation of immune complexes with IgM antibodies in the serum. These immune complexes are deposited in the synovial membrane and initiate a self-perpetuating chronic inflammation of the synovial membrane.

Pathology: Initially the synovium becomes oedematous, filled with fibrin exudates and cellular infiltrates. There is an increase in synovial fluid. As the inflammation persists, the synovium gets hypertrophied and surrounds the periphery of the articular cartilage to form *a pannus*. The articular cartilage loses its smooth shiny appearance. The pannus extends over the cartilage from the periphery and burrows into the subchondral bone. With further progress of the disease, the cartilage becomes worn off and the bone surfaces become raw. The joints gets deformed, initially because of severe muscle spasm associated with pain, but later due to fibrosis of the capsule and other soft tissue structures.

In some cases, adhesions develop between apposing layers of pannus, leading to *fibrous ankylosis,* and later *bony ankylosis.* In an advanced disease, the joint capsule gets distended by the hypertrophied synovium and synovial fluid, and the ligaments supporting the joint are stretched, resulting in subluxation of the joint. Osteoporosis develops in the bones adjacent to the diseased joint. Peri-articular tissues, notably tendons and muscles become oedematous and infiltrated with cells, and may rupture spontaneously.

The *course of the disease* varies from patient to patient. In some, it is no more than a mild arthritis which totally recovers. In others, it may be a severe, chronic debilitating disease, ultimately ending up in deformities. A typical case has a history of spontaneous remissions and exacerbations. Some of the factors known to precipitate an attack are physical exertion, psychological stress, infections and occasionally, trauma.

Stages of rheumatoid arthritis: From clinical viewpoint rheumatoid arthritis can be divided into three stages:

1. *Potentially reversible* soft tissue proliferations: In this stage, the disease is limited to the synovium. There occurs synovial hypertrophy and effusion. No destructive changes can be seen on X-rays.
2. *Controllable but irreversible* soft tissue destruction and early cartilage erosions: X-rays shows a reduction in the joint space, but outline of the articular surfaces is maintained.
3. *Irreversible* soft tissue and bony changes: The pannus ultimately destroys the articular cartilage and erodes the subchondral bone. The joint becomes ankylosed usually in a deformed position (fibrous ankylosis). It may be subluxated or dislocated.

Associated changes: Rheumatoid arthritis is a systemic inflammatory disease which can affect quite a few important organs such as hear, kidney, lungs, etc. With such involvement it may be a potentially fatal disease. There is sometimes evidence of diffuse vasculitis. The most serious lesions occur in the arterial tree; which may be mild non-necrotising arteritis, or severe and fulminant arteritis akin to polyarteritis nodosa. The latter is fatal.

DIAGNOSIS

Clinical features: It occurs between the age of 20 to 50 years. Women are affected about 3 times more commonly than men. Following presentations are common:

a. *An acute, symmetrical polyarthritis:* Pain and stiffness in multiple joints (at least four), particularly in the morning, mark the beginning of the disease. This may be followed by frank symptoms of articular inflammation. The joints affected most commonly are the metacarpophalangeal joints, particularly that of the index finger. Other joints affected commonly are as given in Table 34.3.
b. *Others:* The onset may be with fever, the cause of which cannot be established (PUO), especially in children. Sometimes, visceral manifestations of the disease such as pneumonitis, rheumatoid nodules, etc., may antedate the joint complaints.

Table 34.3: Joints affected in rheumatoid arthritis.	
Common	■ MP joints of hand ■ PIP joints of fingers ■ Wrists, knees, elbows, ankles
Less common	■ Hip joint ■ Temporomandibular joint
Uncommon	■ Atlanto-axial joint ■ Facet joints of cervical spine

Table 34.4: Deformities in rheumatoid arthritis.	
Hand	▪ Ulnar drift of the hand ▪ Boutonniere deformity ▪ Swan neck deformity
Elbow	▪ Flexion deformity
Knee	▪ Early-flexion deformity ▪ Late-triple* subluxation
Ankle	▪ Equinus deformity
Foot	▪ Hallux valgus, hammer toe, etc.

* Flexion, posterior subluxation and external rotation.

On examination, one finds swollen boggy joints as a result of intra-articular effusion, synovial hypertrophy and oedema of the peri-articular structures. The joints may be deformed (Table 34.4).

Joints of the hand show typical deformities as shown in Figure 34.1. There may be severe muscle spasm. Range of motion of the joints may be limited. In later stages, the joints may be subluxated or dislocated. There may be fever, rash and signs suggestive of systemic vasculitis. The rash in rheumatoid arthritis is typically non-pruritic and maculopapular on the face, trunk and extremities.

Extra-articular manifestations of rheumatoid arthritis: Although, rheumatoid arthritis is primarily a chronic polyarthritis, extra-articular manifestations are very common, and sometimes govern the prognosis of a case. These are given in Table 34.5.

Investigations: Following investigations are useful:
1. **Radiological examination:** This consists of X-rays of both hands and of the affected joints. Following features may be present (Fig. 34.2):
   - Reduced joint space
   - Erosion of articular margins

Table 34.5: Extra-articular manifestations of rheumatoid arthritis.	
Vasculitis	▪ Digital arteritis ▪ Raynaud's phenomenon ▪ Fever, skin lesions, chronic leg ulcers ▪ Peripheral neuritis (mononeuritis multiplex) ▪ Necrotising arteritis involving coronary, mesentric or renal vessels
Rheumatoid nodules	▪ Most common site—olecranon ▪ Other sites—dorsal surface of forearm, tendoachilles
Serositis	▪ Lung and pleura - pleurisy, parenchymatous nodules, Caplan's syndrome, Honey comb lung ▪ Heart—cardiomyopathy, pericarditis ▪ Eye—iridocyclitis ▪ Nervous system - peripheral neuritis, carpal tunnel syndrome
Others	▪ Anaemia ▪ Felty's syndrome ▪ Sjogren's syndrome ▪ Amyloidosis

   - Subchondral cysts
   - Juxta-articular rarefaction
   - Soft tissue shadow at the level of the joint because of joint effusion or synovial hypertrophy
   - Deformities of the hand and fingers
2. **Blood:** It shows the following changes:
   - Elevated ESR, CRP, platelet count—all markers of systemic inflammation
   - Low haemoglobin
   - *Rheumatoid factor (RF):* This is an auto antibody directed against the Fc fragment of immunoglobulin G (IgG). RF can belong to any class of immunoglobulins, i.e., IgG-RF, IgM-RF, IgA-RF, or IgE-RF, but commonly done tests

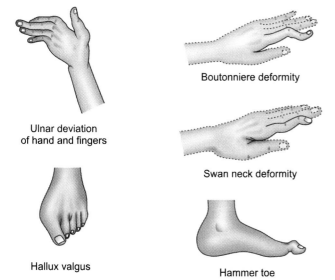

Boutonniere deformity

Ulnar deviation of hand and fingers

Swan neck deformity

Hallux valgus

Hammer toe

Fig. 34.1: Deformities in rheumatoid arthritis.

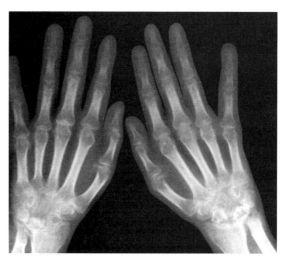

Fig. 34.2: X-rays of both hands, AP view, showing juxta-articular rarefaction.

detect only the IgM type of RF. It can be detected in the serum of the patient by the following tests:

- ◊ *Latex fixation test*: This is an agglutination test where the antibodies are coated to latex particles. Positivity in titres more than 1/20 is significant. Sensitivity is 80 per cent.
- ◊ *Rose-Waaler test*: In this agglutination test *sheep's red blood cells* are used as a carrier. Sensitivity is 60 per cent.
- ◊ *All patients with positive rheumatoid factor do not have rheumatoid arthritis.* Conversely, all patients with rheumatoid arthritis do not have a positive rheumatoid factor. It is the constellation of signs and symptoms, *titre* in which the RF is positive, presence or absence of other positive tests, etc., which determine whether the patient has rheumatoid arthritis or not.
  - ▪ *Anti-CCP* (anti-cyclic citrullinated peptide) test: This is a blood tests, more sensitive to detect rheumatoid arthritis. It should be done in a case suspected of rheumatoid arthritis where rheumatoid factor is negative. People with high titre of anti-CCP have 90% chances of having rheumatoid arthritis. People with positive anti-CCP have more severe variety of rheumatoid arthritis.
- • **Synovial fluid examination**—See Table 22.3 on page 175.
- • **Synovial biopsy:** This can be obtained arthroscopically or by open methods.

DIFFERENTIAL DIAGNOSIS

Rheumatoid arthritis must be differentiated from the following diseases:

a. **Systemic lupus erythematosus (SLE):** In SLE, the joint involvement is not symmetrical; nor are ankylosis and erosions common. Absence of anti-nuclear antibody factor (ANF) is in favour of rheumatoid arthritis, although its presence does not confirm SLE. It is present in 25 per cent cases of rheumatoid arthritis, though in low titres.

b. **Osteoarthritis:** This occurs in older patients. There is complete lack of the systemic features of rheumatoid arthritis such as fever, weight loss, fatigue, etc. Distal interphalangeal joints are often involved. Duration of morning stiffness, joint swelling, ESR, etc., are less compared to rheumatoid arthritis.

c. **Psoriatic arthropathy:** Characteristic skin and nail lesions may be present. Distal interphalangeal joints are usually involved. Rheumatoid factor is negative.

TREATMENT

Principles of treatment: Aims of treatment are as follows:

a. *Induction of remission and its maintenance:* Disease activity is brought under control by drugs. Disease activity is measured by counting the involved joints and level of inflammatory markers.

b. *Preservation of joint functions* and *prevention of deformities* during the activity of the disease and thereafter, by physiotherapy and splinting.

c. *Repair of joint damage* which already exists, if it will relieve pain or facilitate functions. It sometimes requires surgical intervention, e.g., synovectomy.

Methods of treatment: Above mentioned goals can be achieved by medical and orthopaedic treatment.

Medical treatment: Medical treatment essentially consists of antirheumatic drugs. These consist of: (i) non-steroidal anti-inflammatory drugs (NSAIDs); (ii) disease modifying anti-rheumatic drugs (DMARDs); (iii) steroids; (iv) biologicals. For details please refer to a Medicine textbook.

Orthopaedic treatment: Orthopaedic treatment aims at: (a) prevention of joint damage by proper splinting and joint exercises; (b) recovering the lost joint functions by non-operative and operative methods.

Non-operative methods: These consist of the following:

i. *Physiotherapy:* This consists of: (i) splintage of the joints in proper position during the acute phase: (ii) heat therapy – wax bath, hot water fomentation for symptomatic relief; (iii) joint mobilisation exercises to maintain joint functions; and (iv) muscle building exercises to gain strength.

ii. *Occupational therapy:* Role of occupational therapy is to help the patient cope with his occupational requirements despite his/her disability, using appliances.

iii. *Rehabilitation:* Role of rehabilitation is to improve the functions of the patient with the help of devices like braces, walking aids, etc.

Operative methods: Surgical treatment of rheumatoid arthritis can be divided into: (i) preventive surgery; (ii) palliative surgery; (iii) reconstructive surgery; and (iv) salvage surgery.

- • *Preventive surgery:* This is done to prevent damage to the joint and nearby tendons, which could be caused by inflamed, hypertrophied synovium. It consists of synovectomy of the wrist, knee and MP joints, and also tenosynovectomy.

- *Palliative surgery:* This is done in situations where general condition of the patient does not permit corrective surgery, but some relief can be provided by limited surgical procedures such as bone block operations to correct deformity, and tendon lengthening to correct contractures.
- *Reconstructive surgery:* This has revolutionised the putting back to their functions, patients with deformed and painful joints. It includes tendon transfers, interposition arthroplasties and joint replacement. With improvement in surgical techniques and better design of artificial joints, it is now possible to replace practically any joint of the body. The joints where total replacement is most popular are the hip, knee, shoulder, elbow and metacarpophalangeal joints.

Plan of treatment: Management depends upon the stage of the disease, as discussed below:
1. *Potentially reversible* soft tissue proliferation, where drug therapy constitutes the mainstay of treatment.
2. *Controllable* but irreversible soft tissue destruction and early cartilage erosion, where a combination of drug therapy and orthopaedic treatment is required.
3. *Advanced stage of* joint destruction with subluxation or dislocation, where primarily surgical treatment is necessary. Drugs alone are of little use at this stage, though drug therapy needs to be continued to prevent damage to rest of the joints.

Plan of treatment in these three stages is as given in Table 34.6.

Prognosis: Following factors decide the outcome of a patient diagnosed to have rheumatoid arthritis.
- **Natural history of the disease:** It is well known that rheumatoid arthritis is a disease with variable natural history. It may be fulminant, i.e., damaging joints quickly and producing deformities in spite of best care, or more usually a disease with persistent course punctuated with remissions and exacerbations. It is not possible to predict the precise nature of the disease in a particular patient.
- **Sex and age at onset:** Women of child-bearing age with predominant upper extremity involvement have a progressively severe disease. Males, with sparing of upper extremity, where onset of disease is under the age of 30 years, show less severe disease.
- **Type of onset:** It is generally believed that insidous onset disease progresses to have more severe disease.
- **Anaemia:** Anaemia is associated with progressive rheumatoid arthritis. Also, it is believed that unresponsiveness of anaemia to oral iron therapy is a bad prognostic indicater.
- **ESR and C-reactive protein:** High levels are associated with more erosive arthritis.
- **Rheumatoid factor:** A positive rheumatoid factor is associated with more progressive disease. High titres of rheumatoid factor, appearing early in the disease, carry a bad prognosis.
- **Anti-CCP:** Positive anti-CCP correlates with worse disease.
- **Radiological erosions:** Presence of erosions within 2 years of onset of the disease, is a bad prognostic indicator.
- **Histopathological changes:** A case with synovial proliferation, with increased number of synovial cells with DR antigen, carries bad prognosis.

SPONDARTHRITIS (SPA)

These are a group of systemic inflammatory disorders identified by their primary affliction of the spine in addition to joint involvement. These differ from the more common disease of the same group, rheumatoid arthritis, due to: (i) primary spine involvement; (ii) asymmetric involvement of major joints such as hip, knee, ankle and shoulder; (iii) Enthesopathy— pain due to inflammation at tendon to bone junctions. The main disease in this category of diseases is Ankylosing Spondylitis.

ANKYLOSING SPONDYLITIS
(Marie Strumpell Disease)

Ankylosing spondylitis is a chronic disease characterised by a progressive inflammatory stiffening of the joints, with a predilection for the

Table 34.6: Staged therapy in rheumatoid arthritis.			
Stage	**Medical**	**Surgical**	**Physiotherapy**
Stage I	DMARDs* NSAIDs**	Synovectomy	Joint mobilisation
Stage II	NSAIDs DMARDs	Soft tissue repair Arthroplasty	Splints
Stage III	NSAIDs	Arthroplasty (joint replacement) Arthrodesis	Splints and walking aids

* Disease modifying anti-rheumatic drugs
** Non-steroidal anti-inflammatory drugs

joints of the axial skeleton, especially the sacro-iliac joints.

ETIOPATHOLOGY

The exact etiology is not known. A strong association has been found between a genetic marker—HLA-B27 and this disease. Whereas, the incidence of HLA-B27 is less than 1 per cent in general population, it is present in more than 85 per cent of patients with ankylosing spondylitis.

Pathology: Sacro-iliac joints are usually the *first* to get involved; followed by the spine from the lumbar region upwards. The hip, the knee and the manubriosternal joints are also involved frequently. Initially synovitis occurs, followed later by cartilage destruction and bony erosion. Resultant fibrosis ultimately leads to fibrous ankylosis which leads to bony ankylosis. Ossification also occurs in the anterior longitudinal ligament and other ligaments of the spine. After bony fusion occurs, the pain may subside, leaving the spine permanently stiff (burnt-out disease).

CLINICAL FEATURES

Presenting complaints: This is a disease of young adults, more common in males (M : F=10 : 1). The following clinical presentations may be seen:

a. *Classic presentation:* The patient is a young adult 15-30 years old male, presenting with a gradual onset of pain and stiffness of the lower back. Initially, the stiffness may be noticed only after a period of rest, and improves with movement. Pain tends to be worst at night or early morning, awakening the patient from sleep. He gets better only after he walks about or does some exercises. There may be pain in the heel, pubic symphysis, manubrium sterni and costosternal joints. In later stages, kyphotic deformity of spine and deformity of the hips may be prominent features.

b. *Unusual presentations:* Patient may occasionally present with involvement of peripheral joints such as the shoulders, hips and knees. Smaller joints are rarely involved. Sometimes, a patient with ankylosing spondylitis may present with chronic inflammatory bowel disease; the joint symptoms follow.

On examination it is found that the patient walks with a straight stiff back. There may be a diffuse kyphosis. Following clinical signs may be present:

- *Stiff spine:* There may be a loss of lumbar lordosis. Lumbar spine flexion may be limited.
- *Tests for detecting sacro-iliac involvement:* Following tests may be positive in a case with sacro-iliac joint involvement:
- Tenderness, localised to the posterior superior iliac spine or deep in the gluteal region.
- *Sacro-iliac compression:* Direct side to side compression of the pelvis may cause pain at the sacro-iliac joints.
- *Gaenslen's test:* The hip and the knee joints of the opposite side are flexed to fix the pelvis, and the hip joint of the side under test is hyperextended over the edge of the table. This will exert a rotational strain over the sacro-iliac joint and give rise to pain (Fig. 34.3A).
- *Straight leg raising test:* The patient is asked to lift the leg up with the knee extended. This will cause pain at the affected sacro-iliac joint.
- *Pump-handle test:* With the patient lying supine, the examiner flexes his hip and knee completely, and forces the affected knee across the chest, so as to bring it close to the opposite shoulder (Fig. 34.3B). This will cause pain on the affected side.

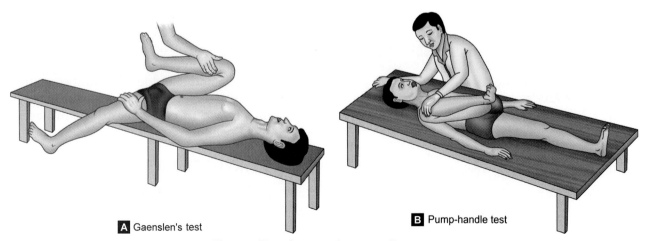

A Gaenslen's test　　**B** Pump-handle test

Fig. 34.3: Tests for sacro-iliac joint affections.

- *Tests for cervical spine involvement:* In advanced stages, the cervical spine gets completely stiff. The Fleche test may detect an early involvement of the cervical spine.
- *Fleche test:* The patient stands with his heel and back against the wall and tries to touch the wall with the back of his head without raising the chin. Inability to touch the head to the wall suggests cervical spine involvement.
- *Thoracic spine involvement:* Maximum chest expansion, from full expiration to full inspiration is measured at the level of the nipples. A chest expansion less than 5 cm indicates involvement of the costovertebral joints.

Extra-articular manifestations: In addition to articular symptoms, a patient with ankylosing spondylitis may have the following extra-articular manifestations:

a. *Ocular:* About 25 per cent patients with ankylosing spondylitis develop at least one attack of acute iritis sometimes during the natural history of the disease. Many patients suffer from recurrent episodes, which may result in scarring and depigmentation of the iris.

b. *Cardiovascular:* Patients with ankylosing spondylitis, especially those with a long-standing illness, develop cardiovascular manifestations in the form of aortic incompetence, cardiomegaly, conduction defects, pericarditis, etc.

c. *Neurological:* Patients may develop spontaneous dislocation and subluxation of the atlanto-axial joint or fractures of the cervical spine with trivial trauma, and may present with signs and symptoms of spinal cord compression.

d. *Pulmonary:* Involvement of the costovertebral joints lead to painless restriction of the thoracic cage. This can be detected clinically by diminished chest expansion, or by performing pulmonary function tests (PFTs). There may also occur bilateral apical lobe fibrosis with cavitation, which remarkably simulates tuberculosis on X-ray.

e. *Systemic:* Generalised osteoporosis occurs commonly. Occasionally, a patient may develop amyloidosis.

INVESTIGATIONS

Radiological examination (Fig. 34.4): In a suspected case, X-rays of the pelvis (AP), and dorso-lumbar spine (AP and lateral) are required. Oblique views of sacro-iliac joints may be required in early stages

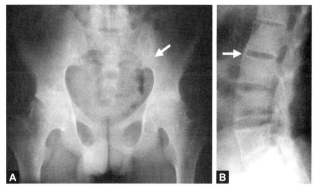

Fig. 34.4: X-rays showing changes in ankylosing spondylitis: (A) X-ray of the pelvis, AP view, showing bilateral SI joint and hip involvement; (B) X-ray of the lumbar spine, lateral view, showing calcification of the ligaments.

to appreciate their involvement. Following changes may be seen on X-ray of the pelvis:
- Haziness of the sacro-iliac joints
- Irregular subchondral erosions in SI joints
- Sclerosis of the articulating surfaces of SI joints
- Widening of the sacro-iliac joint space
- Bony ankylosis of the sacro-iliac joints
- Calcification of the sacro-iliac ligament and sacro-tuberous ligaments
- Evidence of enthesopathy – calcification at the attachment of the muscles, tendons and ligaments, particularly around the pelvis and around the heel.

X-ray of the lumbar spine may show the following:
- **Squaring of vertebrae:** The normal anterior concavity of the vertebral body is lost because of calcification of the anterior longitudinal ligament.
- Loss of the lumbar lordosis.
- Bridging 'osteophytes' (*syndesmophytes*).
- *Bamboo spine* appearance.

In the peripheral joints, X-ray changes are similar to those seen in rheumatoid arthritis, except that there is formation of large osteophytes and peri-articular calcification. Bony ankylosis occurs commonly.

Other investigations: These are the following:
- ESR: elevated
- Hb: mild anaemia
- HLA-B27: positive (to be tested in doubtful cases)

DIFFERENTIAL DIAGNOSIS

In early stages, ankylosing spondylitis may be confused with other disorders, as given in Table 34.7, next page.

Table 34.7: Differential diagnosis of ankylosing spondylitis.

Disease	Clinical	Investigations
Stiffness		
TB spine	Occurs at any age or sex, localised tenderness present, cold abscess present, constitutional symptoms present, family or past history of TB present	• Signs of TB spine on X-rays • Primary lesion in the chest
Fluorosis	• Any age or sex • Dental mottling present • Chest expansion normal	• Posterior longitudinal ligament calcified, seen on X-rays • Interosseous membrane calcification seen on X-rays • Serum and urine fluoride studies – high levels
Back pain		
Lumbo-sacral strain	• Non-specific • Localised tenderness present	• X-rays normal • ESR normal
Disc prolapse	SLRT positive	• No radiological changes • ESR normal
Osteoarthritis	Seen in elderly patients	• Osteophytes present • ESR normal
SI joint diseases		
TB of SI joint	• Any age affected • Generally unilateral • Cold abscess may be seen on CT, ESR high	• Lytic lesions with sclerosis seen on X-ray • Cold abscess present
Osteitis condensans iliac	Bilateral, non-specific sclerosis of ilium, seen in parous women	• ESR normal • Sclerosis of subchondral bone on the illiac side of the SI joint only

OTHER RHEUMATOLOGICAL DISEASES

Gout	Disturbed purine metabolism leading to excessive accumulation of uric acid in the blood—an inherited disorder; or impaired excretion of uric acid by the kidneys. The result is accumulation of *sodium biurate* crystals in some soft tissues. Tissues of predilection are cartilage, tendon, bursa Patient, usually beyond 40 years of age, presents as: (i) arthritis—MP joint of the big toe being a *favourite site,* onset is acute, pain is severe; (ii) bursitis—commonly of the olecranon bursa; or (iii) tophi formation deposit of uric acid salt in the soft tissue, confirmation of diagnosis—urate crystals in the aspirate from a joint or bursa, high serum uric acid levels, treatment—NSAIDs, uricosuric drugs, uric acid inhibitors.
Pseudogout	*Sodium pyrophosphate* crystal deposition, symptoms like those of gout, *meniscus calcification* may be seen on X-rays of the knee, treatment—NSAIDs.
Psoriatic arthropathy	Presentation is like rheumatoid arthritis—a polyarthritis, *distal IP joints* of hands involved (unlike rheumatoid arthritis, where these are spared), classic skin lesions help in diagnosis, treatment is by steroids.
Alkaptonuric arthritis (Ocronosis)	• An inherited defect in enzyme system involved in metabolism of phenylalanine and tyrosine. As a result homogentisic acid is excreted in patient's urine. As a long-term result, it accumulates in the cartilage and other connecting tissues. • Joint symptoms occur after 40 years of age. Spine and shoulder joint are commonly affected. There may be evidence of pigment deposit in the sclera. Homogentisic acid is present in the urine, and results in the colour of the urine turning dark brown on standing (due to oxidation of homogentisic acid on exposure to air) • X-ray—*disc space calcification,* peri-articular calcification in large joints, treatment same as that for osteoarthritis.
Haemophilic arthritis	• Occurs due to a number of bleeding disorders, occurs in males • Joints affected commonly are knee, elbow and ankle • X-ray—non-specific signs including bone resorption, cyst formation, osteoporosis, *widening of intercondylar notch in the knee.* • Treatment—rest during acute stage along with factor VIII supplementation or other deficient factor replacement. In the chronic stage, physiotherapy, bracing, etc., are required. Deformities may be corrected by conservative or operative methods.
Neuropathic arthropathy	• These are changes seen in a neuropathic joint, where repeated strain (Charcot's joint) on a joint due to loss of sensations leads to severe degeneration • Clinically, the joint manifests as painless effusion, deformity or instability • The X-ray changes are those of severe osteoarthritis but without much clinical findings like pain, muscle spasm, etc. • Treatment is difficult. Bracing is usually advised for some joints. Fusion of the joint may be required.

TREATMENT

No specific therapy is available. Aim is to control the pain and maintain maximum degree of joint mobility. This can readily be achieved by life-long pursuit of a structured exercise programme. In some cases surgical intervention is required.

Conservative methods: These consist of: (i) *drugs*— NSAIDs are given for pain relief; Naproxen is effective in most cases; long-acting preparations are preferred. Amongst newer drugs are biologicals; (ii) *physiotherapy* - this consists of proper posture guidance, heat therapy and mobilisation exercises; (iii) *radiotherapy* – in some resistant cases; and (iv) *yoga therapy.*

Operative methods: Role of operative treatment is in correction of kyphotic deformities of the spine by spinal osteotomy, and joint replacement for cases with hip or knee joint ankylosis.

What have we learnt?

- There are two types of arthritis: inflammatory and degenerative.
- Rheumatoid arthritis is a chronic polyarthritis of inflammatory nature, typically affecting peripheral joints.
- Orthopaedic management of rheumatoid arthritis is aimed at prevention of deformity, correction of deformity and joint replacement.
- Ankylosing spondylitis occurs in young men. Treatment is aimed at physiotherapy.

Degenerative Disorders

Competencies

❖ **OR6.1:** Describe and discuss the clinical features, investigations and principles of management of degenerative condition of spine (cervical spondylosis, lumbar spondylosis, PID).

OSTEOARTHRITIS (OSTEOARTHROSIS)

Osteoarthritis (OA) is a degenerative joint disease. Etiology is multifactorial, and still not understood. Commonly it is thought to be wear and tear of joints as one ages. Two types of OA are recognised—primary and secondary.

- **Primary OA:** This occurs in a joint *de novo*. It occurs in old age, mainly in the weight-bearing joints (knee and hip). In a generalised variety, the trapeziometacarpal joint of the thumb and the distal interphalangeal joints of the fingers are also affected. Primary OA is more common than secondary OA.

- **Secondary OA:** In this type, there is an underlying primary disease of the joint which leads to degeneration of the joint, often many years later. It may occur at any age after adolescence, and occurs commonly at the hip (Table 35.1). Predisposing factors are: (i) congenital mal-development of a joint; (ii) irregularity of the joint surfaces from previous trauma; (iii) previous disease producing a damaged articular surface; (iv) internal derangement of the knee, such as a loose body; (v) mal-alignment (bow legs, etc.); and (vi) obesity and excessive weight.

PATHOLOGY

Osteoarthritis is a degenerative condition *primarily affecting the articular cartilage*. The first change observed

Table 35.1: Causes of secondary OA of the hip.

Avascular necrosis

- Idiopathic
- Post-traumatic, e.g., fracture of femoral neck
- Alcoholism
- Post-partum osteonecrosis
- Chronic liver failure
- Patient on steroids
- Patient on dialysis
- Sickle cell anaemia

Coxa vara

- *Congenital dislocation of hip (CDH)*
- *Old septic arthritis of the hip*
- *Malunited fractures*
- *Fractures of the acetabulum*

is an increase in water content and depletion of the proteoglycans from the cartilage matrix. Repeated weight bearing on such a cartilage leads to its *fibrillation*. The cartilage gets abraded by the grinding mechanism at work at the points of contact between the apposing articular surfaces, until eventually the underlying bone is exposed. With further 'rubbing', the subchondral bone becomes hard and glossy *(eburnated)*. Meanwhile, the bone at the margins of the joint hypertrophies to form a rim of projecting spurs known as *osteophytes*. A similar mechanism results in the formation of *subchondral* cysts and sclerosis.

The loose flakes of cartilage incite *synovial inflammation* and thickening of the capsule, leading to deformity and stiffness of the joint. Often one compartment of a joint is affected more than the other. For example, in the knee joint, the medial compartment is affected more than the lateral, leading to a varus deformity (genu varum).

CLINICAL FEATURES

The disease occurs in elderly people, mostly in the major joints of the lower limb, frequently bilaterally. There is a geographical variation in the joints involved, depending probably upon the daily activities of a population. The *hip* joint is commonly affected in a population with western living habits, while the *knee* is involved more commonly in a population with Asian living habits, i.e., the habit of squatting and sitting cross legged.

Pain is the *earliest* symptom. It occurs inter- mittently in the beginning, but becomes constant over months or years. Initially, it is dull pain and comes on starting an activity after a period of rest; but later it becomes worse and cramp-like, and comes after activity. A coarse *crepitus* may be complained of by some patients. *Swelling* of the joint is usually a late feature, and is due to the effusion caused by inflammation of the synovial tissues. *Stiffness* is initially due to pain and muscle spasm; but later, capsular contracture and incongruity of the joint surface contribute to it. Other symptoms are—a feeling of 'instability' of the joint, and 'locking' resulting from loose bodies and frayed menisci.

EXAMINATION

Following findings may be present:
- Tenderness on the joint line
- Crepitus on moving the joint
- Irregular and enlarged-looking joint due to formation of peripheral osteophytes
- Deformity – varus of the knee, flexion-adduction-external rotation of the hip
- Effusion – rare and transient
- Terminal limitation of joint movement
- Subluxation detected on ligament testing
- Wasting of quadriceps femoris muscle

INVESTIGATIONS

Radiological examination: The diagnosis of osteoarthritis is mainly radiological (Fig. 35.1). The following are some of the radiological features:
- Narrowing of joint space, often limited to a part of the joint, e.g., may be limited to medial compartment of tibiofemoral joint of the knee.

- Subchondral sclerosis—dense bone under the articular surface
- Subchondral cysts
- Osteophyte formation
- Loose bodies
- Deformity of the joint

Other investigations are made primarily to detect an underlying cause. These consist of the following:
- Serological tests and ESR to rule out rheumatoid arthritis
- Serum uric acid to rule out gout
- Arthroscopy, if a loose body or frayed meniscus is suspected.

TREATMENT

Principles of treatment: Once the disease starts, it progresses gradually, and there is no way to stop it. Hence efforts are directed, wherever possible, to the following:

a. To *delay the occurrence or stall the progress* of the disease, if the disease has not begun yet. This is done by keeping the weight in check, doing regular fitness exercises, and having a lifestyle favourable to the affected part.

b. To *rehabilitate* the patient, with or without surgery, if his disabilities can be partially or completely alleviated. This is done by the methods discussed below.

Methods of treatment: The following therapeutic measures may be undertaken:

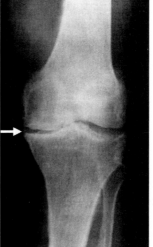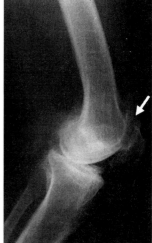

Fig. 35.1: X-rays of the knee, AP and lateral views, showing osteoarthritis of the knee reduction in joint space on the medial side, osteophyte formation—arrow).

a. *Drugs:* Analgesics are used mainly to suppress pain. A trial of different drugs is carried out to find a suitable drug for a particular patient. Long-acting formulations are preferred.

b. *Chondroprotective agents:* A number of products, mostly food supplements have been promoted as chondroprotectic agents. Some of these are: Glucosamine, Chondroitin sulphate and Collegen peptide. Their role as disease modifying agents has yet not been established, but these could be tried in some early cases.

c. *Viscosuplementation:* Sodium Hyaluronan is injected in the joint one injection, to be repeated a few times in a year. It is supposed to improve cartilage functions, and is claimed to be chondroprotective. Effect is variable.

d. *Supportive therapy:* This is a useful and harmless method of treatment and often gives gratifying results. It consists of the following:
   - *Weight reduction,* in an obese patient.
   - *Avoidance of stress* and strain to the affected joint in day-to-day activities. For example, a patient with OA of the knee is advised to avoid standing or running whenever possible. Sitting cross legged and squatting is harmful for OA of the knee.
   - *Local heat* provides relief of pain and stiffness.
   - *Exercises* for building up the muscles controlling the joint help in providing stability to the joint.
   - The local application of *counter-irritants* and liniments sometimes provide dramatic relief.

e. *Surgical treatment:* In selected cases, surgery can provide significant relief. Surgery for OA of the joints (knee or hip) is divided, broadly into two categories—joint preservation surgery and joint replacement surgery.

Joint preservation surgery: These are indicated in early stages of the disease, where a factor likely to hasten the disease progress can be identified (knee deformity, for example). From least invasive to most invasive, these are as follows:

- *Arthroscopic procedures:* Arthroscopic removal of loose bodies, degenerated meniscal tears and other such procedures have become popular for knee OA because of their less invasive nature. In arthroscopic chondroplasty, the degenerated, fibrillated cartilage is excised using a power-driven shaver under arthroscopic vision. Results are unpredictable.

- *Osteotomy:* Osteotomy near a joint has been known to bring about relief in symptoms, especially in arthritic joints with deformities. A high tibial osteotomy for OA of the knee with genu varum

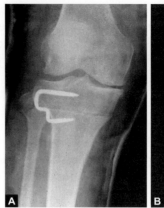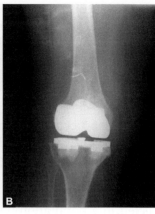

Fig. 35.2: Surgical treatment of osteoarthritis knee; (A) High tibial osteotomy; (B) Total knee replacement.

(Fig. 35.2A), and intertrochanteric osteotomy for OA of the hip have been shown to be useful for pain relief.

- *Joint replacement:* For cases crippled with advanced damage to the joint, total joint replacement operation (Fig. 35.2B) has provided remarkable rehabilitation. These are now commonly performed for the hip and knee. An artificial joint serves for about 10-15 years.

CERVICAL SPONDYLOSIS

This is a degenerative condition of the cervical spine found almost universally in persons over 50 years of age. It occurs early in persons pursuing 'white collar jobs' or those susceptible to neck strain because of keeping the neck constantly in one position while reading, writing, etc.

PATHOLOGY

The pathology begins in the intervertebral discs. Degeneration of disc results in reduction of disc space and peripheral osteophyte formation. The posterior intervertebral joints get secondarily involved and generate pain in the neck. The osteophytes impinging on the nerve roots give rise to radicular pain in the upper limb. Exceptionally, the osteophytes may press on the spinal cord, giving rise to signs of cord compression. Cervical spondylosis occurs most commonly in the lowest three cervical intervertebral joints (the most common is at C_5-C_6).

CLINICAL FEATURES

Complaints are often vague. Following are the common presentations:

- **Pain and stiffness:** This is the most common presenting symptom, initially intermittent but later persistent. Occipital headache may occur if the upper-half of the cervical spine is affected.

- **Radiating pain:** Patient may present with pain radiating to the shoulder or downwards on the outer aspect of the forearm and hand. There may be *paraesthesia* in the region of a nerve root, commonly over the base of the thumb (along the C_6 nerve root). Muscle weakness is uncommon.
- **Giddiness:** Patient may present with an episode of giddiness because of vertebrobasilar syndrome.

EXAMINATION

There is loss of normal cervical lordosis and limitation in neck movements. There may be tenderness over the lower cervical spine or in the muscles of the para-vertebral region (myalgia). The upper limb may have signs suggestive of nerve root compression—usually that of C_6 root involvement. Motor weakness is uncommon. The lower limbs must be examined for signs of early cord compression (e.g., a positive Babinski reflex, etc.).

RADIOLOGICAL FINDINGS

X-rays of the cervical spine (AP and lateral) are sufficient in most cases. Following radiological features may be present (Fig. 35.3):
- Narrowing of intervertebral disc spaces (most commonly between C_5-C_6).
- Osteophytes at the vertebral margins, anteriorly and posteriorly.
- Narrowing of the intervertebral foramen in cases presenting with radicular symptoms, may be best seen on oblique views.

DIFFERENTIAL DIAGNOSIS

The diseases to be considered in differential diagnosis of cervical spondylosis are: (i) other causes of neck pain such as infection, tumours and cervical disc prolapse; and (ii) other causes of upper limb pain like Pancoast tumour, cervical rib, spinal cord tumours, carpal tunnel syndrome, etc.

TREATMENT

Principles of treatment: The symptoms of cervical spondylosis undergo spontaneous remissions and exacerbations. Treatment is aimed at assisting the natural resolution of the temporarily inflamed soft tissues. During the period of remission, the prevention of any further attacks is of utmost importance, and is done by advising the patient regarding the following:
a. *Proper neck posture:* Patient must avoid situations where he has to keep his neck in one position for a long time. Only a thin pillow should be used at night.
b. *Neck muscle exercises:* These help in improving the neck posture.

During an episode of acute exacerbation, the following treatment is required:
- Analgesics
- Hot fomentation
- Rest to the neck in a cervical collar
- Traction to the neck if there is stiffness
- Antiemetics, if there is giddiness

In an exceptional case, where the spinal cord is compressed by osteophytes, surgical decompression may be necessary.

LUMBAR SPONDYLOSIS

This is a degenerative disorder of the lumbar spine characterised clinically by an insidious onset of pain and stiffness and radiologically by osteophyte formation.

CAUSE

Bad posture and chronic back strain is the most common cause. Other causes are, previous injury to the spine, previous disease of the spine, birth defects and old intervertebral disc prolapse.

PATHOLOGY

Primarily, degeneration begins in the intervertebral joints. This is followed by a reduction in the disc space and marginal osteophyte formation. Degenerative changes develop in the posterior facet joints. Osteophytes around the intervertebral foramen may encroach upon the nerve root canal, and thus interfere with the functioning of the emerging nerve.

DIAGNOSIS

Clinical features: Symptoms begin as low backache, initially worst during activity, but later present almost

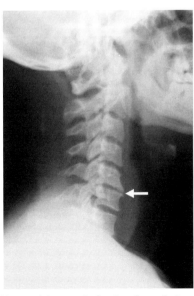

Fig. 35.3: X-ray of the cervical spine, lateral view, showing cervical spondylosis. (Note the lipping of C_5-C_6 vertebrae).

all the time. There may be a feeling of 'a catch' while getting up from a sitting position, which improves as one walks a few steps. Pain may radiate down the limb up to the calf (sciatica) because of irritation of one of the nerve root. There may be complaints of transient numbness and paraesthesia in the dermatome of a nerve root, commonly on the lateral side of leg or foot (L_5, S_1 roots) respectively.

EXAMINATION

The spinal movements are limited terminally, but there is little muscle spasm. The straight leg raising test (SLRT) may be positive if the nerve root compression is present.

RADIOLOGICAL FINDINGS

Good AP and lateral views of the lumbosacral spine (Fig. 35.4) should be done after preparing the bowel with a mild laxative and gas adsorbent like charcoal tablets. It is particularly difficult in obese patients, the ones usually suffering from this disease. Following signs may be present:

- Reduction of disc space
- Osteophyte formation
- Narrowing of joint space of the facet joints
- Subluxation of one vertebra over another

TREATMENT

Principles of treatment: Like cervical spondylosis, lumbar spondylosis also undergoes spontaneous

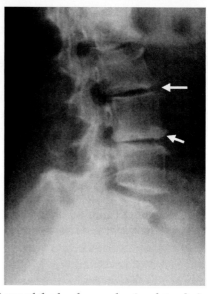

Fig. 35.4: X-ray of the lumbosacral spine, lateral view, showing lumbar spondylosis. (Note reduced disc spaces, osteophytes).

remissions and exacerbations. Treatment is essentially similar to cervical spondylosis. In the acute stage, bed rest, hot fomentation and analgesics are advised. As the symptoms subside, spinal exercises are advised. In some resistant cases, a lumbar corset may have to be used at all times. Spinal fusion may occasionally be necessary.

 What have we learnt?

- Osteoarthritis is a degenerative, progressive disorder. It commonly affects the knee and the back.
- Treatment is preventive, if predisposing factors are known.
- Once progressed, physiotherapy and surgery remain the only options.

Additional information: From the entrance exams point of view

	Osteoarthritis	Rheumatoid arthritis
Characteristic findings	Osteophytes and new bone formation	Juxta-articular osteoporosis, osteophytes and new bone formation usually absent
Joints involved commonly	Distal interphalangeal joints of hand (Heberden's nodes), proximal interphalangeal joints of hand (Bouchard's nodes), 1st carpometacarpal joint, hip, knee	Wrist joint, metacarpophalangeal joints, proximal interphalangeal joints, knee, and hip
Joints not involved	Metacarpophalangeal joints and wrist joint	Lumbar spine, distal interphalangeal joint

- **Type A** synovial cells are phagocytes that engulf joint debris
- **Type B** synovial cells secrete synovial fluid

Affections of the Soft Tissues

Learning Objectives

- ❖ What is bursitis, what are the different sites where it occurs commonly, how is it treated?
- ❖ Discuss etiopathogenesis of frozen shoulder, and its treatment.

BURSITIS

Inflammation may occur in a normally situated bursa or in an adventitious bursa. It may arise from mechanical irritation or from bacterial infection. Accordingly, there are two types of bursitis:

Irritative bursitis: This is the more common of the two types. It is caused by excessive pressure or friction, occasionally due to a gouty deposit. Inflammation of the bursa results in the effusion of a clear fluid within the bursal sac. With prolonged inflammation, the sac gets thickened and may cause pressure erosion on the adjacent bone. Some commonly seen bursites are given in Table 36.1.

Treatment: Most cases respond to analgesics, rest to the part and removal of the causative factor, i.e., friction or pressure. In some resistant cases, the sac is infiltrated with hydrocortisone. Very rarely, excision of the bursa is required.

Infective bursitis: Uncommonly, a bursa may get infected by a pyogenic or tubercular infection. It occurs

Table 36.1: Common bursites.	
Prepatellar bursitis	Housemaid's knee
Infrapatellar bursitis	Clergyman's knee
Olecranon bursitis	Student's elbow
Ischial bursitis	Weaver's bottom
On lateral malleolus	Tailor's ankle
On great toe	Bunion

commonly in trochanteric bursa or prepatellar bursa. Treatment is by surgical drainage and antibacterial drugs.

TENOSYNOVITIS

Inflammation of the thin synovial lining of a tendon sheath (Fig. 36.1) is termed tenosynovitis. It may arise from mechanical irritation or from bacterial infection.

Irritative tenosynovitis is commonly seen in the tendons of the hand and results in pain and swelling. Treatment is by rest, analgesics and ultrasonic

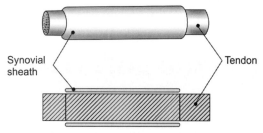

Fig. 36.1: Synovial lining of tendon.

therapy. Some cases need local hydrocortisone infiltration.

Infective tenosynovitis is an infection of the synovial lining of the tendon by pyogenic or tubercular bacteria. Pyogenic infection is common in the flexor tendons of the hand. Tubercular tenosynovitis of the sheaths of the flexor tendons of the forearm at the level of the wrist occurs commonly (compound palmar ganglion).

DUPUYTREN'S CONTRACTURE
(Contracture of the Palmar Aponeurosis)

This is a condition characterised by a flexion deformity of one or more fingers due to a thickening and shortening of the palmar aponeurosis. The cause is unknown, but a hereditary predisposition has been established. There is an increased incidence of the disorder among cirrhotic patients and in epileptics on sodium hydantoin.

PATHOANATOMY

Normally, the palmar aponeurosis is a thin but tough membrane, lying immediately beneath the skin of the palm. Proximally, it is in continuation with the palmaris longus tendon. Distally, it divides into slips, one for each finger. The slip blends with the fibrous flexor sheaths covering the flexor tendon of the finger, and extends up to the *middle* phalanx (Fig. 36.2A). In Dupuytren's contracture, the aponeurosis or a part of it becomes thickened and slowly contracts, drawing the fingers into flexion at the metacarpophalangeal and proximal interphalangeal joints (Fig. 36.2B). The ring finger is the one affected *most* commonly. The contracture is generally limited to the medial three fingers. Sometimes, it may be associated with a thickening of plantar fascia or that of the penile fascia (Peyronie's disease).

CLINICAL FEATURES

In early stages, thickening of the palmar aponeurosis is felt at the bases of ring and little fingers. Later, a flexion deformity of the fingers develops. Dupuytren's contracture can be differentiated from a similar deformity due to contracture of the flexor tendons; in the former only the MP and PIP joints are flexed, unlike the latter where the DIP joints are also flexed.

TREATMENT

An elderly patient with mild contracture does not need any treatment. If the deformity is significant and hampers the activity of the patient, excision of the palmar aponeurosis (subtotal excision) may be required.

TENNIS ELBOW
(Lateral Epicondylitis)

This is a condition characterised by pain and tenderness at the lateral epicondyle of the humerus due to non-specific inflammation at the origin of the extensor muscles of the forearm. Although, it is sometimes seen in tennis players, other activities such as squeezing clothes, carrying a suitcase, etc., are frequently responsible.

CLINICAL FEATURES

One finds tenderness, precisely localised to the lateral epicondyle of the humerus. Pain is aggravated by putting the extensor tendons to a stretch; for example, by palmar-flexing the wrist and fingers with the forearm pronated. Elbow movements are normal. X-ray does not reveal any abnormality.

TREATMENT

The patient is initially treated with analgesics–anti-inflammatory drugs for a week or so. If there is no response, a local injection of hydrocortisone at the point of maximum tenderness generally brings relief.

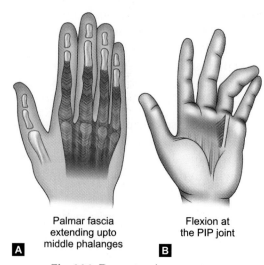

A — Palmar fascia extending upto middle phalanges

B — Flexion at the PIP joint

Fig. 36.2: Dupuytren's contracture.

GOLFER'S ELBOW
(Medial Epicondylitis)

This is a condition similar to tennis elbow where the inflammation is at the origin of the flexor tendons at the medial epicondyle of the humerus. Treatment is on the lines of a tennis elbow.

de QUERVAIN'S TENOSYNOVITIS

This is a condition characterised by pain and swelling over the radial styloid process. It results from inflammation of the common sheath of abductor pollicis longus and extensor pollicis brevis tendons (Fig. 36.3). On examination, the tenderness is localised to the radial styloid process. Pain is aggravated by adducting the thumb across the palm and forcing ulnar deviation and on asking the patient to perform radial deviation against resistance (Finkelstein's test). There may be a palpable thickening of the sheath.

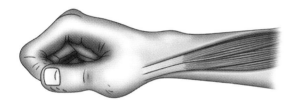

Fig. 36.3: de Quervain's tenosynovitis (affected tendon sheaths).

TREATMENT

In early stage, rest to the wrist in a crepe bandage or a slab, analgesics and ultrasonic radiation may bring relief. In some cases, a local infiltration of hydrocortisone is required. A chronic case may need slitting and excision of a part of the tendon sheath.

TRIGGER FINGER/THUMB

This is a condition resulting from the constriction of the fibrous digital sheath, so that free gliding of the contained flexor tendon does not occur.

CLINICAL FEATURES

Initially, the only symptom is pain at the base of the affected finger, especially on trying to passively extend the finger. As the sheath further thickens, the contained tendon gets swollen proximal to it (Fig. 36.4). The swollen segment of the tendon does not enter the sheath when an attempt is made to straighten the finger from the flexed position. This is called 'locking of finger'. This locking can be overcome either by a strong effort in which case the finger extends with a snap-like trigger of a pistol or by extending the finger passively with other hand.

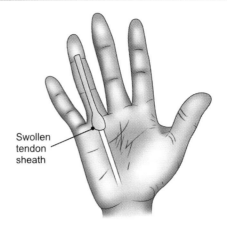

Fig. 36.4: Trigger finger – Pathology.

TREATMENT

In early stages, local ultrasonic therapy provides relief. In a long-standing problem, a local injection of hydrocortisone relieves the pain. In some cases, splitting of the tight tendon sheath may be required.

GANGLION

It is the most common cystic swelling on the dorsum of the wrist. It results from mucoid degeneration of the tendon sheath or the joint capsule. Ordinarily, there are no symptoms other than the swelling itself. Sometimes, a mild discomfort or pain is experienced. The cyst may sometimes be so tense as to resemble a solid tumour of the tendon sheath. Often the cyst is multiloculated. Aspiration of the cyst is performed and an injection of hyalase given. If the cyst recurs, excision may be required.

CARPAL TUNNEL SYNDROME

This is a syndrome characterised by the compression of the median nerve as it passes beneath the flexor retinaculum (Fig. 36.5).

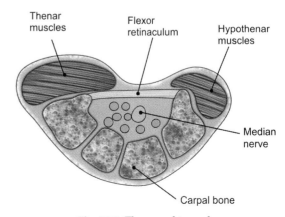

Fig. 36.5: The carpal tunnel.

Table 36.2: Causes of carpal tunnel syndrome	
Idiopathic	The most common cause
Inflammatory causes	Rheumatoid arthritis Wrist osteoarthritis
Post-traumatic causes	Bone thickening after a Colles' fracture
Endocrine causes	Myxoedema, acromegaly

CAUSES

Any space occupying lesion of the carpal tunnel may be responsible. Some of the common causes are given in Table 36.2.

CLINICAL FEATURES

The patient is generally a middle aged woman complaining of tingling, numbness or discomfort in the thumb and radial one and a half fingers, i.e., in the median nerve distribution. Tingling is more prominent during sleep. There is a feeling of clumsiness in carrying out fine movements. On examination, features of low median nerve compression are found (see page 66). Nerve conduction studies show delayed or absent conduction of impulses in the median nerve across the wrist. Treatment is by dividing the flexor retinaculum, and thus decompressing the nerve.

'FROZEN' SHOULDER
(Periarthritis Shoulder)

This is a disease of unknown etiology where the glenohumeral joint becomes painful and stiff because of the loss of resilience of the joint capsule, possibly with adhesions between its folds. Often, there is a history of preceding trauma. The disease is more common in diabetics.

CLINICAL FEATURES

It produces pain and stiffness of the shoulder. In early stages, the pain is worst at night, and the stiffness limited to abduction and internal rotation of the shoulder. Later, the pain is present at all times and all the movements of the shoulder are severely limited.

TREATMENT

This is a self-limiting disease lasting for 6–9 months, after which in most cases, the inflammation subsides, leaving a stiff but painless shoulder. Treatment is by analgesics, hot fomentation and physiotherapy. An intra-articular injection of hydrocortisone may

speed up the recovery. Stiffness can be prevented by continuous shoulder mobilising exercises. Occasionally manipulation under anaesthesia or arthroscopic capsular release is done.

PLANTAR FASCITIS

This is a common cause of pain in the heel. It occurs as a result of inflammation of the plantar aponeurosis at its attachment on the tuberosity of the calcaneum (Fig. 36.6). The pain is worst early in the morning, and often improves with activity. On examination, there is marked tenderness over the medial aspect of the calcaneal tuberosity, at the site of attachment of the plantar fascia.

X-rays sometimes show a sharp bone spur projecting forwards from the tuberosity of the calcaneum. Its significance is doubtful since it is also found in some cases without heel pain. Analgesics, the use of a heel pad and local induction of steroids brings relief in most cases.

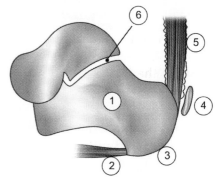

Fig. 36.6: Causes of heel pain: 1. Diseases of calcaneum, 2. Plantar fascitis, 3. Fat pad inflammation, 4. Retrocalcaneal bursitis, 5. Achillis tendinitis, 6. Diseases of subtalar joint.

FIBROSITIS

This is a non-specific condition where there is pain in certain muscles, with tenderness when they are gripped. One can palpate small, firm nodules, mostly over the trapezius and spinal muscles. These nodules are supposed to be trigger points. There are no other objective signs. The patient responds to ultrasonic therapy or local steroid infiltration.

PAINFUL ARC SYNDROME

This is a clinical syndrome in which there is pain in the shoulder and upper arm during the mid-range of of the greater tuberosity or acromion. Treatment consists of ultrasonics to the tender point and anti-inflammatory drugs. Some cases need an injection hydrocortisone in the subacromial space or excision of the anterior, often prominent part of the acromion.

MERALGIA PARAESTHETICA

This is a feeling of tingling, burning, and numbness in the skin supplied by the lateral cutaneous nerve of the thigh as it gets entrapped in the fascia just medial to the anterior superior iliac spine. Treatment is non-specific with analgesics, local hydrocortisone, etc. Sometimes, surgical decompression of the nerve may be required.

FIBROMYALGIA

This is a widespread disease characterised by multiple tender points, affecting both sides of the body—both above and below the waist, lasting more than 3 months. It is known to be associated with irritable bowel, headache, dysmenorrhea and chronic fatigue syndrome. It is an entity, distinct from fibrositis which is a localised disorder. Etiology is not known, but it is proposed to be a part of fatigue syndrome. Diseases like hypothyroidism, SLE, hyperparathyroidism and osteomalacia need to be ruled out by careful investigation. Treatment is by patient counselling, avoidance of aggravating factors, physical therapy and antidepressants.

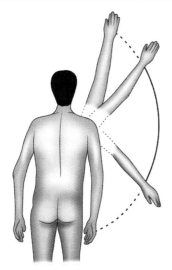

Fig. 36.7: Painful arc syndrome.

glenohumeral abduction (Fig. 36.7). Following are the common causes:

- Minor tears of the supraspinatus tendon
- Supraspinatus tendinitis
- Calcification of supraspinatus tendon
- Subacromial bursitis
- Fracture of the greater tuberosity

In all these conditions, the space between the upper-end of the humerus and the acromion gets compromised, so that during mid-abduction the tendon of the rotator-cuff gets nipped between the greater tuberosity and acromion. X-ray of the shoulder may show calcific deposit, or a fracture

---

 What have we learnt?

- Bursae are deflated balloons around areas which are subjected to friction. They get inflammed and produce pain.
- Dupuytren's contracture is contracture of palmer fascia.
- Tennis elbow and golfer's elbow are epicondylitis.
- de Quervain's disease is tenosynovitis of tendons around the wrist.
- Frozen shoulder is idiopathic capsular inflammation of shoulder, usually responds to physiotherapy.
- Painful arc syndrome occurs because of impingement of rotator-cuff.

Additional information: From the entrance exams point of view

- Types of superficial heat therapy: Hot bath, chemical pack, paraffin wax bath, infrared lamp, moist air cabinet.
- Types of deep heat therapy: Short wave diathermy, microwave therapy, ultrasound therapy.
- 'O' Brien's test done for a tight iliotibial band.
- Dupuytren's contracture: Surgery required if proximal interphalangeal joint contracture >15° and metacarpophalangeal joint contraction >30°.
- Level of tendon sheath constriction in trigger finger is metacarpophalangeal joint (A1 pulley).
- Bursa pes anserinus is between the tendons of the sartorius, gracilis, semitendinosus and the tibial collateral ligament.
- Thoracic outlet syndrome is best diagnosed via clinical examination.
- Athletic pubalgia is due to strain of the rectus abdominus muscle.

Competency

- ❖ **OR7.1:** Describe and discuss the aetiopathogenesis, clinical features, investigation and principles of management of metabolic bone disorders in particular osteoporosis, osteomalacia, rickets, Paget's disease.

CONSTITUTION OF BONE

Osseous tissue is made up of organic and inorganic material along with water. Relative proportions of these constituents are as shown in Flowchart 37.1.

Inorganic constituents of bone: It constitutes 65 per cent of the dry weight of bones. The bulk of this is calcium and phosphate, which in an adult is primarily crystalline (hydroxyapatite crystals). Besides calcium, other minor mineral constituents are Magnesium, Sodium, Potassium, etc. Although, the bone contains a large amount of calcium, only about 65 per cent of it is in an exchangeable form.

Flowchart 37.1: Constitution of bone.

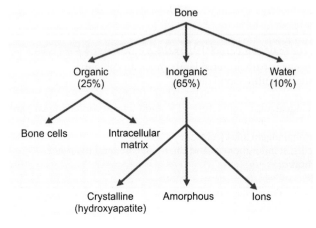

Organic constituents of bone: On a dry weight basis, the organic matrix constitutes 35 per cent of the total weight of human bones. Of this, 95 per cent is collagen; other constituents being polysaccharides (mucoproteins or glycoproteins) and lipids (including phospholipids).

BONE AND CALCIUM

Bone serves as a storehouse for 99 per cent of the body's calcium. Changes in the calcium ion activity in the extracellular fluid affects multiple biological processes. Hence, special regulatory mechanisms are required to provide an overall control of this activity. If for any reason, the serum level of calcium falls below its normal value, the body can react in three specific ways: (i) it may increase intestinal absorption; (ii) it may decrease urinary excretion; or (iii) it may increase the release of calcium from bone. The factors responsible for monitoring these activities are parathyroid hormone (PTH), vitamin D and calcitonin as given in Table 37.1.

In cases with *acute* lowering of the serum calcium level, such as that induced by the administration of calcium complexing substances, the intestinal tract and kidney cannot act swiftly enough to restore the level to normal. In this instance, the first supply of calcium comes from the lacunar and canalicular surfaces of the bone. This effect is believed to be

Table 37.1: Effects of PTH, vitamin D and calcitonin on kidney, GIT and bone.

Agent	Effect on serum levels	Kidney	GIT	Bone
PTH	↑Ca, ↓P	*Direct action* ↑renal phosphate excretion (phosphaturia) ↑resorption of Ca	—	*Direct action* ↑mobilisation of Ca from bone
Vitamin D	↑Ca, ↓P	—	*Direct action* ↑absorption of Ca and P from gut	*Direct action* ↑mobilisation of Ca from bone
Calcitonin	↑Ca, ↓P excretion of Ca	↓urinary	— from bone	↓mobilisation of Ca

an *equilibrium exchange*. It accounts for only a small amount of mineral and lasts for only a few minutes. After this source is depleted, and if the serum level of calcium is still low, parathyroid hormone secretion is stimulated as a direct consequence of the lowered serum level of calcium. This hormone provides a second source of calcium from the bone, from the zone surrounding the osteocytes. This is called *osteocytic osteolysis*. This happens first in cancellous bone and finally in cortical bone. Increase in the number and activity of osteoclasts results in resorption of large amount of bone. This type of resorption is called *osteoclastic resorption*.

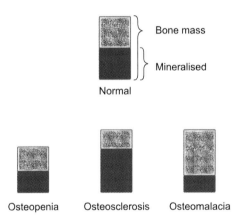

Fig. 37.1: Metabolic bone diseases.

There are four types of metabolic bone diseases (Fig. 37.1).

a. **Osteopenia diseases:** These diseases are characterised by a generalised decrease in bone mass (i.e., loss of bone matrix), though whatever bone is there, is normally mineralised (e.g., osteoporosis).

b. **Osteosclerotic diseases:** These are diseases characterised by an increase in bone mass (e.g., fluorosis).

c. **Osteomalacic diseases:** These are diseases characterised by an increase in the ratio of the organic fraction to the mineralised fraction, i.e.,

the available organic matter is under-mineralised (e.g., osteomalacia).

d. **Mixed diseases:** These are diseases that are a combination of osteopenia and osteomalacia (e.g., hyperparathyroidism).

OSTEOPOROSIS

Osteoporosis is by far the most common metabolic bone disease. It is characterised by a diffuse reduction in the bone density due to a decrease in the bone mass. It occurs when the rate of bone resorption exceeds the rate of bone formation.

CAUSES

Several etiological factors may be operative in a given patient. Most common factor in males is senility and in females is menopause. Table 37.2 gives some of the causes of generalised osteoporosis.

CLINICAL FEATURES

Osteoporosis is an asymptomatic disorder unless complications (predominantly fractures) occur. Loss of bone mass leads to loss of strength so that a trivial trauma is sufficient to cause a fracture. Dorso-lumbar spine is the most frequent site. Pain from these fractures is usually the reason for a person to consult

Table 37.2: Causes of generalised osteoporosis.

- *Senility*
- *Post-immobilisation, e.g., a bed-ridden patient*
- *Post-menopausal*
- *Protein deficiency*
  - Inadequate intake – old age, illness
  - Malnutrition
  - Mal-absorption
  - Excess protein loss (3rd degree burns, CRF, etc.)
- *Endocrinal*
  - Cushing's disease
  - Cushing's syndrome
  - Hyperthyroid state
- *Drug induced*
  - Long-term steroid therapy
  - Phenobarbitone therapy

a physician. Other fractures whose etiology has been linked to underlying osteoporosis are Colles' fracture and fracture of the neck of femur.

On examination, the findings are subtle and can be missed. A slight loss of height and increased kyphosis due to compression of the anterior part of the vertebral bodies is seen in most cases.

RADIOLOGICAL FEATURES

Radiological evidence of decreased bone mass is more reliable, but about 30 per cent of the bone mass must be lost before it becomes apparent on X-rays (Fig. 37.2). Following features may be noticed on X-rays:

- Loss of vertical height of a vertebra due to collapse.
- Cod fish appearance: The disc bulges into the adjacent vertebral bodies so that the disc becomes biconvex.
- Ground glass appearance of the bones, conspicuous in bones like the pelvis.
- Singh's index: Singh et al. graded osteoporosis into 6 grades based on the trabecular pattern of the femoral neck trabeculae. Details are outside the scope of this book.
- Metacarpal index and vertebral index are other methods of quantification of osteoporosis.

OTHER INVESTIGATIONS

These include the following, some of them more recent:
- **Biochemistry:** Serum calcium, phosphates and alkaline phosphatase are within normal limits. Total plasma proteins and plasma albumin may be low.

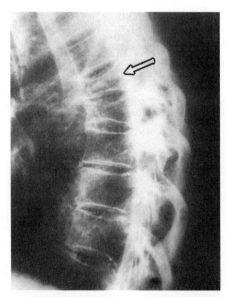

Fig. 37.2: X-ray of the dorsal spine, lateral view, showing marked osteoporosis.

- **Densitometry:** This is a method to quantify osteoporosis. In this method absorption of photons (emitted from gamma emitting isotopes) by the bone calcium is measured. Two types of bone densitometry are available—ultrasound based and X-ray based. DEXA scan is an X-ray based bone densitometry, and is the gold standard in the quantification of bone mass.
- **Neutron activation analysis:** In this method, calcium in the bone is activated by neutron bombing, and its activity measured.
- **Bone biopsy.**

TREATMENT

Since the etiology of osteoporosis is multifactorial and the diagnosis usually delayed, treatment becomes difficult. There are no set treatment methods as yet. The principle objectives of treatment are alleviation of pain and prevention of fractures. Treatment can be divided into medical and orthopaedic.

Medical treatment: This consists of the following:
- *High protein diet:* Many elderly patients suffer from malnutrition. Increasing their protein intake may increase the formation of organic matrix of the bone.
- *Calcium supplementation*: Its role is doubtful, but may be helpful in cases with deficiency of calcium in their diet.
- *Androgens:* These hormones have an anabolic effect on the protein matrix of bone, and in some instances ameliorate symptoms.
- *Estrogens:* Estrogens have been shown to halt the progressive loss of bone mass in post-menopausal osteoporosis.
- *Vitamin D:* This is given, in addition to the above, to increase calcium absorption from the gut.
- *Fluoride:* The use of fluoride is still under study. It is supposed to make the crystallinity of the bone greater; thereby making bone resorption slower.
- *Alandronate:* These are used in once a day dose, empty stomach. Oesophagitis is a troubling complication.
- *Calcitonin:* Parentral administration of calcitonin helps in building up the bone mass and also acts as an analgesic.
- *Teriparatide:* Anabolic agent increasing osteoblastic new bone formation.
- *Denosumab, Strontium:* Antiresorptive agents.

Orthopaedic treatment: This consists of the following:
- *Exercises:* Weight bearing is a major stimulus to bone formation. Increased guarded activity would therefore be of benefit to the patient.

- *Bracing:* Prophylactic bracing of the spine by using an Ash brace or Taylor brace may be useful in prevention of pathological fractures in a severely osteoporotic spine.

RICKETS AND OSTEOMALACIA

Rickets and osteomalacia are the diseases where the organic matrix of the bone fails to calcify properly, leaving large osteoid seams. Manifestations of the two diseases are different only with respect to the stage in life at which they occur. Rickets occurs in the growing bones of children; osteomalacia in the bones of adults. Both conditions are primarily due to a deficiency of vitamin D or a disturbance in its metabolism secondary to renal disease.

Vitamin D and its metabolism: The *endogenous* form of vitamin D, i.e., cholecalciferol, is found in the skin as a product of cholesterol metabolism in a process requiring ultraviolet radiation. The *exogenous* form of the vitamin is usually D_3. The two most important nutritionally useful forms of vitamin D are D_2 (ergocalciferol) and D_3 (cholecalciferol).

Steps in activation: The basic forms, vitamin D_2 and D_3 are inactive until hydroxylated. The first step of hydroxylation (25 hydroxylation) occurs in the liver and the second step (1 hydroxylation) occurs in the kidney. 1,25 dihydroxylated form is the active form and stimulates the intestinal absorption of calcium and also acts on the bone.

Control: The most sensitive of the physiological actions of 1-25 dihydroxy vitamin D is to increase intestinal absorption of calcium. The action of vitamin D metabolites in bone tissue is controversial. To calcify the bone matrix properly, small amounts of the metabolites are necessary along with sufficient calcium.

RICKETS

Rickets is a disease of the growing skeleton. It is characterised by failure of normal mineralisation, seen prominently at the growth plates, resulting in softening of the bones and development of deformities.

CAUSES

There are two types of rickets, i.e., Type I and Type II (Table 37.3). In Type I, there is either a deficiency of vitamin D or a defect in its metabolism. In Type II, the rickets occurs due to a deficiency of phosphates in the extracellular fluid because of defective tubular resorption or diminished phosphate intake.

Table 37.3: Types of rickets.

Type 1

a. *Due to a deficiency of vitamin D*
   - Diminished intake, e.g., malnutrition
   - Diminished absorption, e.g.
     • Mal-absorption syndrome
     • Gastric abnormalities
     • Biliary diseases
     • Lack of exposure to sunlight

b. *Due to disturbance in vitamin D metabolism*
   - Hepatic factor, e.g.
     • Lack of 25 hydroxylation of vitamin D
     • Increased degradation of vitamin D in patients on prolonged anti-convulsant therapy
   - Renal factor, e.g.
     • Lack of 1 hydroxylation (autosomal recessive)
   - Unresponsiveness of target cells to 1-25 dihydroxy vitamin D
   - Renal osteodystrophy

Type 2

a. *Defective absorption of phosphates through renal tubules*
   - Hypophosphataemic rickets (X-linked dominant)
   - Fanconi syndrome
   - Renal tubular acidosis
   - Oncogenic rickets

b. *Diminished intake or absorption of phosphates*

Nutritional deficiency continues to be the *most common* cause of rickets in developing countries because of poor socio-economic conditions.

CLINICAL FEATURES

Nutritional rickets occurs in children about 1 year old. It may occur in older children with mal-absorption syndrome. Following are the clinical features:

- *Craniotabes:* This is the manifestation of rickets seen in young infants. Pressure over the soft membranous bones of the skull gives the feeling of a ping pong ball being compressed and released.
- *Bossing of the skull:* Bossing of the frontal and parietal bones becomes evident after the age of 6 months.
- *Broadening of the ends of long bones,* most prominently around wrists and knees. It is seen around 6-9 months of age.
- *Delayed teeth eruption* is noticed in infants.
- *Harrison's sulcus:* A horizontal depression, along the lower part of the chest, corresponding to the insertion of diaphragm.
- *Pigeon chest:* The sternum is prominent.
- *Rachitic rosary:* The costochondral junctions on the anterior chest wall become prominent, giving rise to appearance of a rosary.
- *Muscular hypotonia:* The child's abdomen becomes protuberant (pot belly) because of marked muscular hypotonia. Visceroptosis and lumbar lordosis occurs.

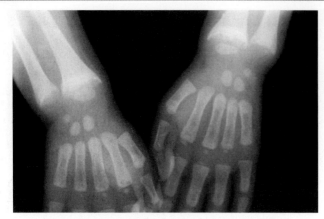

Fig. 37.3: X-ray of the wrists, AP view, showing changes in rickets.

- *Deformities:* Deformities of the long bones resulting in knock knees or bow legs is a common presentation of rickets, once the child starts walking.

RADIOLOGICAL FEATURES

Early radiological changes are observed in the lower ends of the radius and ulna. X-rays of both wrists and knees—antero-posterior views are used for screening a patient suspected of rickets. Following radiological signs may be seen (Fig. 37.3):

- *Delayed appearance of epiphyses.*
- *Widening of the epiphyseal plates:* Normal width of the epiphyseal plate is 2–4 mm. In rickets it is increased because of excessive accumulation of uncalcified osteoid at the growth plate.
- *Cupping of the metaphysis:* Normally, the metaphysis meets the epiphyseal plate as a smooth line of sclerosis (zone of provisional calcification). In rachitic bones, this line is absent and the metaphyseal end appears irregular. The cartilage cells accumulating at the growth plate create a depression in the soft metaphyseal end, giving rise to a cup-shaped appearance (Fig. 37.4).
- *Splaying of the metaphysis:* The end of the metaphysis is splayed because of the pressure by the cartilage cells accumulating at the growth plate.
- *Rarefaction* of the diaphysial cortex occurs late.
- *Bone deformities:* Knock knees, bow legs and coxa vara are common deformities in older children.

OTHER INVESTIGATIONS

Serum calcium is usually normal or low, serum phosphate is low, but serum alkaline phosphatase is high.

TREATMENT

It consists of medical and orthopaedic treatment.

Medical treatment: Administration of vitamin D 6,00,000 units as a single oral dose induces rapid healing. If the line of healing (a line of sclerosis on the metaphyseal side of the growth plate) is not seen on X-rays within 3-4 weeks of therapy, same dose may be repeated. In cases where the child responds to vitamin D therapy, a maintenance dose of 400 IU of vitamin D is given per day. If there is no response even after the second dose, a diagnosis of *refractory rickets* is made. Such patients are evaluated in detail by multispeciality team of nephrologist, endocrinologist and physician.

Orthopaedic treatment: It is required for the correction of deformities by conservative or operative methods.

a. *Conservative methods:* Mild deformities correct spontaneously, as rickets heals. Some surgeons use specially designed splints (mermaid splints) or orthopaedic shoes for correction of knee deformities.

b. *Operative methods:* Moderate or severe deformities often require surgery. This can be performed any time after 6 months of starting the medical treatment. Corrective osteotomies, depending upon the nature of deformities, are performed.

OSTEOMALACIA

Osteomalacia, which means softening of bones, is the adult counterpart of rickets. It is primarily due to deficiency of vitamin D. This results in failure to replace the turnover of calcium and phosphorus in the organic matrix of bone. Hence, the bone content is demineralised and the bony substance is replaced by soft osteoid tissue.

ETIOLOGY

It is common in women who live in *'purdah,'* and lack exposure to sunlight. Other causes are—dietary deficiency of vitamin D, under-nutrition during pregnancy, mal-absorption syndrome, after partial gastrectomy, etc.

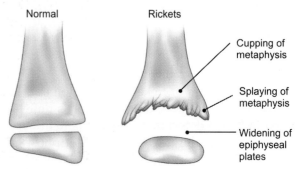

Fig. 37.4: Radiological features of rickets.

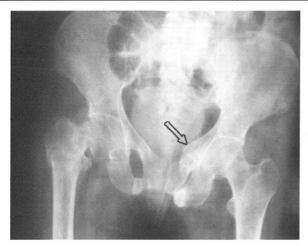

Fig. 37.5: X-ray of pelvis showing 'loosers zones' on the pubic rami.

CLINICAL FEATURES

In its early stages, symptoms and signs are non-specific and the diagnosis is often missed. Following presentations may be seen:

- **Bone pains:** Skeletal discomfort ranging from backache to diffuse bone pains may occur. Bone tenderness is common.
- **Muscular weakness:** The patient feels very weak. He may have difficulty in climbing up and down the stairs. A waddling gait is not unusual. Tetany may manifest as carpopedal spasm and facial twitching.
- **Spontaneous fractures** occur usually in spine, and may result in kyphosis.

INVESTIGATIONS

Following investigations may be carried out:

- **Radiological examination:** Plain X-rays appear to be of 'poor quality', i.e., not sharp and well-defined. Following findings may be present (Fig. 37.5):
  - Diffuse rarefaction of bones.
  - Looser's zone (pseudofractures): These are radiolucent zones occurring at sites of stress. Common sites are the pubic rami, axillary border of scapula, ribs and the medial cortex of the neck of the femur. These are caused by rapid resorption and slow mineralisation and may be surrounded by a collar of callus.
  - Triradiate pelvis in females.
  - Protrusio-acetabuli, i.e., the acetabulum protruding into the pelvis.
- **Bone biopsy:** A bone biopsy from the iliac crest usually confirms the diagnosis. The characteristic histological finding is excessive uncalcified osteoid.

- **Serum:** The serum calcium level is low, the phosphates are low and alkaline phosphatase high.

TREATMENT

When osteomalacia is due to defective intake, vitamin D supplementation therapy, as for rickets, brings dramatic results. Vitamin D in daily maintenance doses of 400 IU is sufficient. If there is mal-absorption, higher dose or intramuscular dose may be needed. In patients with renal disease, alfacalcidol (an activated form of vitamin D) may be used. Calcium supplementation should also be given. In addition, the underlying cause is treated.

HYPERPARATHYROIDISM

Clinical bone disease occurs in less than half of the patients with hyperparathyroidism. For reasons unknown, hyperparathyroidism tends to present either with bone disease or with renal stones, *but not both.*

Before we discuss this topic further, here is a brief account of the action of parathyroid hormone on bone.

Parathyroid hormone and bone: The parathyroid hormone acts directly on the bone to release calcium into the extracellular fluid by stimulating osteoclastic resorption. It activates the adenyl cyclase so that the formation of cyclic AMP is increased, which in turn increases the synthesis of specific lysosomal enzymes. These enzymes break down the organic matrix of bone and release calcium.

CLINICAL FEATURES

The disease can affect either sex, but is more common in women. The majority of cases occur from the third to fifth decades of life. Following are the more common presenting complaints:

- *Bone pains:* This is the most common initial feature. There is tenderness on palpating the bones, especially in the lower limbs and back. Pain is usually associated with general weakness, pallor and hypotonia.
- *Pathological fracture:* Fractures occur with trivial injuries and unite in a deformed position. Common sites of fractures are dorso-lumbar spine, neck of the femur and pubic rami.
- *Brown's tumour:* This is an expansile bone lesion, a collection of osteoclasts. It commonly affects the maxilla or mandible, though any bone may be affected.
- *Anorexia, nausea, vomiting and abdominal cramps* are common presenting complaints.

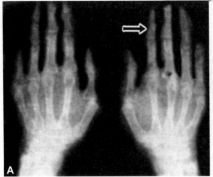
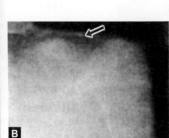
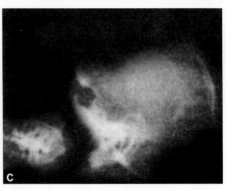

Fig. 37.6: X-rays showing changes in hyperparathyroidism: (A) Subperiosteal resorption in phalanges; (B) Subperiosteal resorption of lateral end of the clavicle; (C) Salt pepper appearance.

- *Occasionally, renal colics* with haematuria, because of renal calculus, may occur.

RADIOLOGICAL INVESTIGATIONS

X-ray examination consists of the lateral view of the skull, dorso-lumbar spine (AP/lateral views), both hands (AP view), pelvis (AP view) and X-ray of the region with symptoms. Following signs may be present (Fig. 37.6):
- Irregular, diffuse rarefaction of the bones.
- *Salt pepper appearance:* The skull bones show a well-marked stippling, but the opaque areas are small pin head size.
- *Loss of lamina dura:* A tooth socket is made up of thin cortical bone seen as a white line surrounding the teeth. This is called the lamina dura. It gets absorbed in hyperparathyroidism.
- *Subperiosteal resorption* of the phalanges is a *diagnostic* feature of hyperparathyroidism (generalised variety). Resorption may also occur at lateral end of the clavicle.
- Spine shows central collapse of the vertebral body and biconvex discs.
- Pelvis and other bones show coarse striations with clear cyst-like spaces.
- *Brown's tumour* is an expansile lytic lesion, which appears like a bone tumour, generally affecting the maxilla/mandible.
- Extraosseous radiological features such as renal calculi, etc. may be present.

OTHER INVESTIGATIONS

- *Serum* calcium is high, phosphates low and alkaline phosphatase high.
- *Urinary* excretion of calcium is low and that of phosphates high, as found on 24-hour urine analysis.
- Investigations for finding the underlying cause of hyperparathyroidism, i.e., CT scan of the neck for parathyroids, and for the evaluation of other organs for ectopic secretion of parathormone.

TREATMENT

It consists of: (i) removal of the basic cause; (ii) orthopaedic treatment; and (iii) urologic treatment.
a. *Treatment* of the basic cause is by surgical excision of the hormone secreting tissue.
b. **Orthopaedic treatment** is directed towards adequate protection of the softened bones from all deforming stress and strain. Once the disease has been arrested and recalcification of bones occurs, the established deformities may be corrected surgically.
c. **Urology treatment:** This is directed towards the removal of calculi and maintenance of renal functions.

FLUOROSIS

Fluorosis is a disease where excessive deposition of calcium occurs in bone and soft tissues. It results from excessive ingestion of fluorides in drinking water. The fluoride content of normal water is less than 1 PPM. In India and parts of south east Asia, large areas have been reported with high water fluoride content. Fluorosis is an endemic disease and a public health problem in some states of India, i.e., Punjab, Andhra Pradesh, Tamil Nadu, etc.

CLINICAL FEATURES

The symptoms and signs may pertain to skeletal system or teeth.
a. **Skeletal fluorosis:** The patient complains of pain in the back and joints. There may be associated stiffness of the spine and paraesthesias in the limbs. In advanced stages, the patient presents with spastic paraparesis and anaemia. Paraparesis occurs because of cord compression resulting from calcification of the posterior longitudinal ligament and subsequent pressure on the cord.
b. **Dental fluorosis:** This is the *earliest* sign of fluorosis. The earliest to occur is mottling of the

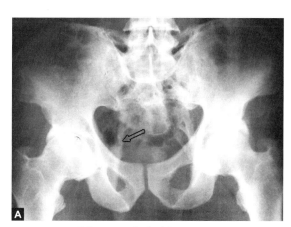

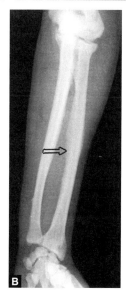

Sclerosis calcified ligaments
(arrow)

Interosseous membrane
calcification

Fig. 37.7: Radiological features of fluorosis.

enamel, best seen in the incisors of the upper jaw. Later the teeth get eroded and fall off.

RADIOLOGICAL INVESTIGATIONS

X-rays of the spine, pelvis and forearms are required in a suspected case. Following features may be seen (Fig. 37.7):
- Spine: Increased density, calcification of the posterior longitudinal ligament.
- Pelvis: Increased density, calcification of the ischiopubic and sacroiliac ligaments.
- Forearm and leg: Interosseous membrane calcification.

OTHER INVESTIGATIONS

- Elevated serum fluoride levels.
- Elevated fluoride levels in urine and drinking water.
- A biopsy shows high fluoride levels in bones.

DIFFERENTIAL DIAGNOSIS

Fluorosis is an osteosclerotic disease, and must be differentiated from other causes of osteosclerosis given in Table 37.4.

Table 37.4: Cause of generalised osteosclerosis.
▪ Fluorosis
▪ Paget's disease of bone
▪ Renal osteodystrophy
▪ Secondaries from prostate, other organs
▪ Marble bone disease (osteopetrosis)
▪ Engelmann's disease

TREATMENT

Prevention is the most important aspect of treatment of this difficult disease. Defluorination of the water is carried out as a public health programme. Patients improve symptomatically once the defluorinated water is used for some time.

DISTURBANCES OF ORGANIC CONSTITUENTS

LATHYRISM

Ingestion of certain agents called lathyrogens causes profound alterations in the collagen of connective tissues and bones. The bones of such individuals are soft, their arteries become weak and develop aneurysms. Treatment is removal of causative factor.

SCURVY

This disease is caused by deficiency of vitamin C (ascorbic acid). The result is decreased production and poor quality collagen. In adults, it presents with swollen gums, gingivitis and abnormal bleeding tendencies typically producing *perifollicular* haemorrhages over the lower part of the thighs. Petechial haemorrhages and spontaneous bruises may occur anywhere in the body, but usually first in the lower extremities. In infantile scurvy, important features are lassitude, anaemia, painful limbs due to subperiosteal haematoma, and scorbutic rosary (bead-like thickening of the ribs due to calcified subperiosteal haematomas). Treatment is by supplementation with vitamin C.

POLYSACCHARIDOSIS

The principle polysaccharide of bone is a mucopolysaccharide—chondroitin-4-sulfate (chondroitin sulfate A). In certain diseases called as mucopolysaccharidosis, there is increased excretion of polysaccharides in the urine. Loss of these polysaccharides from bone and cartilage results in specific skeletal deformities.

 What have we learnt?

- 65% of weight of the bone is inorganic.
- Osteoporosis is deficiency in matrix, whereas osteomalacia is deficiency of mineralisation of bone.
- Rickets and osteomalacia are diseases of deficiency in bone mineralisation.
- Hyperparathyroidism results in mobilisation of calcium from bone.
- Fluorosis is excessive deposition of calcium in bone and soft tissues.

Additional information: From the entrance exams point of view

- Rugger jersey spine is seen in renal osteodystrophy and is due to hyperparathyroidism.
- Milkman fractures are pseudofractures in adults.

Learning Objectives

- What are the causes of avascular necrosis (AVN) of the bone, how to investigate such a case and what are the treatment options?

GENERALISED BONE DISORDERS

ACHONDROPLASIA

This is a condition caused by the failure of normal ossification of bones, mainly the long bones, resulting in dwarfism (Fig. 38.1). Since growth of the trunk is only marginally affected, the *dwarfism is disproportionate;* the limbs being out of proportion with the trunk. Shortening is especially marked in the *proximal* segments of the limbs.

The disease is of autosomal dominant inheritance, but many cases arise from a fresh gene mutation. Intelligence is normal. Typically, the patient has a large skull with a bulging vault and forehead, a flat nose, short limbs, short and stubby fingers and increased lumbar lordosis. These patients lead a near normal life, except for a few who develop spinal canal stenosis. Common causes of dwarfism are given in Table 38.1.

Table 38.1: Common causes of dwarfism.
- Achondroplasia
- Dyschondroplasia
- Diaphyseal aclasis
- Multiple epiphyseal dysplasia
- Cretinism
- Malnutrition
- Morquio's, Hurler's, Hunter's diseases

OSTEOGENESIS IMPERFECTA (FRAGILITAS OSSIUM, VROLIK'S DISEASE)

This is a condition characterised by tendency for *frequent fractures* because of *weak and brittle* bones. It results from defective collagen synthesis, and thus affects other collagen containing soft tissues such as the skin, sclera, teeth, ligaments, etc., as well. The disease is commonly inherited as an autosomal

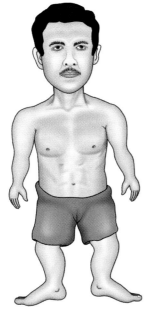
Fig. 38.1: Achondroplasia.

Table 38.2: Causes of tendency for easy fractures.

- Osteogenesis imperfecta
- Osteoporosis
- Osteopetrosis
- Osteomalacia
- Polio limb

dominant disorder, but a severe variant is known to occur where the inheritance is autosomal recessive. Typically, the patient has a tendency for frequent fractures, usually with minimal trauma. Associated features are blue sclera, joint laxity and otosclerosis in adulthood. Patients with the severe type do not survive beyond a few years, but those with the milder disease live their full life interrupted by frequent fractures. The fractures unite normally but deformities secondary to malunion or joint contractures may occur. The tendency to fracture often reduces with age. Some of the common causes of tendency for easy fracture are given in Table 38.2.

DIAPHYSEAL ACLASIS (MULTIPLE EXOSTOSES)

This is a condition characterised by multiple, cartilage-capped *bony outgrowths* from the metaphysis of long bones, and some from flat bones. It is inherited as an autosomal dominant disorder. The basic defect is that of remodelling. The columns of cartilage at the epiphyseal plate grow rapidly and sideways due to poor remodelling forces. X-rays typically show a 'trumpet-shaped' metaphysis and bony projections from it (Fig. 38.2). The problem is of dwarfism, pressure effects of the exostosis, deformities, and a tendency of the exostosis to undergo malignant change. Since, it is impractical to excise all the exostosis, the one causing symptoms is excised.

OSTEOPETROSIS (MARBLE BONE DISEASE, ALBERS-SCHÖNBERG DISEASE)

This is a disorder characterised by *dense but brittle bones* (marble bones). In a less severe, autosomal dominant variety the patient has a tendency to fracture. In a severe, congenital, autosomal recessive variety, the child may have severe anaemia, jaw osteomyelitis and cranial nerve palsies. Most of the patients of the latter type do not survive for long.

PAGET'S DISEASE (OSTEITIS DEFORMANS)

This is a condition characterised by a progressive tendency for one or more bones to bend, get thickened and spongy. Tibia is the bone affected most commonly. The cause is not known, but it is understood to be a defect in the osteoclast functions, so that irregular bone resorption and increased bone turnover occurs. The bone is soft and vascular in the initial stages, but becomes dense and hard later. The disease begins after 40 years of age. Presenting complaints are dull pain, and bowing and thickening of the affected bone. X-rays show multiple confluent lytic areas with interspread new bone formation. Bone scan shows an increased uptake. Serum alkaline phosphatase is elevated. Usual complications are pathological fracture and malignant change. Treatment is by calcitonin or diphosphonate.

NEUROFIBROMATOSIS

A generalised variety of neurofibromatosis (von Recklinghausen's disease) may have skeletal disturbances like scoliosis, solitary bone lesions, pseudarthrosis of the tibia, compressive myelopathy, local gigantism, limb length inequality, etc. In addition, other soft tissue manifestations of the disease may be present. For details, please refer to a Surgery textbook.

HISTIOCYTOSIS X

This comprises of a group of diseases characterised by proliferation of histiocytes in the bones. Three clinical entities are recognised:

a. **Eosinophilic granuloma:** This is a solitary bone lesion, commonly seen in the femur, tibia, spine and ribs. The patient usually presents with a dull pain or a pathological fracture. Treatment is curettage and bone grafting.

b. **Hand-Schuller-Christian disease:** It is a variation of (a), where the lesions are found at multiple sites.

c. **Letterer-Siwe disease:** This is the most severe form. There is involvement of multiple bones. It begins in childhood and progresses rapidly to death.

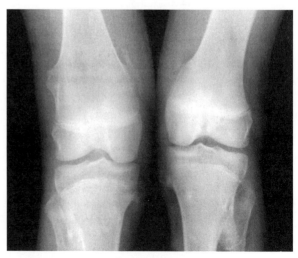

Fig. 38.2: X-ray of both knees, AP view, showing multiple exostoses.

OSTEOCHONDRITIS

These are a group of miscellaneous affections of the growing epiphyses in children and adolescents. Typically, a bony nucleus of the epiphysis affected by osteochondritis becomes temporarily softened; and while in the softened stage it is liable to deformation by pressure. Perthes' disease, the osteochondritis of the epiphysis of the head of the femur is the *most common*. Osteochondritis is sometimes classified into: (i) *crushing type* or osteochondrosis; (ii) *osteochondritis dissecans*; and (iii) *traction osteochondritis* or traction apophysitis. Table 38.3 gives names of some of the common osteochondritis.

Table 38.3: Common osteochondritis.	
Name	**Site affected**
Perthes' disease	Femoral head
Panner's disease	Capitulum
Kienbock's disease	Lunate bone
Osgood-Schlatter's disease	Tibial tubercle
Sever's disease	Calcaneal tuberosity
Köhler disease	Navicular bone
Freiberg's disease	Metatarsal head
Scheuermann's disease	Ring epiphysis of vertebrae
Calvé's disease	Central bony nucleus of vertebral body
Iselin's disease	5th metatarsal

PERTHES' DISEASE
(COXA PLANA, PSEUDOCOXALGIA)

This is an osteochondritis of the epiphysis of the femoral head. In this disease, the femoral head becomes partly or wholly avascular and deformed. The cause is not definitely known, but it is supposed to be due to recurrent episodes of ischaemia of the head in the susceptible age group, probably precipitated by episodes of synovitis. Pathologically, the disease progresses in three ill-defined stages: (i) stage of synovitis; (iii) stage of trabecular necrosis; and (iii) stage of healing.

The disease occurs commonly in boys in the *age group* of 5–10 years. The child presents with pain in the hip, often *radiating to the knee.* There may be limping or hip stiffness. On examination, findings may be minimal—sometimes the only findings being a limitation of abduction and internal rotation and shortening. Radiological examination reveals collapse and sclerosis of the epiphysis of the femoral head. Hip joint space is *increased.* In fact, the contrast between

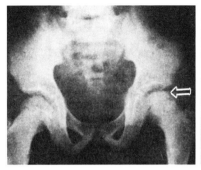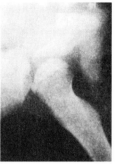

Fig. 38.3: X-rays showing changes of Perthes' disease of the hip. (Both the hips should be included to be able to appreciate early changes).

the paucity of symptoms and signs in the presence of gross X-ray changes is striking (Fig. 38.3). Bone scan may show a decreased uptake by the head of the femur. Four groups have been described by Catterall (1972), depending upon the extent of involvement of the head. He also describes the adverse prognostic signs *(head at risk signs).*

Treatment: Preventing the head from mis-shapening while the bone is in softening phase, is the primary aim of the treatment. The head is required to be kept inside the acetabulum while the revascularisation takes place (head containment). This may be achieved by conservative methods (plaster, splint, etc.) or by operation (containment osteotomy).

AVASCULAR NECROSIS

Avascular necrosis (AVN) of the bone due to loss of a vascularity of a part of the bone occurs commonly after a fracture or dislocation (e.g., AVN of head of the femur in a fracture of the femoral neck). Sometimes, a part of the bone undergoes avascular necrosis spontaneously. The head of the femur is a common site of AVN. It occurs in adults between the ages of 20–40 years. Some of the causes of avascular necrosis of the femoral head are given in Table 38.4.

Diagnosis: The disease is often bilateral (75%). Patient complains of pain in the groin or in front of the thigh. Pain is present at all times, but increases on exertion.

Table 38.4: Causes of avascular necrosis of femoral head.
• Idiopathic – most common
• Alcoholism
• Steroid therapy
• Sickle cell disease
• Patient on renal dialysis
• Patient on anti-cancer drugs
• Post-partum necrosis
• Goucher's disease
• Caisson's disease

X-rays may be normal in early stage; if suspicion is strong, a bone scan may be done. In later stage, an osteolytic lesion can be seen in superolateral part of the head. There may be diffuse osteosclerosis of the head, but the shape of the head may be maintained. In advanced stage, the head collapses (Fig. 38.4). Eventually, changes of secondary osteoarthritis become apparent. MRI scan is the best modality for early diagnosis of avascular necrosis.

Treatment: In early stages, diagnosis is often missed as there are no X-ray findings. Core decompression alone or with additional fibular grafting is done if the head of the femur has not got deformed. Such revascularisation operation are of equivocal importance. In later stages, once the head gets deformed, in some cases with involvement of a part of the head, an intertrochanteric osteotomy has been described. In cases with changes

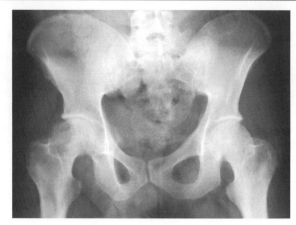

Fig. 38.4: X-rays showing avascular necrosis of head of the femur on the right side.

of advanced osteoarthritis, total hip replacement becomes necessary.

SOME OTHER DEVELOPMENTAL ABNORMALITIES OF ORTHOPAEDIC INTEREST

1.	Ollier's disease (multiple enchondromas) Dyschondroplasia	▪ Not familial ▪ Masses of cartilage in the metaphysis remain unossified ▪ Defective ossification
2.	Melorheostosis	▪ Candle bone disease
3.	Osteopathia striata	▪ Striped bones disease
4.	Osteopoikilosis	▪ Spotted bones disease
5.	Morquio's disease	▪ Familial (autosomal recessive) disease ▪ Gives rise to dwarfism affecting both limbs and trunk ▪ Mental development *normal* ▪ *Corneal opacity* sometimes present ▪ X-ray – typical 'tonguing' of lumbar vertebrae ▪ Keratan sulphate in urine
6.	Hunter's disease	▪ Familial X-linked disease ▪ Defect is the excretion of large amount of keratan sulphate in urine ▪ Dwarf with dorso-lumbar kyphosis, knock-knees, flat feet ▪ Mental deficiency *may* occur ▪ *No* corneal opacity
7.	Hurler's disease (Gargoylism)	▪ Familial (autosomal recessive) disease ▪ Gives rise to dwarfism of both, limbs and trunk ▪ Defect is an error in development of fibroblasts ▪ There is excretion of dermatan sulphate and heparitan sulphate in urine ▪ Typical facial appearance ▪ Mental development *abnormal* ▪ Corneal opacity *present* ▪ X-ray typical 'beak' in 2nd lumbar vertebra
8.	Engelmann's disease	▪ Familial (autosomal recessive) disease ▪ Symmetrical, fusiform enlargement and sclerosis of shafts of the long bones in children. Femur affected commonly ▪ Epiphysis is spared
9.	Caffey's disease (infantile cortical hyperostosis)	▪ Non-familial disease ▪ Starts early in life (before the 5th month) ▪ There is a formation of subperiosteal bone on the shafts of long bones, and on the mandible ▪ *Self-limiting course, resolves by 3 years of age* ▪ Tibia more common than ulna in familial form
10.	Albright's syndrome	▪ Polyostotic fibrous dysplasia and precocious puberty

(Contd...)

(Contd...)

11.	Arthrogryposis multiplex congenita (AMC)	▪ Defective development of muscles ▪ Stiff, deformed joints ▪ Multiple joint dislocations with 'shapeless extremities' ▪ May present as clubfoot
12.	Myositis ossificans progressiva	▪ Ectopic ossification, often beginning in trunk ▪ Short big toe
13.	Multiple epiphyseal dysplasia	▪ Least rare type ▪ Affects all the epiphyses, resulting in stunted growth, deformities (varum, valgum, etc.) ▪ Epiphysis looks ill, defined, irregular on X-rays
14.	Spondyloepiphyseal dysplasia	▪ Spine is also involved in addition to limb epiphyses
15.	Metaphyseal dysplasia (Pyle's disease)	▪ Autosomal recessive ▪ A modelling defect results in 'Erlenmeyer flask' deformity of the distal femur and proximal tibia
16.	Blount's disease	▪ The growth of the medial-half of the proximal tibial epiphysis is retarded, resulting in severe tibia vara deformity in childhood, common in West Indies
17.	Cleidocranial dysostosis	▪ Faulty development of membranous bones ▪ Clavicles are absent ▪ Skull sutures remain open ▪ Coxa vara ▪ Wide foramen magnum
18.	Nail patella syndrome	▪ Familial disorder ▪ Hypoplastic nails and absence of patella
19.	Marfan's syndrome (Arachnodactyly)	▪ Spider fingers ▪ Associated atrial regurgitation ▪ Occular lens dislocation
20.	Apert syndrome	▪ Tower shaped head ▪ Syndactyly

 What have we learnt?

- Achondroplasia produces disproportionate dwarfism.
- Osteogenesis imperfecta is the cause of frequent fractures.
- Diaphyseal aclasis is an autosomal dominant disorder.
- Avascular necrosis commonly affects head of the femur. It is common in patients with sickle cell disease.

Additional information: From the entrance exams point of view

- Investigation of choice to diagnose early Perthe's disease is MRI.
- Vertebra plana seen in eosinophilic granuloma, Ewing's sarcoma, TB, Calve's disease, leukemia and metastasis.
- Trident hand is seen in achondroplasia.
- Osteogensis imperfecta is due to abnormal type I procollagen in the body.
- Muscles most commonly absent congenitally are pectoralis major and minor.
- Osteochondritis dissecans most commonly affects lateral part of medial femoral condyle.

Miscellaneous Regional Diseases

Learning Objectives

- ❖ Describe the developmental deformitities of the knee anf their managerment.
- ❖ Discuss the causes of flat feet and its management.

TORTICOLLIS (Wry Neck)

This is a deformity of the neck where the head and neck are turned and twisted to one side. It may be permanent, temporary, or spasmodic. Spasmodic torticollis is the *most common*. Table 39.1 gives some of the common causes of torticollis. Most often, torticollis is secondary to pain and reflex muscle spasm and recovers once the inflammatory process subsides. Congenital torticollis, a common cause of permanent torticollis, is of orthopaedic interest. Commonly, the presentation is for cosmatic reasons.

Table 39.1: Causes of torticollis.

■ Congenital	Sternomastoid tumour
■ Infection	Tonsillitis
	Atlanto-axial infections
	Labyrinthitis
■ Reflex spasm	Acute disc prolapse (cervical)
■ Neurogenic	Spasmodic condition
	Paralytic condition
■ Ocular	Compensation for squint
■ Others	Rheumatoid arthritis
	Spasmodic torticollis

CONGENITAL TORTICOLLIS (INFANTILE TORTICOLLIS, STERNOMASTOID TUMOUR)

The sternomastoid muscle on one side of the neck is fibrosed and fails to elongate as the child grows, and thus results in a progressive deformity. The cause of fibrosis is not known, but it is possibly a result of ischaemic necrosis of the sternomastoid muscle at birth. Evidence in favour of this theory is the presence of a lump in the sternomastoid muscle in the first few weeks of life, probably a swollen ischaemic muscle. This is termed *sternomastoid tumour*. The lump disappears spontaneously within a few months, leaving a fibrosed muscle. Torticollis occurs more commonly in children with breech presentation.

Diagnosis: The child usually presents at 3-4 years of age, often as late as puberty. The head is tilted to one side so that the chin faces to the opposite side (Fig. 39.1). The sternomastoid is prominent on the side the head tilts, and becomes more prominent on trying to passively correct the head tilt. In cases presenting in the first few weeks of life, a lump may be felt in the sternomastoid muscle. Facial asymmetry develops in cases who present later in life. Radiological

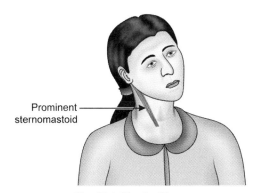

Fig. 39.1: Torticollis.

examination is normal, and is carried out to rule out an underlying bone defect such as scoliosis.

Treatment: In a child presenting with a sternomastoid tumour, progress to torticollis can be prevented by passive stretching and splinting. The same may also be sufficient for mild deformities in younger children. For severe deformities, especially in older children, release of the contracted sternomastoid muscle is required. It is usually released from its lower attachment, but sometimes both attachments need to be released. Following surgery, the neck is maintained in the corrected position in a *Callot's cast.*

CERVICAL RIB

This is an additional rib which arises from the 7th cervical vertebra. It is usually attached to the first rib close to the insertion of the scalenus anterior muscle, and is present in less than 0.5 per cent of the population. It may be a complete rib, but more often it is present posteriorly for a short distance only; the anterior part being just a fibrous band. The cervical rib is usually unilateral and is more common on the right side.

CLINICAL FEATURES

In 90 per cent of cases, there are no symptoms; an extra rib is detected on an X-ray made for some other purpose. In others, it produces symptoms after the age of 30 years, probably because with declining youth the shoulders sag, increasing the angulation of the neurovascular structures of the upper limb as they come out of the neck. It is more often symptomatic in females. A patient may present with the following symptoms:

a. **Neurological symptoms:** Tingling and numbness along the distribution of the lowest part of the brachial plexus (T_1 the dermatome), along medial border of the and hand, is the most common complaint. There may be weakness and wasting of the hand muscles and clumsiness in the use of the hand.

b. **Vascular symptoms:** These are uncommon. Compression of the subclavian artery may result in an aneurysm distal to constriction. This is a potential source of tiny emboli to the hand and may cause gangrene of the finger tips. There may be a history of pain in the upper limb on using the arm or elevating the hand (claudication).

c. **Local symptoms:** Occasionally, the patient presents with a tender supraclavicular lump (the anterior end of the cervical rib) which, on palpation, is bony hard and fixed.

RADIOLOGICAL EXAMINATION

X-ray examination may show a well-formed rib articulating posteriorly with transverse process of C_7 vertebra. It is attached anteriorly to middle of the 1st rib. More often there is no fully developed cervical rib but merely an enlargement of the transverse process of the seventh cervical vertebra (Fig. 39.2).

DIFFERENTIAL DIAGNOSIS

A patient with cervical rib is to be differentiated from those presenting with pain radiating down the upper limb due to other causes. Some of these causes are as follows:

a. **Carpal tunnel syndrome:** The symptoms are in the median nerve distribution. Nocturnal pain is characteristic.

b. **Cervical spine lesions:** In cases with cervical disc prolapse and spondylosis, pain radiates to the *outer* side of the arm and forearm. Associated limitation of neck movement and characteristic X-ray appearance may help in diagnosis.

c. **Spinal cord lesions:** Syringomyelia or other spinal cord lesions may cause wasting of the hand, but

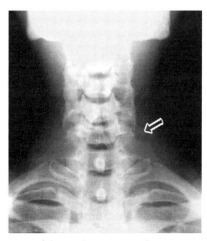

Fig. 39.2: X-ray of the neck, AP view, showing a cervical rib.

other neurological features help in reaching a diagnosis.

d. **Ulnar neuritis** may mimic this lesion but can be differentiated on clinical examination or by electrodiagnostic studies.

TREATMENT

Conservative treatment is usually rewarding. It consists of 'shrugging the shoulder' exercises to build up the muscles, and avoidance of carrying heavy objects like shopping bag, bucket full of water, suitcase, etc. Occasionally, surgical excision of the *first rib* may be required to relieve compression on the neurovascular bundle of the upper limb.

OBSERVATION HIP
(Transient Synovitis)

This is a non-specific synovitis of the hip seen in children 4-8 years of age. It results in a painful stiffness of the hip which subsides after 2-3 weeks of rest and analgesics. X-ray examination and the erythrocyte sedimentation rate (ESR) are normal. It is termed 'observation hip' because it must be 'observed' and differentiated from the following conditions:

a. **Early infective arthritis:** Some cases of early tuberculosis or septic arthritis may have features similar to observation hip. A high ESR, systemic symptoms, and persistent signs may necessitate a biopsy; especially in countries where tuberculosis is common.

b. **Chronic synovitis:** A monoarticular rheumatoid arthritis may resemble an 'observation hip'.

c. **Perthes' disease:** In its early stages, before X-ray findings appear, Perthes' disease may resemble a transient synovitis, but further follow up shows characteristic X-ray changes of the former.

Treatment: It consists of bed rest and analgesics. Recovery occurs within a few weeks.

COXA VARA

Coxa vara is a term used to describe a reduced angle between the neck and shaft of the femur. It may be congenital or acquired.

INFANTILE COXA VARA

This is coxa vara resulting from some unknown growth anomaly at the upper femoral epiphysis. It is noticed as a painless limp in a child who has just started walking. In severe cases, shortening of the leg may be obvious. On examination, abduction and internal rotation of the hip are limited and the leg

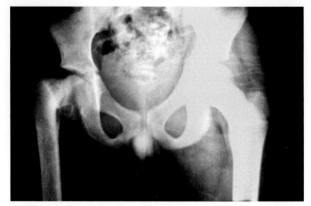

Fig. 39.3: X-ray of the pelvis, AP view, showing coxa vara of the hip. (Note reduction of neck-shaft angle of the femur).

is short. X-rays will show a reduction in neck-shaft angle (Fig. 39.3).

The epiphyseal plate may be too vertical. There may be a separate triangle of bone in the inferior portion of the metaphysis, called Fairbank's triangle (Fig. 39.4). Treatment is by a subtrochanteric corrective osteotomy.

SLIPPED CAPITAL FEMORAL EPIPHYSIS

In this condition, the upper femoral epiphysis may get displaced at the growth plate, usually postero-medially, resulting in coxa vara. The slip occurs gradually in majority of cases, but in some it occurs suddenly.

CAUSES

Etiology is not known but it is thought to be a result of trauma in the presence of some not yet understood underlying abnormality. It occurs more commonly in unduly fat and sexually underdeveloped; or tall, thin sexually normal children.

CLINICAL FEATURES

Following are the salient clinical features:
- **Age:** It occurs at puberty (between 12-14 years).
- **Sex:** It is more common in boys.

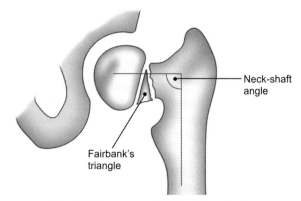

Fig. 39.4: Coxa vara – Fairbank's triangle.

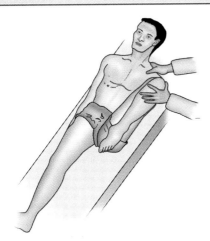

Fig. 39.5: Clinical examination in slipped capital femoral epiphysis. The knee points towards axilla.

- **Side:** It occurs on both sides in 30 per cent of cases.
- There is a definite history of *trauma* in some cases.
- It is *more common* in patients with endocrine abnormalities.

Presenting symptoms: Pain in the groin, often radiating to the thigh and the knee is the common presenting complaint. Often in the initial stages, the symptoms are considered due to a 'sprain', and are disregarded. They soon disappear only to recur. Limp occurs early and is more constant.

Examination: The leg is found to be externally rotated and 1-2 cm short. Limitation of hip movements is characteristic—there is limited abduction and internal rotation, with a corresponding increase in adduction and external rotation. When the hip is flexed, the knee goes towards the ipsilateral axilla (Fig. 39.5). Muscle bulk may be reduced. Trendelenburg's sign may be positive.

RADIOLOGICAL FEATURES

X-ray changes are best seen on a lateral view of the hip. The following signs may be present:
- **On AP view:** The growth plate is displaced towards the metaphyseal side. A line drawn along the superior surface of the neck remains superior to the head unlike in a normal hip where it passes bisecting the head – Trethowan's sign (Fig. 39.6).
- **On lateral view:** The head is angulated on the neck. This can be detected early.

TREATMENT

It is based on the following considerations:
a. **Treatment of an acute slip:** This is by closed reduction and pinning, as for a fracture of the neck of the femur.

b. **Treatment of a gradual slip:** This depends upon the severity of the slip present. If it is less than 1/3 the diameter of the femoral neck, the epiphysis is fixed internally *in situ*. If the slip is more than 1/3, a corrective osteotomy is performed at the inter-trochanteric region.

c. **Treatment of the unaffected side** in unilateral cases: Since the incidence of bilateral involvement is 30 per cent, prophylactic pinning of the unaffected side in a case with unilateral slip is justified.

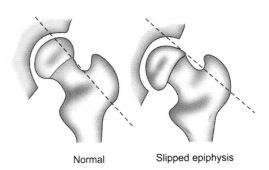

Normal   Slipped epiphysis

Fig. 39.6: Trethowan's sign.

DEFORMITIES OF THE KNEE

KNOCK KNEES (GENU VALGUM)

This is a condition where the knees are abnormally approximated and the ankles abnormally divergent (Fig. 39.7A).

Causes (Table 39.2): The most common type is developmental, almost invariably bilateral. The

Table 39.2: Causes of genu valgum.
Idiopathic
Post-traumatic   ■ Fractures of the lateral femoral or tibial condyles   ■ Damage to the lateral side of the lower femoral or upper tibial epiphyses or epiphyseal plates
Post-inflammatory   ■ Damage to the lateral side of the lower femoral or upper tibial epiphyses or epiphyseal plates by infection
Neoplastic causes   ■ A tumour causing a growth disparity at the epiphyseal plate e.g., chondroblastoma
Bone softening   ■ Rickets and osteomalacia   ■ Bone dysplasias   ■ Rheumatoid arthritis
Stretching of joints   ■ Charcot's disease   ■ Paralytic disease
Cartilage thinning   ■ OA of the lateral compartment of the knee

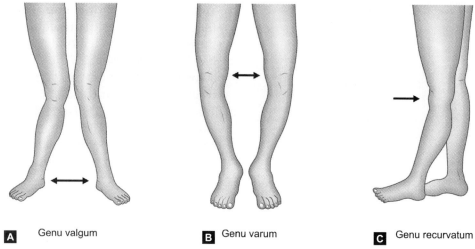

A Genu valgum   **B** Genu varum   **C** Genu recurvatum

Fig. 39.7: Deformities of the knee.

deformity basically results from the unequal growth of two sides of the growth plate of the lower femoral epiphysis or upper tibial epiphysis.

Clinical features: Physiological genu valgum appears at the age of 2-3 years and nearly always corrects by the age of 6. It may be associated with flat feet. The degree of deformity is estimated by measuring the intermalleolar distance, with the child lying supine, with the knees in contact. In genu valgum secondary to a disease such as rickets, there will be findings suggestive of the primary disease.

Treatment: Spontaneous recovery occurs in most idiopathic cases. A medial shoe raise (3/16 inch) is sometimes prescribed. It has no proven scientific rationale but does help in satisfying anxious parents. If the intermalleolar distance is 10 cm or more by the age 4, genu valgum may not correct by itself, and may need an operation. Surgery for genu valgum falls in the following categories:

Growth modulation surgery: In this, One plays with the growing part of the bone (the physis of distal femur) in such a way that growth of the medial side of the physis is stopped temporarily by putting a plate (8 plate) across the physis. In few months of years, due to stoppage of growth on one side, and continuing growth of the other side, the deformity gets corrected. This can only be done in a child of growing age (between 12-14 years).

Corrective osteotomy: In this surgery, the deformed bone is cut at a suitable location and the ends aligned in desired way, thus correcting the deformity. There is a cosmetic way of doing this surgery, called *percutaneous osteotomy* performed through 1 cm incision. The other method is doing correction by formal *open surgery* and fixing the same by plate and screw.

BOW LEGS (GENU VARUM)

This is a condition where the knees are abnormally divergent (bow like) and the ankles abnormally approximated (Fig. 39.7B).

Causes: Idiopathic is the most common type. In others, causes similar to those for genu valgum can be identified, except that the defective growth is on the medial side of the epiphyseal plate. Blount's disease is a special type of genu varum where the posteromedial part of the proximal tibial epiphysis fails to grow during the first 3 years of life.

Clinical features: An ugly deformity is the main complaint. Severity of deformity can be estimated by measuring the distance between the two knees with the ankles held together. If the distance is more than 8 cm, further investigations for an underlying cause are required.

Treatment: Idiopathic type usually corrects spontaneously. Shoes with an outer raise (3/16 inch) are usually prescribed, but have no proven value. If significant bowing persists beyond childhood, surgical correction may be required. This is done by growth modulation or by corrective osteotomy.

GENU RECURVATUM (FIG. 39.7C)

This means hyperextension at the knee joint. It may be congenital or acquired. Polio is the most common cause of acquired genu recurvatum. Others causes are: (i) diseases known to produce lax ligaments (Marfan's syndrome, Charcot's arthropathy); (ii) epiphyseal growth defects; and (iii) malunited fractures.

Treatment: It is difficult. Generally, support with braces is required. In some cases, upper tibial corrective osteotomy may be required.

POPLITEAL CYST

This follows a synovial rupture or its herniation in the popliteal region. It may be osteoarthritic (Morrant-Baker's cyst) or secondary to rheumatoid arthritis. The lump is in the midline and fluctuant, but is not tender. It may shrink following knee aspiration if it is connected to the knee, or may leak or rupture so that the fluid tracks down the calf. Arthroscopic excision is the treatment of choice for symptomatic cases not responding to conservative treatment.

LOOSE BODIES IN JOINTS

This is a common problem, seen most frequently in the knee joint. A fractured osteophyte, becoming loose in an osteoarthritic, is the most common cause. Other causes are knee osteochondritis, osteochondral fractures, synovial chondromatosis, etc. In synovial chondromatosis, the number of bodies is more than 50-60. The complaint of a patient with a loose body in the joint is sudden locking of the joint. Often he can feel the loose body within the joint. Most loose bodies are radiopaque and can be seen on plain X-rays. In some, an arthroscopic examination may be required. Treatment is removal of the body arthroscopically or by opening the joint.

FLAT FOOT

This is a foot with less developed longitudinal arches.

Relevant anatomy: A normal foot has longitudinal and transverse arches. The longitudinal arch consists of medial and lateral components resting on a common pillar posteriorly—the tuberosity of the calcaneum (Fig. 39.8). The talus is the keystone of the arches. It receives the body weight and transmits it to the arches below. Through the arches, the weight is transmitted to the ground via the tuberosity of the calcaneum and the heads of first and fifth metatarsals.

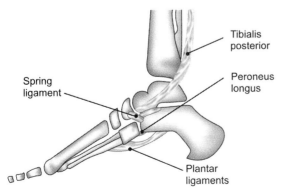

Fig. 39.8: Arches of the foot—anatomy.

Table 39.3: Causes of flat foot.

Biomechanical causes
Congenital
- Infantile or physiological
- Congenital vertical talus

Acquired
- Occupational
- Obesity
- Postural
- Secondary to anatomical defect elsewhere
- External rotation of the limb
  Genu valgum
  Equinus deformity of the ankle
  Varus deformity of the foot

Others

Paralytic	Flaccid flat foot
Spasmodic	Due to peroneal spasm
Arthritic	Rheumatoid arthritis
Traumatic	Fracture calcaneum

The integrity of the arches is maintained by the plantar ligaments, the plantar aponeurosis, the extrinsic and intrinsic muscles and the structure of the bones of the foot. Ligaments are the most important of these structures; especially the spring ligament, long plantar ligament, short plantar ligament, interosseous ligaments and plantar aponeurosis. Of the muscles, tibialis posterior and peroneus longus are more important.

Causes: Idiopathic flat foot is the most common. There are factors related to the anatomical development of the foot which predispose to formation of a flat foot. Some common causes of flat foot are given in Table 39.3.

CONGENITAL FLAT FOOT (VERTICAL TALUS)

The feet of all newborns appear flat because the postural tone of the intrinsic muscles has not yet developed; but in some, the foot is not only flat but also its undersurface is convex (rocker-bottom foot). Such a foot may be in severe valgus. This is due to a congenital anomaly where the talus lies in a vertical position rather than the normal horizontal (Fig. 39.9). Diagnosis can usually be confirmed by taking an X-ray of the foot (lateral view), on which one can see the head of the talus facing vertically downwards. The navicular, along with rest of the foot, rests on the dorsal surface of the talus. Treatment is difficult. In mild cases, the footwear is modified to provide an arch support at mid-foot. In severe cases, corrective surgery is required.

INFANTILE FLAT FOOT

This is the most common type. The child is brought usually soon after he starts walking with

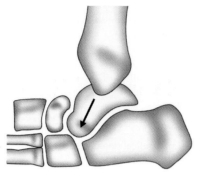

Fig. 39.9: Congenital vertical talus.

the complaints that he walks on flat feet. There is sometimes a tendency for frequent falls. Arches develop as the child grows, and no special treatment is required. In some children, the feet may remain flat but there are no symptoms. Either of the parents usually have flat feet. Such individuals lead a normal life except that they are prone to developing foot strain and are unfit for joining professions requiring high levels of physical fitness (e.g., army). Foot exercises are taught and arch support is given in the shoes. In late adulthood, pain in the foot and stiffness after physical exertion are common complaints.

ACQUIRED FLAT FOOT

These are *static* flat feet, where there has been a structural change in the foot, e.g., flail foot in a fat person, post-traumatic flat foot following a fracture

of the calcaneum, flat foot secondary to genu valgum, etc. The other type is *spasmodic* flat foot where there is a spasm of the peronei muscles due to some painful condition of the foot such as rheumatoid arthritis, tuberculosis, intertarsal bar, etc.

DEFORMITIES OF THE TOES

HALLUX VALGUS

It is the lateral deviation of the great toe at the metatarsophalangeal joint. Causes are many, but it is commonly due to rheumatoid arthritis, wearing pointed shoes with high heels, idiopathic, etc. Usually there are no symptoms. If symptoms are present, surgical correction may be necessary. Common operations performed are: (i) osteotomy of neck of the first metatarsal (Mitchell's osteotomy); (ii) excision of the metatarsal head (Mayo's operation); and (iii) excision of the base of the proximal phalanx (Keller's operation).

HALLUX RIGIDUS

This means a stiff big toe due to OA of the metatarsophalangeal joint of the great toe. It is usually a result of old trauma, arthritis, etc.

HAMMER TOE

It is a fixed flexion deformity of an interphalangeal joint of the toe, usually with callosity over the prominent proximal joint.

 What have we learnt?

- Fibrosis of sternomastoid muscle is the cause of torticollis.
- Cervical rib arises from 7th cervical vertebra.
- In infantile coxa vara, neck-shaft angle is reduced.
- Slipped capital femoral epiphysis is a disease of adolescence, commonly associated with endocrine disorders.
- Genu valgus, genu varum, flat foot are developmental disorders which often get corrected with growth.

Additional information: From the entrance exams point of view

- Steel's metaphyseal blanch sign and Scham's loss of dense triangular appearance of inferomedial articular neck is seen in SCFE.
- Phocomelia is a defect in the development of long bones.
- Madelung's deformity is seen in the wrist.
- Congenital pseudoarthrosis of the tibia and fibula and musculoskeletal deformities are seen in neurofibromatosis type II. They are treated by internal fixation and bone grafting.

Learning Objectives

- ❖ What are the types of amputation, common reasons for amputating the limb, and principle of post-amputation care?
- ❖ Discuss prosthesis and orthosis used in orthopaedic practice.

AMPUTATIONS

Amputation is a procedure where a part of the limb is removed through one or more bones. It should be distinguished from *disarticulation* where a part is removed through a joint. For simplifying this discussion, the term 'amputation' is applied to both these procedures. Amputation of lower limb is more commonly performed than that of upper limb; however, partial amputation of fingers or hand is common in developing countries, mainly as a sequelae of farm and machine injuries.

INDICATIONS

Overall, injury is the most common cause of amputation in developing countries. The injury may be sustained in traffic accidents, in agriculture fields during harvesting season, in riots, etc. Upper limb amputations occur commonly by *kutti* chopper or thresher machines. Train accidents, at a level railway crossing, unaware of a coming train, is a common cause of lower limb amputation. Some common indications for amputation are given in Table 40.1.

Indications for amputation vary in different age groups. In the *elderly* (50-75 years), peripheral vascular disease with or without diabetes is the main cause. In *younger adults* (25-30 years), amputation is

Table 40.1: Indications for amputation.
▪ Injury
▪ Peripheral vascular disease, including diabetes
▪ Infections, e.g., gas gangrene
▪ Tumours
▪ Nerve injuries
▪ Congenital anomalies

most often secondary to injury or its sequelae. In *children*, limbs may be deficient since birth. Amongst the acquired causes, injury and malignancy top the list.

TYPES

Guillotine or Open Amputation

This is where the skin is not closed over the amputation stump, usually when the wound is not healthy. The operation is followed, after some period, by one of the following procedures for constructing a satisfactory stump:

- **Secondary closure:** Closure of skin flaps after a few days.
- **Plastic repair:** Soft tissues are repaired without cutting the bone and skin flaps are closed.
- **Revision of the stump:** Terminal granulation tissue and scar tissue, as well as a moderate amount of bone is removed and the stump reconstructed.

- **Re-amputation:** This is amputation at a higher level, as if an amputation is being performed for the first time.

Closed Amputation

This is where the skin is closed primarily (e.g., most elective amputations).

SURGICAL PRINCIPLES–FOR CLOSED TYPE

Amputation surgery is a very important step in the rehabilitation of an amputee, and must be approached as a plastic and reconstructive procedure. Following are some of the basic principles to be followed meticulously:

a. **Tourniquet:** Use of a tourniquet is highly desirable *except* in case of an ischaemic limb.

b. **Exsanguination:** Usually a limb should be squeezed (exsanguinated) by wrapping it with a stretchable bandage (Esmarch bandage) before a tourniquet is inflated. It is *contraindicated* in cases of infection and malignancy for fear of spread of the same proximally.

c. **Level of amputation:** With modern techniques of fitting artificial limbs, strict levels adhered to in the past are no longer tenable. Principles guiding the level of amputations are as follows:

   - *The disease:* Extent and nature of the disease or trauma, for which amputation is being done, is an important consideration. One tends to be conservative with dry-gangrene (vascular) and trauma, but liberal with acute life-threatening infections and malignancies.

   - *Anatomical principles:* A joint must be saved as far as possible. These days, it is possible to fit artificial limbs to stumps shorter than 'ideal' length, as long as the stump is well-healed, non-tender and properly constructed.

   - *Suitability for the efficient functioning of the artificial limb:* Sometimes, length is compromised for efficient functioning of an artificial limb to be fitted on a stump. For example, a long stump of an above-knee amputee may hamper with optimal prosthetic fitting.

Classification of amputation on the basis of its level is given in Table 40.2.

Skin flaps: The skin over the stump should be mobile and normally sensitive, but atypical skin flaps are preferable to amputation at a more proximal level.

Muscles: Muscles should be cut distal to the level of bone. Following methods of muscle sutures have been found advantageous:

Table 40.2: Nomenclature of amputation by levels.

Name	Part of the limb removed
Upper limb	
Forequarter amputation	Scapula + lateral 2/3 of clavicle + whole of the upper limb
Shoulder disarticulation	Removal through the gleno-humeral joint
Above elbow amputation	Through the arm
Elbow disarticulation	Through the elbow
Below elbow amputation	Through the forearm bones
Wrist disarticulation	Through the radiocarpal joint
Ray amputation	Removal of a finger with respective metacarpal from carpometacarpal joint
Krukenberg's amputation	Making 'forceps' with two forearm bones
Lower limb	
Hindquarter amputation	Whole of the lower limb with one side of the ilium removed
Hip disarticulation	Through the hip
Above knee amputation	Through the femur
Knee disarticulation	Through the knee
Below knee amputation	Through the tibia-fibula
Syme's amputation	Through the ankle joint
Chopart's amputation	Through talonavicular joint
Lisfranc's amputation	Through intertarsal joints

- *Myoplasty,* i.e., the opposite group of muscles are sutured to each other.
- *Myodesis,* i.e., the muscles are sutured to the end of the stump.

These are contraindicated in peripheral vascular diseases.

Nerves are gently pulled distally into the wound, and divided with a sharp knife so that the cut end retracts well proximal to the level of bone section.

Large nerves such as the sciatic nerve contain relatively large vessels and should be ligated before they are divided.

Major blood vessels should be isolated and *doubly* ligated using non-absorbable sutures. The tourniquet should be released before skin closure and meticulous haemostasis should be secured.

Bone level is decided as discussed earlier. Excessive periosteal stripping proximally may lead to the formation of 'ring sequestrum' from the end of the bone. Bony prominences which are not well padded by soft tissues should be resected. Sharp edges of the cut bone should be made smooth.

Drain: A corrugated rubber drain should be used for 48-72 hours post-operatively.

After treatment: Treatment, from the time amputation is completed till the definitive prosthesis fitted, is important if a strong and maximally functioning stump is desired. Following care is needed:

- *Dressing:* There are two types of dressings used after amputation surgery: (i) conventional or soft dressing; and (ii) rigid dressing. The latter has been found to be advantageous for wound healing and early prosthetic fitting.
  Soft dressing: This is conventional dressing using gauge, cotton and bandage.
  Rigid dressing: In this type of dressing, after a conventional dressing, a well moulded PoP cast is applied on to the stump at the conclusion of surgery. This helps in enhancing wound healing and maturation of the stump. In addition, the patient can be fitted with a temporary artificial limb with a prosthetic foot (pilon) for almost immediate mobilisation.
- *Positioning and elevation of the stump:* This is required to prevent contracture and promote healing.
- *Exercises:* Stump exercises are necessary for maintaining range of motion of the joint proximal to the stump and for building up strength of the muscles controlling the stump.
- *Wrapping* the stump helps in its healing, shrinkage and maturation. This can be done with a crepe bandage.
- *Prosthetic fitting and gait training:* This is started usually 3 months after the amputation.

COMPLICATIONS

1. **Haematoma:** Inadequate haemostasis, loosening of the ligature and inadequate wound drainage are the common causes. Haematoma results in delayed wound healing and infection. It should be aspirated and a pressure bandage given.
2. **Infection:** The cause generally is an underlying peripheral vascular disease, diabetes or a haematoma. Wound breakdown and occasionally spread of infection proximally may necessitate amputation at a higher level. A wound should not be closed whenever the surgeon is in doubt about the vascularity of the muscles or the skin at the cut end. Any discharge from the wound should be treated promptly.
3. **Skin flap necrosis:** A minor or major skin flap necrosis indicates insufficient circulation of the skin flap. It can be avoided by taking care

at the time of designing skin flaps that as much subcutaneous tissues remain with the skin flap as possible. Small areas of flap necrosis may heel with dressings but for larger areas, redesigning of the flaps may be required.

4. **Deformities of the joints:** These results from improper positioning of the amputation stump, leading to contractures. A mild or moderate contracture is treated by appropriate positioning and gentle passive-stretching exercises. Severe deformity may need surgical correction.
5. **Neuroma:** A neuroma always forms at the end of a cut nerve. In case a neuroma is bound down to the scar because of adhesions, it becomes painful. Painful neuroma can usually be prevented by dividing the nerves sharply at a proximal level and allowing it to retract well proximal to the end of the stump, to lie in normal soft tissues. If it does form, it is to be excised at a more proximal level.
6. **Phantom sensation:** All individuals with acquired amputations experience some form of phantom sensation, a sensation as if the amputated part is still present. This sensation is most prominent in the period immediately following amputation, and gradually diminishes with time. Phantom pain is the awareness of pain in the amputated limb. Treatment is difficult.

SPECIAL FEATURES OF AMPUTATIONS IN CHILDREN

Amputations in children have the following special features:

- Children may have amputation since birth.
- A *disarticulation is preferred* to an amputation through the shaft of a long bone at a more proximal level. This is because disarticulation preserves the epiphysis distally, and therefore growth of the stump continues at the normal rate.
- As the child grows, terminal overgrowth of the bone occurs and needs frequent revisions.
- A child needs frequent changes in the size of the artificial limb.
- Children tolerate artificial limbs much better and get used to wearing it more quickly.

PROSTHESES IN ORTHOPAEDIC PRACTICE

Prosthetics is a unit of rehabilitation medicine dealing with the replacement of whole or a part of a missing extremity with an artificial device. The device so manufactured is called a prosthesis.

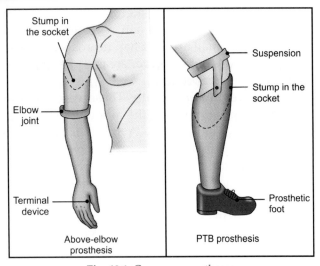

Stump in the socket

Elbow joint

Terminal device

Above-elbow prosthesis

Suspension

Stump in the socket

Prosthetic foot

PTB prosthesis

Fig. 40.1: Common prostheses.

b. An above-knee amputee with 45 degrees flexion contracture at the hip.
c. A below-elbow amputee with a flail elbow and shoulder.
d. Bilateral above-knee amputee with short stumps.

Parts of a prosthesis: The prosthesis consists of a *socket*, designed to be in close contact with the stump; a *suspension* to hold the socket to the stump; a *prosthetic extension* with substitute joints; and a *terminal device* Fig. 40.1). The sockets are shaped according to the shape of the stump. These could be *end bearing sockets* – where end of the stump bears the weight, or *total contact socket* – where the weight is distributed evenly throughout the surface of the socket. The socket is the fundamental component to which the remaining components are attached. Most sockets are double-walled. A plaster cast moulding of the stump is used to fabricate the socket for optimal fit, function and comfort.

Traditionally, the terminal device of a lower limb prosthesis is a prosthetic foot, called SACH* foot. It is a simple device that has a wooden core surrounded by a solid rubber foot. This permits a combination of stiffness with pliability. The cushioned heel absorbs the impact of heel strike. In India, at Jaipur, SACH foot has been modified in a number of ways to make it suitable for barefoot walking. Essentially, these modifications are:
i. Appearance of the foot is that of a normal foot; and
ii. It allows movement at forefoot and midfoot, making walking on uneven surfaces easier. Similarly, for an above-knee amputee, a prosthesis has been developed at AIIMS, New Delhi, which permits squatting and sitting cross-legged. Upper limb prostheses are named by the level of amputation. Some of the commonly used prostheses are given in Table 40.3.

Recently, electrically operated prostheses have been developed. These have opened up a new world of freedom and function for persons with amputation, but these are very expensive. There have been a number of advances in designing of prosthesis. With the help of computers, the socket can be so designed keeping in mind particular areas over which pressure could be relieved.

Uses of prostheses: A prosthesis may be used to replace a body part externally (e.g., an artificial limb) or internally (e.g., an artificial hip joint). During the past two decades considerable progress has occurred in prosthetics and rehabilitation of an amputee. Improved materials, new designs, and better evaluation and fitting techniques have resulted in prostheses that are lighter and stronger, and provide improved function, cosmesis and comfort. By and large, prosthetic replacement of the lower limb offers excellent restoration of function, and the cosmetic appearance is satisfactory. However, providing prosthesis for the upper limb is more difficult. It is almost impossible for a mechanical device to reproduce the versatility, dexterity and appearance of the natural hand. One of the most important aspect of a rehabilitation programme for a patient with amputation is to orient the patient realistically as to what the prosthesis can and cannot do.

A prosthesis can be: (i) cosmetic—to provide normal appearance or (ii) functional—to provide function of the missing part. The prosthesis does not have sensation, proprioception or muscle power. The power is provided to a prosthesis by forces arising from movement of the residual or other side limb. These are called *body powered prostheses;* in others an external source of power, usually rechargeable batteries is used.

In general, more distal the amputation, more functional the individual is with the use of a prosthesis. Poor candidates for functional prosthetic fitting are the following:
a. A lower limb amputee with ischaemic limb, with an open or poorly healed wound.

* Solid Ankle Cushioned Heel.

Table 40.3: Commonly used prostheses.	
Above-knee amputation	Quadrilateral socket prosthesis
Below-knee amputation	PTB (Patellar Tendon Bearing) prosthesis
Syme's amputation	Canadian Syme's prosthesis
Partial foot amputation	Shoe fillers

ORTHOSES IN ORTHOPAEDIC PRACTICE

Orthotics is the unit of rehabilitation which deals with improving function of the body by the application of a device which aids the body part. The device so manufactured is called an orthosis.

NOMENCLATURE OF ORTHOSES

Until recently, the terms braces, calipers, splints, and corsets, used to name and describe orthoses were not uniform. Now a logical, easy to use system of standard terminology has been developed. This system uses the first letter of the name of each joint which the orthosis crosses in correct sequence, with the letter O (for orthosis) attached at the end. Some of the commonly used orthoses are given below:

- AFO   Ankle Foot Orthosis
          (previously called below-knee caliper)
- KAFO   Knee-Ankle-Foot Orthosis
          (previously called above-knee caliper)
- HKAFO   Hip-Knee-Ankle-Foot   Orthosis
          (previously called above-knee caliper with pelvic band)
- KO   Knee Orthosis (previously called knee brace)
- CO   Cervical Orthosis
          (previously called cervical collar)
- WHO   Wrist Hand Orthosis
          (previously called cock up splint)
- CTLSO   Cervico-Thoraco-Lumbo-Sacral Orthosis
          (previously called body brace)

- FO   Foot Orthosis
          (previously called surgical shoes)

Orthoses can be divided into static and dynamic types. *Static orthoses* are used: (i) to support an arthritic joint or a fractured bone; (ii) to prevent joint contractures in a paralytic limb; and (iii) for serial splinting of a joint to correct contracture. *Dynamic orthoses* are used to apply forces to a joint which is damaged by arthritis or when the muscles that normally control the joint are weak.

USES OF ORTHOSES

Orthoses are used for the following functions:
- To immobilise a joint or body part, e.g., a painful joint
- To prevent a deformity, e.g., in a polio limb
- To correct a deformity, e.g., in Volkmann's contracture
- To assist movement, e.g., in a polio limb
- To relieve weight bearing, e.g., in an ununited fracture
- To provide support, e.g., to a fractured spine.

Some common clinical conditions requiring orthoses are cervical spondylosis or whiplash injury [common cervical collar or cervical orthosis), wrist drop (WHO), foot drop (AFO), poliomyelitis (orthosis depending upon muscle power), rheumatoid arthritis, and spinal injury, Fig. 40.2]. Some surgical shoe modifications made for different orthopaedic conditions are given in Table 40.4.

In recent years, quality of orthosis has improved with availability of better material and designing facilities.

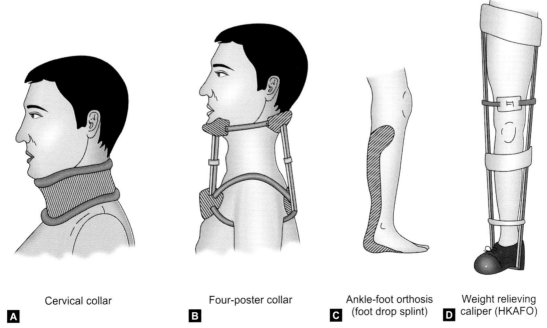

A	B	C	D
Cervical collar	Four-poster collar	Ankle-foot orthosis (foot drop splint)	Weight relieving caliper (HKAFO)

Fig. 40.2: Common orthoses.

For polio, traditional calipers can now be replaced by aesthetic plastic inserts which can go inside the shoes and can be worn under clothes (Fig. 40.2c). More and more orthoses are made available in 'ready to use' designs; these can be adjusted to fit individual patients. Also, custom made components of orthosis are available. These can be assembled and a caliper/orthosis made, thus saving time. In newer designs, adjustment of height of the orthosis is possible in growing children.

Contributed by: Dr Sanjay Wadhwa
Professor
Department of Physical Medicine
All India Institute of Medical Sciences, New Delhi

Table 40.4: Surgical shoes.	
■ Shoe with Thomas heel (C and E heel*)	Flat foot
■ Shoe with arch support	Flat foot
■ CTEV shoes	Clubfoot
■ Shoe with heel pad	Plantar fascitis
■ Shoe with metatarsal pad	Corns
■ Shoe with metatarsal bar	Metatarsalgia
■ Shoe with medial raise	Genu valgum
■ Shoe with lateral raise	Genu varun
■ Shoe with universal raise	Short leg

* Crooked and Elongated heel

What have we learnt?

- Amputations are named according to their level.
- Well-constructed stump and well-fitted prosthesis are key to good functions.
- Modern nomenclature of orthoses is based on the joints the orthosis is supposed to control.
- Shoe modifications help settle foot disorders.

Arthroscopic Surgery

Learning Objectives

- ❖ What is arthroscopic surgery, what are the different joints on which this can be performed, and what are the common indications?

Sports medicine has become a fast growing subspeciality of orthopaedics. Initially, it was to do with the knee injuries in competitive athletes, but now it has expanded to include the overall care of an athlete at every level. The speciality consists of care of the injured athlete, his pulmonary and cardiovascular build up, training techniques, nutrition, etc. Hence, it has become a speciality with multi-disciplinary approach involving trainers, physical therapists, cardiologists, pulmonologists, orthopaedic surgeons and general practitioners.

Arthroscopy is a technique of surgery on the joints in which tip of a thin (4 mm diameter) telescope called arthroscope is introduced into a joint, and the inside of the joint examined (Fig. 41.1). This is called *diagnostic arthroscopy*. Once the diagnosis is made, necessary correction can be done, there and then, by introducing micro-instruments through another small skin puncture. This is called *arthroscopic surgery*. Today, most operations on the joints, particularly on the knee and shoulder, can be carried out arthroscopically. This technique has revolutionised the treatment of joint disorders.

ADVANTAGES OF ARTHROSCOPIC SURGERY

- **Minimally invasive technique:** The operation is performed through small punctures, without cutting open the joint. There is almost no blood loss.
- **Day-care surgery:** The surgery is performed on day-care basis, which means that the patient is admitted on the morning of the operation and sent home the same evening.
- **Little immobilisation required:** The only immobilisation of the knee is in the form of a small dressing for 48 hours. It allows the knee to be bent. It is possible for the patient to be up and about in the house within 48 hours. Very little or no physiotherapy is required.

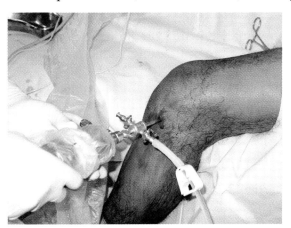

Fig. 41.1: Knee arthroscopic surgery.

- **Barely visible scars:** Since the whole operation is performed through multiple small punctures, the scars are barely visible.
- **Possible under local anaesthesia:** In selected cases, it is possible to perform the operation under local anaesthesia. The patient can literally walk into the operation theatre and walk out of it.
- **Better assessment of the joint:** Arthroscopy is the best modality for diagnosing a joint pathology. Even MRI, which is a close next to arthroscopy gives only limited information. MRI, being a sensitive investigation, can sometime pick up lesions which may not be clinically significant (false positive), and also may miss lesions which are better picked up by actually seeing them and probing them (false negative).
- **Dynamic assessment of the joint possible:** Since it is possible to move the joint while arthroscopy is being performed, one can actually see how the structures inside the joint appear when the joint is moved. A new group of abnormalities in the joint have come to light due to the possibility of dynamic assessement. For example, an abnormal tracking of the patella (patella not moving concentrically in the trochlear notch) may be seen very convincingly arthroscopically.
- **New diagnostic possibilities:** A number of new diagnostic possibilities have come to knowledge since the availability of arthroscope. A whole new group of conditions in the knee called *Plicas* have been understood to be associated with patient's symptoms. Similarly, some lesions such as *SLAP** lesions, which cause shoulder pain, can be diagnosed only arthroscopically.
- **Research possibility:** Being a minimally invasive procedure, arthroscopy offers the possibility of studying the changes in the intra-articular structures, e.g., changes in an implanted artificial ligament and its process of acceptance by the body.

INDICATIONS FOR ARTHROSCOPIC SURGERY

Arthroscopy may be done to confirm a diagnosis in case it has not been possible to do so otherwise. In most cases, a provisional diagnosis is made before proceeding with arthroscopic surgery. Once the diagnosis is confirmed arthroscopically, necessary corrective measures are taken. Some of the common procedures which can be successfully performed arthroscopically are as shown in Table 41.1.

---

* Superior Labrum Anterior-Posterior

Table 41.1: Indications for arthroscopic surgery.

Knee Joint
- Loose body removal
- Partial or complete menisectomy
- Chondroplasty (repair or removal of degenerated cartilage)
- Excision of plicas, the thickened synovial folds in the knee
- Correction of patellar maltracking
- Synovial biopsy
- Synovectomy
- Release of a stiff knee (arthrolysis)
- Ligament reconstruction
- Fusion of the knee (arthrodesis)

Shoulder Joint
- Loose body removal
- Debridement of loose labrum glenoidale
- Diagnosis of the cause of shoulder pain
- Arthroscopic shoulder stabilisation in recurrent dislocation of the shoulder
- Excision of AC joint
- Subacromial decompression
- Release of a frozen shoulder
- Rotator-cuff repair

Ankle Joint
- Loose body removal
- Correction of anterior impingement
- Chondroplasty
- Synovectomy
- Synovial biopsy
- Arthrodesis

Elbow
- Release of stiff elbow
- Removal of loose body
- Synovectomy

Wrist
- Diagnosis of wrist pain
- Debridement of torn triangular cartilage
- Synovial biopsy and synovectomy

EQUIPMENT

Arthroscopic surgery is an equipment dependent surgery. Most of the equipment is imported and expensive. The following equipment is necessary.

a. **To visualise inside the joint:** Arthroscope, light source, fibre-optic cable, video camera and TV monitor.

b. **To perform basic operations:** Hand instruments such as a probe, cutters, graspers, scissors, knives, etc.

c. **To perform complex operations:** Instruments such as motorized shaver, underwater cutting cautery, etc. Some special instruments are required for particular operations such as anterior cruciate ligament (ACL), posterior cruciate ligament (PCL) reconstructions.

An arthroscope is a 4 mm telescope having a 30° forward oblique angle (Fig. 41.2). This obliquity

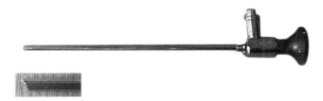

Fig. 41.2: An arthroscope.

helps in increasing the field of vision. Smaller size arthroscope is used for smaller joints.

PROCEDURE

One needs to develop special psychomotor skills to be able to perform arthroscopic surgery. Following are the commonly scoped joints.

KNEE ARTHROSCOPY

Procedure on the knee is done with the patient under spinal or general anaesthesia. A tourniquet is applied on the thigh. The knee is cleaned and draped as would be done for any other major knee operation. The arthroscope and instruments are introduced through small cuts called portals, as shown in Figure 41.3. The most common portal is anterolateral portal located just lateral to the patellar tendon, at the level of the joint. This is the one through which the arthroscope is introduced. A small video camera is attached to the arthroscope, and the inside of the knee can be seen on the TV monitor. The arthroscope can be moved to different parts of the joint, and all the structures inside the joint are thoroughly examined. A second portal is used for introducing probe or other instruments. The portal used commonly for this purpose is made on the medial side of the patellar tendon (anteromedial portal). The crux of performing arthroscopic surgery is the ability to bring the tip of the instruments in front of the telescope (triangulation).

Ligament Surgery: The Anterior Cruciate Ligament (ACL) and Posterior Cruciate Ligament (PCL) when torn are reconstructed by making new ligaments using spare tendons in the body (MC hamstring and patellar tendon) (autografts) or from cadavers (allograft) and rarely synthetic ligaments. Tunnels are drilled arthroscopically on the femur and tibia at specific origins and insertions of these ligaments, the newly prepared ligament is then inserted through these tunnels and fixed at either end using specialised devices like buttons and screws.

Meniscus Surgery: The meniscus has three parts the anterior horn, body and posterior horn. When torn from the body or posterior horn they can either be partially/totally removed (menisectomy) or repaired back to their position (meniscus repair).

CARTILAGE SURGERY

Chondroplasty: In this technique the degenerated cartilage is debrided till the subchondral bone is reached to stimulate healing with fibrocartilage.

Microfracture: In this technique small holes are made in the subchondral bone to stimulate healing in cartilaginous defects.

Mosaicplasty: In this technique articular cartilage is harvested from a non-articular part of the knee and transplanted to the cartilaginous defect.

Artificial Chondrocyte Implantation: In this technique pieces of articular cartilage are taken from a non-articular part of the knee arthroscopically and cultured in a laboratory. They are then mixed with a medium and put back into the cartilaginous defect to stimulate healing.

Loose pieces of bone/cartilage floating in the knee obstructing the smooth gliding of the surfaces of the knee can be removed arthroscopically.

SHOULDER ARTHROSCOPY

It is very useful in making a correct diagnosis in shoulder problems. The usual approach to arthroscopic shoulder examination is via a posterior portal. This is located 2 cm below and medial to the posterolateral angle of the acromian. Other instruments such as a probe, are passed from anterior portals, all of which are lateral to the coracoid process. In order to ensure clear visibility, and since a tourniquet cannot be used,

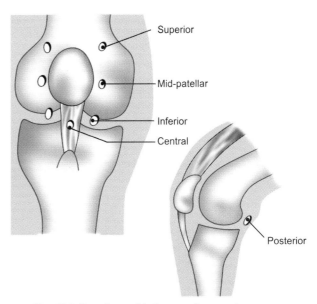

Fig. 41.3: Portals used in knee arthroscopic surgery.

clarity is maintained by inflating the joint with saline and maintaining it under pressure with the help of a fluid pump.

Bankart Repair: Labral tears especially on the antero-inferior region of the glenoid (Bankart lesions) can be repaired arthroscopically using suture anchors (small platic/metallic screws with threads attached to them that are placed on the glenoid surface. The threads are then used to stitch back the labrum in place.

Rotator Cuff Repair: Rotator cuff tendons comprising the supraspinatus infraspinatus, teres and subscapularis may tear in sporting individuals or the elderly (degenerative). They are repaired back in place using suture anchors placed on the humeral head (near the footprint of these tendons).

LIMITATIONS OF ARTHROSCOPIC SURGERY

CASE SUITABILITY

Arthroscopic surgery is not a panacea for each and every joint disorder. It has no role where the disease is too early and can be managed with medicines and physiotherapy. Sometimes the damage is beyond arthroscopic repair. In the knee, arthroscopic procedures have failed to produce significant relief in advanced stages of osteoarthritis. Also, a stiff knee with quadriceps scarring and adhesions cannot be managed only arthroscopically, and open surgery is required.

In the shoulder, arthroscopy is not effective if the exact cause of pain has not been diagnosed before surgery. Arthroscopy has limited role in treatment of shoulder osteoarthritis, massive rotator-cuff tears and multidirectional instability. The fascinating aspect of arthroscopic surgery is that what its limitation is today, may not remain so in future as advances in technology makes it possible.

LEARNING CURVE

Arthroscopy has a steep learning curve. One has to work within a confined space, and manoeuvering the scope as well as instruments is difficult. Rough movements can cause damage to the intra-articular structures and breakage of the rather delicate instruments.

EQUIPMENT

The equipment used for arthroscopy is expensive. The instruments being delicate, need continuous care and replenishment. A number of procedure specific instruments are necessary. One has to keep a big inventory of instruments and implants. There is no role of make-shift (*Jugaad*) in arthroscopic surgery.

What have we learnt?

- Arthroscopy is a fast developing field of orthopaedics with a steep learning curve.
- Most operations on joints can be performed by keyhole surgery. It is particularly useful for knee and shoulder.

Additional information: From the entrance exams point of view

- Microfracturing is done for osteochondral defects.

Joint Replacement Surgery

Learning Objectives

❖ What are the different types of joint replacement of the hip, what are the indications and possible complications?
❖ Discuss the philosophy behind knee replacement, what are the indications, types, complications?

Joint replacement is a procedure whereby one or both the components forming a joint are replaced with artificial components (called prosthesis). The prostheses are made up of special metal alloy or special high density polyethylene. A lot of research has gone into choice of the material, designing of the prosthesis and technique of their implantation. But, even till today, no artificial joint is as good as God given joint. Following are some of the commonly performed joint replacement procedures.

HEMIARTHROPLASTY
(Partial Joint Replacement)

This means replacing only one side of a joint. For instance, the head of the femur is replaced with an artificial component while the acetabulum is left as it is. Hemiarthroplasty is indicated in situations where only one half of the joint is affected, e.g., fracture neck of the femur in the elderly. A variety of prostheses are used—it could be a single piece (*monopolar*) or two piece (*bipolar*) prosthesis (Fig. 42.1 on next page). In the latter, motion occurs between the two parts of the prosthesis itself. The prosthesis could be modular, where the prosthesis could be assembled on the table from a choice of combination of stem and head sizes. The prosthesis could be cemented (bonded to the host bone by bone cement), or uncemented (a press-

fit design where natural bonding occurs between the host bone and the prosthesis). The operative technique consists of exposing the hip, dislocating the hip, resecting the ends, preparing the medullary canal for receiving the prosthesis, implanting the prosthesis in the canal, reducing the hip and closing the wound. Post-operative rehabilitation is very important. A similar hemiarthroplasty operation is also done in the shoulder where the damaged head of the humerus is replaced with a prosthesis.

TOTAL JOINT REPLACEMENT

This means that both the components of the joint are replaced, e.g., the head as well as the acetabulum are replaced in a total hip replacement operation. This procedure is often required in patients suffering from arthritic afflictions of the joint. The procedure was first developed by Sir John Charnley in 1960. It has proved to be a successful operation giving 15-20 years of good function. Success of this operation depends upon the skill of the surgeon, his understanding of the basic biomechanics and the functional status of the joint before surgery.

These are expensive operations because good quality artificial joints are imported. Just for an idea, the cost of the artificial joint itself is approximately ₹ 30,000–100,000 (variable). Good quality Indian joints have

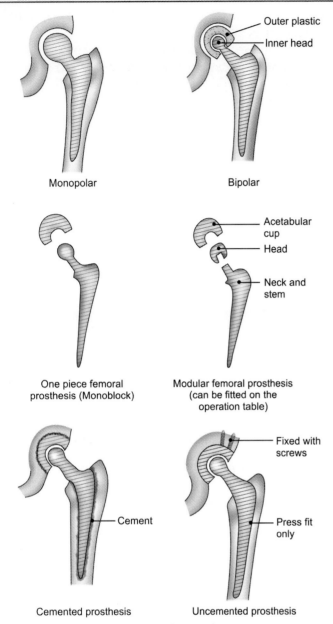

Fig. 42.1: Types of hip replacement.

become available and give satisfactory results in the hands of those using them. Apart from the joint, training of the surgeon, standard of the operation theatre and post-operative care constitute essential ingredients to making this operation successful.

Total joint replacement operations started with hip replacement, quickly went on to the knee, the shoulder, the elbow, etc. Today, almost all joints of the body have been replaced with varying degree of success. Two most popular replacement operations are the hip and the knee replacement.

TOTAL HIP REPLACEMENT

This is an operation where both, the acetabulum and the head of the femur are replaced with artificial components. For the acetabulum, a cup made of high density polyethylene is used, and for the head a specially designed prosthesis made of metal alloy (cobalt-chromium alloy) is used. Both components are fixed in place with or without bone cement (Fig. 42.2).

Indications: An overall indication of total hip replacement is incapacitating arthritis of the hip, severely affecting patient's functions. It could result from a variety of reasons such as rheumatoid arthritis, osteoarthritis, etc. Before considering a hip for replacement, full non-operative treatment should have been tried. Also should have been taken into consideration, other less invasive joint preserving procedures such as osteotomy, joint debridement and hemiarthroplasty. An arthrodesis may be a more suitable option in some cases.

Choice must be made between cemented and uncemented joint replacement. In general, cemented arthroplasty is used in elderly people with expected life of 10-15 years and uncemented in younger people.

Complications: It is a highly demanding operation. The following complications can occur:

a. **Deep venous thrombosis (DVT):** This occurs due to inadvertent manipulation of the thigh during surgery, venous stasis in the limb due to immobility, and some inherent factors in the patient which put him at a higher risk for developing DVT. Treatment consists of prevention of DVT by pharmacologic agents such as heparin and its newer derivatives, and by mechanical means such as continuous exercises of the leg, compression garments, elevation of the leg, etc.

b. **Nerve palsies:** These are relatively infrequent. Sciatic nerve is the most commonly affected, particularly in procedures requiring complex hip reconstruction.

c. **Vascular injury:** This is uncommon, but can occur mainly due to technical reasons.

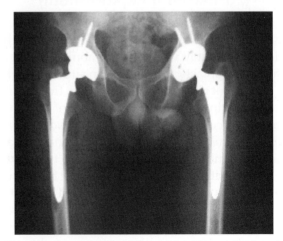

Fig. 42.2: X-ray showing bilateral total hip replacement.

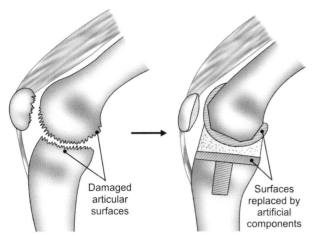

Fig. 42.3: Total knee replacement is actually only a resurfacing operation.

d. **Fracture:** These may occur during the process of implantation of the prothesis, mainly on the femoral side, or later due to stress concentration. The latter usually occurs just distal to the tip of the femoral stem. Treatment depends upon the site and type of fracture, and it does prolong the rehabilitation.

e. **Dislocation:** The rate of dislocation of an artificial hip joint is between 1-8 per cent. It is primarily due to mal-positioning of the limb during early post-operative period, malposition of the replaced components, and later, loosening of the components.

f. **Infection:** This is the most serious of all complications. Prevention is the best way.

g. **Heterotrophic bone formation:** New bone formation around the components occurs in some cases such as ankylosing spondylitis, and results in decreased range of joint movements.

TOTAL KNEE REPLACEMENT

This is a relatively newer operation. In true sense, the term total knee replacement is a misnomer, since unlike the hip replacement where a part of the head and neck are actually removed and replaced with similar shaped artificial components, in the knee only the damaged articular surface is sliced off to prepare the bone ends to take the artificial components which 'cap' the ends of the bones. In a way, this could be more appropriately called a knee resurfacing operation (Fig. 42.3).

Indications: Like in the hip, painful disabling arthritis is the main indication of doing a total knee arthroplasty. It is contraindicated if there is a focus of sepsis, extensor mechanism is insufficient or if the joint is neuropathic. Relative contraindications are: a younger patient (less than 50 years), obesity and those in physically demanding profession where results may not be as good.

The Implant and the Procedure: The artificial knee joint consists of the following parts (Fig. 42.4):
a. A U-shaped femoral component to 'cap' the prepared lower end of the femur.
b. A tibial base plate to cover the cut flat surface of the upper end of the tibia. Either both cruciates or only anterior cruciate is excised.
c. A plastic tray inserted between the above two metallic components.
d. A patellar button made of polyethylene to replace the damaged surface of the patella.

The *procedure* consists of a series of steps based on specially designed jigs. These jigs are used in a step by step manner. The whole idea is to prepare the ends of tibia and femur to take the artificial components. The important goal of the procedure is to achieve optimal alignment of the leg and soft tissue balance between ligaments around the knee. This provides crucial stability to the artificial joint (Fig. 42.5). New developments are happening every year, directed towards better biomaterials, better component designs, better surgical techniques, better postoperative pain management and rehabilitation.

It is fair to expect 15-20 years of excellent functions after a properly executed total knee replacement. The success of this operation depends upon proper selection of the patient, technically perfect execution of the procedure and sincere rehabilitation effort.

Complications: Following complications can occur:
1. **Infection:** Infection could be minor in the form of wound breakdown, or a major infection necessitating another operation to clean up the joint. Sometimes the infection may not be controlled, and removal of the prosthesis and fusion of the joint may become necessary.

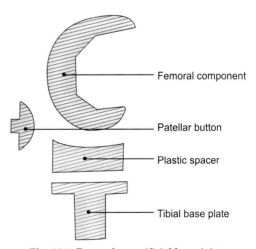

Fig. 42.4: Parts of an artificial knee joint.

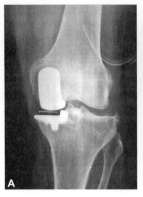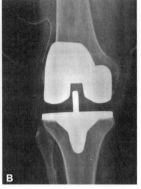

Fig. 42.5: X-ray of the knee, AP view showing: (A) Partial knee replacement; (B) Total knee replacement.

2. **Deep venous thrombosis (DVT):** It occurs as a result of immobility. Treatment is on lines as discussed in hip section.

3. **Nerve palsy:** Common peroneal nerve palsy sometimes occurs in cases requiring dissection on the lateral side of the knee. Spontaneous recovery occurs in most cases.

4. **Fractures:** Fractures may occur while performing the operation, particularly in osteoporotic bones of a bedridden rheumatoid patient. Fractures may occur late through the bones near the prosthesis due to stress concentration in that area.

5. **Extensor mechanism complications:** Handling of extensor mechanism is required during the course of the operation. These may occur due to avulsion of the patellar tendon, inadvertent cutting of the tendon, etc.

6. **Knee stiffness:** The patient may not be able to regain range of motion due to heterotopic bone formation or intra-articular adhesions.

PARTIAL KNEE REPLACEMENT
(Unicondylar Replacement)

This is a newer operation, done for a knee where only a part is damaged (partial damage). Here the knee is opened using a small incision, a cap is put on top of the damaged part without removing any ligaments, muscles, etc. In selected cases, this works as well as the more invasive total knee replacement. It is indicated in strictly partially damaged knee.

SHOULDER REPLACEMENT

Shoulder replacement has become an established operation over the years. This operation has limited indications because, compared to knee and hip, osteoarthritis of the shoulder is an uncommon condition.

There are different types of shoulder replacement (Fig. 42.6): (a) *Partial replacement*, where only the head of the humerus is addressed, by either resurfacing (putting a metal cap on the native head), stemless head replacement or stemmed head replacement: (b) *Total shoulder replacement*, which can be *anatomic shoulder replacement* (both the glenoid and the head are replaced with similar artificial components) or (c) *reverse shoulder replacement* where the articulation is reversed, which means, the head is placed on the glenoid side and the cup is placed on the humerus side.

TOTAL ELBOW REPLACEMENT

This is indicated in stiff and painful elbows due to rheumatoid arthritis and as a fall out of elbow injuries. The techniques have now got established to ensure good functions for 10-15 years.

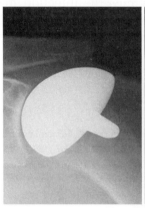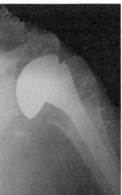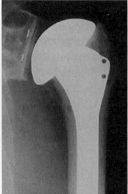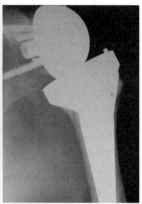

Fig. 42.6: Types of shoulder replacement arthroplasties.

What have we learnt?

- Joint replacement surgery is well-established with practically all joints of the body having been replaced.
- Hip, knee and shoulder replacement are common.
- Joint replacement can be partial or total depending upon whether one or both articulating surfaces are replaced.

Imaging Modalities in Orthopaedics

Learning Objectives

- ❖ Discuss the different imaging modalities used in orthopaedics, and their indications.

X-RAYS

These are a type of electromagnetic radiation when projected onto a surface like bone, the calcium in the bone absorbs most of the radiation which reduces the level reaching the film (detector) thus giving a clear image of the bone on a radiograph.

USES

This is a basic investigation that is used to diagnose injuries to the joints and bones. They lend information mainly about fractures, dislocations, certain types of tumours along with advanced degeneration of the joint. In injuries X-ray should always be done of the joint above and below and done in 2 planes. When in doubt an X-ray of the opposite normal limb helps in diagnosis.

COMPUTED TOMOGRAPHY SCANS

Combine X-rays with computer technology to produce a more detailed cross-sectional image of the body part. Computed tomography (CT) gives a 3-dimensional perception of the bone/joint that makes it superior to X-rays in imaging of fractures (Fig. 43.1).

USES

They are especially useful in fractures communicating with the joint (intra-articular fractures) as they need to be reduced anatomically. They thus aid in surgical planning.

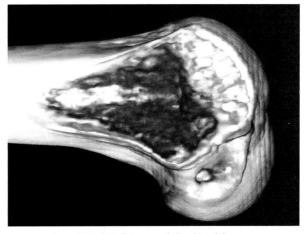

Fig. 43.1: 3D CT scan of the distal femur.

CT's are especially useful in diagnosing bony tumours and their extent. 3D CT scans are useful in planning surgery for bone tumours too to decide the extent of resection. Interventions like biopsies of tumorous lesions can be done CT guided to reach the exact location.

MAGNETIC RESONANCE IMAGING

Is a non-invasive method to visualise structures. The technique involves subjecting the atoms in the part of the body to a magnetic force that causes them to align in a north/south direction. When the force is removed the atoms emit energy that is fed into the computer and a signal to a computer that uses a mathematical

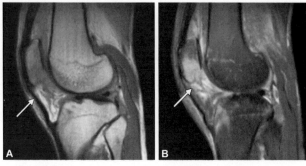

Fig. 43.2: MRI of the knee: (A) T1; (B) T2 weighted images.

formula to convert it into an image (Fig. 43.2). Two types of images are produced broadly:
T1: fat appears bright, fluid dark
T2: fluid appears bright and fat dark
Three sections are taken sagittal, coronal and axial.

USES

Magnetic resonance imaging (MRI) is better for soft tissue pathologies like tumours, ligament injury, cartilaginous injuries and tendon injuries.

BONE SCAN

It is a test that detects bone activity by injecting certain radiopharmaceutical substances, e.g. technetium-99 (99^{Tc}).

Increased uptake in a certain part means bone forming activity and decreased uptake a bone destroying activity (lytic lesion).

There are three phases in the process:
  i. Flow phase that starts 60 seconds after IV injection of the substance through the vein. It lasts for 2-5 minutes and the substance perfuses an area.
 ii. Blood pool phase starts 5 minutes later followed by the delayed phase which is 2-4 hours later.

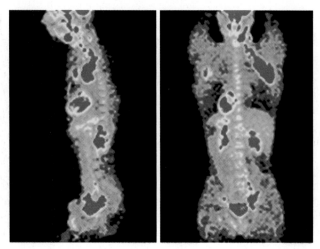

Fig. 43.3: PET scan of the body.

iii. This delayed phase scans differentiate cellulitis from osteomyelitis.

USES

These are in primary tumours of the bone, staging tumours, response to chemo/radiation therapy, complex regional pain syndrome, stress fractures and metastatic bone disease.

POSITRON EMISSION TOMOGRAPHY (PET) SCAN

This is a test where a short lived radioactive isotope (Fig. 43.3) [Fluorodeoxyglucose (FDG)] is injected into the body. The substance is a sugar and cancer cells consume, it more rapidly than normal cells thus showing up more prominently on imaging. The subject is placed in an imaging scanner that records tissue concentration of the substance with time.

USES

Diagnose soft tissue sarcomas, metastasis and infection.

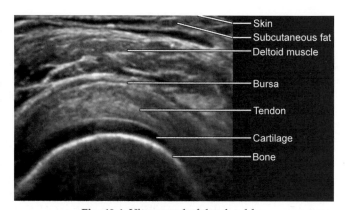

Fig. 43.4: Ultrasound of the shoulder.

ULTRASOUND

This is a dynamic testing modality that uses serial ultrasound waves in the body are reflected by interfaces to give the depth of the reflecting surface (Fig. 43.4). Diagnostic ultrasound uses waves in the range of 2.5-14 MHz.

USES

To assess functioning of a joint/tendon/ligament in motion and rest. It is mainly used to check for effusion in joints, tendons tears in the shoulder and as an adjunct to therapeutic procedures like intra-articular injections and aspirations that can be done ultrasound guided.

Clinical Methods

GENERAL

The art of clinical methods can be mastered only in the ward. It essentially consists of the following:

Developing a rapport with the patient: The patient should be made comfortable in a chair or on a couch. Initial general talking will make the patient feel at home, and give the examiner an idea of the mental status of the patient. Patients usually feel at ease with one of their relatives with them. Patients have a concept that doctors are extremely busy people, and forget half the things when they face a doctor. It is the duty of a doctor to present himself as a well-composed, well-dressed, full of concern, not-in-a-hurry person.

Establishing communication with the patient so that you can understand what he says and means. Patients have their own concepts about diseases and their causes. Do not get carried away by what they say. Ascertain what they mean by intelligent cross questioning.

History taking: This consists of two parts. The first part is the presenting complaint i.e., what complaint has brought the patient to the hospital. The second part is the history of present illness i.e., the sequence of events starting from the onset of the problem till the time of presentation. It is best to let the patient say whatever he has to, or whatever he feels about his illness. You can always extract relevant information by moderating history.

Examination: This consists of examining the patient to look for salient features which may be in support of or against the diagnosis. It is best to arrive at some differential diagnoses on the basis of the history, before beginning the examination.

Therefore, the aims of clinical history and examination are as follows:
a. *To arrive at a diagnosis* i.e., to find out the cause of the problem.
b. To find out whether the basic disease has produced *any complication*. For example, a patient with chronic osteomyelitis may have developed shortening of the bone due to effect of the disease on the growth plate.
c. To determine what way has the disease or its complication, if any, affected the *functions of the patient*. For example, in the case of a patient with affection of the lower limb there may be decreased ability to walk – there may be limp, or support may be needed for walking.

The last part of the work-up—the functional disability, is the most important in orthopaedics. It represents the way the disease has affected the functions of the patient; and it is this that concerns us and the patient the most. Upon it depends the treatment planning.

HISTORY TAKING

History taking is not merely a record of what the patient says, but it is an art of understanding and collecting information regarding what happened to the patient, what could have caused it, what

way the patient has been affected by it, what treatment has the patient taken for it, and ultimately, what functional level of activity does the patient possess. For extracting relevant information, background knowledge of different diseases, their presentation, their complications, etc., are necessary. The following discussion is only to form concepts in clinical orthopaedics. There is no 'always' in medicine. At places the reader may find over-emphasis; these are only meant to highlight some concepts.

Broadly, the history tells us about the disease etiology (i.e., whether it is infection, tumour, etc.), and the examination about the site of involvement (i.e., whether it is the bone or joint or the tendon, etc., the tissue affected).

GENERAL INFORMATION

First note the name, age, sex, address and occupation of the patient. Some of this information may be helpful in thinking about the possible diagnosis, as discussed below:

Table 1: Diseases which occur at a particular age.	
Polio	1-2 years
Rickets (Nutritional)	1-2 years
Perthes' disease	5-10 years
Slipped capital epiphysis	12- 16 years
Acute Osteomyelitis/arthritis	<15 years
Bone malignancies	10-20 years
PIVD	20-40 years
Rheumatoid arthritis	20-40 years

Age: There are fractures which occur more commonly in children, others occur more often in adults or in the elderly. Hence by knowing the age, one can think of possible injuries which could occur at that age. Patients with congenital malformations such as CDH present early in life. Infections and bone tumours are common in children. Degenerative diseases occur at an older age. Some diseases occur in a particular age group and age consideration becomes very important in the diagnosis of these diseases (Table 1).

Sex: Some diseases are more common in males; some others in females. Table 2 lists some of these diseases. In general, all type of injuries are nearly as frequent in males as in females.

Table 2: Sex predisposition in orthopaedic diseases.	
CDH	Females
Slipped epiphysis	Males
Rheumatoid arthritis	Females
Ankylosing spondylitis	Females
Osteomalacia	Females

Occupation: What the patient does has a lot of relevance in orthopaedics in two ways: (a) a number of complaints can be traced back to the kind of occupation. For example a patient, who is required to bend forward and lift heavy weight in the course of his job, may develop back strain; (b) in cases where cure is not possible, physical requirements of the patient become the basis for deciding the treatment. For example, a little limp due to instability, at the cost of gaining movements at the hip, may be acceptable for a housewife. The same may be severely disabling for a heavy manual worker, who may prefer a stiff but stable hip. Similarly the living style of a patient (e.g., the habit of sitting on the floor), may become an important consideration in planning the treatment.

PRESENTING COMPLAINTS

History taking begins with asking the patient what exactly bothers him (i.e., what is his complaint?), and for how long. It takes a little while to be able to understand what and for how long has the problem been. One should let the patient say what he has to say, rather than obstructing his flow of thoughts and trying to fit them into the 'sequence of questions' you have learnt in the 'book'. Often, the patient's story is required to be guided by some clarification and direct questions. The following are some of the common complaints of an orthopaedic patient.

- Pain
- Difficulty in using the limb (usually upper limb)
- Inability to walk (patient is brought in a wheel chair, trolley, in the lap)
- Limp
- Deformity of a limb
- Swelling
- Stiffness
- Weakness
- Discharging sinus
- Altered sensation

There are usually more than one presenting complaints. If so, note the sequence in which they appeared.

HISTORY OF PRESENTING ILLNESS

One must give the patient time to settle down. A general greeting, or a nonspecific talk will make the patient at ease. One should let the patient narrate the 'story' of his illness. The following points need to be brought out from patient's account:

Onset of Symptoms: Broadly, orthopaedic diseases can be divided into two groups – trauma related and nontrauma related. Hence, the first question to be asked is whether or not there was a trauma preceding the onset of symptoms. A number of patients may falsely implicate an unrelated episode of trauma as the cause of their disease. A detailed inquiry into the nature of the injury, the period between the injury and onset of the symptoms, etc., can help in deciding whether injury did play a role in causing the disease or not. The following leading questions help in this assessment.

a. When did the injury occur in relation to the onset of symptoms i.e., immediately preceding, or a few days or weeks before*.
b. How did the injury occur? i.e., to assess whether severity of the trauma was sufficient to cause whatever the patient complains of, and also to know the exact mode of the injury.
c. Did the patient have symptoms (such as pain, swelling, etc.) immediately following the trauma or did they occur 'after a few days or weeks'?
d. Was the patient able to carry out his activities despite the injury or in the case of a child, did the child continue to play after

* It is a fact that sometimes there may be a long period between the injury and onset of symptoms (of course unrelated).

the 'injury'? Obviously, if this was so, the episode of trauma is unlikely to be related to the symptoms.

e. Was the patient given any treatment? Did he get any X-ray done at that time? These suggest that the injury was serious enough.

In case one is sure that the disease is not related to trauma inquire into the type of onset of the symptoms – whether acute, subacute or chronic.

Progress of the disease: This consists of finding out how the symptoms progressed over a period of time. The questions one must ask are: Whether it is a progressively worsening disease? Is it a disease with remissions and exacerbations? Is it a disease which came rather suddenly and subsided over a period of time?, etc. Any treatment carried out during this period and its effect should also be noted. At the end, one should make an assessment of the current status of the patient, his functional activity, severity of pain, etc. (Table 3).

Table 3: Sample history.

After a history taking session, a student should be able to arrange the sequence of events in this way:
The patient was all right till .... when he noticed .... There was no* history of trauma related to the onset. The symptom appeared slowly**. Gradually the patient noticed additional symptoms such as (.......). He consulted .... and was prescribed .... There was some*** relief with that treatment. In the meanwhile, the symptoms worsened.**** The patient could not do .... things. Now the patient can not do ....

* or yes, ** or suddenly *** or no relief, ****or improved/did not change.

COMMON COMPLAINTS OF AN ORTHOPAEDIC PATIENT

The following is an account of some of the common complaints of an orthopaedic patient and the way they are analysed.

Pain: This is the most common complaint. The pain may be at the site of the disease or it may be a pain referred from some other part. The following details about the pain need to be elicited.

a. What is the *exact site* of the pain? Try to be as specific as possible. It helps to ask the patient to point to the site of pain.
b. Does the pain *radiate* to some other area? It is common in limbs to have pain originating in one part and radiating to another part (Table 4).

Table 4: Radiation of pain.

Site from	Radiation to
Neck	Shoulder, arm
Shoulder	Arm
Elbow	Forearm and hand
Thoracic spine	Girdle pain
Lumbar Spine	Loin
Lumbo-sacral spine	Gluteal region
SI joint	Back of thigh and knee
Hip	Front of thigh and knee
Thigh	Knee
Knee	Shin of tibia

c. Is the pain *present at all times*? A pain due to neoplasia is present at all times; it may fluctuate, but is persistent. A pain due to trauma is maximum within 4 to 6 hours of injury and then starts subsiding. A pain of inflammatory origin builds up rather suddenly and then subsides. Remissions and exacerbations are seen in pain due to chronic inflammatory diseases such as rheumatoid arthritis. A sudden appearance of pain in a rather painless disease is an indication of change in the nature of the disease. For example, it could be malignant change in a benign swelling, or a pathological fracture through a bone affected with some disease.

d. What *aggravates or relieves the pain*? A pain of mechanical origin becomes worse with activity, and improves with rest. On the other hand, a pain of chronic inflammation like osteoarthritis and rheumatoid arthritis comes up after a period of rest, and improves with activity.

e. What *term can best describe the pain*? This sometimes helps in localising the cause of the pain. A dull ache usually arises from a deeper structure; a shooting pain may indicate a neurogenic pain or that due to acute inflammation.

f. Are there any *other symptoms associated* with the pain? In most painful conditions of inflammatory, neoplastic or traumatic origin, pain is associated with the swelling, though in some cases it may not be clinically detectable. A referred pain or a pain of neurogenic origin may not have any local symptoms.

Difficulty in using the limb: This is usually a result of the pain. Sometimes, stiffness of joints deformity or muscle weakness may be responsible for the difficulty in using the limb.

Inability to walk: The cause of this is the same as above. It is important to know at what rate has the disease progressed to cause whatever limitation of walking i.e. whether it has been sudden, over days, over weeks, etc.

Limp: This is a common early symptom in a patient with lower limb disease. Limp is of two types – painful or painless. Causes of limp are as given in Table 5.

Table 5: Causes of limp.
● *Painful limp*
- Any traumatic condition of the limb
- Any inflammatoiy condition of the limb, e.g., TB hip
- Osteoarthritis hip
● *Painless limp*
- Polio affecting lower limb
- Coxa vara deformity of the hip
- CDH
- Deformity of a joint or bone
- Fused hip, knee or ankle

Deformity: It is required to know the onset of the deformity. A deformity following an episode of injury could be due to subluxation or dislocation of a joint, or malunion or nonunion of a fracture. It may be as a result of a complication related to the trauma (e.g., VIC following a fracture). In an acute painful condition the deformity comes up due to the muscle spasm initiated by the pain. Later, contractures of the muscles and capsule develop. Gradual progress of the deformity occurs in chronic infections, growth related disorders, or in gradually worsening diseases. It is important to know whether the deformity is progressive or static; and what does the deformity not allow the patient to do.

---

* Sometimes, a neoplastic swelling may reduce in size due to tumour degeneration.

Swelling: Swelling. with or without pain, is a common complaint. When without or with a little pain it is due to a benign growth or a low grade malignant growth. Swelling following a fracture may be due to callus formation or displacement at the fracture site. Swelling associated with pain is due to inflammatory or neoplastic disorders. The way the swelling progresses indicates its etiology. A neoplastic swelling keeps on growing, whatever the rate may be. On the other hand, an inflammatory swelling has remission after an initial rapid onset. The key question is whether the swelling ever reduced in size – if it did, suggests that it is not a neoplastic swelling*. Swellings at more than one site are seen in diseases like neurofibromatosis, multiple exostosis, multifocal tuberculosis or polyarthritis, etc.

Stiffness: Stiffness is a symptom of joint involvement. In early stages of the disease, stiffness occurs due to protective spasm of the muscles around the joint. This is nature's way of avoiding movement at a painful joint. In late stages the joint becomes stiff due to intra-articular and extra-articular adhesions. In advanced stages, severe limitation of joint movement occurs. This is called ankylosis of the joint. The cause of ankylosis could be intra-articular or extra-articular (Table 6). In inflammatory diseases like rheumatoid arthritis and ankylosing spondylitis, stiffness increases after rest (e.g., after an overnight sleep) but improves with activity.

Table 6: Causes of ankylosis.
● *Intra-articular*
- TB
- Septic arthritis
- Viral arthritis
● **Extra-articular**
- Myositis
- Arthrogryposis multiplex congenita
- Burn contracture
- Scleroderma and other such diseases

Weakness: Weakness of a limb is due to loss of muscle power. This could be secondary to disuse atrophy of the muscle or due to some neurological condition. The cause of neurological weakness may be affection of the brain, (e.g., a stroke), spinal cord (e.g., poliomyelitis), nerve (e.g., neuropathy), neuro-muscular junction (e.g., myasthenia) or muscle (e.g., myopathy). If there is no associated sensory loss, the cause may be either myopathy, neuropathy of a motor nerve, polio, or other motor neurone diseases. The onset of weakness may be sudden as in injury; or insidious as in myopathy, leprosy, etc. Weakness is progressive in neuropathy and myopathy, but it improves with time (in the first few months) in polio.

Discharging sinus: A sinus discharging pus over a period of time, not healing with usual treatment, may indicate deeper infection. This could be an underlying bone infection. History of discharge of a piece of bone (sequestrum) from the sinus is a sure evidence of bone involvement. Other causes of a persistent discharging sinus are as listed in Table 7.

Table 7: Causes of persistent discharging sinus.
● Generalised disease like diabetes
● Resistant bacteria
● Fungal infection
● Osteomyelitis
● Foreign body
● Epithelialisation of the sinus
● Scar tissue around the sinus
● Malignant change in the sinus

PAST ILLNESS

Some illnesses in the past may give rise to symptoms years after apparent 'healing' of the disease.

Some of these are as follows:

- An old injury: Osteoarthritis, presenting with pain and stiffness, is common many years after a joint is damaged due to injury or infection.
- In an old infection, recurrence may occur years after apparent healing of the infection.
- An old tubercular lesion anywhere in the body, may present as TB in the bone or joint.

PERSONAL HISTORY

The occupation of the patient, his living style, the kind of physical activity he is required to do, etc., have a bearing on his treatment.

FAMILY HISTORY

This may be relevant in a genetically transmitted disorder and in tuberculosis.

EXAMINATION

Before beginning the examination of a patient, the doctor must ensure the following:

a. Patient is *comfortably lying* on a couch, or sitting on a chair.
b. The part to be examined is exposed, and also the opposite limb, in the case of examination of a limb. This provides an opportunity of comparing the involved limb with the opposite, normal one.
c. *Things required* to examine a patient are available. These are as follows:
    - An inch tape
    - Patellar hammer
    - Cotton wool, pins, a tuning fork
    - Skin marking pen
    - Goniometer to measure angles

General examination: A general review of the different systems of the body, as is done in any other case, is performed.

Regional examination: This differs from region to region, and will be discussed subsequently.

Gait Analysis: Evaluation of gait constitutes an important part of orthopaedic examination for the following reasons:

a. It gives a clue to the cause of gait abnormality and hence the diagnosis.

b. It gives an idea of the extent of disability caused by the abnormal gait so that the treatment could be aimed at correction of the gait.

Gait can be evaluated by observing a person walk in slow motion. Normal gait has a definite pattern. It is made up of a number of gait cycles (Fig. 1). One gait cycle constitutes the period from heel strike of a leg to its next heel strike. Gait cycle can be divided into two phases:

a. Stance phase
b. Swing phase

Stance phase: This is the part of the gait cycle when the foot is on the ground. It starts with heel strike and ends with toe off. It constitutes 60 percent of the gait cycle and consists of essentially three events.

- Heel strike – when heel strikes the ground
- Mid stance – when the whole foot is flat on the ground, and
- Push off – when the body is propelled by taking a push from the foot; first the heel goes off the ground, and finally the toes.

Swing phase: This is the part of the gait cycle when the foot is off the ground. It starts with toe off and finishes when the foot is ready to strike the ground again. It constitutes 40 percent of the gait cycle, and consists of essentially the following events:

- *Acceleration:* Once the foot is off the ground, the leg moves forward with the help of hip flexors.
- *Mid swing:* This is the mid part of the swinging leg.
- *Deceleration:* The swinging leg is slowed down to get the foot ready for heel strike.

Normal gait: In normal walking, each leg goes through a stance phase and a swing phase alternately. The rhythmic repetition of such cycles provides grace to the gait. Normal gait is mechanically efficient, and therefore, only minimal energy is consumed while walking. In case the rhythm of the gait is disturbed due to any reason, one lands up using extra energy for walking, and thus gets easily tired.

Abnormal gait: There are number of reasons for abnormality of gait. Usually there are a combination of factors. Some of the typical abnormal gaits which are of value in making a diagnosis are as shown in Table 8.

EXAMINATION OF THE HIP

The hip joint is special in the following ways:

a. It is a joint thickly covered with soft tissues, thus making it difficult to elicit signs.

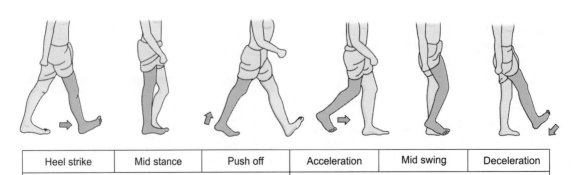

Heel strike	Mid stance	Push off	Acceleration	Mid swing	Deceleration
Stance phase—60%			Swing phase—40%		

Fig. 1: Gait cycle.

Table 8: Abnormal gaits.

Gait	Pattern	Cause
Antalgic or painful gait	Time taken on the affected leg is reduced. Body weight is shifted quickly to the normal leg.	Painful condition of the leg
Stiff hip gait	Lifts the pelvis, and swings it forward with leg in one piece	TB hip, Rheumatoid hip, Ankylosing Spondylitis
Stiff knee gait	The leg is circumducted and brought forward in order to get clearance.	TB knee, Painful stiff knee
Short limb gait	Becomes apparent only if the limb is shorter than 2 inches. The body on the affected side moves up and down every time the weight is borne on the affected leg.	Congenital short femur, Shortening secondary to fracture
Trendelenburg gait or Gluteus medius gait	The body swings to the affected side every time weight is borne on that side	Dislocated hip, CDH Congential coxa vara Fracture neck of femur Gluteus medius paralysis
Gluteus maximus lurch	The body swings backwards every time weight is borne	Gluteus maximus paralysis in polio
Quadriceps lurch	The person walks by hyperextending, and thereby locking the knee	Quadriceps paralysis
Hand-knee gait	The person walks with hand on the knee to prevent the knee from buckling in a quadriceps deficient knee with flexion deformity.	Polio
High stepping gait or Foot drop gait	Due to drop of the foot, the leg is lifted more in order to get clearance. First to touch the ground is the forefoot, and not the heel.	Common peroneal nerve palsy, sciatic nerve palsy
Scissor gait	Legs are crossed in front of each other while walking due to spasm of the adductors of the hip	Cerebral palsy

b. There are a number of diseases exclusive to the hip, for example, Perthes' disease, slipped femoral epiphysis.

c. The compensatory mechanisms mask the deformities at the hip, e.g., the flexion deformity is masked by forward tilting of the pelvis.

d. It is near the private parts, hence proper exposure and cooperation of the patient becomes difficult.

HISTORY TAKING

Presenting Complaints: As the hip is a deep joint, the patient often cannot localize the site of his problem. Rather, he complains of what he finds difficult to do. Common complaints of a patient with hip disease are as follows:

Pain in the groin, in the front of the thigh or sometimes in the knee*. Pain in the groin can be a referred pain from upper lumbar spine.

Inability to squat: This is due to stiffness of the hip. The stiffness may be due to painful spasm of the muscles around the hip or because of the adhesions within or around the hip.

Limb: This may be painless as in CDH or coxa vara, or painful as in early arthritis.

---

* A pain from the hip is often referred to the knee.
** Pain in the gluteal region is not from the hip, it is usually from LS spine or SI joints.

Inability to walk: This may be due to a painful condition or due to mechanical failure in the region of the hip (e.g., fracture neck of the femur, polio, etc.)

Swelling: A swelling arising from the hip comes to notice very late, except when it is from the greater trochanter or pubic bone.

Deformity: Deformity of the hip may be the presenting symptom. The patient walks with a bend at the hip. The cause of the deformity could be the hip joint per se or the structures around the hip (e.g., psoas spasm due to inflammatory lesion in the vicinity of the psoas).

HISTORY OF PRESENTING COMPLAINTS

Pain: When pain is the major presenting complaint, the following details need to be elicited.

- Where is the pain? In the groin, in front of the thigh, outer side of the hip, back of the hip**.
- Does the pain radiate? Pain from the hip radiates to the knee, but not beyond. If the pain radiates beyond, its origin could be from the spine.
- Duration of the pain: Short duration pains are due to trauma, acute infections, acute arthritis, etc. Long duration pains are due to chronic infections, chronic arthritis, secondary osteoarthritis, tumours, etc.
- Onset and progress of the pain: The main idea is to find out whether there was any trauma at the time of onset of the pain, and whether there is remission and exacerbation of the pain.

- What exaggerates or relieves the pain?: This may give a clue to the nature of the disease.

EXAMINATION

Exposure: Proper exposure is essential for examination of the hip. The part of the body below the mid-thorax should be exposed, except for the area of the private parts, which should be covered with a small cloth. In Indian culture, especially in a female patient, such an exposure may not be socially acceptable. It is a must to have a female attendant/nurse while examining the hip of a female patient. While examining a patient with hip disease, the examination couch should be away from the wall. This makes it possible to go to both sides of the body to examine the respective hip. It also allows space for abduction of both the hips.

Gait: Observe the gait of the patient. The following are some of the common gait patterns in hip diseases. A combination of these may be present.

Antalgic gait: In a painful hip disease, the patient can hardly bear weight on the affected side. So, he quickly takes the weight off the affected limb to the normal limb. Hence, he keeps the affected limb on the ground for a shorter time than the normal side.

Trendelenburg gait: In a hip disease, where the hip joint is not stable, (i.e., the abductor mechanism of the hip is not effective) in order to avoid falling, the torso of the patient tilts to the affected side. In case of a bilateral unstable hip, the swing may be bilateral – the so called waddling gait (e.g., in bilateral CDH).

Short limb gait: If the affected limb has become short due to some disease, when the patient walks, the whole affected side of the body dips down in order to make it possible for the patient to bring the foot to the ground. It is the 'up and down' movement of the half of the body, which is characteristic of a short limb gait as against the 'sideways lurching' seen in a Trendelenburg gait.

Circumduction gait: When the hip is 'fixed' in abduction, there occurs apparent lengthening of the limb. In order to walk in such a situation, the patient has to take the affected 'long limb', in a round about fashion, and thus take the step forward.

In flexion deformity: With mild flexion deformity of the hip, the patient manages to walk 'straight' by compensatory lumbar lordosis. If the deformity is more than 30°, the patient can no longer compensate, and is required to stoop forward at the hip to be able to walk. This also happens in patients with ankylosing spondylitis, where compensatory lumbar lordosis is not possible due to stiffness of the spine.

EXAMINATION WITH THE PATIENT STANDING

The patient should be examined first in standing position. The examiner observes him from front, from the side and from the back. The following points are noted:

Any obvious deformity – flexion, abduction, adduction or rotation deformity at the hip.

Any compensatory mechanism – increased lumbar lordosis to compensate for the flexion deformity, and pelvic tilt (as noted by position of the ASISs on the two sides) to compensate for the abduction or adduction deformities.

Gross shortening can be observed when the patient, trying to keep the leg on the ground produces plantar-flexion at the ipsilateral ankle or by keeps the opposite normal knee flexed.

Wasting of muscles on the affected side: This is an index of disuse atrophy of the muscles, and indicates long duration of the illness. Note especially the gluteal muscles and the quadriceps.

Any swelling: Note especially in the gluteal region, in the region of greater trochanter and in the groin. The greater trochanter may appear more prominent due to its proximal migration in some hip diseases.

Any active sinus or a scar of a healed sinus or previous operation: Scar of a healed sinus is puckered as against that of a superficial skin infection.

Trendelenburg's test: This is a test to establish the stability of the hip. A hip is stable if the abduction mechanism of the hip is effective in preventing the pelvis from dipping on the opposite side, when weight is borne on the limb. The test and its explanation are as follows:

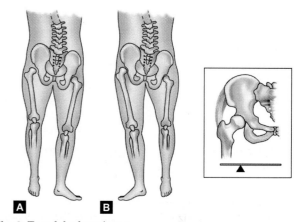

Fig. 2: Trendelenburg's test.
(A) The patient stands on the normal limb, the opposite ASIS goes up; (B) The patient stands on the affected limb, the opposite ASIS dips down. Box shows the abductor mechanism.

- *Test:* The ASISs of both sides should be exposed. The patient is asked to stand on the normal leg. As he does so, the opposite ASIS will be lifted up i.e., the pelvis will be tilted towards the side bearing weight (Fig. 2). Now, the patient is asked to stand on the affected side. If the hip on this side is not stable, the opposite ASIS will dip down. In order to avoid falling, the patient will tilt his torso to the affected side and thus balance himself.
- *Explanation:* When a person stands on both legs, the centre of gravity falls in between the two feet (the base). As soon as one leg is lifted off the ground, the centre of gravity of the body falls outside the base (single foot this time). The pelvis on the opposite side tends to dip. This is prevented by the balancing done by the body by tilting the pelvis toward the side on which the person is standing. The tilting is possible due to 'effective contraction' of the abductor muscles of the hip (mainly gluteus medius). This abductor mechanism can be compared to a lever (Fig. 2, box). The fulcrum of the lever is the centre of the hip, the load is the weight of the body trying to tilt the pelvis down. This load is counter-acted by the abductor muscle force which acts through the lever-arm (the neck of the femur). Any failure in the effectivity of the abductor mechanism causes dipping of the ASIS on

the opposite (normal) side. This could occur if: (a) there is no fulcrum, e.g., dislocation of the hip, destruction of the head; (b) ineffective lever-arm (the neck of the femur), e.g., fracture of the neck of the femur; (c) ineffective contraction of abductor muscles, e.g., weakness of the muscles due to polio or abductor muscles acting ineffectively through a short lever-arm (as in coxa vara).

EXAMINATION WITH THE PATIENT LYING ON THE COUCH

Inspection: Ask the patient to lie as straight as he can and observe the following:

Position of the ASIS on the affected side, if it can be distinctly seen. Normally, with the patient lying straight, both the ASISs should be square (i.e., at the same level). If the ASIS on the affected side is more proximal, an adduction deformity may be present. The reverse of this may occur in abduction deformity.

Lumbar lordosis: An exaggerated lumbar lordosis may be a result of tilt of the pelvis to compensate for the flexion deformity.

The patient may be keeping the hip flexed. There may be a rotational deformity of the hip as noticed by in or out turning of the patella.

Palpation: Following points are noted on palpation.

Temperature especially of the groin and over the swelling, if any.

Tenderness especially in the groin, over the greater trochanter. Tenderness in the gluteal region is usually due to sciatic pain arising from the spine.

Abnormal swelling: Any abnormal swelling is examined with regard to its site of origin, size, shape, surface, consistency, tender or not, margins, fixity to the bone and other structures.

Thickening of the greater trochanter: Greater trochanter is the most lateral, bony structure around the hip. It is often difficult to feel it in an obese person. The way is to palpate the shaft of the femur, and move the hand up. The most prominent bony structure at the proximal end of the thigh is the greater trochanter. It can be confirmed by moving the thigh – it should move with the thigh. Another bony prominence which can often be mistaken as ASIS is the ischeal tuberosity, but can be differentiated as the latter does not move with the movement of the thigh. A dislocated head or a myositic mass around the hip, if present, can be confused as the trochanter. The trochanter is thickened in diseases involving the trochanter as in – malunited inter-trochanteric fracture, fibrous dysplasia and trochanteric bursitis.

Proximal migration of the greater trochanter: In diseases of the hip where the head of the femur is dislocated or damaged, or if there is a fracture of the neck of the femur, the greater trochanter is proximal than on the opposite side. This can be roughly judged by keeping the thumb at the ASISs and feeling the greater trochanters with middle finger so as to appreciate the distance between the two on two sides (Fig. 3). The other method of finding this out is by drawing a Bryant's triangle as discussed subsequently:

Swelling: Whether the swelling is in relation to the pelvis or the femur can be found by observing whether it moves with the femur. A dislocated head may be palpable in the gluteal region (in posterior dislocation of the hip) or in the groin (in anterior dislocation of the hip). A swelling in relation to the trochanters similarly moves on moving the thigh.

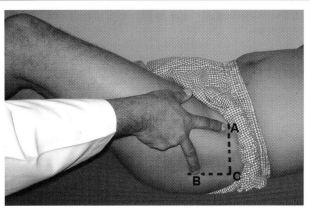

Fig. 3: Proximal migration of the greater trochanter. A is ASIS, B is greater trochanter, C is an imaginary point, and gives an idea about position of the trochanter.

Deformity and Range of Movements: Hip deformities are often not apparent because of compensatory mechanisms. It is customary to look for the deformity and test for range of motion simultaneously. In a normal person the position of complete extension is taken as zero position. In cases with deformities, the arc of movement from the deformed position of the hip to whatever further movement is possible, is noted. The following are the methods of finding out the extent of different deformities of the hip.

Flexion deformity: This is the most common deformity of the hip, probably because the flexors of the hip are stronger than the extensors. When there is spasm of the muscles, the stronger flexors pull the hip in flexion. The test to evaluate the degree of the flexion deformity is called Thomas' test, as discussed below:

Thomas' Test: Aim of the test is to remove the compensatory lumbar lordosis so that the flexion deformity becomes obvious and can be measured. The patient is asked to lie supine on a hard surface, with legs straight. He may be able to do so despite the flexion deformity by producing excessive lumbar lordosis. The same can be appreciated by the examiner passing his hand behind the patient's lumbar spine. Now, the sound hip of the patient is flexed gradually. After the hip flexion is complete, the pelvis begins to tilt (Fig. 4). This obliterates the lumbar

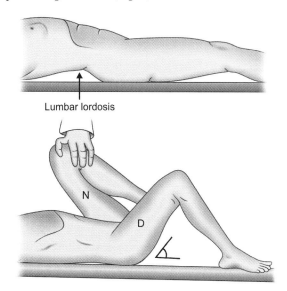

Lumbar lordosis

Fig. 4: Thomas' test. Note that to measure the deformity, the compensatory effect of the lumbar lordosis is to be removed.

lordosis, as can be felt by the hand under the lumbar spine. As this happens, the affected hip will automatically come to be in the deformed position (flexion position). The angle between the affected thigh and the bed is the degree of flexion deformity. One must be careful not to overflex the normal hip, as this results in excess tilting of the pelvis anteriorly, thereby falsely exaggerating the flexion deformity.

Problems of Thomas' test: These are as follows:
- It is difficult to perform in a female patient as proper exposure is not always possible.
- It is difficult to perform in fat patients as in them lordosis cannot be appreciated.
- In a painful hip, the patient may be hurt during the test and thus may become uncooperative.
- It is difficult to perform this test if both the hips are affected or if the ipsilateral knee is stiff and deformed. In the case of bilateral hip deformity, better method is to put the patient prone at the edge of the couch in such a way that the body is on the couch with the legs hanging out (Fig. 5). The lumbar spine is seen straight (no lordosis) and flexion deformity at the hip becomes obvious. With the palm of the hand stabilising the lumbar spine, the hip is extended gently, till the lordosis starts showing up. The angle between the body and the thigh indicates the flexion deformity at the hip.

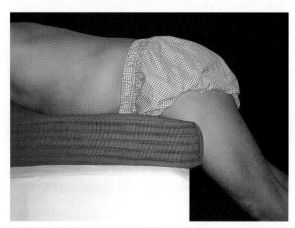

Fig. 5: Method of assessing the flexion deformity when both the hips are deformed. In prone lying position, the lumbar lordosis is automatically obliterated.

Range of Flexion: Once the flexion deformity is measured the patient is asked to hold the normal knee flexed, the examiner keeping his one hand under the lumbar spine. The affected hip is now gently flexed further, beyond the position of the deformity. The arc of motion (from deformed position to the position of possible flexion) constitutes the range of motion of the hip. Normally, it is possible to flex the hip so much that the front of thigh touches the abdomen. In cases, where the hip flexion is limited, the pelvis will start tilting as the hip is forced beyond the limit of flexion. This becomes apparent as the hand under the lumbar spine can feel the movement at the spine. Hence we write that the range of hip flexion is from 20°–120° (150°). The figure in the bracket shows the ROM on the normal side. It is important to keep one hand over the ASIS so as to detect tilting of the pelvis while performing this test. It is possible to 'flex' a completely fused hip by 30°–40°, the movement actually occurring at the spine.

Abduction Deformity: A patient with abduction deformity compensates, and may appear 'straight' by tilting the pelvis

movement which may be present is movement in the direction of the deformity. This is again measured as arc of movement from deformity position to whatever further movement is possible. For example, it could be 20° of abduction deformity with further abduction from 20° to 50°. It is noted as 'abduction deformity 20°, with ROM 20°–50° (60°)'. The figure in the bracket is the range

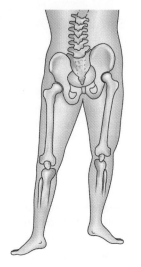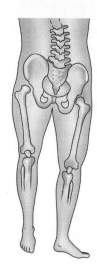

Fig. 6: Compensation of adduction and abduction deformities.

(Fig. 6). In abduction deformity, the pelvis on the affected side tilts down (hence the ASIS is lower). The opposite of this occurs in adduction deformity (i.e., ASIS on the affected side goes up). By removing the compensatory affect of the pelvic tilt one can make the deformity obvious, and measure it. This is done in the following way:

Test for detecting adduction and abduction deformities: Let the patient lie as straight as he can with both the legs parallel to each other. In doing so, in case an abduction or adduction deformity is present, the patient will tilt the pelvis depending upon the deformity and conceal it. The examiner first palpates the ASISs on the two sides. This is done by moving his thumb from the groin laterally, and the first bony prominence detected is the ASIS. These are marked. Possibilities are that: (a) both the ASISs are at the same level (pelvis is square) which means that there is no abduction or adduction deformity; (b) ASIS on the affected side is higher (more proximal) than that on the normal side, which means that there is adduction deformity, compensated by the pelvic tilt; (c) ASIS on the affected side is lower than that on the normal side, which means that there is abduction deformity compensated by the pelvic tilt. Once it is known that the pelvis is not square, we know which deformity is present. The next step is to square the pelvis to be able to measure the deformity. This is done as follows:

Depending upon which deformity is present, the only thing one has to do is to produce that very deformity. As this is being done, the ASIS on the affected side will move up or down as the case may be, and the pelvis will be squared (Fig. 7). This is checked by feeling the two ASISs and joining them with a measuring tape. The angle between the long axis of the body and that of the leg is the degree of abduction–adduction deformity.

Range of Adduction and Abduction: Once the adduction-abduction deformity is measured, the next step is to see how much further adduction-abduction movement is possible. One must remember that if a hip has an adduction deformity, no abduction movement will be possible and vice versa. The only

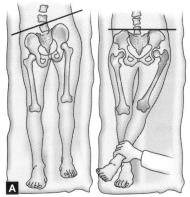
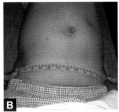

Fig. 7: (A) Method of detecting adduction–abduction deformities of the hip; (B) Use of a measuring tape is a useful method of checking that the pelvis is square.

of abduction on the normal side. The precaution required while measuring the range of abduction and adduction movement is that the pelvis should not be allowed to move while this is being done. This is checked by keeping one hand over the opposite ASIS while moving the hip, and detecting any movement of the ASIS, (and hence that of the pelvis).

Problem of the test: Sometimes, squaring is not possible due to fixed pelvic tilt, as may occur in a patient with lumbar scoliosis. It may also not be possible to square a pelvis with old injury where the normal anatomy is disturbed.

Rotation Deformity: Gross rotational deformities may be noticed by looking at the patella or the foot. Normally, the patella faces 5° to 10° outward. If it faces inwards compared to the opposite side, internal rotation deformity is present and vice-versa for the external rotation deformity. Minimal internal or external rotation deformities become more noticeable when one observes from the foot end of the patient's bed. Comparing the two sides is important for this. Rotational deformities cannot be compensated or concealed.

Range of Rotations: Range of motion of rotation can be measured with the hip in extension or in flexion. With the hip extended, the leg is held by the thigh and the knee. The leg is gently turned inward and outward. This gives an idea whether there is any gross limitation of rotations. Precise measurements can be made by testing rotations with the hips in flexion. This is done on one leg at a time. The leg is held at the knee with one hand and at the ankle with the other hand (Fig. 8A). The hip and knee are flexed to 90°. The rotation movement is produced at the hip by moving the leg as a lever. The arc made by the leg shows the amount of internal or external rotation. This can be compared with the same on the opposite side. Range of rotations can be tested on the two sides simultaneously (Fig. 8B). This gives an instant idea of limitation of rotation on the affected side.

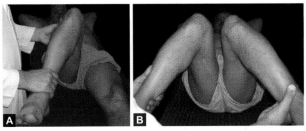

Fig. 8: Method of measuring range of rotations: (A) Using one leg at a time; (B) Using both the legs together.

Range of movement in other positions: Range of hip movements is tested in other positions as discussed: Abduction-in-flexion: This is a good, quick method of comparing abduction movement on the two sides. The hips are flexed to 45° with the knees and ankles together.

Both the knees are now 'opened apart' so as to allow the outer side of the knees to touch the couch. A limitation of abduction becomes obvious as the knee on the affected side remains at a higher level (Fig. 9).

Limb Length Measurement: Shortening of the limb is common in hip diseases. Some of the shortening is compensated by the patient by: (a) tilting the pelvis down on that side; (b) plantar flexing the foot; and (c) flexing the knee on the normal side. While examining for shortening, it is important to note: (a) whether shortening is present; (b) if yes, whether it is true or apparent shortening; (c) if it is true shortening, whether it is from the hip (supra-trochanteric) or from some other part of the limb. It is customary to measure the apparent length (the length of the limb with compensatory mechanisms allowed) and true length (the actual length of the limb after removing the compensatory mechanism). Accordingly, after comparing the lengths on the two sides, apparent and true shortenings are calculated. It is the apparent shortening which concerns the patient i.e., the shortening which remains even after compensation by the body. True shortening is of significance to the clinician for diagnosis, as it is the shortening produced by the disease due to actual destruction or shortening of the bone.

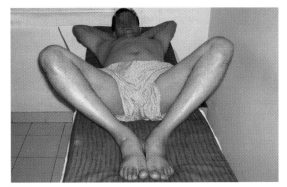

Fig. 9: Measuring abduction-in-flexion on both the sides simultaneously.

There may be a situation where all bones and joints are all right, but the limb is 'short'. This will be due to deformity at the hip, and will be called apparent shortening. There will be no true shortening in this situation. On the other hand, there may be true shortening of the bones, but the body, by compensating this shortening, may make the leg appear equal. Hence, there will be no shortening effectively (no apparent shortening), although true shortening is present, and can be detected by unmasking the compensatory mechanism.

- **Measurement of apparent length:** This is simpler to measure. The patient lies supine on the couch, as straight as he can. Both the legs should be parallel and in alignment with the body. Measurement is taken from any fixed point in the midline of the trunk (e.g., Xiphisternum, suprasternal notch, etc.) upto the prominent tip of the medial malleolus. No attempt is made to correct any deformity while measuring the apparent length.
- **Measurement of true length:** The patient lies supine. The first step is to check whether the pelvis is square. If yes, the length is measured from ASIS to the tip of the medial

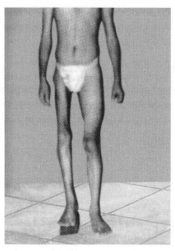

Fig. 10: Leg length measurement in standing position.

malleolus. If the pelvis is not square, the same is done first (as discussed on page 342). As the pelvis is square, the hip deformity will show up. The limb length, from ASIS to tip of the medial malleolus is measured in the deformed position of the limb. When the normal limb is being measured for comparison, it is necessary that it be placed in the position as that of the affected limb. Hence, before measuring the normal limb, the pelvis must be squared, and the limb should be in a position, identical to that of the affected limb.

- **Leg length measurement in standing position:** In a hip without deformity, a quick and accurate method of measuring true shortening is as follows: The patient is asked to stand against a wall, facing the examiner. The pelvis may be tilted due to shortening of the limb. The examiner puts wooden blocks under the foot on the shorter side, one after another, till the ASISs on the two sides are level (Fig. 10). The thickness of the blocks is measured. This indicates the amount of true shortening. Similarly, if the affected limb is longer, insert wooden blocks under the foot on the normal side, till the pelvis is square. The height of the wooden blocks indicates true lengthening of the affected limb. CT scanogram is the radiological method of accurately measuring the limb length.
- **Supra-trochanteric shortening:** Any disparity in length (true length) of the limb has to be further examined to find out as to which segment of the limb is short, i.e., whether the leg is short, the thigh is short or the shortening is above the trochanter. The last one is called supra-trochanteric shortening and is important in the diagnosis of hip diseases.
- *Measurement of supra-trochanteric shortening:* A quick assessment of supra-trochanteric shortening can be made by feeling the greater trochanters in relation to respective ASISs. The patient lies supine. The examiner places his hands on both the hips as shown in the Fig. 3. page 341. The thumbs are placed on ASISs, the tips of the middle fingers over the tips of the trochanters and tip of the index finger over an imaginary point at the intersection of two perpendiculars – one dropped from ASIS over the bed and the other from tip of the greater trochanter on to the first one. This gives a rough idea about proximal migration of the greater trochanter mostly* due to supra-trochanteric shortening. Supra-trochanteric shortening can be accurately measured by drawing Bryant's triangle (Fig. 11).

Bryant's Triangle: The patient lies supine with the pelvis square and the limbs in identical position. The tips of the greater trochanters and ASISs on both the sides are marked. A perpendicular is dropped from each ASIS on to the bed. From the tip of the greater trochanter, another perpendicular is dropped on to the first one. The tips of the greater trochanters are joined to the ASISs on the respective sides. This forms a triangle ABC. Each side of the triangle is compared with its counterpart on the normal side. The side BC of the triangle measures supra-trochanteric shortening. This may be due to: (a) dislocation of the hip; (b) central fracture-dislocation of the hip; (c) destruction of the head or acetabulum or both; (d) fracture of the neck of the femur; (e) coxa vara deformity of the hip; and (f) malunited inter-trochanteric fracture.

Some other tests have been described to roughly assess the position of the greater trochanter, but as these are difficult to perform and are not accurate, these are no longer used. Some of these are as follows:

- *Nelaton's line:* With the hip in 90° of flexion, a line joining ASIS and ischeal tuberosity passes through the tip of the greater trochanter on that side. Therefore, in cases with supra-trochanteric shortening, the trochanter will be proximal to this line.
- *Shoemaker's line:* With the patient lying supine, the line joining ASIS and tip of the greater trochanter is extended on the side of the abdomen on both sides.
- Normally, these lines meet in the midline, above the umbilicus. In case one of the greater trochanter has migrated proximally, the lines will meet on the opposite side of the abdomen, and below the umbilicus.
- *Chiene's lines:* With patient lying supine, lines are drawn joining the two ASISs and the two greater trochanters. Normally, these make two parallel lines. In case one of the trochanter has moved proximally, the lines will converge on that side.
- *Morris' bistrochanteric test:* This is used for detecting inward migration of the greater trochanter, as may occur in a central fracture-dislocation of the hip. It is no longer used.

Telescopy: It is to test stability of a hip. The patient lies supine on the couch, with the affected side towards the examiner. Keep one hand (the right hand for examination of the left hip) to stabilise the pelvis using the thenar eminence over the ASIS and the fingers of this hand on the greater trochanter (Fig. 12). The knee and the hip

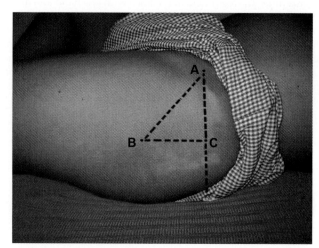

Fig. 11: Bryant's triangle: A. ASIS, B. Greater trochanter
C. Junction of the two perpendiculars.

---

* Sometimes, the trochanter is pointed as in coxa vara.

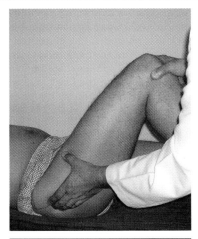

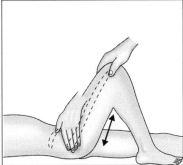

Fig. 12: Telescopy test.
Note, the fingers are at the greater trochanter to feel the up and down movement of the trochanter while the pull and push force is applied by the other hand.

are flexed to 90°. With the other hand holding the knee, a gentle push and pull force is applied along the long axis of the thigh. An up and down movement of the greater trochanter can be felt by the fingers in case the hip is unstable. A positive telescopy means that either the head is out of the acetabulum, or there is a fracture of the neck of the femur. In bulky individuals, it is difficult to perform this test and also to feel the greater trochanter. The whole limb may have to be gripped between the chest wall and the arm to be able to apply push and pull force. It is easy to perform this test in young children with CDH, in which it is a very useful test.

OTHER EXAMINATION

Examination of the ipsilateral knee, the contralateral hip, the spine and neurovascular status of the limb must always be done in a case with hip disease. A per rectal examination may be required if it is a suspected case of TB hip, central fracture-dislocation or pathological condition affecting the acetabulum. An examination of the abdomen, to look for any intra-abdominal cause for the deformity of the hip (e.g., a psoas abscess) may be done. Examination of the inguinal lymph nodes should be done.

DIFFERENTIAL DIAGNOSIS

The most important sign, the key to the diagnosis of a hip disease is movements of the hip. If movements are markedly restricted in all directions (ankylosis), the disease could be a severely damaging arthritis such as septic arthritis, tuberculosis, rheumatoid arthritis, etc. If the hip movements are well preserved but there is pain and terminal limitation of movements, a secondary OA of the hip is more likely. Some movements may be more limited than others if the head is deformed, as may occur in avascular

necrosis, old Perthes' disease, etc. Limitation of movement in only one direction usually indicates an extra-articular cause. For example, a child with psoas spasm due to infective focus in the vicinity of the psoas may have flexion deformity of the hip (hence no extension possible), but other movements, especially rotations, will be normal. Similarly, in coxa vara deformity of the hip, abduction is limited but with increased abduction (actually it is merely a change in the arc of motion). Hip movements may be increased in all directions in a case of non-union of fracture of the femoral neck or in a case of old Tom-Smith arthritis.

The other important sign of hip disease is stability of the hip as seen by performing telescopy or by Trendelenburg's test. If positive, it narrows the possibilities of diagnosis to a few.

The third important sign is the amount of true supra-trochanteric shortening. Only a little true shortening occurs in most hip diseases. Greater amount of shortening occurs in a dislocated hip, a non-union of fracture of the femoral neck, Tom-Smith arthritis, etc. Classic deformities at the hip may also help in diagnosis.

Examination of a patient with hip disease
Inspection
Patient standing
- Gait
- Obvious deformity
- Compensating mechanism - lordosis, pelvic tilt
- Shortening
- Wasting of muscles
- Swelling all around
- Sinus, scar
- Trendelenburg's test

Patient lying
- ASISs on two sides
- Lumbar lordosis

Palpation
- Temperature
- Tenderness
- Swelling - details of swelling
- Greater trochanter
  - Thickening
  - Proximal migration

Measurement
- Degree of deformities: Flexion, Add.–Abd., Rotation
- Range of movement: Flexion, Add.–Abd., Rotation
- Apparent shortening/lengthening
- True shortening/lengthening, and in which component of the leg is it?
- Bryant's triangle

Telescopy
Ipsilateral knee
Contralateral hip
Spine
Neurovascular structures of the limb
Examination of the abdomen, if needed

EXAMINATION OF THE KNEE

The knee joint is special in the following ways:
a. It is the major weight bearing joint of the body, hence its diseases are very disabling.
b. It is a superficial joint, hence more prone to injuries.

c. It is a joint whose stability is dependent primarily on the ligaments, and hence ligament injuries are common.

d. The joint has intra-articular structures like the menisci, a common source of knee symptoms.

e. The joint has a large synovial space, hence it is commonly involved in the diseases affecting the synovium.

A number of orthopaedic diseases such as osteomyelitis and sarcoma occur around the knee.

The knee is therefore, affected in a wide variety of orthopaedic conditions. Broadly, these can be divided into trauma-related and non-traumatic. While examining a patient with knee complaints, one must think of the conditions affecting the knee joint *per se* (e.g., arthritis); those affecting the bones constituting the joint (tumours around the knee); and diseases elsewhere, which may present with pain in the knee (e.g., a referred pain from a disease of the hip, presenting as pain in the knee).

HISTORY TAKING

Presenting Complaints: Following are the usual presenting complaints:

- Pain in the knee
- Swelling
- Deformity
- Stiffness
- Mechanical symptoms such as a give-way, something getting stuck, a catch, etc.

History of Present Illness: A detailed account of the presenting complaints, looking at since when is it present; how it started; how the other symptoms have added on; how activity makes a difference, if any; how any treatment has made a difference; natural progress of the symptoms (whether intermittent, gradually progressive, gradually subsiding, etc.) will constitute the contents of the history of presenting complaints. Most deformities related to arthritis are painful. Painless deformities may occur in paralytic diseases (e.g., polio, CP) or if the joint is completely destroyed and fused. Deformity in arthritis is the flexion deformity; varus (bowing of legs) and valgus (knock knees) deformities may be present. Recurvatum (hyperextension) deformity may occur in polio or due to a fracture in the region of the knee.

EXAMINATION

The patient should be examined in the lying down position: first in supine position and then in prone position. Always compare the affected knee with the opposite, normal knee.

Exposure: The whole limb on the affected as well as unaffected side should be exposed. It is difficult to examine the knee when the thigh is half covered by tightly rolled up trousers or pyjama.

Gait: Observe the gait of the patient. A deformity of the knee will be obvious. Recurvatum deformity can be best appreciated when the patient walks. A patient with weakness of the quadriceps muscles may walk with 'hand-knee gait' i.e., he supports his knee on the front with his hand when he takes weight on the leg, and thus 'prevents the knee from buckling'.

Inspection: The following points are noted on inspection:

Deformity and attitude: Flexion deformity is the most common. Initially, it occurs due to spasm of the hamstring muscles in any painful condition of the knee. Later, the capsule and other structures around the knee develop contracture, and the deformity becomes permanent. A slight flexion deformity (basically an inability to extend the knee completely) is often

termed as 'locking'. True locking means inability to extend the knee for terminal 15° to 20°, but, flexion from there is possible. This kind of block to extension, if due to meniscus tear, is more springy'. Locking due to hamstring spasm, osteoarthritis or loose body (pseudo-locking) is not springy. Locking due to loose body occurs in different positions of the knee, and gets locked and unlocked early. Flexion movement from the position of locking may not be free and complete in osteoarthritis.

In advanced stages of arthritis, the capsule and ligaments of the knee become lax. This leads to flexion, posterior subluxation and lateral rotation of the tibia, the so-called triple displacement. The leg may be abnormally abducted (valgus) or adducted (varus).

Swelling: An early swelling of the knee can be appreciated on inspection. Comparison of the two knees will show that hollows, normally present on each side of the patella have been filled up. The swelling may be diffuse – which indicates an intra-articular pathology; or localized to one part of the joint. In the latter case, depending upon the location, it could be: (a) an inflamed bursa; (b) a tumour arising from within or in the vicinity of the knee; or (c) a malunited fracture of one of the bones constituting the knee. Different bursae in relation to the knee, which may present as swelling are: (a) semi-membranosus bursa causes painless oval swelling at the postero-medial aspect of the knee; (b) infra-patellar bursa (Clergyman's knee) lying deep to the ligamentum patellae; (c) pre-patellar bursa (Housemaid's knee) lying in front of the patella; (d) Morrant-Baker's cyst – a posterior herniation of the synovial membrane in the popliteal fossa. A swelling can be seen distending the suprapatellar pouch, giving rise to a horseshoe shaped swelling, and is suggestive of effusion into the knee. Thickening of the capsule and bones can only be appreciated on palpation, specially on comparing it with the opposite, normal side. An extra-articular swelling of diffuse nature (e.g., cellulitis), extends all over the knee, over the patella, patellar tendon, and also far beyond the anatomical limits of the knee joint.

Muscle wasting: Wasting of the thigh muscles is indicative of significant knee pathology. It can be appreciated on inspection when both thighs are exposed, side by side. Wasting of the leg muscles should also be noted.

Skin over the knee: It may be stretched and shiny in an inflammatory disease. There may be an active sinus or a scar of a healed sinus, indicating an infective pathology. A scar of an old injury may suggest a direct hit on the knee.

Palpation: Palpation is carried out to find the following:

Temperature of the overlying skin.

Swelling: If there is swelling, its nature i.e., fluid, synovial thickening or bony swelling, should be made out as discussed below:

a. *Fluid within the joint:* Fluid within the joint can be detected by one of the following tests:

- *Cross fluctuation test:* When there is adequate fluid in the joint, it fills up the supra-patellar pouch. With one hand over the pouch and the other on the sides of the patellar tendon, one can feel cross-fluctuation between the fluid in the supra-patellar pouch and that on the side of the patella.

- *Patellar tap:* With the knee fully extended, the supra-patellar pouch is emptied by pressing it with one hand. The fluid comes to lie between the patella and femoral condyles, and thus 'lifts' the patella. Now one can, with a gentle tap on the patella, feel it hitting the femoral condyle and springing back. This sign may be negative

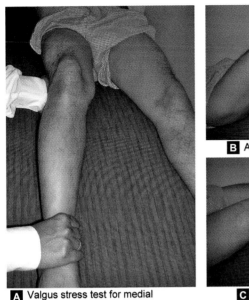

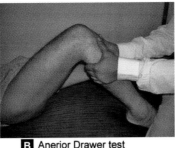

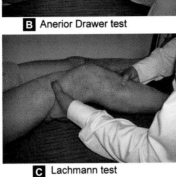

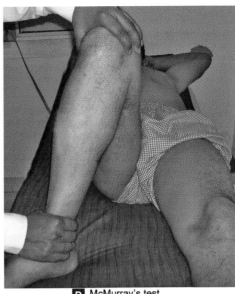

A Valgus stress test for medial collateral ligament

B Anerior Drawer test

C Lachmann test

D McMurray's test

Fig. 13: Methods of testing for ligament and meniscus injuries.

even in the presence of fluid if: (a) either there is very large, tense effusion not allowing the patella to hit the femoral condyles: or (b) if it is too little to be able to lift patella enough. It will also be negative if there is a flexion deformity of the knee. Hence, it is not a very reliable test. The fluid within the joint could be effusion, blood or pus. What exactly it is, can be guessed from history of onset of the symptoms and associated symptoms. Haemarthrosis builds up quickly, effusion slowly. In case there is pus inside the joint, signs of inflammation may be prominent.

b. *Synovial thickening:* Hypertrophied synovium and thickened capsule is a feature of chronic arthritis. The thickening may be appreciated in the suprapatellar pouch where it feels like a boggy swelling. Minimal synovial thickening can be appreciated by rolling one's fingers over the medial femoral condyle where one can feel a 'chord like' structure, suggestive of the thickened synovium and capsule.

c. *Bony thickening:* Bony thickening can be appreciated by palpation of the swelling. The swelling may be all around due to osteophytes, or localised to one of the condyles — as may occur in a bone tumour. In order to appreciate an early bony swelling, one should feel the bones forming the knee on both sides, and appreciate any difference in thickness, smoothness, etc.

Tenderness: The joint may be diffusely tender, as in cases of infective arthritis. Tenderness may be localised to a particular area. Joint line tenderness, on medial or lateral side occurs in meniscus tears or osteoarthritis. With the knowledge of surface anatomy, different parts of the bones, patellar tendon, medial and lateral collateral ligaments are pressed systematically with tip of the thumb, and tenderness correlated with the underlying structure.

Muscle wasting: Wasting of the muscles can be measured by measuring the girth of the thigh and that of the leg at fixed points from the pole of patella. Obtain the measurement on both sides and compare.

Deformity: Full extension of the knee is taken as zero degree, and from there how much it is bent constitutes the flexion deformity. Attempt at gently correcting the deformity may give a 'springy' feel (indicative of locking). or it may result in muscle spasm in a painful knee. The block may be bony as occurs in an osteoarthritic knee. Any varus or valgus deformity can be measured with the help of a goniometer. Posterior subluxation of the tibia becomes obvious when one looks at the knee from side.

Range of Movement: Active range of movement shows the capability of the patient to use his muscles within the constraints of pain. It may be diminished if the muscles are weak. Passive range of movements show how much the destruction of joint articulating surfaces, and resultant adhesions have occurred. Limitation of joint movement, both flexion and extension suggests intra-articular pathology. Sometimes, there may be extra-articular block to flexion (due to bony mass behind the knee) or due to tight quadriceps muscle holding the knee on the front (as occurs in quadriceps fibrosis). Normally, the range of flexion is enough to bring the heel in contact with the buttock, but comparison with the opposite normal knee is the best. A few degrees of hyperextension is possible in a normal knee.

Tests for integrity of the ligaments: There are four main ligaments in the knee. The medial collateral ligament (MCL), lateral collateral ligament (LCL), anterior cruciate ligament (ACL) and posterior cruciate ligament (PCL). Integrity of these can be tested by the following tests.

*   **Medial and lateral collateral ligaments (Fig. 13A):** With the patient lying supine, the leg is lifted and held in the axilla. The knee is kept in 20° to 30° of flexion*. Gentle adduction (to test LCL) and abduction (to test MCL) force is applied, as if one is trying to 'force open' the joint on one or the other side. The fingers over the joint line can appreciate 'opening-up' of the joint. Even if the joint does not open up but an attempt to do so produces pain at the ligament, it indicates a partial tear of the ligament being tested.

*   **Anterior cruciate ligament:** This is the most frequently injured ligament of the knee. It can be tested by the following methods:

    ▪   *Anterior drawer test* (Fig. 13B): The patient lies supine. The knee is flexed to 90° with the foot flat on the couch. The

---

* With the knee in flexion (20-30°). the main restrain to medio-lateral instability are the collateral ligaments.

examiner sits lightly on the foot to stabilise it. The upper end of the tibia is held between two hands in such a way that fingers are behind the knee, the thenar eminences over the tibial condyles and the tips of the thumbs, one on each femoral condyle. The fingers behind the knee check for relaxation of the hamstrings when this test is being performed. A gentle pull is applied on the upper end of tibia and forward movement of the tibia in relation to the femoral condyles appreciated. Normally, there is a glide of upto half a centimeter. Anything more than this is suggestive of ACL laxity.

- *Lachmann test:* This test is considered better than anterior drawer test. In this test, the knee is kept in 15 to 20° of flexion. One hand supports the thigh just above the knee and the other grasps the upper end of the tibia (Fig. 13C). The extent of anterior glide indicates integrity of anterior cruciate ligament. This test is difficult to perform in bulky, muscular individuals, as in them it is difficult to hold the thigh and tibia.

- **Posterior cruciate ligament:** This ligament is injured uncommonly. One can suspect such an injury by carefully observing backward sagging of the upper end of the tibia. It can be further confirmed by the following test:

  - *Posterior drawer test:* It is like anterior drawer test except, one has to make a note of how much is it possible to push the tibia backwards.

Tests for meniscus injury: These are as follows:

- **McMurray's test (Fig. 13D):** With the patient lying on a couch, the surgeon stands at the side of the injured limb. He grasps the foot firmly with one hand and the knee with the other. The knee joint is completely flexed. The foot is rotated externally and the leg abducted. The joint is now slowly extended keeping the leg externally rotated and abducted. As the torn cartilage gets caught during this manoeuvre, the patient will experience pain or a click may be heard and felt. The angle at which these symptoms occurs indicates the position of the tear. The more posterior the tear, the more flexed position of the knee is, when the sign becomes positive. A similar test with the foot internally rotated and leg adducted is carried out for lateral meniscus tears.

- **Apley's grinding test:** The patient lies prone on the couch. The surgeon places one hand on the back of the thigh, and with the other hand flexes the knee is flexed to 90°. The surgeon now applies compression along the long axis of the tibia while rotating it on the femur (grinding movement). Pain during this movement indicates a meniscal tear. Pain on lateral rotation indicates a medial meniscal tear while that on medial rotation indicates a lateral meniscal tear.

Examination with the patient lying prone: In prone position, one looks for any tenderness over the muscle attachments (sprain), any swelling over site for semimembranosus bursa, any swelling in the popliteal fossa (due to Morrant-Baker's cyst or lymph nodes, etc.).

Examination of the neurovascular structures of the limb distal to the knee is carried out in all cases. The ipsilateral hip may be examined in case no significant abnormal findings are evident on examination of the knee, as the knee pain could be a pain referred from the hip. The opposite knee should also be examined, as often knee diseases are bilateral.

DIFFERENTIAL DIAGNOSIS

Patient with knee swelling: A non-traumatic knee swelling could be due to arthritis of the knee. If it involves only one joint (monoarthritis), the usual causes are tuberculosis, septic arthritis, villo-nodular synovitis, chronic traumatic synovitis and haemophiliac arthritis (see relevant sections of the book for details). In children, it could be a presentation of juvenile chronic polyarthritis – monoarticular type. Bilateral knee symptoms may be due to osteoarthritis (in elderly people), rheumatoid arthritis (in younger, usually females), gout, osteo-chondritis, etc.

Patient with deformity: The cause of the flexion deformity could be arthritis affecting the joint, in which case there will be painful limitation of movements. If the deformity is due to 'burnt out' arthritis or due to polio, it is painless. A severe limitation of movement usually indicates an infective arthritis either tubercular or pyogenic. Valgus and varus deformities of the knee occur commonly. The causes of these are as discussed on page 315–316.

Pain in the knee: It is a very complex symptom. The causes can be divided broadly into traumatic (meniscus tear, ligament tears, fracture, etc.) or inflammatory (arthritis group). Lack of significant generalised signs and presence of specific signs go in favour of traumatic causes. Often, it is difficult to diagnose the cause, and such a case is broadly termed as "Internal Derrangement of the Knee" or IDK.

Examination of a patient with knee disease

Inspection
- Deformity and attitude
- Swelling
- Muscle wasting
- Skin over the knee

Palpation
- Temperature
- Tenderness
- Swelling—whether fluid, synovium or bone
- Muscle wasting

Deformity
Range of movements
Testing for integrity of ligaments
Testing for meniscal injury
Examination with patient lying prone
- Swelling
- Tenderness

Ipsilateral hip
Contralateral knee
Neurovascular structures of the limb

EXAMINATION OF THE ELBOW

The elbow joint is special in the following ways:
a. It is superficial joint
b. A number of important neurovascular structures lie in close proximity of the elbow, and are prone to damage in disorders of the elbow.
c. Bones around the elbow are commonly injured during childhood.
d. The elbow is very prone to stiffness.

HISTORY TAKING

Presenting complaints: Following are the usual presenting complaints:

Pain: This occurs commonly in the arthritis affecting the elbow. The elbow is one of the joint affected in a polyarticular disease, but uncommonly it could be involved alone, e.g., in tuberculosis of the elbow. More commonly, the pain around the elbow is due to extra-articular diseases such as lateral epicondylitis (tennis elbow); medial epicondylitis (golfer's elbow); olecranon bursitis (student's elbow, etc.).

Swelling: Pain and swelling usually occur together. With limitation of movements of the joint, an arthritic condition is more likely. A swelling without much pain may point to a neoplasm in the elbow region. History of remissions is an important indicator of inflammatory pathology.

Stiffness: This is a common and disabling symptom. It hampers the utility of the hand by restricting its reach. It is usually as a result of painful arthritis and associated muscle spasm. In late conditions. intra-articular and extra-articular adhesions contribute to stiffness. Elbow joint is highly prone to develop post-traumatic stiffness due to myositis.

Deformity: Flexion deformity occurs in any arthritic condition, or as a result of post-traumatic stiffness. Varus or valgus deformities occur, usually following fractures around the elbow. Cubitus varus occurs commonly due to a malunited supracondylar fracture of the humerus. Cubitus valgus occurs in fracture of the lateral condyle of the humerus. Hyperextension deformity occasionally occurs in a supracondylar fracture malunited in extension.

Past history: In a case with an old elbow injury, details of injury and treatment received are important. One must ask for history of massage, in particular. This is often the cause of stiffness due to myositis ossificans.

EXAMINATION

Exposure: The whole upper limbs on both the sides should be exposed.

Inspection: Following points are to be noted:

Deformity and attitude: Flexion deformity is obvious on putting the affected limb next to the normal limb. Varus and valgus deformities become apparent only in full extension of the elbow, because it is only in full extension that the deformed part of the lower end of the humerus articulates with the forearm bones. Hyperextension deformity is usually mild and can be appreciated by looking from the side.

Swelling: Early swelling of the elbow joint may be noticed on looking at the elbow from behind with the patient sitting on a stool with his hands on the thigh (elbow in about 30° flexion). Fullness on the two sides of the triceps tendon indicate fluid in the joint. A swelling just proximal to the joint, or on one side of the joint may be due to a malunited fracture, callus formation, myositis ossificans or a tumour.

Muscle wasting: This can be appreciated on exposing the other arm. Wasting of the arm muscles and that of the shoulder muscles should be noticed.

Skin over the elbow: Any healed sinus, scars of operation may be present.

Palpation: Following points should be noticed:

Temperature: This is increased in arthritic conditions or inflammatory conditions.

Tenderness: Diffuse tenderness indicates arthritis. Localised tenderness may occur in tennis elbow (over lateral epicondyle), in golfer's elbow (over medial epicondyle), and in students' elbow (over the tip of the olecranon).

Muscle wasting: The severity of muscle wasting can be measured at a fixed distance from a bony point, and compared with the opposite normal side.

Stability: Medio-lateral stability of the elbow is ascertained by alternatively stressing the elbow.

Three bony point relationship: This is an important sign. It is helpful in diagnosing different traumatic conditions around the elbow. With the elbow in 90° flexion, the three bony points around the elbow, i.e., the medial epicondyle, lateral epicondyle and tip of the olecranon form a near-isosceles triangle (page 93). The base of the triangle is formed by the line joining the two epicondyles and the apex by the tip of the olecranon. In a supracondylar fracture the relationship of three bony points is maintained (normal). In posterior dislocation of the elbow, the triangle is reversed. In intercondylar fractures of the elbow, and in malunited fracture of lateral condyle of the humerus, the base of the triangle is broadened.

Sometimes, identification of the three bony points becomes difficult due to a number of other bony prominences – either from a malunited fracture, or due to myositic masses of bone. It is therefore, best to identify the three bony points as follows: Palpate the medial and lateral supracondylar ridges of the humerus, about 4 to 5 cm proximal to the elbow. The most prominent points, as one follows the ridges, are the epicondyles. For identifying the tip of the olecranon, one follows the subcutaneous border of the ulna proximally.

Deformity: Flexion deformity of the elbow is measured considering full extension as zero. Varus, valgus deformities can be measured as an angle between the long axis of the arm and that of the forearm, with the forearm supinated. Hyperextension deformity is measured with full extension as the zero reference point.

Range of movement: of flexion is measured from zero position or from the position of the deformity — up to as much flexion possible. It is noted as flexion 20° to 80° (150°), with the range in the bracket being the movement on the normal side. Any pain, muscle spasm, crepitus during movement is noted. The nature of limitation of flexion; soft in arthritis, and 'bony block' in malunion and myositis may be appreciated.

SOME SPECIAL TESTS

Wringing test: When the patient is asked to wring a towel, pain is felt at the lateral epicondyle in tennis elbow.

Cozen's test: With the forearm pronated, ask the patient to make a tight fist. The examiner now holds the fist and palmar-flexes the wrist. Pain will be felt at the lateral epicondyle in a case of tennis elbow.

Ipsilateral hand and shoulder should be examined in a case of elbow disease as there may be secondary involvement of these joints.

Distal neurovascular structures: Like elsewhere in the limb, all the peripheral pulses and nerves should be examined.

Examination of a patient with elbow disease
Inspection
- Deformity and attitude
- Swelling
- Muscle wasting
- Skin over the elbow

Palpation
- Temperature
- Tenderness

- Muscle wasting
- Stability of the elbow
- Three bony point relationship

Deformity

Range of movement

Special tests - Wringing test, Cozen's test

Ipsilateral shoulder and hand

Neurovascular structures of the limb

EXAMINATION OF THE SHOULDER

The shoulder joint is special in the following ways:

a. It is a joint complex made up of mainly two joints — the gleno-humeral joint (shoulder joint proper), and the scapulo-thoracic joint.

b. It is a very unstable joint because the ball (the head of the humerus) is bigger than the cup (the glenoid). The capsule is lax, and thus allows a large range of movement.

c. The shoulder is prone to stiffness, primarily because the lax capsule has a tendency to develop contracture whenever immobilised.

HISTORY TAKLNG

Presenting complaints: The following are some of the common presenting complaints:

- Pain
- Stiffness
- Instability
- Swelling

HISTORY OF PRESENTING COMPLAINTS

Pain: A shoulder pain may be of traumatic origin, when it is sudden onset with a history of clear cut trauma. It could be a fracture in the region of the shoulder, a subluxation or dislocation of the shoulder, or tear of one of the soft tissues around the shoulder (e.g., rotator-cuff tear, deltoid contusion, etc). Pain without a history of antecedent trauma could be from the shoulder joint *per se* – as may occur in periarthritis of the shoulder; or from structures around the shoulder – as may be due to rotator-cuff tendinitis, biceps tendinitis, acromio-clavicular (AC) joint arthritis, etc. An important cause of pain in the shoulder is referred pain. It could be from cervical spine disease, visceral pathologies such as angina, cholecystitis, etc.

Location of the pain may point toward its etiology. Pain at the top of the shoulder is usually from the AC joint. The patient can, more or less point to the site of pain with a finger. Pain at the lateral side of the arm, in the region of the deltoid is usually from rotator-cuff disease or a disease from deep shoulder joint. The patient points to the pain with whole of his palm over the deltoid. Pain in the front of the shoulder and forearm is usually due to biceps tendinitis or subacromial bursitis.

Stiffness: It is a very disabling symptom, and makes it difficult for the patient to take his hand in different directions, particularly while changing clothes. The shoulder joint is very prone to get stiff. Stiffness could be due to pain and the associated muscle spasm – as occurs in acute painful conditions. It could be primarily stiffness with not much pain, as in chronic conditions such as periarthritis. Shoulder commonly gets stiff following trauma or immobilisation due to any reason. Stiffness in all directions, specially limitation of rotations points to intra-articular pathology (e.g., periarthritis); limitation in only one direction (e.g., limitation of mainly abduction) points to a localised, extra-articular cause (e.g., rotator-cuff tendinitis). In cases of visceral diseases presenting as pain in the shoulder, the range of movement of the shoulder is normal.

Instability: The patient presents with symptom that the shoulder 'comes out'. Less frequently the complaint is more vague – such as a sudden onset pain or the arm dropping 'dead' (dead arm syndrome). Symptoms occur while throwing something or doing some overhead activity. A careful history into the first episode is important. The history about what happened and how it was treated helps. An X-ray taken, if any, at the time of the first episode may leave no doubt whether the ' instability' is due to recurrent dislocation or not.

EXAMINATION

Exposure: The patient is examined sitting on a stool, so that it is possible to go around the shoulder. The trunk is exposed (except the brassiere in a female patient).

Inspection: The shoulder is inspected from front, from side, and from behind. Following findings are noted:

Contour of the shoulder: Normally, the shoulder is round — the roundness contributed by the head of the humerus and the bulky deltoid. The shoulder may appear flat if the head is not in place (i.e., dislocated) or destroyed; or if the deltoid has got wasted due to diseases such as polio, tubercular arthritis, etc. The shoulder may appear swollen due to effusion into the joint or due to subdeltoid bursitis. If it is due to effusion, the swelling extends all around; and also, fullness can be seen (and later felt) in the axilla. Swelling may also be due to old injury or a tumour in the region of the shoulder; in which case, the swelling will be localised to one side. The AC joint may be unusually prominent in cases with AC joint subluxation or arthritis.

Muscle wasting: This occurs in any chronic problem of the shoulder. It is more marked in the region of supraspinatus and infraspinatus when there is a rupture of the rotator-cuff. In long standing cases, the deltoid and the arm muscles may also be wasted.

Skin over the swelling may be inspected for stretching and engorged veins, or any healed or active sinuses, particularly in the axilla, in an infective pathology.

Attitude: In most affections of the shoulder, the arm is held by the side of the chest. Any deviation from normal can be noticed by comparing the two sides. An attitude of internal rotation may be present in a case with posterior dislocation of the shoulder. Sometimes the shoulder girdle appears elevated due to a high scapula (Sprengle's shoulder).

Palpation: Following points are noted on palpation:

Temperature rise, if any, of the skin overlying the shoulder should be noted.

Tenderness: Different bones forming the shoulder are examined for tenderness. Start from the sterno-clavicular joint, shaft of clavicle, lateral end of the clavicle, AC joint, acromion, spine of the scapula and borders of the scapula. The base of the neck, rotator-cuff area just distal to the margin of the acromion process, biceps tendon, and the deltoid are also examined for tenderness. A diffuse tenderness is present in an arthritis of the shoulder. Localised tenderness may indicate a disease of the underlying structure.

Swelling: If there is a diffuse, fluctuant swelling, the cause could be fluid in the joint. It is best felt in the axilla. A cystic swelling beneath the acromion, without any fullness in the axilla occurs in subacromial bursitis. The swelling may be localised to lateral end of the clavicle (due to AC joint arthritis), subacromial area (subacromial bursitis), below the coracoid (in a dislocated shoulder), or any other place (due to a tumour).

Range of movement: The movements present at the shoulder joint are flexion, extension, abduction, adduction, internal and external rotations, and circumduction. Abduction and adduction movements occur in the plane of the scapula. Thus, in abduction, the arm is carried not only laterally but also forward. Flexion and extension occur in a plane perpendicular to that in which adduction – abduction occur. It is important that the movements at the shoulder joint (the gleno-humeral joint) are tested in isolation. This is done by stabilising the scapula. Movement of the scapula may be wrongly considered as that at the shoulder, by a novice. A 'good' range of movement may be possible even in the presence of a stiff shoulder as a result of movement of the scapula. Following are the methods of testing passive and active shoulder movements:

Passive movements: The patient sits on the stool. The examiner stands behind him, stabilises his scapula with one hand (Fig. 14A), and holds his flexed elbow with the other. The arm is gradually abducted till the scapula starts moving (this can be made out by the hand stabilising the scapula). Normally, up to 100° of abduction is possible at the gleno-humeral joint. Abduction beyond 100° occurs at the shoulder girdle. Adduction can be carried out only up to neutral position because the arm very soon comes in contact with the chest wall. The arm is brought in flexion and extension. Normal range of flexion is 75° and that of extension is 45°. For testing rotations, with one hand the scapula is stabilised, with the other, the elbow is held flexed. The forearm acts as a pointer, showing how much range of internal and external rotation is present (Fig. 14B). Normally, about 90° of internal and external rotation are present. External rotation of the two sides can be compared by doing the above manoeuvre on both sides simultaneously (Fig. 14C).

Active movements: The importance of examining active range of movements lies in the fact that these may be limited in patients with normal passive movements. This occurs in paralytic diseases of the shoulder, and incomplete tear of the supraspinatus tendon. Active abduction may be limited due to pain caused by impingement in the subacromial space, commonly due to supraspinatus tendinitis. In diseases of the AC joint, the *extreme* of shoulder abduction may be limited due to pain.

Measurement: This involves measuring the length of the arm, a circumference of the arm (for muscle wasting). Length of the

arm is measured from the angle of acromion process to tip of the lateral condyle of the humerus. The angle of the acromion is felt as follows: one feels the spine of the scapula and palpates laterally. The angular prominence felt is the angle of the acromion. Muscle bulk is measured on both the arms at a fixed distance from the point of acromion.

Examination of a patient with shoulder disease
Inspection
• Contour of the shoulder
• Muscle wasting
• Swelling
• Skin over the swelling/shoulder
• Attitude of the arm
Palpation
• Temperature
• Tenderness
• Swelling and its details
Deformity
Measurements
• Arm shortening
• Muscle wasting
Range of movements – active and passive
Special signs
• Painful arc
• Drop-arm sign
• Apprehension test

SPECIAL SIGNS

Painful arc: This is a test to detect subacromial impingement of the rotator-cuff as a cause of shoulder pain. The patient is asked to gradually abduct his shoulder with the arm rotated internally. It will be noticed that the pain starts at around 40° to 50° of abduction, and disappears at about 120° abduction. This is because the rotator-cuff gets impinged between the head of the humerus and the acromion between this arc of abduction.

Drop-arm sign: This is a sign suggestive of complete tear of the rotator-cuff. The examiner abducts the arm of the patient, while stabilising the scapula with the other hand. Once 90° of abduction is achieved, the patient is asked to hold the arm in the air as the examiner leaves the elbow. In case there is a complete tear of the rotator-cuff, the patient will not be able to hold the arm, and it will drop by the side of the trunk.

Apprehension sign: This is a test to detect an unstable shoulder. The shoulder is abducted and externally rotated. As the examiner

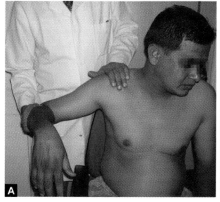
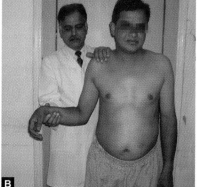
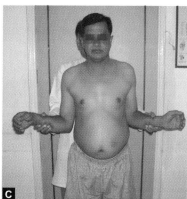

Fig. 14: Testing passive movements at the shoulder.
Note. (A) the scapula has to be slabilised all through; (B) the forearm acts as a pointer for rotations at the shoulder; (C) comparing external rotation on two side.

loads the shoulder along the long axis of the arm, the patient becomes apprehensive, and tries to resist any further movement by using his hand or by making the shoulder stiff by muscle spasm.

EXAMINATION OF A PATIENT WITH OLD FRACTURE

Examination of a patient with an old fracture is carried out with an aim to find out the following:

a. Whether the fracture has united or not: If it has united, whether the union has occurred in proper position or not. When a fracture has united but not in acceptable position, it is called as malunion. If the fracture has not united, it is judged whether it is on way to union (delayed union), or there are signs suggestive of non-union, as will be discussed subsequently.

b. What secondary effects has the fracture produced on the limb as a whole (e.g., joint stiffness. muscle wasting or myositis).

c. Whether there is any damage to the neurovascular structures of the affected limb, with the injury or due to treatment.

HISTORY TAKING

Usually, the patient gives a history of clear trauma. Often, there is an underlying disease in the bone to have lead to the fracture and subsequent problem in union. So it is wise to ask a direct question whether the patient was alright before the episode of injury. Details of the type of fracture (whether open or not); details of treatment especially whether the immobilisation was sufficient; and finally, what the patient is not able to do because of the fracture; should be brought out in the history.

EXAMINATION

Exposure: The patient should be seated comfortably, with the limb supported. The whole of the limb should be exposed, as also the opposite, normal limb.

Inspection: Important features to be noted are as follows:

Gross deformity and shortening: A comparison with the opposite limb is important.

Swelling may be due to malposition of the fracture fragments or due to callus formation.

Any scar, suggestive of a compound fracture in the past. Wasting of the muscles and deformity of the joints may be present.

Palpation: Following features are noted on palpation:

Tenderness at the site of the fracture: This is an important sign of an un-united fracture.

Palpation of bone ends: This is to examine whether the alignment and apposition of the bone is alright. Any bony irregularity in the form of a gap, a sharp elevation or a bend indicates an improper position of the bone. This is a definite sign of old fracture.

Abnormal mobility at the fracture site: This is a pathognomonic sign of non-union of a fracture. Mobility should be tested in both antero-posterior and medio-lateral planes. It is often difficult to appreciate minimal mobility in an obese person or if the fracture is close to a joint. Presence of a crepitus while looking for abnormal mobility and also any pain on stressing the fracture site are important signs of an un-united fracture.

Absence of transmitted movements: This test is another way of judging whether the fracture has united or not. It is useful in fractures of the shaft of femur, tibia and humerus. One end of the bone is rotated with one hand, while with the other, the

movement is felt at the other end. If there is no transmitted movement, the fracture is mobile.

Limb length measurement: It is important to keep the following in mind while measuring the limb length.

a. Did the patient have any pre-existing limb length discrepancy?

b. The normal limb must be placed in the same position as the affected limb.

Limb length is measured from any two prominent bony points of the affected bone. Shortening indicates the amount of overlapping at the fracture site.

Examination of the joints proximal and distal to the affected bone to detect any deformity, swelling, limitation of movements should be done. There may be an associated injury to the nearby joint.

Examination of nerves and vessels going across the fracture site is carried out by examining the part of the limb distal to the fracture.

Any complication of the fracture, such a dystrophy, etc., are noted.

DIFFERENTIAL DIAGNOSIS

A fracture presenting late could be one of the following:

a. **United:** No mobility, no pain on stressing, no deformity or shortening.

b. **Malunited:** No mobility, no pain on stressing but with deformity and/or shortening.

c. **Un-united:** Abnormal mobility with or without pain at the fracture site. If there is mobility without pain, it is called pseudarthrosis. In some cases, there may be no appreciable abnormal mobility, but only pain on stressing the fracture site. Some cases of non-union appear clinically united except that the patient cannot bear weight on the limb. It is difficult to differentiate these from a delayed union, and diagnosis is made only on X-rays.

Examination of a patient with old fracture

Inspection
- Deformity
- Shortening
- Swelling
- Wasting
- Scar

Palpation
- Temperature
- Tenderness
- Palpation of bone ends
- Abnormal mobility
- Absence of transmitted movements

Measurement
- Shortening
- Muscle wasting

Range of movement of adjacent joints
Ipsilateral joints
Neurovascular bundle

EXAMINATION OF A PATIENT WITH BONY LESION

HISTORY TAKING

Following are relevant in the history:

Age: Bone tumours occur at specific ages as shown in Table 28.7, page 238. Osteomyelitis is common in children, but may present any time in life.

Sex: Some tumours are more common in females, and others in males. Males develop osteomyelitis more commonly than females.

Presenting complaints: It may be only pain in early stages of malignant tumours, but pain and swelling may be present together. Benign tumours generally have little pain until a pathological fracture occurs through the tumour (e.g., through a bone cyst).

Following are the common presenting complaints of patients presenting with bony lesion:
- Pain
- Swelling
- Pain and swelling
- Inability to use the limb, due to weakness, pain or pathological fracture.

HISTORY OF PRESENTING COMPLAINTS

Onset of symptoms and their progress is important in considering differential diagnosis. Most tumours are insidious in onset, but often the patient gives a history of antecedent trauma at the onset. On detailed questioning, it can be ascertained whether the trauma was related; usually it is not. An insidious onset disease which comes rather suddenly, is usually inflammatory while an insidious onset progressive disease suggests a neoplasm or a chronic infection. Course of the disease is progressive in case of a neoplasm, howsoever slow it may be. On the other hand, an inflammatory swelling has remissions and exacerbations. The various symptoms of a patient presenting with a bony lesion should be evaluated in this light.

Pain: This is the most common symptom. Onset of pain is insidious, but sometimes, a history of trauma (mostly insignificant or unrelated) is present. Pain is constant at all times in a neoplastic swelling.

Swelling: Benign tumours present with swelling and little or no pain. In some benign tumours like osteoid osteoma, pain is the main presenting symptom. Onset of the swelling is insidious. The swelling grows at a slow rate (over months or years) or remains static. Benign swellings such as an osteochondroma is related to growth of the patient, and stop growing once the child attains maturity. A change in the rate of growth of a pre-existing swelling is ominous – there may be a malignant change in the swelling. Similarly, appearance of pain in a painless swelling may indicate a malignant change, or a complication such as a pathological fracture.

A swelling from the bone expands usually in all directions. Some swellings from the bone grow eccentrically (e.g., GCT). Swelling arising from structures other than the bone are localised to one side of the limb. Swelling near a joint may produce limitation of joint movements; either by producing a mechanical block to motion, or due to the pain associated with motion. Swelling may produce pressure on the adjacent neurovascular bundle of the limb, and produce symptoms thereof. The latter does not occurs in benign swellings. If a swelling appears benign on the basis of the history, inquire about similar swellings elsewhere (e.g., diaphyseal achlasis).

Pain and swelling: This is a common complaint, mostly in malignant tumours. The appearance of pain first or swelling first, is of academic significance only. It has to be differentiated from pain and swelling of inflammatory origin. One key question is whether the pain and swelling ever subsided completely or significantly. This occurs in inflammatory disorders, and not in neoplastic disorders.

Inability to use the limb: Inability to walk is usually a complaint in tumours of the lower limb. A pathological fracture, often without any trauma at all, may occur in a tumour which is primarily an osteolytic lesion (e.g., GCT). The other reason for not being able to use the limb may be paralysis of the limb muscles due to a tumour pressing on some nerve or a tumour arising from a nerve.

Associated complaints such as fever may be present in some sarcomas. It is a common symptom in Ewing's sarcoma, and can create confusion in differentiating it from an inflammatory swelling.

EXAMINATION

Position: A patient with suspected lower limb tumour should be made comfortable on a couch and the affected leg should be well-supported. A patient with upper limb swelling can be examined, sitting on a stool. A patient with swelling of the hand should be asked to rest his hands on the table.

Exposure: Exposure of the whole of the involved limb is essential. It should permit examination of the most proximal part of the limb (e.g., axillary lymph nodes in case of upper limb). It is wise to have the following questions in mind before proceeding for examination.
a. From which structure of the limb is the swelling arising: Is it from the bone, joint, muscle, fascia, nerve or vessel?
b. Whether the swelling is benign or malignant?
c. Whether the swelling has produced any secondary effects such as restriction of joint movement, pathological fracture, etc.
d. Whether there is any evidence of regional (to lymph nodes) or distal metastasis (to lungs, etc.)?
e. Whether the neurovascular status of the limb is okay?

Whatever sequence of examination is adopted, at the end, the examiner should be able to get answers to the above questions.

Inspection: Begin with something most striking. It could be swelling, a deformed joint, muscle wasting, etc.

Swelling: Following features are noted on inspection:
- *Site:* Be precise about the site of the swelling, especially whether it involves the ends* of the bone or away from the ends. Is the appearance nodular? Is the swelling all around the limb or more on one side than the other? A swelling in all directions is usually malignant. A swelling on one side may be an eccentrically growing bone swelling such as GCT, osteochondroma, etc.; or it could be a swelling arising from structures outside the bone.
- *Shape and size:* An approximate size; whether the swelling is diffuse or well-defined; whether it is spherical, fusiform or irregular should be noted.
- *Surface:* Whether the surface appears smooth or lobulated should be noted.
- *Skin over the swelling:* Whether the skin over the swelling has any signs suggestive of infection – these are discharging sinuses, redness and oedema of the skin.
  The skin becomes tense, glossy, and often red over a rapidly growing large tumour such as an osteosarcoma. The subcutaneous veins get engorged. There may be scar of the previous biopsy or an operation.
  Any pressure effects on the limb, such as oedema of the distal limb, nerve palsy, etc. should be noted.

---

* A swelling at the end of the bone right next to the joint line means that it is originating from the epiphysis (as occurs in GCT)

Any deformity of the joint: Joints develop deformities as an after effect of osteomyelitis – either due to direct involvement of the joint (see page 167), or secondary to its effect on the growth plate. In tumour, deformity may occur due to its effect on the growth plate or due to painful contracture of the joint as a result of painful spasms of the muscles around the joint. Flexion deformity at the knee is common in tumours around the knee. Varus or valgus deformities occur at different joints due to irregularity at the growth plate, as may occur in an osteochondroma or osteomyelitis.

Wasting of the group of muscles around the swelling may be noted.

Any signs suggestive of involvement of the distal neurovascular structures, e.g., loss of hair, shriveled up skin, ulcer, trophic changes in the nails, etc. should be noted.

Palpation: Before examining the patient, ensure that he is comfortable, and has gained the confidence that you are not going to suddenly press or move the already painful part. Start examining from the least painful area to the most painful area. Keep talking to the patient to divert his attention, and thus allay his fears. One can never be too gentle in handling a patient! It is suggested to follow a defined order while palpating; otherwise, important findings may be missed. But, at the end, answers to questions mentioned above is sought – you may like to look for some specific signs; otherwise missed.

Local temperature: Local rise of temperature is best felt with the back of the fingers. A comparison with the other side or the nearby normal skin may be useful. A local rise of temperature is a characteristic finding of an inflammatory swelling, but the skin over a sarcoma may have a rise in temperature due to increased vascularity of the tumour.

Tenderness: It is best to ask the patient to point to the most tender area, and avoid palpating that area till the end (if at all necessary). Do not just keep palpating here and there with no aim. Look at the face of the patient. He will wince with pain if the area being palpated is tender. There is no need to ask the patient about 'pain'. Tenderness is more marked in an inflammatory swelling than in a neoplastic swelling.

Ulcers and sinuses: To be able to say that the ulcer or sinus is related to the underlying bone, one must be able to demonstrate its fixity to the bone.

Details of the Swelling: Visual impression of the swelling is now corroborated. If it is a diffuse bony swelling, it could be due to osteomyelitis. A more localised swelling occurs in a neoplasm. Following points are considered in connection with any bony swelling:

- *Size of the swelling:* Measure in two directions (e.g., length and breadth), or simply, so many by so many cms.
- *Location:* For swelling arising near a joint, one has to make out whether it is from the joint itself, very near the joint (from epiphyseal region) or a little away from the joint (from metaphyseal region). For this, it is required to be able to define the joint line clearly.
- *Extent:* Look at the extent of the swelling – whether it is growing all around, or on one side; whether it is a pedunculated or sessile swelling.
- *Surface:* Note whether the swelling is smooth, or nodular. Malignant swellings are smooth, ill-defined as against the benign swellings which may be smooth or nodular, but well-defined.
- *Margins:* Palpate the margins of the swelling. Are these well defined, or is it that the swelling merges with the surrounding tissues rather imperceptibly?

- *Consistency:* The swelling may be bony hard, as in a case of benign bony swelling such as osteochondroma. The swelling may be firm as in most sarcomas. The consistency may be variable from soft to hard in a malignant growth. In swelling due to GCT, it may be possible to elicit 'ping pong' type of crepitus what is called egg shell crackling. This is due to ping pong ball-like springiness of the thin rim of bone surrounding the tumour. A soft swelling is usually due to fluid in a bursa, a cold abscess, or just a lump of fat.
- *Fixity to the surrounding structures:* First thing to decide is whether the swelling is fixed to the underlying bone. Grip the swelling carefully between your fingers and appreciate mobility in more than one directions. Beware of the feeling of 'movement' of the muscles over the swelling as that of the swelling. A swelling fixed to the bone is usually taken as arising from the bone or periosteum. Rarely, a swelling from outside the bone may be deep, and may appear to be 'fixed' to the bone.

  If the swelling is from a bone, assess whether it has invaded the surrounding muscles, skin, nerve or vessels as discussed below. Fixity to the surrounding structures is an important sign to differentiate between a benign and a malignant swelling.

  a. *Fixity to the muscles:* A swelling infiltrating into a muscle will restrict flexibility of that muscle, and hence, there will be checkrein type of limitation of the joint motion. Also, the power of the involved muscle will be reduced.

  b. *Fixity to the skin:* Skin is 'fixed' early in a malignant growth from a subcutaneous bone such as the tibia. If this doesn't happen, the growth is most likely benign. In other areas, where the bone is deep, it may take long before skin fixity occurs. The skin may sometime get stretched over a huge underlying tumour, and appear fixed to it.

  c. *Fixity to the nerve or vessel* will cause signs of nerve palsy or vascular insufficiency distal to the tumour. A malignant tumour in the vicinity of a nerve will nearly always infiltrate the nerve if it has reached a reasonable size.

If it is clear that the swelling is not fixed to the bone (i.e., it is not arising from the bone), make out from which structure is it arising. First step is to decide whether it is deep to the muscles within the muscles or superficial to it. For this, the patient is asked to contract the concerned muscle against resistance. A tumour which is deep to the muscle becomes less prominent; a tumour superficial to the muscle becomes more prominent; and the one in the muscle remains same. Also, the tumour superficial to the muscle remains as mobile as it was before the muscle contracted; whereas the one within the muscle becomes 'immobile' due to fixity provided by the contracted muscle belly.

A swelling originating from a nerve is suspected if there is a major branch of a nerve in that area. Also, tapping such a swelling may produce paraesthesias in the region of sensory distribution of the nerve. A swelling in relation to the vessel may elicit pulsation, either transmitted or expansile depending upon the exact nature of the swelling.

Other signs: Presence of a thrill on palpation or a bruit on auscultation may indicate a highly vascular tumour or an arteriovenous malformation.

Any deformity of the limb: Abnormal mobility due to pathological fracture or any limb length discrepancy should be looked for.

Movement of the neighbouring joints: Regional lymphadenopathy and distal neurovascular status should always be examined.

A **general examination** of the patient, to look for secondaries in a suspected case of malignancy, should be done. Also, a general review of all systems is made to assess the overall health status of the person.

DIFFERENTIAL DIAGNOSIS

Diagnosis of bone tumours depends upon: (i) age of the patient; (ii) the bone affected; and (iii) the site (epiphysis, metaphysis or diaphysis). Characteristic clinical features of some of the common bone tumours are discussed below (for details consult relevant text).

Osteosarcoma

- Age group: 15 to 25 years, and after 45 years
- Bones: Around the knee, upper humerus
- Site: Metaphysis
- Others features: Usually short duration (3–6 months); pain and swelling present; signs of a malignant swelling such as diffuse margins, fixity to muscle and skin, dilated veins, etc. present.

Ewing's Sarcoma

- Age group: 10 to 15 years, occasionally up to 30 years
- Bones: Tibia, femur, also flat bones – ileum, scapula, ribs
- Site: Diaphysis
- Others features: Usually short duration (1–2 months); may present with fever, pain and swelling and thus confused with infection. Signs of a malignant swelling present.

Chondrosarcoma

- Age group: 20 to 50 years
- Bones: Upper femur, flat bones
- Site: Diaphysis or metaphysis
- Others features: Variable duration (few months to few years), usually slow growing. History of an underlying osteochondroma, usually well defined with a little pain.

Osteoclastoma (Giant cell tumour)

- Age group: 20 to 40 years (after fusion of epiphysis)
- Bones: Around the knee, lower end of radius
- Site : Epiphysis
- Others features: Variable duration of pain (3–6 months), often presents with sudden-onset pain due to pathological fracture. Usually well-capsulated, smooth, eccentric growth, not infiltrating the nearby tissues.

Osteochondroma: The most common benign tumour (tumour-like swelling) of the bone.
- Age group: 10 to 20 years (during growth period)
- Bones: Around the knee or upper humerus (if a solitary osteochondroma). Around the knee, shoulder, and wrist (in multiple osteochondromas)
- Site: Metaphysis or diaphysis
- Other features: Long duration (months to year), slow growing, grows as long as the child grows. A well defined, painless benign swelling may produce mechanical block to movement of the adjacent joint. Deformity or distal neural deficit, may present with complications.

ENCHONDROMA

- Age group: 15 to 30 years
- Bones: Small bones of the hand (phalanges, metacarpals, etc., usually multiple
- Site: Diaphysis

- Others features: Long duration, benign swellings. Swelling is the main complaint.

Examination of a patient with bony lesion
Inspection
- Swelling
  - Site
  - Shape and Size
  - Surface
  - Skin over the swelling
  - Pressure effects
- Deformity of the adjacent joint
- Muscle wasting
- Signs suggestive of distal neurovascular involvement

Palpation
- Temperature
- Tenderness
- Ulcer, sinuses
- Details of the swelling
  - Size-measure it
  - Site
  - Extent
  - Surface
  - Margins
  - Consistency
  - Fixity to the surrounding structures

Other Signs
- Thrill, bruit over the swelling

Deformity of the limb
Neurovascular status of the limb

EXAMINATION OF THE SPINE

A patient with spine disorder presents either with pain usually in the cervical or lumbo-sacral region; or with a deformity. The deformity may be a kyphosis (stooping forward) or scoliosis (sideways bending). Sometimes, there may be no or minimal symptoms in the back, but are primarily in the limbs: upper limb pain in cervical disorders (brachialgia), and lower limb pain in lower limb disorders (sciatica).

At times, the presenting symptom of a patient with spine disorder is neurological deficit — quadriplegia, paraplegia or paraesthesias and weakness pertaining to one or more nerve roots.

HISTORY TAKING

Presenting complaints: Following are the common presenting complaints:

Pain in the neck or back.

Radiating pain in the upper limb, girdle pain along the trunk, or sciatic pain along the back or front of the leg.

Paraesthesia and weakness in a part of the limb due to involvement of one or more nerve roots.

More extensive weakness of limbs, e.g., paraplegia or quadriplegia.

HISTORY OF PRESENTING ILLNESS

Pain: Pain is a common symptom. It is mostly non-specific but following are some characteristic pains indicating a specific diagnosis.

- Sharp, shooting pain down the limb, which is exaggerated by coughing or on minimal movements. This indicates a disc prolapse.
- Dull boring pain which increases on exertion and gets relieved on rest is due to osteoarthritis.
- Pain in a young male, associated with stiffness, more early in the morning, which wears off as the person gets involved in daily chores, could be seronegative spondarthritis (SSA).
- Backache associated with pain and numbness, radiating down the leg, especially on exertion and gets relieved on rest is indicative of spinal canal stenosis. Such a symptom is called neurological claudication.
- Back pain in the dorso-lumbar region in the young may be due to traumatic or infective pathology.

Neurological symptoms: Complaints such as weakness, numbness and paraesthesias are often associated with spinal disorders. Symptoms localised to one limb usually indicate disc pathology. Bilateral lower limb weakness and loss of sensation occurs usually in dorsal and dorso-lumbar spine diseases. A cauda equina syndrome presentation occurs in lumbar spine diseases. Neurological symptoms in TB spine and in tumours are gradual in onset; in disc prolapse these are rather sudden.

EXAMINATION

Exposure: A proper exposure of the whole spine is crucial. A female patient should be asked to change and wear a gown open from the back. A female attendant/nurse should be present when examining a female patient.

Position: A patient with cervical spine disease is examined sitting on a stool, so that the examiner can observe from front, side or back. A patient with lumbar spine or dorso-lumbar spine disease is examined first standing, then lying supine and then lying prone.

Inspection: Following points are noted on inspection:

Gait: Observe the gait as the patient walks into the room. A side lurching gait may suggest a scoliosis. A patient with painful condition of the spine walks rather cautiously, with short steps and a stiff spine. A patient with acute disc prolapse has a forward stoop and sideways tilt of the torso on the pelvis.

Deformity: Normally, the neck has lordosis (forward curve), the dorsal spine is kyphotic and lumbar spine lordotic. The nape of the neck is in a straight line above the natal cleft. The position of the shoulder, scapular blades, lumbar hollows and iliac wings is symmetrical. Any deviation could be due to a disease.

A diffuse kyphosis occurs in ankylosing spondylitis, Schuermann's disease, osteoporosis, etc. A localised kyphosis may be very sharp due to collapse of one vertebra (a knuckle type) or localised to collapse of 2 to 3 vertebrae (gibbus type). Loss of lumbar and cervical lordosis occurs in painful conditions of that part of the spine. Scoliosis may be obvious, or may be detected on carefully comparing the symmetry of the spine as discussed above. A transverse deep furrow, more like a step, may be seen in the lumbo-sacral region in spondylolisthesis. Swelling in the paravertebral region or a little away could be due to a cold abscess. Prominence of one spinous process (knuckle) occurs in traumatic spine. Prominence of more than two spinous processes (gibbus) occurs commonly in Pott's spine.

Palpation: Following points are noted:

Tenderness: Ask the patient to point to the site of pain. A general localisation of the site of disease can be made by gently hitting the

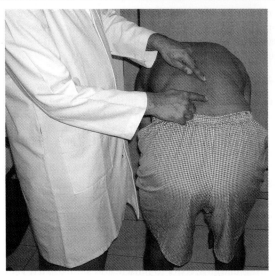

Fig. 15: While testing flexion, normally there should be movement between two adjacent spinous processes.

spine from top to bottom with a fist. More specific localisation is made by pressing the spinous processes with the thumb.

Movements: Following movements of the spine are noted:
- **Flexion:** The patient is asked to bend forward and touch his feet. While he does so, the examiner feels the movement between the spinous processes, away from one another (Fig. 15). Also, one should look for spasm of the erector spinae muscles on both sides of the spine, when flexion is being tested.
- **Side flexion:** The patient is asked to bend sideways, and any limitation noted.
- **Rotations:** The patient is asked to sit on a stool and side rotations are examined.

Neurological testing: A complete neurological examination of the limb, especially if there are symptoms such as radiating pain, paraesthesia or weakness, is necessary. This consists of the following.
- **Stretch test** (Fig. 16): These are SLRT and femoral stretch test for root compression in a disc prolapse as discussed below:
  - *Straight Leg Raising Test (SLRT):* This test indicates nerve root compression. With the patient lying on a couch, his affected leg is lifted gradually with the knee straight. As this is done, the patient complains of pain or 'stretching' at the back of the thigh or in the calf (not back of the knee). The angle at which this occurs is noted. A positive SLRT at 40° or less is suggestive of root compression. The leg is now lowered a little till the 'stretching' becomes less. At this angle if the ankle is passively dorsiflexed, the pain at the back of thigh or in the calf will again be felt. This is called reinforcement positive (Bragard's sign). Sometimes, a SLRT performed on the unaffected side, may give rise to pain on the affected side. This is termed a contralateral positive SLRT and is a very specific sign of root compression, possibly by a disc prolapse.

Examination of a patient with spine disease
Inspection
- Gait
- Posture
- Deformity
- Swelling
- Paravertebral muscle spasm

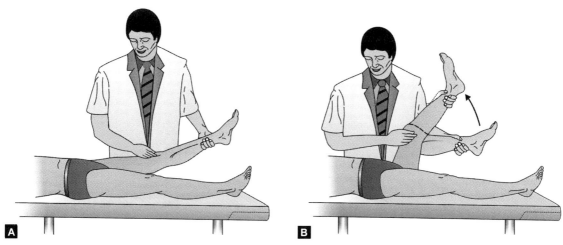

Fig. 16: Clinical tests for detecting nerve root compression: (A) Straight leg raising test (SLRT); (B) Lasegue test.

Palpation
- Tenderness
- Swelling
- Prominence of the spinous processes

Range of movements
Neurological testing of the legs
- Motor
- Sensory
- Reflexes

SI joint examination
Examination of abdomen, chest

- *Lasegue Test:* This is a modification of SLRT where first the hip is lifted to 90° with the knee bent. The knee is then gradually extended by the examiner. If nerve stretch is present, it will not be possible to do so, and the patient will experience pain in the back of the thigh or leg.
- **Motor power:** These are examined in different muscle groups of the limb, especially that of EHL, ankle dorsiflexors in a case of disc prolapse.

- **Sensory Loss:** These are examined dermatome-wise, especially in L_4, L_5, S_1 dermatomes.
- **Reflexes:** The deep and superficial reflexes, and Babinski reflex are examined.

Examination of the lower limb: Length of both the legs should be measured. Sometimes, a disparity is the cause of scoliosis. Both the hips should be examined, as there could be simultaneous involvement of the hips and spine; or the hip disease may be responsible for the spine deformity.

General examination: Following examination should be done in a case with spine disease:
- Look for cold abscesses away from the site of tuberculosis of the spine (see page 187).
- Chest should be examined to look for a tubercular focus there or to rule out an old chest disease as a cause of scoliosis.
- Examination of the breast, kidney, prostate, thyroid and abdomen is necessary if secondaries are being suspected in the spine.

Orthopaedic Terminology

FRACTURES

Fracture: A break in the continuity of bone
- **Avulsion:** bone piece pulled off by attached muscle or ligament
- **Burst:** vertebral body fracture where fragments burst out in different directions
- **Chip:** just a sliver of bone chipped off
- **Closed (Simple):** the skin over the fracture intact
- **Comminuted:** fracture in multiple pieces
- **Complicated:** fracture associated with a complication such as a vascular injury
- **Compression:** vertebral body fracture where the body is compressed
- **Displaced:** fragments separated
- **Greenstick:** fracture in children where one cortex breaks and the other cortex bends
- **Impacted:** fracture where one fragment gets jammed with the other fragment
- **Open (Compound):** the fracture communicates with outside through a rent in the skin and overlying soft tissues.
- **Pathological:** the broken bone had an underlying weakness
- **Segmental:** fracture at two levels in the same bone
- **Stress (Fatigue):** fracture caused due to repeated stress at one point
- **Traumatic:** cause of the fracture is injury
- **Undisplaced:** not displaced, only a crack

FRACTURES WITH EPONYMS

- **Aviators:** fracture of the neck of the talus
- **Barton's:** distal radius, intra-articular fracture
- **Bennett's:** fracture of base of the 1st metacarpal, intra-articular
- **Boxers':** fracture of neck of 5th metacarpal
- **Bumper:** comminuted fracture of lateral condyle of the tibia
- **Chauffer's:** radial styloid fracture
- **Colles':** distal radius, extra-articular fracture with *dorsal* tilt of the distal fragment
- **Cotton's:** trimalleolar ankle fracture
- **Galleazzi:** fracture of distal 1/2 of the radius with dislocation of *distal* radio-ulnar joint
- **Hangman's:** fracture pedicle-lamina of C_2 vertebra
- **Jone's:** fracture of the base of the 5th metatarsal
- **Malgaigne's:** pelvic ring disruption with both pubic rami and sacro-iliac injury on the same side
- **Mallet:** avulsion of attachment of ext tendon from base of the distal phalanx
- **March:** stress fracture of shaft of 2nd metatarsal
- **Monteggia:** fracture of proximal 1/2 of the ulna with dislocation of head of the radius
- **Night stick:** isolated fracture shaft of the ulna
- **Pott's:** bimalleolar ankle fracture
- **Rolando:** fracture of base of 1st metacarpal, extra-articular

- **Smith's:** distal radius fracture, extra-articular with volar tilt of the distal fragment

DISLOCATIONS

Dislocation: Complete separation of joint surfaces
Subluxation: Incomplete separation of joint surfaces
- **Congenital:** present at birth
- **Acquired:** develop later in life
  - **Habitual:** occurs every time the joint is moved
  - **Pathological:** occurs due to some disease of the joint, e.g. sepsis.
  - **Recurrent:** occurs again and again
  - **Traumatic:** due to Injury

DISLOCATIONS WITH EPONYMS

- **Chopart's:** dislocation through talo-navicular joints
- **Divergent:** elbow dislocation where ulna and radius dislocate in opposite directions
- **Lisfranc's:** dislocation through inter-tarsal joint
- **Lunate:** wrist injury where lunate bone comes out to lie in front of other carpal bones
- **Luxatio erecta:** inferior dislocation of shoulder
- **Otto pelvis:** gradual shift of the acetabulum into the pelvis (e.g., in osteomalacia)
- **Perilunate:** wrist injury where the lunate remains in its place and the other carpal bones dislocate around it dorsally
- **Spondylolisthesis:** movement of one vertebra over another (usually L_4 over L_5)
- **Sprain:** A break in the continuity of a ligament
- **Strain:** A break in muscle fibres

SIGNS AND TESTS

- **Adson's test:** for thoracic outlet syndrome
- **Allen's test:** for testing patency of radial and ulnar arteries
- **Alli's test:** for CDH
- **Anvil test:** for testing tenderness of the spine
- **Ape thumb:** for median nerve injury
- **Apley's grinding test:** for meniscus injury
- **Apprehension test:** for recurrent dislocation of the shoulder
- **Barlow's test:** for CDH
- **Blue sclera:** Osteogenesis imperfecta
- **Bryant's test:** for anterior dislocation of the shoulder
- **Callaways' test:** for anterior dislocation of the shoulder
- **Chovstek's sign:** for tetany
- **Claw hand:** for ulnar nerve injury
- **Coin test:** for dorso lumbar tuberculosis of spine
- **Cozen's test:** for tennis elbow
- **Drawer test:** for ACL and PCL injuries
  - **Anterior:** for ACL injury
  - **Posterior:** for PCL injury
- **Finkelstein's test:** for de Quervain's tenovaginitis
- **Foot drop:** for common peroneal nerve injury
- **Froment's sign:** for ulnar nerve injury

- **Gaenslen's test:** for SI joint involvement
- **Galleazzi sign:** for CDH
- **Gower's sign:** for muscular dystrophy
- **Hamilton ruler test:** for anterior dislocation of the shoulder
- **Kanavel's sign:** for infection in ulnar bursa
- **Lasegue's test:** for disc prolapse
- **Lachmann test:** for ACL injury
- **Ludloffs sign:** for avulsion of lesser trochanter
- **McMurray's test:** for meniscus injury
- **Nagffziger test:** for disc prolapse
- **Ober's test:** for tight ilio-tibial band (e.g., in polio)
- **O'Donoghue triad:** triad of MCL, ACL and medial meniscus injuries occurring together
- **Ortolani's test:** for CDH
- **Pivot shift test:** for ACL injury
- **Policeman tip:** for Erb's palsy
- **Runner's knee:** patellar tendinitis
- **Sulcus sign:** for inferior dislocation of the shoulder
- **Thomas' test:** for hip flexion deformity
- **Trendelenburg's test:** for unstable hip due to any reason (e.g., CDH)
- **Tinel's sign:** for detecting improving nerve injury
- **Volkmann's sign:** for ischaemic contracture of forearm muscles
- **Wrist drop:** for radial nerve injury

- **NCV** Nerve conduction velocity
- **NWB** Non-weight bearing
- **OA** Osteoarthritis
- **ORIF** Open reduction internal fixation
- **PCL** Posterior cruciate ligament
- **PIP** Proximal inter-phalangeal
- **PIVD** Prolapsed intervertebral disc
- **PoP** Plaster of Paris
- **PSS** Peripheral systemic sclerosis
- **PTB** Patellar tendon bearing
- **PWB** Partial weight bearing
- **RA** Rheumatoid arthritis
- **RoM** Range of motion
- **SI** Sacro-iliac
- **SLAP** Superior labrum anterior posterior tear
- **SLE** Systemic lupus erythematosus
- **SLRT** Straight leg raising test
- **SOS** If necessary
- **SSA** Sero-negative spond-arthritis
- **SWD** Short-wave diathermy
- **THR** Total hip replacement
- **TJ** Tendon jerk
- **TKR** Total knee replacement
- **US** Ultrasonic waves
- **WNL** Within normal limit

SOME ABBREVIATIONS USED IN ORTHOPAEDICS

- **Abd** Abduction
- **ACL** Anterior cruciate ligament
- **Add** Adduction
- **ADL** Activities of daily living
- **AE** Above elbow
- **AJ** Ankle jerk
- **AK** Above knee
- **AP** Antero-posterior
- **ASIS** Anterior superior iliac spine
- **B/L** Bilateral
- **BB** Both bones
- **BE** Below elbow
- **BJ** Biceps jerk
- **BK** Below knee
- **Bx** Biopsy
- **CDH** Congenital dislocation of the hip
- **CP** Cerebral palsy
- **CTEV** Congenital talipes equino-varus
- **DIP** Distal inter-phalangeal
- **DVT** Deep vein thrombosis
- **EMG** Electromyography
- **FDP** Flexor digitorum profundus
- **FDS** Flexor digitorum superficialis
- **FFD** Fixed flexion deformity
- **# D** Fracture-dislocation
- **#** Fracture
- **HLA** Human leukocyte antigen
- **IDK** Internal derrangement of the knee
- **KJ** Knee jerk
- **Lat.** Lateral
- **LM** Lateral meniscus
- **LS** Lumbo-sacral
- **MM** Medial meniscus
- **MP** Metacarpo-phalangeal
- **MWD** Micro wave diathermy

SOME ORTHOPAEDIC TERMS

- **Arthrocentesis:** aspiration of a joint
- **Arthrodesis:** fusing a joint
- **Arthrography:** imaging a joint with dye inside it
- **Arthrolysis:** releasing a stiff joint
- **Arthroplasty:** creating a new joint
- **Arthroscopy:** looking into a joint with a telescope
- **Arthrotomy:** opening up a joint
- **Closed reduction:** setting a fracture in position by manipulation
- **Epiphysiodesis:** knocking out an epiphyseal plate to stop its growth
- **Fenestration:** removing ligamentum flavum (from in-between the laminae)
- **Hemi-laminectomy:** removing half of the lamina
- **Laminectomy:** removing whole of the lamina
- **Laminotomy:** making a hole in the lamina
- **Neurectomy:** cutting a nerve (as in CP)
- **Neurolysis:** releasing a tight nerve
- **Neurorraphy:** repairing a nerve
- **Open reduction:** setting a fracture by operation
- **Osteoclasis:** rebreaking a uniting fracture (to obtain better reduction)
- **Osteogenesis:** new bone formation
- **Osteosynthesis:** reconstructing a fractured bone
- **Osteotomy:** making a cut in the bone
  - Derotation osteotomy for CDH
  - Dimon-Houston osteotomy for inter-trochanteric fracture
  - Dwyer's osteotomy for CTEV
  - French osteotomy for cubitus varus deformity
  - High tibial osteotomy for OA knee with varus
  - McMurray's osteotomy for fracture neck femur
  - Pauwel's osteotomy for fracture neck femur
  - Pemperton osteotomy for CDH
  - Salter's osteotomy for CDH
  - Sandwitch osteotomy for slipped epiphysis
  - Spinal osteotomy for ankylosing spondylosis
  - Wilson's osteotomy for congenital coxa vara

- **Tendon transfers:** changing the direction or action of a tendon
- **Tenodesis:** attaching a tendon to another tendon or bone
- **Tenolysis:** releasing a tendon from adhesions
- **Tenotomy:** cutting a tendon

IMPLANTS AND THEIR USES

- **Austin-Moore prosthesis:** for fracture neck of the femur
- **Baksi's prosthesis:** for elbow replacement
- **Buttress plate:** for condylar fractures of the tibia
- **Charnley prosthesis:** for total hip replacement
- **Condylar blade plate:** for condylar fractures of the femur
- **DHS:** for inter-trochanteric fracture
- **Ender's nail:** for fixing inter-trochanteric fracture
- **GK nail:** for femoral or tibial shaft fracture
- **Gamma nail:** for inter or sub-trochanteric fractures
- **Harrington rod:** for fixation of the spine
- **Hartshill rectangle:** for fixation of the spine
- **Insall Burstein prosthesis:** for total knee replacement
- **Interlocking nail:** for femoral or tibial shaft fractures
- **Kirschner wire:** for small bone fixation
- **Kuntscher nail:** for fracture shaft of the femur
- **Luque rod:** for fixation of the spine
- **Moore's pins:** for fracture neck of the femur
- **Neer's prosthesis:** for shoulder replacement
- **Rush nail:** for diaphyseal fractures of the long bone
- **SP nail with McLaughlin's plate:** for inter-trochanteric fracture
- **SP nail:** for fracture neck of the femur
- **Seidel nail:** for fracture of the shaft of humerus
- **Soutter's prosthesis:** for elbow replacement
- **Steffi plate:** for fixation of the spine
- **Steinmann pin:** for skeletal traction
- **Swanson prosthesis:** for finger joint replacement
- **Talwalkar nails:** for fracture of radius and ulna
- **Thompson prosthesis:** for fracture neck of the femur

OPERATIONS BY NAME

- **Bankarts' procedure:** for recurrent dislocation of the shoulder
- **Bristow's procedure:** for recurrent dislocation of the shoulder
- **Dilwyn Evan's operation:** for correction of CTEV
- **Dwyer's osteotomy:** for varus of heel in CTEV
- **Girdlestone arthroplasty:** for TB hip
- **Grice Green operation:** for subtalar arthrodesis
- **Hauser's operation:** for recurrent dislocation of patella
- **Jone's operation:** for foot deformity in polio
- **Keller's operation:** for hallux valgus correction
- **Lambrinudi operation:** for correcting equinus deformity of the foot
- **Meyer's operation:** for fracture neck of the femur
- **Putti-Plat procedure:** for recurrent dislocation of the the shoulder
- **Soutter's release:** for flexion deformity of the hip in polio
- **Steindler's release:** for cavus deformity of the foot
- **Tension-band wiring:** for fracture patella, olecranon
- **Turco's procedure:** for CTEV
- **Wilson's release:** for flexion deformity of the knee
- **Yount's release:** for flexion deformity of the knee in polio

ANATOMICAL POSITIONS AND DIRECTIONS

PLANES

- **Coronal:** side-to-side, dividing into anterior and posterior portions
- **Horizontal:** transverse, dividing into superior and inferior portions
- **Sagittal:** antero-posterior, dividing into left and right portions

JOINT MOTION

- **Abduction:** movement of a part away from the body
- **Adduction:** movement of a part towards the body
- **Apposition:** being in close contact
- **Eversion:** turning the foot outward
- **Extension:** straightening a joint
- **External rotation:** outward rotation, e.g., patella facing outward
- **Flexion:** bending a joint
- **Internal rotation:** inward rotation, e.g., patella facing inward
- **Inversion:** turning the foot inward
- **Pronation:** twisting inward, e.g., palm facing down
- **Supination:** twisting outward, e.g., palm facing up

RADIOLOGICAL SIGNS

SPECIAL VIEWS

- **Judet views:** for acetabular fracture
- **Mortice view:** for ankle injuries
- **Oblique view of the wrist:** for fracture scaphoid
- **Shenton's line:** hip X-ray in CDH
- **Sunset view:** for patello femoral dysplasia
- **Von Rosen view:** for CDH

ANGLES

- **Bohler's angle:** fracture of the calcaneum
- **Carrying angle:** elbow
- **Kite's angle:** talo-navicular angle in CTEV
- **Neck-shaft angle:** of the femoral neck
- **Pauwel's angle:** fracture neck of the femur

CLASSIC FEATURES

- **Aneurysmal sign:** TB spine (anterior type)
- **Febella:** sesamoid bone in the lateral head of gastronemius
- **Onion-peel appearance:** Ewing's Sarcoma
- **Patchy calcification:** Chondrosarcoma
- **Risser's sign:** Epiphysis of iliac bone
- **Sagging rope sign:** Perthes' disease
- **Shepherd Crook deformity:** Fibrous dysplasia
- **Soap-bubble appearance:** Osteoclastoma
- **Spondylolisthesis:** slip of one vertebra over other
- **Spondylolysis:** break in posterior elements (at pars inter-articularis)
- **Spondylosis:** degenerative spine disease
- **Sun-ray appearance:** Osteosarcoma
- **Tonguing of vertebra:** Morquio-Brails disease
- **Trethowan's sign:** Slipped capital femoral epiphysis
- **Wormian bones:** Osteogenesis imperfecta

GAITS

- **Antalgic gait:** occurs in painful condition of lower limb
- **Charlie Chaplin gait:** occurs in tibial torsion
- **Circumduction gait:** occurs in hemiplegia
- **Duck waddling gait:** occurs in bilateral CDH
- **High stepping gait:** occurs in foot drop
- **Sailor's gait:** occurs in bilateral CDH
- **Scissoring gait:** occurs in CP
- **Stiff hip gait:** occurs in ankylosis of the hip
- **Trendelenburg gait:** occurs in an unstable hip due to CDH, gluteus medius weakness, etc.

CLASSIFICATIONS

- **Garden's:** for fracture neck of the femur
- **Gustilo's:** for open fractures
- **Lauge-Hansen:** for ankle injuries
- **Neer's:** for upper end of humerus fractures
- **Pauwel's:** for fracture neck of the femur
- **Salter and Harris:** for epiphyseal injuries

MISCELLANEOUS

- **Bone grafting:** A technique where 'spare' bone is taken from some part and put where required.

- **Delayed union:** A fracture not uniting in expected time
- **Image intensifier:** A modified portable X-ray machine, where a much clearer X-ray image of a part can be seen on a TV screen. Radiation exposure is much less than a conventional X-ray exposure.
- **Malunion:** A fracture united in unacceptable alignment.
- **Nail:** A rod made of steel, usually hollow, used for internal fixation of fractures
- **Non-union:** Failure of a fracture to unite
- **Osteoarthritis:** Wear and tear arthritis
- **Osteophyte:** A bony spur at the margin of an osteoarthritic joint
- **Plate:** A thick strip of a metal (usually steel) with holes, used for internal fixation of fractures
- **Pseudarthrosis:** Painless, mobility at a fracture due to non-union (as if a 'false' joint has formed)
- **Spica:** is a plaster cast in which a limb and a part of the trunk are included (e.g., shoulder spica)
- **Valgus deformity:** The distal part goes outwards (e.g., knock knee – Genu valgus).
- **Varus deformity:** The distal part goes inwards (e.g., bow legs – Genu varum)

Orthopaedic Instruments and Implants

INSTRUMENTS

PERIOSTEUM ELEVATOR

The periosteum elevator is used to elevate the periosteum. Elevation of the periosteum is necessary in all operations on the bone because all the important structures such as vessels, nerves, tendons, etc., are outside the periosteum, and therefore, once the periosteum is elevated, the surgeon is in a safe plane. All the muscles of the extremity are attached to the periosteum, and are lifted off the bone with periosteum.

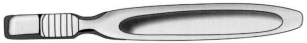

Fig. 1: Periosteum elevator (Farabeauf).

The periosteum is not elevated in some operations such as excision of osteochondroma, where the periosteum is excised with the osteochondroma to avoid recurrence. Periosteum elevators are of different shapes and sizes depending upon their uses (Fig. 1).

BONE LEVER

It is used to lever out a bone from the depth of a wound after the periosteum has been elevated (Fig. 2). It is placed between the bone and the periosteum, and thus retracts the soft tissues.

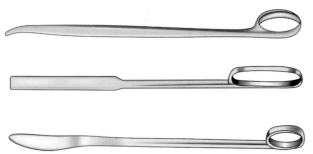

Fig. 2: Different types of bone levers.

BONE NIBBLER

It is used for nibbling the bone (Fig. 3A). It is available in various sizes and with different angle of the nose. Some of the common bone nibblers are: (i) straight nibbler – for general use; (ii) curved nibbler – for spinal surgery; and (iii) double action nibbler – straight or curved. The double-action nibblers are mechanically superior.

BONE CUTTER

It is used for cutting a bone into small pieces, e.g., for cutting bone grafts (Fig. 3B). It is also available with straight or curved ends, and with double-action type.

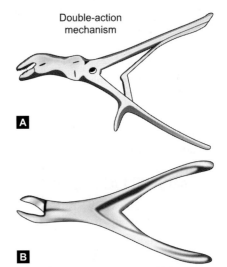

Double-action mechanism

Fig. 3: (A) Double-action bone nibbler (Rounger); (B) Double-action bone cutter.

OSTEOTOME

It is used for osteotomy – cutting a bone. Its both edges are bevelled (Fig. 4A). It is available in different widths of the blade. Some of the osteotomies commonly performed are: (i) McMurray's osteotomy for fracture of the neck of the femur; (ii) corrective osteotomy for deformities such as genu varum (bow legs), genu valgum (knock knees), etc.

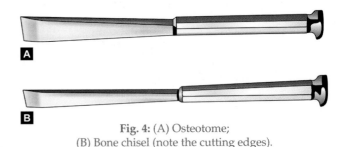

Fig. 4: (A) Osteotome; (B) Bone chisel (note the cutting edges).

BONE CHISEL

It is like an osteotome except that only one of its surfaces is bevelled (Fig. 4B). It is used for removing a protruding bone or levelling a bone surface, e.g., for levelling excessive callus, removing an osteochondroma, etc.

MALLET

It is used for hammering osteotome, chisel, etc. (Fig. 5).

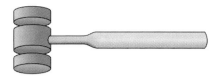

Fig. 5: Mallet.

BONE CURETTE

This is used for curetting a cavity in the bone or for removing fibrous tissue from fracture ends of an old fracture (Fig. 6). Curettage is performed for: (i) benign tumours such as enchondroma, giant cell tumour; and (ii) infections such as tubercular cavity of the bone, osteomyelitis, etc.

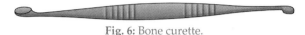

Fig. 6: Bone curette.

BONE GOUGE

This is a concave bladed chisel used for cutting on round bone surfaces (Fig. 7), or sometimes for making a round hole in the bone.

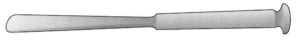

Fig. 7: Bone gouge.

BONE AWL

This is a pointed thin instrument for making a hole in the bone (Fig. 8). There is an eye at its tip to thread a wire through the bone, e.g., for tendon attachment.

Eye

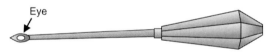

Fig. 8: Bone awl.

BONE HOLDING FORCEPS

There are different types of forceps for holding a bone (Fig. 9). These are: (i) Lane's forceps – for holding the femur, tibia, etc.; (ii) lion-toothed forceps; and (iii) self-retaining – AO type forceps.

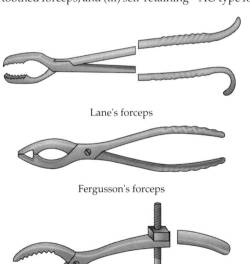

Lane's forceps

Fergusson's forceps

AO type forceps

Fig. 9: Bone holding forceps.

Plate-holding forceps: Once the reduction is achieved, a plate of suitable size is placed over the fracture and held with the help of the following plate holding forceps: (i) Lowman's clamp; and (ii) AO type self-retaining forceps (Fig. 10).

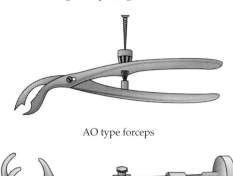

AO type forceps

Lowman's clamp

Fig. 10: Plate-holding forceps.

TRACTION INSTRUMENTS

Kirschner wire: This is thin, straight steel wire, of diameter ranging from 1 to 3 mm (Fig. 11A). It is used (i) for internal fIxation of small bones; (ii) for giving traction, e.g., for applying traction through the olecranon; (iii) for fixing fractures in children; and (iv) for Ilizarov's fixation system.

Steinmann pin: This is a stout, straight steel rod, of diameter ranging from 3 to 6 mm (Fig. 11B). It is used for skeletal traction—common sites being upper end of tibia, supracondylar region of the femur and calcaneum.

Bohler's stirrup: This is a device used for holding a Steinmann pin and applying traction (Fig. 11C). The screws on the sides of the stirrup are used to hold the pin. It is possible to change the direction of traction without moving the pin inside the bone, thus avoiding loosening of the pin.

K-wire stirrup with tensioner: When skeletal traction is to be applied with the help of K-wire, the strength of the wire is increased by subjecting it to an axial tension by a tensioner (Fig. 11D).

Skull traction tongs: These are tongs to apply skull traction in cases of cervical spine injury or disease (Fig. 11E). Examples are Crutchfield tongs, Blackburn tongs, etc.

IMPLANTS

NAILS

Nails are devices used for the intramedullary fixation of fractures of long bones. Some of the nails used commonly are as follows:

- **Kuntscher's nail:** This is used for internal fixation of fracture of the femoral shaft.
- **Smith-Petersen nail (SP nail):** This is used for internal fixation of fracture of the femoral neck.
- **V nail:** This is used for internal fixation of fracture of the tibial shaft.
- **Talwalkar nail:** This is used for fractures of forearm bones.
- **Rush nail:** This is used for some special situations in long bone fractures.
- **Ender's nail:** This is used for internal fixation of inter-trochanteric fractures of the femur.

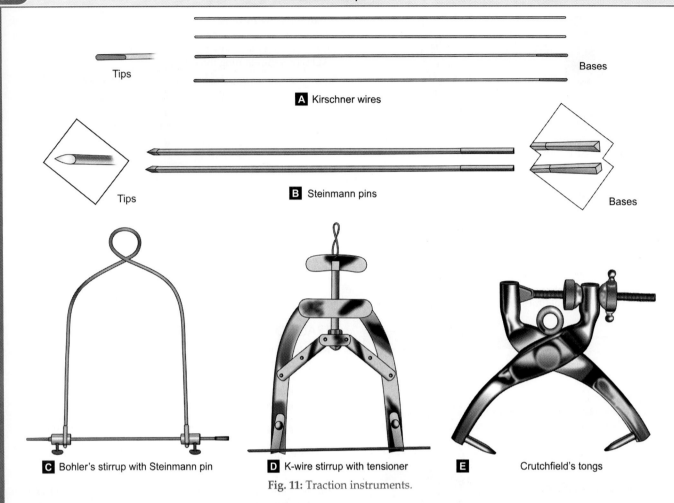

Fig. 11: Traction instruments.

Kuntscher's cloverleaf intra-medullary nail (K-nail): Kuntscher, a German surgeon devised the intramedullary nail for internal fixation of femoral fractures. The nail is a hollow tube with a slot on one side (Fig. 12). It is *cloverleaf shape* in cross section. The fixation by K-nailing is based on the concept of three point fixation i.e., when a straight rod passes through the curved medullary cavity of the femur, it fixes the bone at three points — at either ends and at the isthmus (Fig. 12A). The cloverleaf shape is designed to give good rotational stability to the fracture (Fig. 12B). The nail has an 'eye' at its either end; in which the hook of the extractor is introduced while removing the nail (Fig. 12C).

The size of a *K-nail* required for a particular case is found by determining the length and diameter of the nail required. The length is measured from the tip of the greater trochanter to the lateral joint line of the knee, and subtracting 2 cm from it. The diameter is determined on an X-ray, from the width of the medullary cavity at the isthmus.

The nail can be inserted by two techniques. In the first technique, the nail is inserted from the fracture site, and is hammered proximally till it comes out of the trochanter. The fracture is reduced and the nail driven back into the distal fragment. This is called *retrograde nailing*. In the second technique, the nail is introduced from the greater trochanter over a guide-wire passed from the fracture site. Once, the nail comes up to the fracture site, the guide-wire is removed, the fracture reduced under vision, and the nail driven home. About 2 cm nail is left protruding at the trochanter to facilitate removal usually a minimum two years after operation. For this, the hook of an extractor is engaged into

the nail at the 'eye' and the nail pulled out by outward stroking of the extractor.

Some common complications of K-nailing are: (i) nail getting stuck; (ii) splintering of the cortex while hammering the nail; (iii) proximal migration of the nail, leading to bursitis over its protruding end; (iv) distal migration of the nail leading to stiffness of the knee; and (v) infection.

Smith-Peterson nail (SP nail): Smith-Peterson (Fig. 12) cannulated triflanged nail is an implant used for internal fixation of a fracture of the neck of the femur. The advantages of its triflanged shape are that: (a) it prevents axial rotation of the fragments; and (b) it cuts only a little bone to provide good stability. The nail is cannulated because it is threaded over a guide-wire introduced at the correct site under X-ray control. It can be used along with a McLaughlin's plate for the fixation of inter-trochanteric fractures (Fig. 12).

Dynamic Hip Screw (DHS): This is a device used for the internal fixation of trochanteric fractures (Fig. 12). It has two components – the lag screw and the barrel. The lag screw slides freely inside the barrel, so that if there is collapse at the fracture site, the screw does not cut out of the cortex; it telescopes into the barrel.

PLATES AND SCREWS

These are used for fixing two bony fragments. Different types of plates are available; these may be heavy duty broad and narrow plates or semi-tubular plate (Fig. 13).

Screws may be used alone or in combination with a plate. Different types of screws used in orthopaedic practice are as shown in

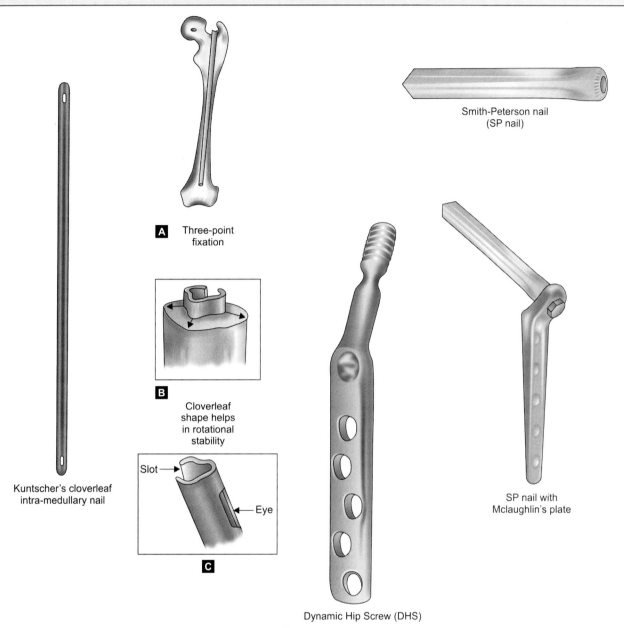

A Three-point fixation

B Cloverleaf shape helps in rotational stability

C Slot → ← Eye

Kuntscher's cloverleaf intra-medullary nail

Smith-Peterson nail (SP nail)

SP nail with Mclaughlin's plate

Dynamic Hip Screw (DHS)

Fig. 12: Common implants.

Figure13. In the past, machine screws (self-tapping screws) were used, but now AO screws (non-tapping screws) are used. A non-tapping screw is better than a self tapping screw because in the latter, while tightening, heat is produced at the bone–screw interface causing necrosis of the bone, and thus loosening of the screws. For a non-tapping screw, threads are cut in the bone with a special instrument, called a *bone tap* (Fig. 14).

PROSTHESES

Austin-Moore prosthesis: This is used for replacement of femoral head in a case of fracture of the neck of the femur in elderly persons. The prosthesis has a head with a small neck and a stem (Fig. 15A). It is available in head sizes ranging from 35 to 59 mm (odd numbers). There is a small hole at the top of the stem for the hook of the extractor, used while removing the prosthesis. The stem has two fenestrations in its middle, through which the bone supposedly grows and helps in fixation of the prosthesis.

This prosthesis can thus be used only without cement because the use of cement would make its removal, if required, difficult.

Thompson prosthesis: This is a prosthesis for the head of the femur, similar to AM prosthesis (Fig. 15B). It is especially indicated in cases where the neck of the femur is absorbed, e.g. in old fractures of the femoral neck. It can be used with or without cement.

Charnley's total hip prosthesis: This is a prosthesis for the replacement of both, the acetabulum and the head of the femur. The acetabulum is replaced by a plastic (polyethylene) acetabulum cup, and the head by a steel component. The diameter of the head of the prosthesis is 22 mm. Both the components are fixed to respective bones by bone cement (Polymethylmethacrylate).

Muller's total hip prosthesis: It is essentially similar to Charnley's prosthesis except that the size of the head of this prosthesis is 32 mm, and the stem is available in different thicknesses.

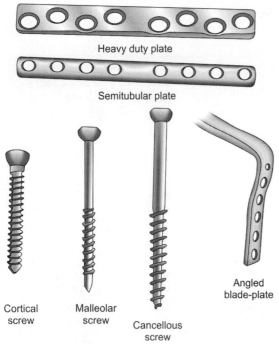

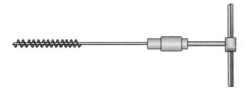

Fig. 13: Plates and screws of different types.

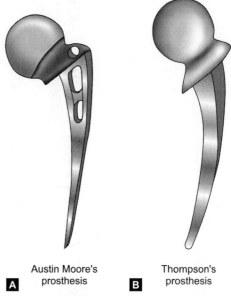

Fig. 15: Common hip prosthesis.

Fig. 14: A bone tap.

Total knee prosthesis: Thare several designs available (Fig. 16). Total condylar designs are most popular. In this type, the articular surfaces of femur, tibia and patella are replaced by metallic (for femur) and polyethylene (for tibia and patella) prosthesis. Common prosthesis used are Insall-Burstin knee, Freeman-Samuelson knee, etc.

IMPLANT MATERIAL IN ORTHOPAEDICS

A number of implants are used in orthopaedics. These may be used as a temporary device, e.g., a steel rod used for fixation of a fracture; or as a permanent, device, e.g. a total hip prosthesis used for replacing a damaged hip joint. The material used for these implants is foreign for the body, and is subjected to harsh chemical environment of the body. A usual foreign body, subjected to this environment shall evoke a reaction from the body which may range from a benign to a chronic inflammatory response. To avoid this, the implant materials used in our body are so designed that they have suitable mechanical strength and are biocompatible. Implant materials can be divided in the following categories:

Metals: These have been used for fixation of fractures, for a long time. The most common one is stainless steel. The surgical grade stainless is SS 316L. Other metal used for fracture fixation is titanium based alloy. Titanium is stronger and lighter than steel. For manufacturing components for joint replacement, cobalt based alloys are preferred as these have high resistance to corrosion.

Non-metals: The most common non metal material is some form of plastic. Following non-metals are commonly used:

- **Ultra high density polyethylene (UHDPE):** This is used for making acetabular cup for total hip, and the plastic insert for knee replacement.
- **Bone cement:** This is used as an anchoring agent to fix metallic components to the bone. Chemically it is polymethylmethacrylate. On mixing the monomer, powder form of polymethacrylate with liquid methylmethacrylate, a dough like material is formed which sets in 5 to 7 minutes into a hard material. It is something like an ordinary cement which sets on adding water. This process is exothermic and irreversible.
- **Ceramics:** Ceramics have been used to design articulating surfaces of artificial joints. These are more resistant to wear, but disadvantage is that these are brittle.
- **Silicon:** Silicon implants are used for artificial inter-phalangeal joints in the form of silicon elastomer (silastic).
- **Polyester fibre:** This is used for manufacturing artificial ligaments.

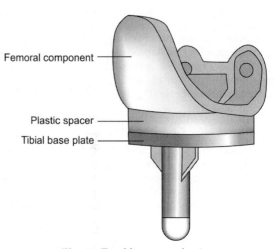

Fig. 16: Total knee prosthesis.

Index

Page numbers followed by *f* refer to figure, *fc* refer to flowchart, and *t* refer to table.